Operative Techniques in
Hand and Wrist Surgery

Operative Techniques in
Hand and Wrist Surgery

Kevin C. Chung, MD, MS

EDITOR-IN-CHIEF
EDITOR, HAND AND WRIST

Chief of Hand Surgery, Michigan Medicine
Director, University of Michigan Comprehensive Hand Center
Charles B. G. de Nancrede Professor of Surgery
Professor of Plastic Surgery and Orthopaedic Surgery
Assistant Dean for Faculty Affairs
Associate Director of Global REACH
University of Michigan Medical School
Ann Arbor, Michigan

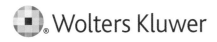

Philadelphia • Baltimore • New York • London
Buenos Aires • Hong Kong • Sydney • Tokyo

Executive Editor: Brian Brown
Development Editor: Ashley Fischer
Editorial Coordinator: John Larkin
Marketing Manager: Julie Sikora
Senior Production Project Manager: Alicia Jackson
Senior Designer: Joan Wendt
Artist/Illustrator: Body Scientific International
Senior Manufacturing Coordinator: Beth Welsh
Prepress Vendor: SPi Global

Printed in China

Cataloging-in-Publication Data available on request from the Publisher.
ISBN 978-1-9751-2737-4

To Chin-Yin and William.

—KCC

Contributors

Sonya Paisley Agnew, MD
Assistant Professor
Loyola University Medical Center
Chicago, Illinois

Shoshana W. Ambani, MD
Plastic Surgeon
Medical Director of Plastic Surgery
Henry Ford Allegiance Hospital
Jackson, Michigan

Neal C. Chen, MD
Assistant Professor
Harvard Medical School
Interim Chief
Department of Orthopaedic Surgery
Hand and Upper Extremity Service
Massachusetts General Hospital
Boston, Massachusetts

Kevin C. Chung, MD, MS
Chief of Hand Surgery, Michigan
  Medicine
Director, University of Michigan
  Comprehensive Hand Center
Charles B. G. de Nancrede Professor of
  Surgery
Professor of Plastic Surgery and
  Orthopaedic Surgery
Assistant Dean for Faculty Affairs
Associate Director of Global REACH
University of Michigan Medical School
Ann Arbor, Michigan

Rafael J. Diaz-Garcia, MD
Attending Surgeon
Medical Operations Officer
Department of Surgery
Allegheny Health Network
Clinical Assistant Professor
Department of Plastic Surgery
University of Pittsburgh School of
  Medicine
Pittsburgh, Pennsylvania

Kyle R. Eberlin, MD
Assistant Professor of Surgery
Associate Director, MGH Hand
  Surgery Fellowship
Division of Plastic and Reconstructive
  Surgery
Massachusetts General Hospital
Harvard Medical School
Boston, Massachusetts

Kate Elzinga, MD, FRCSC
Plastic Surgeon
Department of Surgery
University of Calgary
Calgary, Alberta, Canada

John M. Felder, MD
Assistant Professor of Surgery
Division of Plastic Surgery
Washington University in
  St. Louis
St. Louis, Missouri

John R. Fowler, MD
Assistant Dean for Medical Student
  Research
Assistant Professor, Department
  of Orthopaedics
University of Pittsburgh School of
  Medicine
Pittsburgh, Pennsylvania

Thomas B. Hughes, MD
Clinical Associate Professor of
  Orthopaedic Surgery
Orthopaedic Specialists,
  UPMC
School of Medicine
University of Pittsburgh
Pittsburgh, Pennsylvania

Matthew L. Iorio, MD
Associate Professor
Co-Director of Hand Surgery, &
  Extremity Microsurgery
Associate Program Director
Division of Plastic Surgery
University of Colorado Hospital
Aurora, Colorado

Robert A. Kaufmann, MD
Associate Professor, Orthopaedics
University of Pittsburgh
Pittsburgh, Pennsylvania

Grant M. Kleiber, MD
Assistant Professor
Department of Plastic Surgery
MedStar Georgetown University
  Hospital
Washington, District of
  Columbia

Jason H. Ko, MD
Associate Professor
Division of Plastic and Reconstructive
  Surgery
Department of Orthopedic Surgery
Feinberg School of Medicine
Northwestern University
Chicago, Illinois

Emily Krauss, MD, MSc, FRCSC
Clinical Instructor
University of British Columbia and the
  University of Victoria
Victoria, British Columbia, Canada

Brian I. Labow, MD, FACS, FAAP
Associate Professor of Surgery
Harvard Medical School
Boston Children's Hospital
Boston, Massachusetts

John R. Lien, MD
Assistant Professor
Department of Orthopaedic Surgery
  and Section of Plastic Surgery
University of Michigan Health System
Ann Arbor, Michigan

Angelo B. Lipira, MD, MA
Assistant Professor of Plastic and
  Reconstructive Surgery
Oregon Health & Science University
Portland, Oregon

Jacques A. Machol IV, MD
Plastic, Hand, and Microsurgery
Department of Plastic Surgery
Southern California Permanente
  Medical Group
West Los Angeles & Los Angeles
  Medical Centers
Clinical Assistant Professor
Division of Plastic Surgery
University of Southern California
Los Angeles, California

Mary Claire Manske, MD
Pediatric Hand and Upper Extremity
  Surgery
Department of Orthopaedic Surgery
Shriners Hospital for Children
  Northern California
University of California
Davis Sacramento, California

Amy M. Moore, MD
Assistant Professor of Surgery
Chief, Section of Hand
    Surgery
Program Director, Hand, Nerve and
    Microsurgery Fellowship
Washington University School of
    Medicine
St. Louis, Missouri

Mark Morris, MD
Joseph H. Boyes Hand Surgery
    Fellow
University of Southern California
Los Angeles, California

Shelley S. Noland, MD
Hand & Peripheral Nerve Surgery,
    Division of Plastic Surgery
Assistant Professor, Plastic &
    Orthopedic Surgery
Associate Program Director, Division of
    Plastic Surgery
Mayo Clinic College of Medicine
Phoenix, Arizona

Donato Perretta, MD
Orthopedic Surgery
Hand Surgery
Private Practice
New York Presbyterian—Hudson
    Valley Hospital
Cortlandt, New York

Joseph Pirolo, MD
Orthopaedic Surgeon
Seattle, Washington

Paymon Rahgozar, MD
Assistant Professor
Division of Plastic and Reconstructive
    Surgery
University of California San Francisco
San Francisco, California

Patrick Reavey, MD, MS
Assistant Professor
Section of Plastic and Reconstructive
    Surgery
Department of Surgery
Department of Orthopedic Surgery and
    Rehabilitation
University of Chicago Medicine
Chicago, Illinois

**James T. W. Saunders, BSc, MD,
FRCSC**
Division Head of Plastic and
    Reconstructive Surgery
Lions Gate Hospital, North Vancouver
Clinical Professor at the University of
    British Columbia
North Vancouver, British Columbia,
    Canada

Ketan Sharma, MD, MPH
Resident Physician
Barnes-Jewish Hospital
Washington University St. Louis
St. Louis, Missouri

Michael Smith, MD
Director of Hand and Upper Extremity
    Surgery
Grandview Medical Center
Birmingham, Alabama

Amir H. Taghinia, MD, MPH, MBA
Assistant Professor of Surgery
Harvard Medical School Staff
    Surgeon
Department of Plastic and Oral
    Surgery
Boston Children's Hospital
Boston, Massachusetts

Richard Tosti, MD
Hand, Wrist, Elbow, and Microvascular
    Surgeon
Philadelphia Hand to Shoulder
    Center
Assistant Professor of Orthopaedic
    Surgery
Thomas Jefferson University
King of Prussia, Pennsylvania

Joseph Upton, MD
Clinical Professor for Surgery
Harvard Medical School
Chestnut Hill, Massachusetts

Mark A. Vitale, MD, MPH
ONS Foundation for Clinical Research
    and Education, ONS, P.C.
Greenwich, Connecticut

David Wei, MD
Attending Orthopaedic Surgeon
Department of Orthopaedic
    Surgery
Greenwich Hospital, Yale-New Haven
    Health
ONS Foundation for Clinical
    Research and Education, ONS, P.C.
Greenwich, Connecticut

Preface

The elegant anatomy of the hand and wrist presents a tremendous challenge to surgeons. Surgeons treating hand surgery patients must understand the functional anatomy, which not only restores the architecture but also achieves movement and strength. This textbook is designed to provide the needs of all surgeons, whether their background training is in orthopedic surgery, plastic surgery, or general surgery, who are committed to understanding the complexity of hand and wrist disease and injuries. Rather than presenting a list of options for a particular problem, the authors strive to share their preferred procedure that has been proven to yield predictable and safe outcomes.

Each operation is organized in a highly illustrated, sequential fashion for efficient learning. I have edited every chapter, and I am proud to present to you an outstanding product that not only shares my personal experience but also leverages the collective expertise of noted authorities in this specialty. I hope that you will embrace this textbook for its simplicity, elegance, and directness in achieving the results to which you aspire. I am grateful for your support and confidence in adding this textbook to your collection.

Kevin C. Chung, MD, MS
Chief of Hand Surgery, Michigan Medicine
Director, University of Michigan Comprehensive Hand Center
Charles B. G. de Nancrede Professor of Surgery
Chief of Hand Surgery, Michigan Medicine
Professor of Plastic Surgery and Orthopaedic Surgery
Assistant Dean for Faculty Affairs
Associate Director of Global REACH
University of Michigan Medical School
Ann Arbor, Michigan

Contents

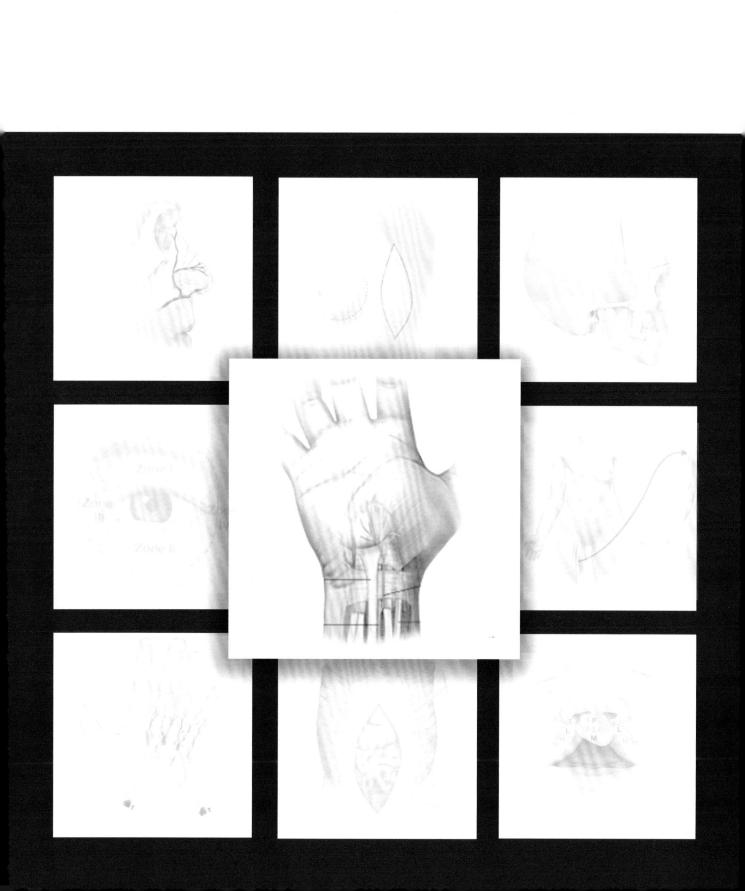

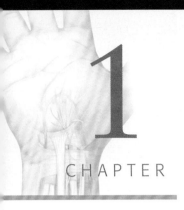

Section I: Anesthesia and Emergency Procedures

Anesthesia and Emergency Procedures

John R. Lien and Kevin C. Chung

DEFINITION

- Wrist and digital blocks are essential for patient anesthesia in the operating room and during emergency room procedures.
- Nerve blocks assist with postoperative pain control.
- Wide-awake local anesthesia no tourniquet (WALANT) involves local injection of epinephrine with lidocaine for hemostasis and anesthesia instead of applying a tourniquet and sedation. This technique is useful for minor hand procedures as well as tendon surgery.

ANATOMY

- Median nerve
  - At the distal forearm/wrist, the median nerve lies between the palmaris longus (PL) and flexor carpi radialis (FCR) tendons (**FIG 1**).
  - The palmar cutaneous branch (PCB) usually passes subcutaneously between the FCR and PL tendons.

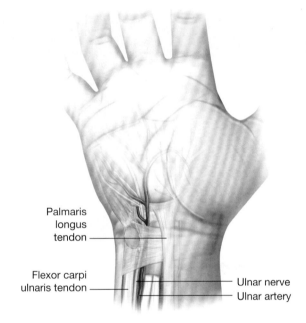

FIG 2 • Ulnar neurovascular bundle anatomy at volar wrist.

- Ulnar nerve
  - At the wrist level, the ulnar nerve is radial and dorsal to the flexor carpi ulnaris (FCU) tendon (**FIG 2**).
  - The ulnar artery is adjacent to the radial aspect of the ulnar nerve.
  - The dorsal cutaneous branch (DCB) originates from the ulnar nerve approximately 5 cm proximal to the ulnar styloid. It crosses from palmar to dorsal near the styloid process.[1]
- Superficial branch of the radial nerve
  - The superficial branch of the radial nerve (SBRN) becomes subcutaneous approximately 9 cm proximal to the radial styloid.[2]
  - At the radial styloid, there are two to three branches of the SBRN in the subcutaneous tissue (**FIG 3**).
- Digital nerves
  - Four nerve branches (two palmar, two dorsal) provide sensation to each digit.
  - The common digital nerves bifurcate to the proper digital nerves at the level of the distal palmar crease.

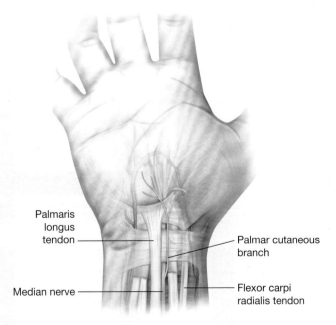

FIG 1 • Median nerve anatomy at volar wrist.

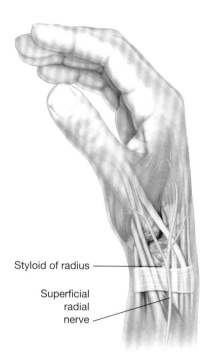

FIG 3 • Superficial branch of the radial nerve anatomy at the radial wrist.

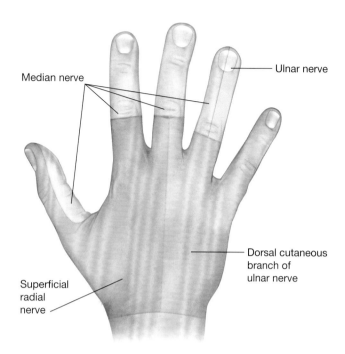

FIG 4 • Dorsal hand sensory innervation.

- The dorsal digital nerves of the thumb and small finger extend to the tip of the dorsal digit.
- The volar digital nerves supply dorsal sensation distal to the proximal interphalangeal joint in the index, middle, and ring fingers (**FIG 4**).

SURGICAL MANAGEMENT

Preoperative Planning

- Materials
  - Syringe
  - 27-gauge needle
  - Commonly used local anesthetic agents and additives
    - Lidocaine is commonly used due to its rapid onset (within 2–5 minutes of injection) and medium duration of action (2 hours for digital block).[3]
    - Bupivacaine has a slower onset of action (5–10 minutes) but longer duration of action (12 hours for digital block).[3]
    - Epinephrine additive induces vasoconstriction, which promotes hemostasis, prolongs duration of anesthesia, and reduces the systemic toxicity of the local anesthetic agent.
    - Sodium bicarbonate 8.4% additive buffers the low pH of lidocaine, decreasing injection pain.

Positioning

- Whether the procedure is in the operating room or emergency department, the patient should lie comfortably supine to minimize patient movement during the procedure.
- Hand table or Mayo stand.

Approach

- Digital block
  - Volar subcutaneous approach: This is our preferred technique as it only requires one injection and is shown to be less painful than the transthecal approach.[4]
  - Dorsal transmetacarpal approach
  - Transthecal approach
- Wrist block
  - Median nerve
  - Ulnar nerve
  - Superficial branch of radial nerve
- WALANT
  - Use 1% lidocaine with 1:100 000 epinephrine
  - Buffer the lidocaine and epinephrine in a 10:1 ratio with 8.4% sodium bicarbonate
  - Allow adequate time for the vasoconstrictive effect of epinephrine to take effect (25 minutes).[5]
- Volume of injection depends on the site of surgery (**FIG 5**).[6]

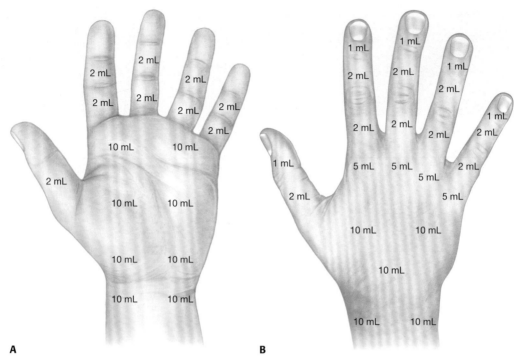

FIG 5 • Palmar **(A)** and dorsal **(B)** hand injection volumes.

■ Digital Nerve Block

Volar Subcutaneous Block

- Insert a 27-gauge needle at the distal palmar crease at the level of the A1 pulley (**TECH FIG 1**).
- Inject 3 mL of local anesthetic into the subcutaneous tissue. The anesthetic should cause tumescence and flow of anesthetic solution radial and ulnar to the flexor tendon

sheath (see **FIG 5A**). If there is significant resistance to injection, withdraw the needle slightly.

Dorsal Transmetacarpal Block

- Identify the metacarpal head of the digit of interest.
- At this level, introduce a 27-gauge needle from the dorsal web space and advance toward the palm (**TECH FIG 2**).

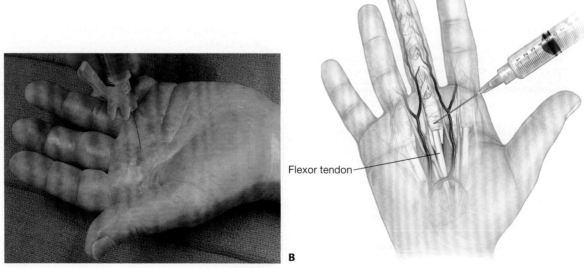

Flexor tendon

TECH FIG 1 • Middle finger volar subcutaneous block. Note tumescence radial and ulnar to the flexor tendon sheath in **A**. Note the needle is in the subcutaneous tissue superficial to the flexor tendon sheath in **B**.

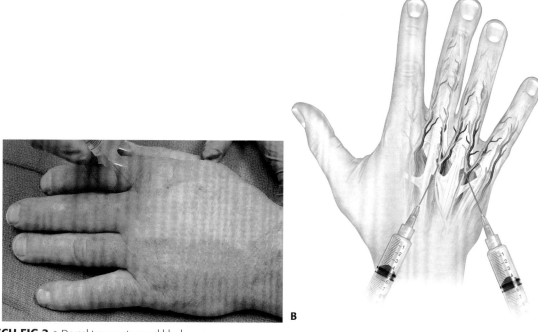

A **B**

TECH FIG 2 • Dorsal transmetacarpal block.

■ Inject 2 mL of local anesthetic into the radial and ulnar web space to anesthetize each digital nerve. Periodically aspirate the syringe to prevent intravascular injection.

Transthecal Digital Block

■ Palpate the flexor tendon sheath at the palmar digital crease.

■ Insert a 25-gauge needle through the flexor tendon at this level until contact with bone.
■ After bone contact, slowly withdraw the needle with gentle pressure on the syringe (**TECH FIG 3**).
■ When the needle is withdrawn 1 to 2 mm, anesthetic will enter the sheath.
■ Inject 2 mL of local anesthetic.

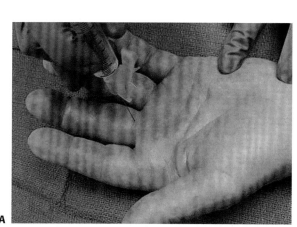

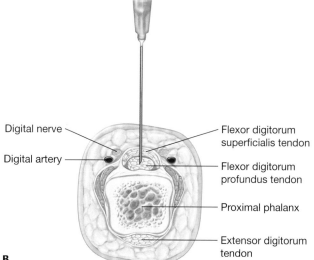

Digital nerve

Digital artery

Flexor digitorum superficialis tendon

Flexor digitorum profundus tendon

Proximal phalanx

Extensor digitorum tendon

A **B**

TECH FIG 3 • **A.** Transthecal digital block. **B.** Cross-section view.

■ Wrist Block

Median Nerve Block

- Identify the FCR and PL tendons at the proximal wrist crease.
- Insert the needle just proximal to the wrist crease and penetrate the flexor retinaculum (**TECH FIG 4**).
  - In the absence of PL tendon, insert the needle on the ulnar side of the FCR tendon.
- Inject 5 mL of local anesthetic around the nerve.

Ulnar Nerve Block

- Identify the FCU tendon at the proximal wrist crease.
- Introduce a 25-gauge needle ulnar and dorsal to the FCU, aiming the needle radially (**TECH FIG 5**). From this approach, the ulnar nerve is encountered first. Avoid pushing the needle too far; the ulnar artery is radial to the nerve.
- Inject 5 mL of local anesthetic around the ulnar nerve, taking care to intermittently aspirate.
- Infiltrate the subcutaneous dorsoulnar wrist with 5 mL of local anesthetic to anesthetize the dorsal cutaneous branch (DCB) of the ulnar nerve.

Superficial Branch of Radial Nerve Block

- Palpate the styloid process of the radius.
- Insert a 25-gauge needle and inject 5 mL of local anesthetic into the subcutaneous tissue overlying the first through third dorsal compartments.

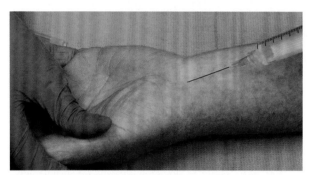

TECH FIG 4 • Median nerve block at wrist.

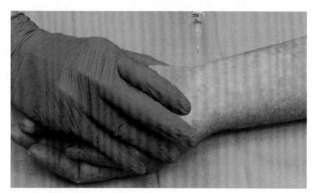

TECH FIG 5 • Ulnar nerve block at wrist.

■ WALANT: Trigger Finger Release Example

- Prepare a mixture of 1% lidocaine and 1:100 000 epinephrine buffered with 8.4% bicarbonate. For trigger finger, we inject a total of 10 cc locally.
- Warm the local anesthetic solution to body temperature.
- Distract the patient to look away from the injection site.
- Use a 27-gauge needle to inject 0.5 mL of the anesthetic perpendicularly subdermally over the A1 pulley (**TECH FIG 6**).
- Stabilize the syringe and pause until the patient reports he/she does not feel the needle pain.
- Inject an additional 2 mL prior to moving the needle.
- Move antegrade slowly with a tumescent wheal of local anesthetic visible ahead of the needle.
- Prior to incision, wait at least 25 minutes for the vasoconstrictive effect of epinephrine to take place. There is excellent hemostasis without the use of tourniquet (**TECH FIG 7**).

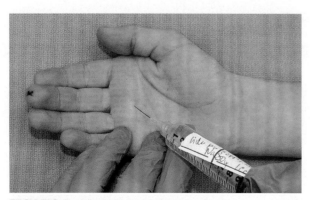

TECH FIG 6 • WALANT injection for trigger finger.

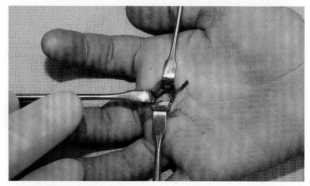

TECH FIG 7 • Trigger finger release demonstrates hemostasis without tourniquet.

PEARLS AND PITFALLS

Physical exam	▪ Do not forget to carefully document the sensory and motor exam prior to administration of local anesthetic.
Technique	▪ Avoid intravascular injection by careful intermittent aspiration. ▪ Palpate the flexor tendon sheath prior to digital block. The flexor tendon sheaths and neurovascular bundles are ulnar to midline in the thumb and radial to midline in the small finger. ▪ Injection of small boluses of local anesthetic followed by brief periods of observation is a safe way to prevent intravascular systemic toxicity. ▪ Inject slowly to decrease pain.
Local anesthetic dosage	▪ The maximum adult dose of plain lidocaine is 4–5 mg/kg.[7] ▪ The maximum adult dose of plain bupivacaine is 2.5 mg/kg.[7]

POSTOPERATIVE CARE

▪ Postoperative care will depend on the procedure performed.

OUTCOMES

▪ A systematic review compared six local anesthetic preparations (lidocaine, lidocaine with epinephrine, bupivacaine, bupivacaine with epinephrine, lidocaine with bupivacaine, and ropivacaine). All provided benefits in digital nerve blocks.[3]
  ▪ Lidocaine demonstrated the shortest mean onset of anesthesia (3.1 minutes), whereas bupivacaine was the longest (7.6 minutes).
  ▪ Lidocaine also had the shortest mean duration of anesthesia (1.8 hours), whereas ropivacaine had the longest duration (21.5 hours).

COMPLICATIONS

▪ Amino esters (chloroprocaine, procaine, tetracaine, cocaine) are more likely to cause allergic reactions than amino amide compounds (lidocaine, bupivacaine, ropivacaine, mepivacaine).
▪ Systemic toxicity is extremely rare with hand and wrist local anesthesia but can occur with intravascular injection.
  ▪ Central nervous system manifestations can include facial numbness, metallic taste, light-headedness, tinnitus, and seizure.
  ▪ Cardiac depression can culminate in cardiovascular collapse (ventricular tachycardia or fibrillation).
  ▪ Primary therapy in the setting of cardiac arrest involves advanced cardiovascular life support (ACLS).
  ▪ Consider intravenous lipid emulsion therapy in the treatment of local anesthetic systemic toxicity.[8,9]

▪ Although the authors have never encountered digital infarction with use of epinephrine, it is important to know that local phentolamine injection reverses epinephrine-induced vasoconstriction.[10]

REFERENCES

1. Puna R, Poon P. The anatomy of the dorsal cutaneous branch of the ulnar nerve. *J Hand Surg Eur Vol.* 2010;35E(7):583-585.
2. Abrams RA, Brown RA, Botte MJ. The superficial branch of the radial nerve: an anatomic study with surgical implications. *J Hand Surg [Am].* 1992;17(6):1037-1041.
3. Vinycomb TI, Sahhar LJ. Comparison of local anesthetics for digital nerve blocks: a systematic review. *J Hand Surg [Am].* 2014;39(4):744-751.
4. Hung VS, Bodavula VK, Dubin NH. Digital anaesthesia: comparison of the efficacy and pain associated with three digital nerve block techniques. *J Hand Surg Eur Vol.* 2005;30B(6):581-584.
5. McKee DE, Lalonde DH, Thoma A, et al. Optimal time delay between epinephrine injection and incision to minimize bleeding. *Plast Reconstr Surg* 2013;131:811-814.
6. Lalonde DH, Martin A. Tumescent local anesthesia for hand surgery: improved results, cost effectiveness, and wide-awake patient satisfaction. *Arch Plast Surg.* 2014;41(4):312-316.
7. Katz RD, LaPorte DM. Use of short-acting local anesthetics in hand surgery patients. *J Hand Surg [Am].* 2009;34(10):1902-1905.
8. Cordell CL, Schubkegel T, Light TR, Ahmad F. Lipid infusion rescue for bupivacaine-induced cardiac arrest after axillary block. *J Hand Surg [Am].* 2010;35(1):144-146.
9. Neal JM, Mulroy MF, Weinberg GL. American Society of Regional Anesthesia and Pain Medicine checklist for managing local anesthetic systemic toxicity: 2012 version. *Reg Anesth Pain Med.* 2012;37(1):16-18.
10. Nodwell T, Lalonde D. How long does it take phentolamine to reverse adrenaline-induced vasoconstriction in the finger and hand? A prospective, randomized, blinded study: the Dalhousie project experimental phase. *Can J Plast Surg.* 2003;11(4):187-190.

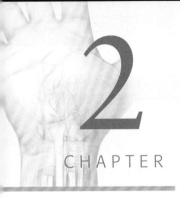

2

CHAPTER

Fasciotomy for Compartment Syndrome of the Hand and Forearm

John R. Lien and Kevin C. Chung

DEFINITION

- Compartment syndrome occurs when interstitial tissue pressure rises to levels that impair blood flow and cellular function.

ANATOMY

- The hand contains 10 muscular compartments as well as the carpal tunnel and digital compartments (Table 1, **FIG 1**).
- The forearm consists of three myofascial compartments: volar, dorsal, and the mobile wad (Table 2, **FIG 2**).

PATHOGENESIS

- If there is swelling within the fascial compartments, intracompartmental pressure will rise.
- Increased compartment pressure can result in tissue ischemia and necrosis.
- Causes of compartment syndrome:
  - Intracompartmental swelling: Bleeding/soft tissue injury from trauma, anticoagulation, infection, high-pressure injection injury, reperfusion injury, intravenous fluid infiltration.
  - External compression: Burn eschar, prolonged syncope with pressure on the limb, tight dressings or casts.
- Major limb replantation/revascularization requires prophylactic fasciotomy due to risk of reperfusion injury and compartment syndrome.

NATURAL HISTORY

- Irreversible muscle damage occurs within 6 to 8 hours of ischemia.
- Rhabdomyolysis from myonecrosis can result in acute renal failure and electrolyte abnormalities.
- Left untreated, permanent nerve deficit and muscle fibrosis of the forearm can result in secondary Volkmann contracture.

PATIENT HISTORY AND PHYSICAL FINDINGS

- Understand the mechanism of injury and have a high clinical suspicion—compartment syndrome is a clinical diagnosis.
- Remove any constrictive dressings or clothing.
- Physical exam findings:
  - Tense, swollen compartment, blistering (**FIG 3**)
  - Pain with passive stretch of the compartment muscles
  - Paresthesias
  - Paralysis of the involved compartment muscles develops after nerve paresthesias.
  - Pallor and pulselessness are late findings.

DIAGNOSTIC STUDIES

- Compartment syndrome is usually a clinical diagnosis; diagnostic studies may complement the diagnosis.
- If there is a history of trauma, plain radiographs are indicated to assess for fracture or dislocation.
- Other advanced imaging (ultrasound, MRI) is rarely indicated. Time-consuming studies should not preclude emergent fasciotomy if there is high clinical suspicion for compartment syndrome.
- Laboratory studies (complete blood count, coagulation panel, basic metabolic panel, creatine phosphokinase, serum and urine myoglobin) are obtained.

Table 1 Hand Compartments

Compartment	Muscle	Nerve
Thenar	Abductor pollicis brevis, opponens pollicis, flexor pollicis brevis	Recurrent motor
Hypothenar	Abductor digiti minimi, opponens digiti minimi, flexor digiti minimi	Ulnar
Adductor	Adductor pollicis	Ulnar
Interosseous (7)	4 dorsal and 3 palmar interossei	Ulnar
Carpal tunnel	Flexor digitorum superficialis, flexor digitorum profundus, flexor pollicis longus (tendons)	Median
Digit		Digital

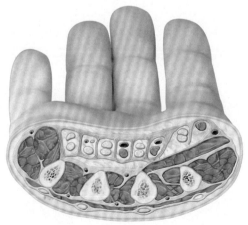

FIG 1 • Midpalmar cross-section of hand compartments.

Table 2 Forearm Compartments

Compartment	Muscle	Nerve
Volar		
Superficial	Flexor digitorum superficialis, pronator teres, palmaris longus, flexor carpi radialis, flexor carpi ulnaris	Median, ulnar
Deep	Flexor digitorum profundus, flexor pollicis longus, pronator quadratus	Anterior interosseous
Dorsal		
Superficial	Extensor digitorum communis, extensor digiti minimi, extensor carpi ulnaris	Posterior interosseous
Deep	Abductor pollicis longus, extensor pollicis brevis, extensor pollicis longus, extensor indicis proprius, supinator	Posterior interosseous
Mobile wad	Brachioradialis, extensor carpi radialis brevis, extensor carpi radialis longus	Radial

- If clinical diagnosis is equivocal or the patient is obtunded, compartment pressure measurements should be obtained. We use a commercially available Stryker manometer.
  - An acute compartment syndrome is assumed if the compartment pressure is within 30 mm Hg of the diastolic blood pressure.[1] If the compartment measurement is measured under anesthesia, the pressure should be compared to the preinduction diastolic blood pressure.
  - If measurements are not consistent with compartment syndrome, close monitoring and repeat clinical examination with serial compartment pressures may be indicated.

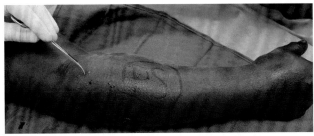

FIG 3 • Forearm gunshot wound with dorsal compartment swelling and skin blistering.

SURGICAL MANAGEMENT

- If there is high clinical suspicion or objective manometric evidence supporting the diagnosis of compartment syndrome, perform emergent fasciotomy.
- The goal of fasciotomy is to reduce compartment pressure and allow for tissue perfusion.

Preoperative Planning

- In the setting of trauma, review radiographs and prepare for skeletal stabilization if necessary.
- Consider reversal of anticoagulation if indicated.

Positioning

- Patient is positioned supine with a hand table.
- A tourniquet is applied to the arm; we do not inflate the tourniquet unless there is difficulty with visualization.

Approach

- The standard approach for the volar forearm involves a curvilinear incision extending from the medial epicondyle to the proximal wrist crease, creating a flap of skin over the distal forearm to cover the flexor tendons and median nerve (**FIG 4A**).

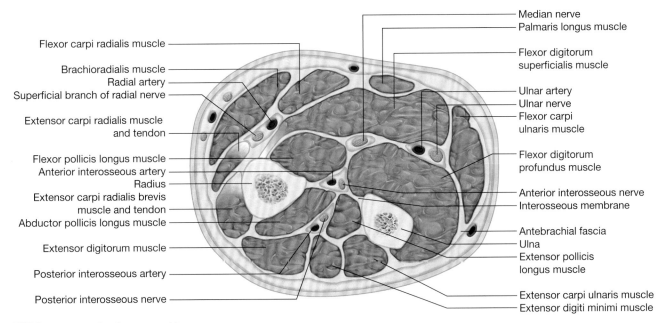

Flexor carpi radialis muscle
Brachioradialis muscle
Radial artery
Superficial branch of radial nerve
Extensor carpi radialis muscle and tendon
Flexor pollicis longus muscle
Anterior interosseous artery
Radius
Extensor carpi radialis brevis muscle and tendon
Abductor pollicis longus muscle
Extensor digitorum muscle
Posterior interosseous artery
Posterior interosseous nerve

Median nerve
Palmaris longus muscle
Flexor digitorum superficialis muscle
Ulnar artery
Ulnar nerve
Flexor carpi ulnaris muscle
Flexor digitorum profundus muscle
Anterior interosseous nerve
Interosseous membrane
Antebrachial fascia
Ulna
Extensor pollicis longus muscle
Extensor carpi ulnaris muscle
Extensor digiti minimi muscle

FIG 2 • Cross-sectional anatomy of forearm.

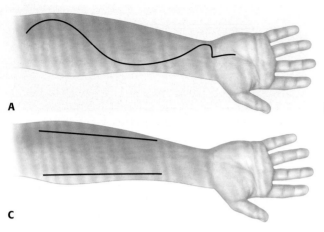

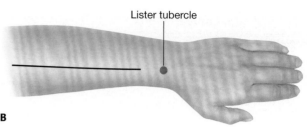

A

B

C

FIG 4 • A. Volar forearm curvilinear approach. **B.** Dorsal forearm longitudinal approach. **C.** Alternative parallel forearm incision approach.

- The dorsal forearm and mobile wad are decompressed through a longitudinal dorsal forearm incision (**FIG 4B**).
- An alternative forearm fasciotomy with two parallel longitudinal incisions (**FIG 4C**)

- A volar radial incision allows access to the volar compartment and mobile wad without exposure of the median nerve or flexor tendons.
- An ulnar incision allows access to the dorsal compartment.

■ Fasciotomy of the Hand

Dorsal Hand Compartment Release

- Identify the second and fourth metacarpals dorsally.
- Perform longitudinal incisions on the radial border of the second and fourth metacarpal down to the level of the extensor tendons (**TECH FIG 1A**). Avoid incisions directly over the metacarpals; if the wound is left open, the tendon will desiccate. Avoid injury to the sensory branches of the radial and ulnar nerves.
- The incision over the fourth metacarpal is used to decompress the third and fourth dorsal interossei (**TECH FIG 1B**).
- The incision over the second metacarpal is used to decompress the first and second interossei.
  - Dissect bluntly through the dorsal interossei to decompress the three palmar interosseous muscles.
- Release the adductor compartment through the incision over the second metacarpal.

Thenar Compartment Release

- Palpate the radial border of the first metacarpal and make an oblique longitudinal incision (**TECH FIG 2**, line A).
- Identify the thenar fascia overlying the abductor pollicis brevis (APB) and incise it longitudinally.

Hypothenar Compartment Release

- Make a longitudinal incision just volar to the ulnar border of the fifth metacarpal and hypothenar eminence (see **TECH FIG 2**, line B).
- Identify the hypothenar fascia overlying the abductor digiti minimi (ADM) and incise it longitudinally.

Carpal Tunnel Release

- Make an incision over the carpal tunnel in line with the radial border of the fourth ray between the thenar and hypothenar compartments (see **TECH FIG 2**, line C).

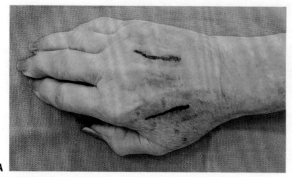

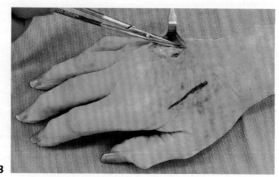

A

B

TECH FIG 1 • A. Dorsal hand compartment release incisions. **B.** Decompression of the fourth dorsal interosseous compartment.

T E C H N I Q U E S

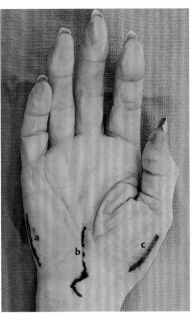

TECH FIG 2 • Palmar hand fasciotomy incisions: hypothenar (*a*), carpal tunnel (*b*), and thenar (*c*).

- Identify the longitudinal fibers of the palmar aponeurosis and split them longitudinally.
- Longitudinally divide the transverse fibers of the transverse carpal ligament from the level of the sentinel fat pad to the antebrachial fascia, taking care to protect the median nerve and its motor branch.
- This incision may be incorporated into a volar forearm fasciotomy.

Digital Compartment Decompression

- Approach the digit on its noncontact side (ulnar incision for the index, long, and ring fingers, radial incision for the thumb and small finger).
- Make a midaxial incision (dorsal to the neurovascular bundles) and divide Cleland ligaments.

Wound Management

- Place loose tagging sutures as indicated over the carpal tunnel incision and over any areas with concern for tendon exposure.
- Apply a bulky dressing and splint in a functional position.

■ Fasciotomy of the Volar Forearm With Curvilinear Incision

- Design a curvilinear incision from the ulnar wrist crease to the medial antecubital fossa (**TECH FIG 3A**).
- If a carpal tunnel release is performed, extend the proximal carpal tunnel incision ulnarly at the wrist flexion crease.
  - This creates a radially based flap that prevents desiccation of the median nerve and flexor tendons.
- Curve the incision radially in the mid forearm and then toward the medial elbow.
- Release the forearm fascia overlying the superficial and deep compartments of the volar forearm (**TECH FIG 3B**).

- Release the lacertus fibrosus at the medial elbow (**TECH FIG 3C**).
- Inspect each muscle and release individual muscle fascia if necessary.
  - Debride any devitalized muscle.
- The mobile wad can be released through the volar or dorsal incision.
- Loose sutures may be placed to secure skin flaps over the median nerve and flexor tendons. Leave the rest of the wound open, as significant swelling will usually prevent skin closure (**TECH FIG 3D**).
- Apply a loose bulky dressing and splint.

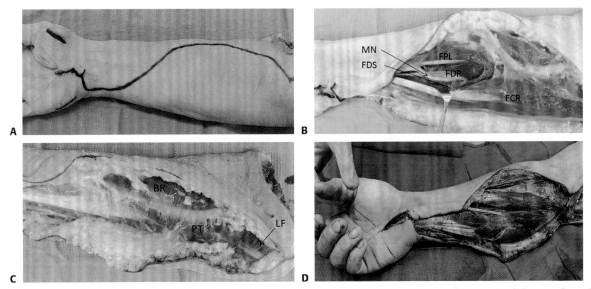

TECH FIG 3 • **A.** Volar forearm curvilinear incision. **B.** Exposure of deep volar muscle compartment. FCR, flexor carpi radialis; FDS, flexor digitorum superficialis; FDP, flexor digitorum profundus; FPL, flexor pollicis longus; MN, median nerve. **C.** Identification of lacertus fibrosus at medial elbow. LF, lacertus fibrosus; PT, pronator teres; BR, brachioradialis. **D.** Clinical image after volar forearm fasciotomy, with significant swelling preventing primary wound closure.

■ Fasciotomy of the Dorsal Forearm

- Re-evaluate for the need for dorsal fasciotomy. After volar forearm and mobile wad compartment release, the dorsal forearm may have been indirectly decompressed.
- Make a longitudinal dorsal incision starting 3 to 4 cm distal to the lateral epicondyle extending toward Lister tubercle (**TECH FIG 4A**).

- Release the fascia over the dorsal compartment and the mobile wad.
- Inspect each muscle and release individual muscle fascia if necessary (**TECH FIG 4B**).
  - Debride any devitalized muscle.
- Perform any secondary procedures such as skeletal fixation.
- The wound is left open. A loose dressing and splint are applied.

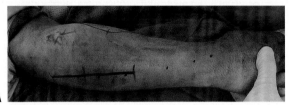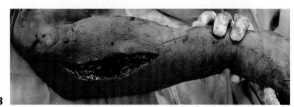

TECH FIG 4 • A. Dorsal forearm compartment incision. **B.** Dorsal forearm compartment release and debridement. In this case, devitalized extensor muscle from gunshot wound was debrided.

■ Fasciotomy of the Forearm With Two Longitudinal Incisions

- Make a longitudinal incision on the volar radial forearm along the ulnar border of the brachioradialis (**TECH FIG 5A**).
- Undermine the ulnar aspect of the incision to gain access to the superficial volar forearm fascia.
- Release the underlying volar forearm fascia longitudinally.
- Access to the deep volar compartment is through a volar Henry approach between FCR and brachioradialis (**TECH FIG 5B**).
- Undermine the proximal ulnar aspect of the incision to gain access and release the lacertus fibrosis.

- The mobile wad can be released from the radial aspect of the incision.
- Make a longitudinal incision along the ulnar forearm and release the dorsal forearm compartment (**TECH FIG 5C**).
- Inspect each muscle and release individual muscle fascia if necessary.
  - Debride any devitalized muscle.
- The wound is left open and a loose dressing and splint are applied.
  - This double incision allows decompression without exposure of the median nerve or tendons at the distal forearm.

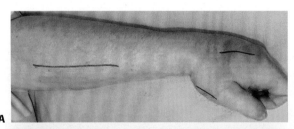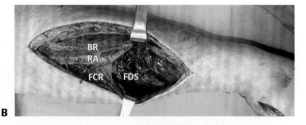

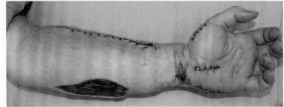

TECH FIG 5 • A. Alternative volar radial longitudinal incision. **B.** Access to superficial and deep volar compartments. BR, brachioradialis; RA, radial artery; FCR, flexor carpi radialis; FDS, flexor digitorum superficialis. **C.** Ulnar longitudinal approach for dorsal forearm compartment release.

PEARLS AND PITFALLS

Indications	▪ Have a low threshold to proceed with compartment release.
Examination	▪ Pain out of proportion to injury an early finding in patients with compartment syndrome.[2]
Technique	▪ Attempt to preserve cutaneous nerves and veins whenever possible. ▪ Debride any devitalized muscle. ▪ Release any restrictive epimysium that can subcompartmentalize muscle groups (flexor digitorum profundus). ▪ Do not close fascia. ▪ Loose sutures can be used to hold skin flaps over exposed nerve or tendon—initial wound closure should prioritize coverage of neurovascular structures and tendons. ▪ Wounds generally should be left open in the acute setting; return for delayed primary closure vs skin grafting or flap coverage as clinically indicated.
Postoperative management	▪ If there is concern for delayed presentation and muscle necrosis, serial debridement may be necessary.

POSTOPERATIVE CARE

- After initial fasciotomy the limb should be splinted in a functional position.
- Intravenous antibiotics are administered while the wound is open.
- Monitor electrolyte and renal function closely; myoglobinemia can result in acute renal failure.
- Return to operating room is planned within 48 hours for interval debridement and assessment of the wound bed.
- Once the wound bed is stabilized, perform delayed primary closure or split-thickness skin graft (**FIG 5**). Rarely, flap coverage is indicated for exposed tendon or nerve.
- Edema management with elevation and loose dressings proximal to the involved site
- Begin range of motion as soon as reasonable to prevent joint contractures and decrease swelling.

OUTCOMES

- Patient outcomes are dependent on the timing of fasciotomy.
- Early recognition and expedient treatment generally results in favorable outcomes.
- Late recognition and delayed treatment may result in irreversible nerve and muscle injury with limited functional recovery.
- The mechanism and severity of initial injury also influence prognosis.

COMPLICATIONS

- Untreated compartment syndrome will result in nerve dysfunction as well as Volkmann ischemic contracture (**FIG 6**).

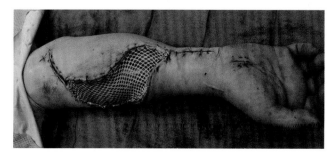

FIG 5 • Split-thickness skin graft application to volar forearm.

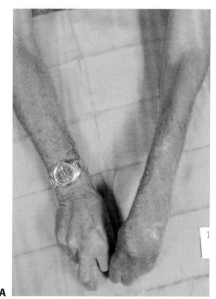

A

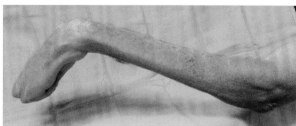

B

FIG 6 • Untreated compartment syndrome with Volkmann contracture.

- Rhabdomyolysis can result in acute renal failure.
- Incomplete release of the deep volar compartment can result in extrinsic flexor contractures.

REFERENCES

1. Leversedge FJ, Moore TJ, Peterson BC, Seiler JG III. Compartment syndrome of the upper extremity. *J Hand Surg [Am]*. 2011;36(3): 544-560.
2. Codding JL, Vosbikian MM, Ilyas AM. Acute compartment syndrome of the hand. *J Hand Surg [Am]*. 2015;40(6):1213-1216.

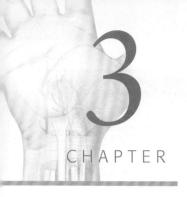

3
CHAPTER

Revision Amputation and Shortening of the Digit

John R. Lien and Kevin C. Chung

DEFINITION

- Fingertip injuries involve trauma to the digit distal to the insertion of the flexor and extensor tendons.
- The primary goal of treatment is a painless fingertip with supple and sensate skin coverage.
- The method of treatment should be individualized to the patient and injury pattern.
- This chapter will focus on revision amputation and shortening of the digit. The principles discussed can be applied to finger amputations more proximal than the fingertip.
- Refer to Chapter 60 for flap coverage options of fingertip injuries.

ANATOMY

- The nail complex (perionychium) consists of the nail plate and surrounding tissues[1] (**FIG 1**):
  - Eponychium: Skin proximal to the nail plate, covering the nail fold
  - Paronychium: Skin lateral to the nail plate
  - Hyponychium: Skin immediately distal and palmar to nail
  - Nail bed: Germinal matrix and sterile matrix

- Germinal matrix: Soft tissue deep and proximal to nail plate, responsible for majority of nail growth. Distal margin is the lunula.
- Sterile matrix: Tissue distal to lunula, responsible for nail adherence
- Nail fold: Consists of dorsal roof matrix and proximal germinal matrix.
- Lateral matrix horns: The proximal lateral corners of the matrix, formed by the confluence of the germinal matrix, dorsal roof matrix, and lateral nail fold.
- The terminal extensor tendon insertion on the distal phalanx is approximately 1.2 mm proximal to the germinal matrix.[2]
- The pulp of the fingertip consists of fibrofatty tissue stabilized by septae extending from the dermis to the palmar periosteum of the distal phalanx.
- The proper digital nerve lies palmar to its corresponding digital artery. The nerve trifurcates at the level of the distal interphalangeal (DIP) joint (**FIG 2**).

PATHOGENESIS

- Traumatic mechanisms of injury: sharp, crush, avulsion

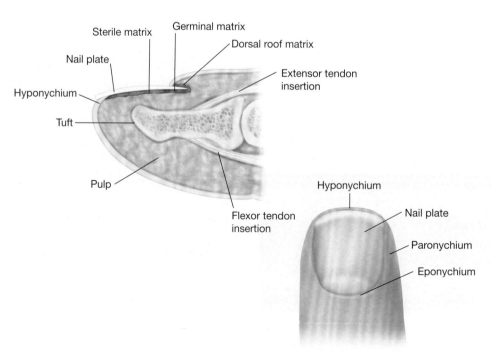

FIG 1 • Sagittal and dorsal views of the distal phalanx and nail complex.

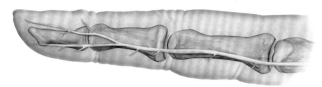

FIG 2 • Digital nerve anatomy. The nerve arborizes at the level of the distal interphalangeal joint.

PATIENT HISTORY AND PHYSICAL FINDINGS

- History:
  - Age
  - Handedness
  - Occupation
  - Medical comorbidities
  - Mechanism of injury
  - Timing of injury
  - Tobacco use
  - Tetanus status
- Physical exam:
  - Identify the level of amputation; fingertip vs more proximal.
  - Assess for nail bed injury.
  - Assess for exposed bone. If there is significant exposed bone, healing by secondary intention will not be successful.
  - Morphology of fingertip injury: transverse, dorsal oblique, palmar oblique, radial/ulnar oblique.
  - Assess residual soft tissue: Can it be closed primarily with minimal tension?

IMAGING

- Radiographs of the digit

NONOPERATIVE MANAGEMENT

- Fingertip injuries without exposed bone will heal by secondary intention with local wound care.
- Irrigation and primary closure can be considered only if there is adequate skin resulting in a tensionless closure.

SURGICAL MANAGEMENT

Preoperative Planning

- Fingertip and amputations distal to the metacarpophalangeal joint with exposed bone and inadequate soft tissue coverage are candidates for bone shortening and primary closure.
  - Amputations at the level of the eponychium and proximal are usually best suited for revision amputation.
  - For fingertip injuries with exposed bone involving the mid-portion of the nail bed, consider flap coverage depending on injury morphology and patient factors (see Chapter 60).
  - For finger amputations presenting with an amputated piece, consider replantation (see Chapter 68).
- Uncomplicated finger amputation can be performed in the emergency department.
- If there is a nail bed injury, prepare to repair the nail bed with chromic suture or Dermabond (Ethicon, Inc., Somerville, NJ).[3]
- If the revision amputation will result in removal of over two-thirds of the nail matrix and/or its underlying bony support, prepare to ablate the nail bed.
- Perform a digital block and gather instruments and dressings prior to starting the procedure.

Positioning

- Patient is positioned supine with hand table or Mayo stand.

Approach

- Goals of this procedure are a painless, sensate fingertip, preservation of as much length as possible and avoidance of nail dystrophy.
- The decision to proceed with bone shortening and primary closure should take injury characteristics and patient factors into account. For example, if a patient with a volar oblique fingertip amputation is a smoker and a laborer who must return to work as soon as possible, we would recommend revision amputation with shortening and primary closure as opposed to a homodigital island flap or cross-finger flap.

■ Revision Amputation With Primary Closure

- Administer a digital block prior to sterile preparation.
- Apply a finger tourniquet.
- Debride contaminated or devitalized tissue sharply.
- If there is nail matrix involvement, consider ablation vs nail bed repair.
- Mobilize the soft tissue around the level of bony exposure (**TECH FIG 1A,B**).
- Use a rongeur to shorten and contour the bone (**TECH FIG 1C**).
  - Bone should be shortened for tension-free closure.
  - Remove articular cartilage if performing a disarticulation.
- If the amputation is through or proximal to the DIP joint, identify the radial and ulnar digital nerves and shorten them to prevent neuroma being caught in the incision that will be painful (**TECH FIG 1D,E**).
- Reassess skin flaps to ensure tension-free closure and round fingertip by removing the dog ear over either side of the incision to create a round tip rather than a boxy tip.
- Close skin flaps with 5-0 nonabsorbable suture (**TECH FIG 1F**).
- Release the finger tourniquet to ensure adequate perfusion of the skin flaps. If the flaps appear tight or ischemic, consider additional bony shortening.
- Apply a sterile dressing.

TECHNIQUES

T E C H N I Q U E S

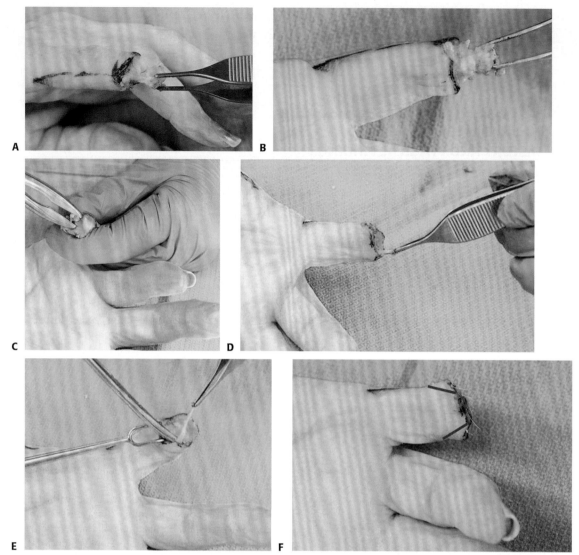

TECH FIG 1 • Revision amputation through middle phalanx. **A,B.** Mobilization of the viable soft tissue around the amputation site. **C.** Bone contouring of middle phalanx head at amputation site. **D,E.** Digital nerve identification and shortening to prevent symptomatic neuroma. **F.** Amputation wound closure without tension. The boxy appearance should be rounded by removal of dog ears as marked.

■ Nail Ablation

- If the revision amputation will result in removal of over two-thirds of the nail matrix and/or its underlying bony support, prepare to ablate the nail bed (**TECH FIG 2A**).
- Administer a digital block prior to sterile preparation.
- Apply a finger tourniquet.
- Remove the nail plate (if it remains) with a Freer elevator and hemostat.
- Make periungual incisions, perpendicular to the radial and ulnar margins of the eponychium, but do not incise through the dorsal roof matrix (**TECH FIG 2B,C**).
- Use methylene blue or a surgical marker to stain the germinal matrix and dorsal roof matrix from within the nail fold[4] (**TECH FIG 2D**).

- Use a scalpel to raise the eponychial skin from the dorsal roof matrix. Separate these layers to the proximal extent of the germinal matrix (**TECH FIG 2E,F**).
- Avoid injury to the terminal extensor tendon. It inserts on the distal phalanx 1.2 mm proximal to the germinal matrix.[2]
- Identify the radial and ulnar lateral horns of the matrix, as these define the radial and ulnar limits of ablation.
- Excise the germinal and sterile matrix from the underlying periosteum of the distal phalanx (**TECH FIG 2G,H**).
- The proximal confluence of the lateral nail fold, germinal matrix, and dorsal roof matrix forms a pocket of tissue (lateral horns of the matrix) that should be excised en bloc. All marked tissue should be contained within this pocket.
- Perform bony shortening as indicated.
- Close with 5-0 nonabsorbable suture (**TECH FIG 2I,J**).

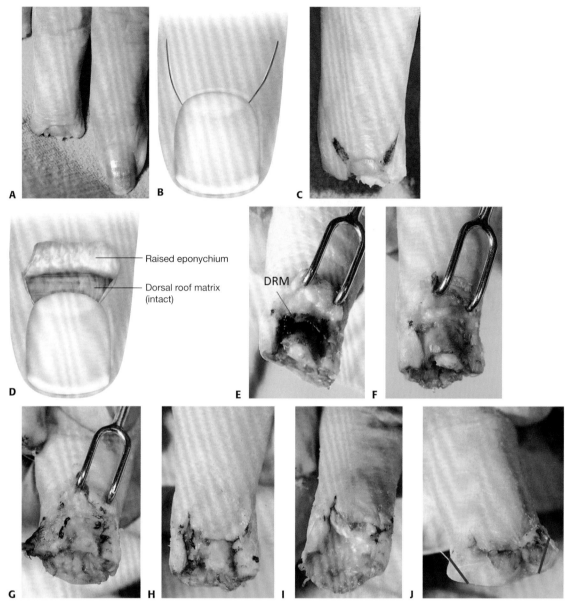

TECH FIG 2 • A. Fingertip amputation with significant loss of sterile matrix and bony support. **B,C.** Incisions for nail ablation. **D.** Use of a surgical marker or methylene blue helps define the extent of the nail fold for ablation. DRM, dorsal roof matrix. **E,F.** Elevation of the eponychial skin from the dorsal roof matrix. **G,H.** Nail ablation completed. **I,J.** Wound closure after nail ablation and bone shortening. The closure is contoured by removing dog ears as marked.

PEARLS AND PITFALLS

Preparation	▪ Gather all instruments and dressings prior to starting the procedure.
	▪ Perform the digital block prior to gathering supplies. This allows time for the anesthetic to take effect.
Revision amputation technique	▪ If the flexor or extensor tendon insertion is injured, strongly consider DIP joint disarticulation. The residual digit will be more stable with little sacrifice of length.
	▪ Ensure shortening of digital nerves to prevent painful neuroma formation at the fingertip.
Nail ablation technique	▪ Complete removal of the germinal matrix is easier if the dorsal roof matrix is left in continuity with the germinal matrix. This allows for a "pocket" of matrix to be removed en bloc.
	▪ Handle the thin dorsal eponychial skin with care when elevating from the underlying dorsal matrix.
Wound closure	▪ Tension-free closure is a necessity. Shorten bone further if needed.
	▪ Contour skin edges to minimize dog ears.

POSTOPERATIVE CARE

- A nonadherent soft dressing is applied over the digit.
- Oral antibiotics may be routinely prescribed postprocedure.
- Nonabsorbable sutures are removed 2 weeks postprocedure.
- After revision amputation, hand therapy is useful for fingertip desensitization, contouring, and early motion.

OUTCOMES

- Average static two-point discrimination after revision amputation is 3.8 mm.[5]
- Overall, revision amputation results in better static two-point discrimination when compared to local flaps.
- Good functional outcomes can be expected, with 95% of total active motion preserved.[5]
- Cold intolerance is common after revision amputation, with a 77% incidence.[5]

COMPLICATIONS

- Infection
- Cold intolerance and hypersensitivity are common.
- Painful neuroma
- Poor wound healing may be a result of closure under tension.
- Stiffness can result if early motion is not encouraged.
- Nail remnants may grow at the site of incomplete nail ablation.

REFERENCES

1. Peterson SL, Peterson EL, Wheatley MJ. Management of fingertip amputations. *J Hand Surg [Am]*. 2014;39(10):2093-2101.
2. Shum C, Bruno RJ, Ristic S, et al. Examination of the anatomic relationship of the proximal germinal nail matrix to the extensor tendon insertion. *J Hand Surg [Am]*. 2000;25(6):1114-1117.
3. Strauss EJ, Weil WM, Jordan C, et al. A prospective, randomized, controlled trial of 2-octylcyanoacrylate versus suture repair for nail bed injuries. *J Hand Surg [Am]*. 2008;33(2):250-253.
4. Baran R, Haneke E. Matricectomy and nail ablation. *Hand Clin*. 2002;18(4):693-696.
5. Yuan F, McGlinn EP, Giladi AM, et al. A systematic review of outcomes after revision amputation for treatment of traumatic finger amputation. *Plast Reconstr Surg*. 2015;136(3):99-113.

Drainage of Septic Flexor Tenosynovitis

John R. Lien and Kevin C. Chung

CHAPTER 4

DEFINITION

- Pyogenic flexor tenosynovitis is a bacterial infection in the flexor tendon sheath of the fingers or the thumb.

ANATOMY

- The flexor tendon sheath extends from the A1 pulley to the distal interphalangeal joint (**FIG 1**).
- The thumb flexor tendon sheath and radial bursa are contiguous.
- The small finger flexor tendon sheath and ulnar bursa are contiguous.
- The radial and ulnar bursae communicate through the space of Parona, which lies between the fascia of the pronator quadratus and flexor digitorum profundus tendon sheath.

PATHOGENESIS

- Most infections are caused by a penetrating injury to the tendon sheath.
- The most common organism responsible for disease is *Staphylococcus aureus*.[1]

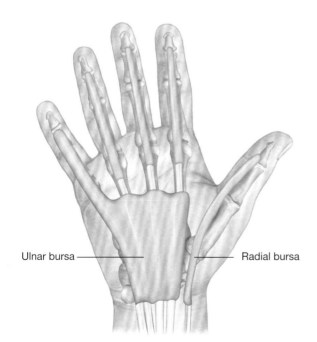

FIG 1 • Flexor tendon sheaths of the hand. There is potential communication between the thumb and small finger sheaths with the radial and ulna bursae, respectively.

Ulnar bursa — — Radial bursa

- Hematogenous disease can be caused by disseminated gonococcal infection.
- Inoculated bacteria use the synovial fluid within the sheath as nutrition.
  - Bacterial growth leads to increased volume and pressure within the tendon sheath.
- Horseshoe abscess: Thumb or small finger flexor tenosynovitis can extend proximally into the space of Parona and track back up distally the opposite side flexor sheath.

NATURAL HISTORY

- Left untreated, the infection creates adhesions within the tendon sheath, resulting in stiffness and loss of tendon gliding.
- Increased pressure obstructs extrinsic vincular blood supply to the tendon, contributing to tendon necrosis and rupture.

PATIENT HISTORY AND PHYSICAL FINDINGS

- History of penetrating trauma. Evaluate for puncture wound on the palmar aspect of the digit.
- Assess the timing of injury and onset of symptoms.
- Diagnosis is clinical. Kanavel's four cardinal symptoms and signs are useful in diagnosis[1]:
  - Exquisite tenderness along the flexor tendon sheath
  - Semiflexed position of the digit
  - Fusiform swelling of the digit
  - Pain with passive extension of the digit
- Examine the thenar and hypothenar eminences to assess for proximal extension of thumb or small finger tenosynovitis.
- Examine the distal forearm; tenderness or fullness of the volar wrist may indicate extension to the space of Parona (**FIG 2**).

IMAGING

- Radiographs should be obtained to assess for foreign body, pyarthrosis, or osteomyelitis.
- Laboratory evaluation with CBC, ESR, and CRP is helpful to monitor the disease process.

DIFFERENTIAL DIAGNOSIS

- Felon
- Paronychia
- Herpetic whitlow
- Gout
- Local abscess
- Septic arthritis
- High-pressure injection injury

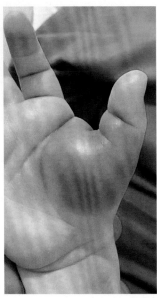

FIG 2 • Thumb flexor tenosynovitis with extension into the space of Parona. Note swelling and erythema in radial volar forearm.

- Nonseptic acute flexor tenosynovitis from an inflammatory process such as rheumatoid arthritis

NONOPERATIVE MANAGEMENT

- Early infection (less than 24–48 hours after inoculation) in immunocompetent patients with mild symptoms may be treated with intravenous antibiotics, immobilization, and elevation.[1]

- If symptoms do not improve within the first 12 to 24 hours of antibiotic therapy, surgical treatment is warranted.

SURGICAL MANAGEMENT

- Indications for surgical management:
  - Patients presenting with symptoms for more than 24 to 48 hours
  - Immunocompromised or diabetic patient
  - Failure of symptom improvement with nonoperative management.

Preoperative Planning

- Plan for carpal tunnel decompression and extension to the distal forearm if there is concern for proximal involvement.

Positioning

- Supine with hand table
- General anesthesia
- Tourniquet without Esmarch exsanguination

Approach

- Closed tendon sheath irrigation is preferred for acute infections.[2] The limited incisions prevent tendon desiccation and minimize postoperative scarring.
- Extensile open debridement of the flexor tendon sheath through a longitudinal midlateral incision is used in the setting of subacute or chronic infection with thick purulence and phlegmon. The volar skin should not be disturbed to avoid wound separation, leading to exposure of the flexor tendon sheath that will require flap coverage to avoid tendon desiccation.

■ Closed Tendon Sheath Irrigation (Acute Presentation)

Debridement and Exposure

- Thoroughly irrigate and debride any wounds.
- Distal exposure of the flexor tendon sheath
  - Make a 1-cm midaxial skin incision on the noncontact side of the digit overlying the A5 pulley (**TECH FIG 1A**).
  - Deepen the incision by dividing Cleland ligaments, dorsal to the neurovascular bundle.

- Bluntly elevate the volar flap of the incision in order to visualize the A5 pulley of the flexor tendon sheath (**TECH FIG 1B**).
- Incise the A5 pulley longitudinally and send any purulent or cloudy material for culture and sensitivity.
- Proximal exposure of the flexor tendon sheath
  - Make a chevron or oblique incision in the palm overlying the A1 pulley (see **TECH FIG 1A**).
  - Bluntly dissect the soft tissue overlying the flexor tendon sheath, taking care not to injure the neurovascular bundles.

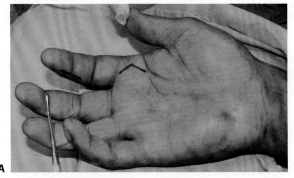
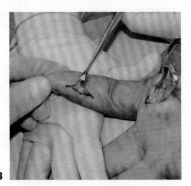

A   **B**

TECH FIG 1 • **A.** Incision markings for index finger tendon sheath exposure. **B.** Distal portal exposure of A5 pulley. The incision is dorsal to the neurovascular bundle and away from the contact surface of the distal pulp.

- Identify the A1 pulley.
- The A1 pulley does not have to be incised to perform tendon sheath irrigation. However, if there is thickened tenosynovium at this level, debride and send cultures.
- In the thumb, proximal exposure is performed through a thenar crease incision with release of the distal centimeter of transverse carpal ligament. The irrigation catheter is inserted along the flexor pollicis longus tendon.

Tendon Sheath Irrigation

- Place a 16-gauge intravenous catheter or 5F pediatric feeding tube in the proximal flexor sheath under the A1 pulley.
- From the proximal catheter, irrigate the tendon sheath with sterile saline until the effluent is clear (**TECH FIG 2**). We typically irrigate at least 500 mL of fluid.
- If resistance is met, place a second catheter distally to facilitate irrigant egress.
- If irrigant is exiting through a debrided wound proximal to the distal catheter, irrigate thoroughly and then replace the proximal catheter in the distal aspect of the debrided wound to complete distal irrigation of the tendon sheath. Be sure that the saline is not injected into the subcutaneous tissue to avoid pressure necrosis of the soft tissue.

Wound Management

- Release the tourniquet and achieve hemostasis.
- Place small drains such as a 0.25 in. Penrose in the proximal and distal incisions.

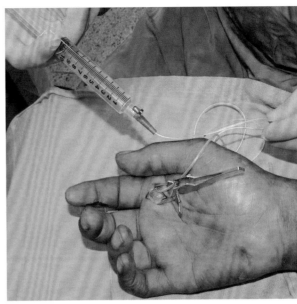

TECH FIG 2 • Irrigation of flexor tendon sheath with pediatric feeding tube.

- Loose sutures are placed only to prevent tendon exposure and desiccation. The wounds should be left open otherwise.
- Apply a forearm-based splint with the hand in resting position.

■ Open Debridement of Flexor Tendon Sheath (Subacute or Chronic Presentation)

Debridement and Exposure

- Thoroughly irrigate and debride any wounds.
- Make a midlateral incision from the distal interphalangeal flexion crease to the metacarpophalangeal flexion crease.

- Elevate a full-thickness palmar flap over the flexor tendon sheath. Extend the incision with oblique Bruner incisions distally and proximally if necessary.
- Identify the proximal extent of the flexor sheath system at the A1 pulley either through a separate chevron incision or by oblique proximal extension of the midlateral incision (**TECH FIG 3A**).
- Debride purulent and unhealthy appearing tenosynovium. Typically, this tissue cannot be washed away with closed sheath irrigation.

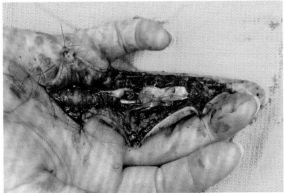

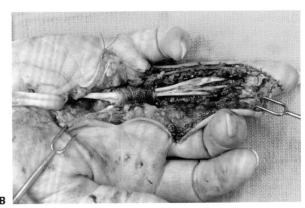

A **B**

TECH FIG 3 • **A.** Extensile exposure of flexor tendon sheath in setting of extensive purulence. **B.** Debridement of ruptured necrotic flexor digitorum profundus tendon.

- Necrotic tendon and/or pulley may need to be debrided (**TECH FIG 3B**).
- Send tissue for culture and sensitivities.
- Thoroughly irrigate the wound.

Wound Closure

- Release the tourniquet and obtain hemostasis.
- The palmar flap may be loosely closed over the flexor tendon sheath; compared to a standard Bruner approach, the midlateral approach minimizes the risk of tendon desiccation (**TECH FIG 4**).
- Leave drains in place to allow for fluid egress.
- Apply a forearm-based splint with the hand in resting position.

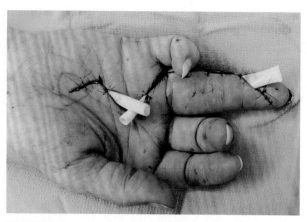

TECH FIG 4 • Wound closure to cover the flexor tendons.

PEARLS AND PITFALLS

Diagnosis	▪ Prompt clinical diagnosis is essential to initiate early treatment.
Incision placement	▪ Plan incisions so they may be incorporated into extensile exposures if needed. ▪ Avoid injury to the neurovascular bundle. The digital nerve trifurcates at the distal interphalangeal joint crease. ▪ Inadequate exposure may fail to drain the infection.
Culture	▪ Obtain stains, cultures, and sensitivities for aerobic, anaerobic, fungal, acid-fast bacillus, and atypical mycobacterial organisms. ▪ If a hematogenous source is suspected, obtain blood cultures and gonococcal tests.
Tendon sheath irrigation	▪ Avoid high-pressure injection if there is resistance to syringe irrigation. Reposition the entrance and egress catheters if necessary. ▪ If there is extensive infection, indicated by thick phlegmon or viscous drainage from the tendon sheath, extensile exposure may be necessary. ▪ Continue irrigation until there is clear effluent.
Postoperative	▪ Return for interval irrigation and debridement if there is no clinical improvement within 24–48 h.

POSTOPERATIVE CARE

- Elevate the extremity.
- Continue empiric antibiotics while cultures are pending. Include methicillin-resistant *S aureus* coverage.
- Remove the dressing postoperative day one and begin soaks 3 times daily.
- Initiate early motion of the digits to minimize stiffness.
- If symptoms do not improve within the first 24 to 48 hours, return to the operating room for additional irrigation and debridement.
- In the setting of severe infection with persistent infection and/or tendon necrosis, discuss amputation with the patient.

OUTCOMES

- Patients average 70% to 80% recovery of total active motion.[3]
- Risk factors for failure of surgical treatment resulting in amputation include[3]:
  - Age over 43 years
  - Diabetes mellitus, peripheral vascular disease, or renal failure
  - Presence of subcutaneous purulence
  - Ischemic changes at presentation
  - Polymicrobial infection

COMPLICATIONS

- Finger stiffness
- Persistent infection
- Digital nerve injury
- Tendon desiccation and rupture

REFERENCES

1. Draeger RW, Bynum DK. Flexor tendon sheath infections of the hand. *J Am Acad Orthop Surg.* 2012;20(6):373-382.
2. Neviaser RJ. Closed tendon sheath irrigation for pyogenic flexor tenosynovitis. *J Hand Surg [Am].* 1978;3(5):462-466.
3. Pang HN, Teoh LC, Yam AT, et al. Factors affecting the prognosis of pyogenic flexor tenosynovitis. *J Bone Joint Surg Am.* 2007;89(8):1742-1748.

Distal Phalanx Fractures

John R. Fowler and Thomas B. Hughes

5

CHAPTER

DEFINITION

- Distal phalanx fractures can be divided into several main categories (**FIG 1**):
  - Extensor tendon injuries, including soft tissue–only extensor tendon avulsions and "bony mallet" injuries that involve avulsion of a fragment of the distal phalanx. Bony mallet injuries may cause volar subluxation of the distal phalanx.
  - Distal phalanx fractures without involvement of the ligaments or tendons
  - Open epiphyseal fracture with nail bed laceration (Seymour fracture)
- A fracture is present in one-third of all mallet fingers.[1]
- Mean age is 30, and the middle finger is most commonly involved.[2]
- Mallet injuries may be classified using the Wehbe and Schneider classification[2]
  - Type I: No subluxation at DIP joint
  - Type II: DIP joint subluxation

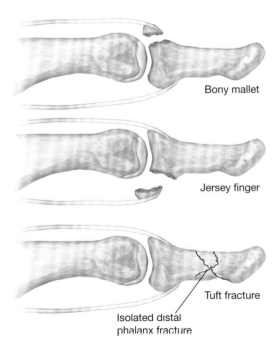

FIG 1 • Type of distal phalanx fractures. **A.** Bony mallet fractures. **B.** Jersey finger—avulsion of the flexor digitorum profundus from the base of the distal phalanx. **C.** Distal phalanx shaft/epiphyseal fracture or tuft fracture.

Bony mallet

Jersey finger

Tuft fracture

Isolated distal
phalanx fracture

- Type III: Epiphyseal injury
- The types are further subdivided based on the amount of articular surface that is involved:
  - Type A involves less than 1/3 of the articular surface.
  - Type B involves 1/3 to 2/3 of the articular surface.
  - Type C involves greater than 2/3 of the articular surface.

ANATOMY

- The terminal tendon inserts on the distal phalanx articular edge and has a footprint of approximately 12 mm.[3]
- The terminal tendon insertion is, on average, 1.4 mm proximal to the leading edge of the germinal matrix.[3]
- The extensor tendon inserts on the epiphysis, and flexor tendon inserts on the metaphyseal portion of the distal phalanx.[4] This results in a flexed posture for epiphyseal fractures.

PATHOGENESIS

- The classic mechanism for a mallet injury is a ball striking the tip of the finger, causing eccentric flexion, resulting in tendon rupture and/or distal phalanx fracture.
- Subluxation of the joint may occur with large fracture fragments as the collateral ligaments are attached to the fracture fragment and the flexor digitorum profundus then has unopposed pull.[1]
  - Biomechanical studies have found that fractures involving less than 43% of the joint surface do not result in joint subluxation, whereas fractures involving over 52% of the joint surface do result in joint subluxation.[5]
- Seymour fractures are more commonly caused by a crushing mechanism resulting in distal phalanx epiphyseal fracture with nail bed laceration.[4] This is an open fracture that requires immediate debridement, reduction, nail bed repair, and pinning.

NATURAL HISTORY

- Bony mallet injuries without volar subluxation of the joint have excellent healing rates.
- The average extensor lag with nonoperative treatment is 7 degrees.
- Seymour fractures that are not treated with formal irrigation and debridement historically have a high infection rate and risk for osteomyelitis.[4]

PATIENT HISTORY AND PHYSICAL FINDINGS

- Patients typically present after a "jamming"-type injury of the finger with a chief complaint of inability to extend the finger at the distal interphalangeal joint.
- The distal interphalangeal joint is often swollen and erythematous. There is a variable amount of nail plate ecchymosis depending on the specific fracture type.

IMAGING

- AP and lateral radiographs of the finger are obtained.

NONOPERATIVE MANAGEMENT

- Conservative treatment in a DIP extension splint is indicated for soft tissue mallet fingers and bony mallet injuries involving less than 40% of the articular surface and injuries without volar subluxation.
  - The DIP extension splint is worn continuously for 6 weeks and then only at night for an additional 2 weeks.
- The vast majority of fractures without volar subluxation of the distal phalanx should be treated nonoperatively. K-wire fixation is a secondary solution.

SURGICAL MANAGEMENT

- Indications for surgical management
  - Open fracture (Seymour fracture or open bony mallet)
  - More than 40% articular surface involvement
  - Volar subluxation of the distal phalanx
  - A relative indication is a patient who is a professional (such as a surgeon) who cannot wear an extension splint continuously for 6 weeks. They require pinning, with the pin buried under the skin and removed after 6 weeks.

Positioning

- The patient is placed in the supine position with the arm on a radiolucent table.
- The surgeon sits so that the dominant hand can drill the K-wires retrograde into the finger. For right-handed surgeons, this is at the head of the table.

Approach

- Mallet fingers are treated percutaneously. Seymour fractures require open debridement and pinning.

TECHNIQUES

■ Closed Reduction and Pinning

- First, a closed reduction is performed under live fluoroscopy by hyperextending the distal interphalangeal joint by 5 to 10 degrees.
- If this results in apposition of the bony mallet fragment and distal phalanx, a 0.045 in. K-wire is placed from the fingertip, through the distal phalanx, and across the distal interphalangeal joint (**TECH FIG 1**).

- The pin can be cut and bent above the skin for removal in the office or buried and removed at a later time.
- If the dorsal bony fragment remains significantly displaced, the finger is flexed, and under live fluoroscopy, a 0.045 in. K-wire is placed 1 to 2 mm proximal to the avulsion fragment and then drilled into the head of the middle phalanx.[6]

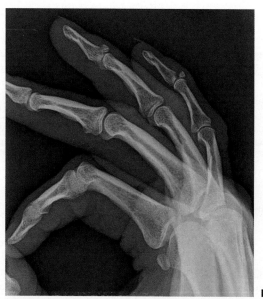 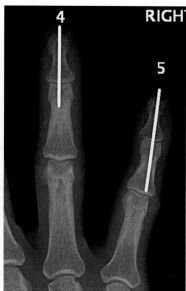

TECH FIG 1 • A. Oblique radiograph demonstrating bony mallet fractures of the small and ring finger distal phalanges. The joint reduced with extension of the distal phalanx, and the avulsion fragments became closely opposed. Postoperative **(B)** and lateral **(C)** AP demonstrate near anatomic overall alignment.

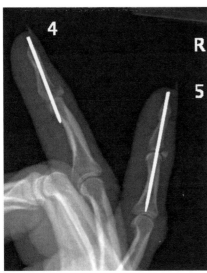

TECH FIG 1 (Continued)

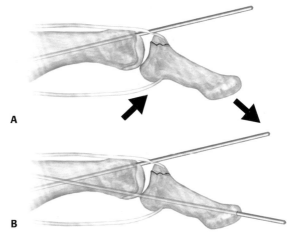

TECH FIG 2 • A. After a K-wire is placed just proximal to the avulsion fragment, the distal phalanx is extended to reduce the avulsion fragment to the distal phalanx. **B.** A second K-wire is placed across the DIP joint to hold the distal phalanx in extension.[6]

- The finger is then fully extended (**TECH FIG 2A**), and a second 0.045 in. K-wire is placed from the fingertip, through the distal phalanx, and across the distal interphalangeal joint (**TECH FIG 2B**).[6]

- The starting point for this K-wire is just volar to the nail bed. One must be careful not to be too dorsal because nail deformities can occur if the K-wire is driven through the nail bed.

■ Open Reduction and Internal Fixation

- An H-shaped incision is made dorsally, over the distal interphalangeal joint.
- Thick flaps are raised proximally and distally to expose the terminal tendon.

- The fracture is reduced and held in place with a 0.035 in. K-wire.
- Depending on the size of the fragment, two 1.3- to 1.5-mm mini-fragment screws are placed to stabilize the fracture.
  - The reduction is indirect as visualization is blocked.

■ Open Treatment of Seymour Fractures

- The nail bed is carefully removed using a combination of a Freer elevator and a hemostat. Care is taken to not injure the underlying nail bed.
- There is usually a transverse laceration in the nail bed at the level of the germinal matrix.
- It may be necessary to make a longitudinal incision on either edge of the eponychium to lift the eponychium up "like a car hood" to allow better visualization of the germinal matrix.
- The finger is flexed to expose the open epiphyseal fracture. The interposed soft tissue is carefully removed and the bone is well irrigated. Excessive debridement

of the bone is not performed as this would risk epiphyseal closure.
- The fracture is reduced and a 0.045 in. K-wire retrograde across the fracture and then across the DIP joint (**TECH FIG 3**).
- The nail bed is repaired using 5-0 chromic suture. The eponychial fold incisions are repaired using 5-0 chromic as well.
  - The nail plate is trimmed, washed, and replaced under the eponychial fold to prevent scarring to the nail bed. Alternatively, the foil wrapper from the chromic suture package is cut in the shape of a nail and placed under the eponychial fold.

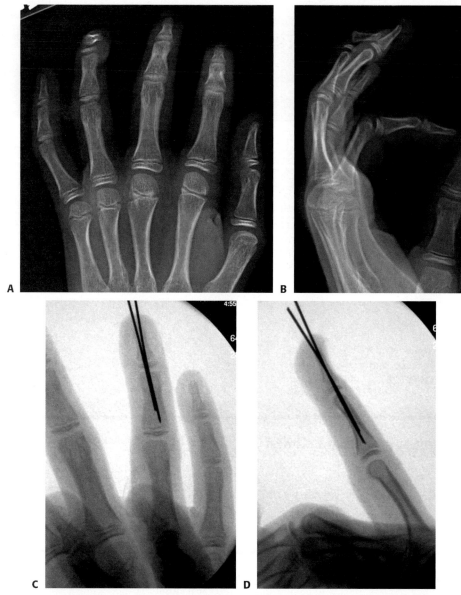

TECH FIG 3 • Preoperative AP **(A)** and lateral **(B)** radiographs demonstrating an open distal phalanx epiphyseal fracture. The fracture site was debrided and reduced. **C,D.** Two 0.045 in. K-wires were then drilled retrograde across the fracture and across the DIP joint for stability.

PEARLS AND PITFALLS

Indications	■ Classic indications include volar subluxation of the distal phalanx and/or a fracture involving more than 40% of the joint surface.
Seymour fractures	■ Early irrigation, debridement, and pinning are essential to successful outcomes. These fractures have a high risk of osteomyelitis if not appropriately treated.
Treatment	■ Attempt to avoid skin incisions and treat percutaneously, if possible, to avoid dorsal skin necrosis.

POSTOPERATIVE CARE

- Patients are immobilized in a DIP extension splint, leaving the PIP joint free.
- Early active motion of the PIP joint is encouraged to prevent stiffness and contracture.

OUTCOMES

- Hofmeister et al.[7] reported on 24 fingers that underwent extension block pinning at a mean follow-up of 74 weeks.
  - Mean time to union was 35 days.
  - Mean extension was –4 degrees.
  - Mean flexion was 78 degrees.
  - Three fingers had a superficial pin site infection that resolved with oral antibiotics.
  - Two fingers had loss of reduction less than 2 mm.
- Darder-Prats and colleagues[8] reviewed 22 mallet fractures that underwent extension block pinning at mean follow-up of 25 months. All patients reported a good or excellent result.
- Krusche-Mandl et al.[9] reviewed 24 patients with Seymour fractures and noted that 23/24 obtained full range of motion and there were no chronic infections. However, 5 patients had distal phalanx growth disturbances and 6 had limited nail dystrophies.

COMPLICATIONS

- The majority of distal phalanx fractures (with the exception of Seymour fractures) should be treated nonoperatively due to the high complication rate associated with operative treatment.
- King et al.[10] reported complications in 41% of operatively treated mallet fractures in their series. The most common complication was dorsal skin necrosis. Other complications included osteomyelitis, pin tract infection, nail deformity, and recurrent extensor lag.

- Stern and Kastrup[11] reported a 53% complication rate for operatively treated mallet fractures. The complications included nail deformity, pin infection, and joint incongruity.
- Superficial pin site infections usually resolve with pin removal and oral antibiotics.
- Patients may have persistent extensor lag at the DIP joint despite operative treatment. Additionally, surgical intervention may result in permanent decreased DIP flexion.

REFERENCES

1. Wada T, Oda T. Mallet fingers with bone avulsion and DIP joint subluxation. *J Hand Surg Eur Vol.* 2015;40(1):8-15.
2. Wehbe MA, Schneider LH. Mallet fractures. *J Bone Joint Surg Am.* 1984;66(5):658-669.
3. Schweitzer TP, Rayan GM. The terminal tendon of the digital extensor mechanism: part I, anatomic study. *J Hand Surg [Am].* 2004;29(5):898-902.
4. Abzug JM, Kozin SH. Seymour fractures. *J Hand Surg [Am].* 2013;38(11):2267-2270; quiz 2270.
5. Husain SN, Dietz JF, Kalainov DM, Lautenschlager EP. A biomechanical study of distal interphalangeal joint subluxation after mallet fracture injury. *J Hand Surg [Am].* 2008;33(1):26-30.
6. Ishiguro T, Yabe Y, Itoh Y, Hashizume N. Extension block with Kirschner wire for fracture dislocation of the interphalangeal joint. *Tech Hand Up Extrem Surg.* 1997;1(2):95-102.
7. Hofmeister EP, Mazurek MT, Shin AY, Bishop AT. Extension block pinning for large mallet fractures. *J Hand Surg [Am].* 2003;28(3):453-459.
8. Darder-Prats A, Fernandez-Garcia E, Fernandez-Gabarda R, Darder-Garcia A. Treatment of mallet finger fractures by the extension-block K-wire technique. *J Hand Surg Br.* 1998;23(6):802-805.
9. Krusche-Mandl I, Kottstorfer J, Thalhammer G, et al. Seymour fractures: retrospective analysis and therapeutic considerations. *J Hand Surg [Am].* 2013;38(2):258-264.
10. King HJ, Shin SJ, Kang ES. Complications of operative treatment for mallet fractures of the distal phalanx. *J Hand Surg Br.* 2001;26(1):28-31.
11. Stern PJ, Kastrup JJ. Complications and prognosis of treatment of mallet finger. *J Hand Surg [Am].* 1988;13(3):329-334.

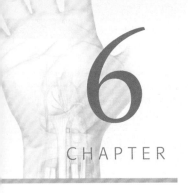

6
CHAPTER

Proximal Phalanx Fractures

John R. Fowler

DEFINITION

- Proximal phalanx fractures represent 23% of all hand and forearm fractures.[1]
- These fractures can be classified by
  - Location
    - Extra-articular
    - Intracondylar
    - Base/epiphyseal
  - Fracture pattern
    - Oblique
    - Transverse
    - Comminuted

ANATOMY

- The proximal phalanx is the longest phalanx in each finger and has a mild palmar concavity.[2]
- The head of the proximal phalanx has two convex condyles and a central shallow depression.[2]
- Proximal phalanx shaft fractures typically assume an apex volar angulation.[2]
  - The intrinsic muscles insert on the proximal phalanx base.
  - The central slip pulls the distal fragment into extension.
- The extensor mechanism (**FIG 1**) is in direct contact with the proximal phalanx. Therefore, fracture hematoma and resulting fibrosis may greatly inhibit gliding of the extensor mechanism.
  - One must consider this close relationship if considering the use of dorsal hardware.

PATHOGENESIS

- Phalanx fractures occur through several common mechanisms of injury:
  - Axial load (jamming type injury)
  - Rotational torque
  - Medial/lateral angular force
  - Crush or direct blow
- The injury mechanism is important for the type of fracture that is created. Rotational torque typically produces an oblique fracture, while crush/direct blow mechanisms produce a transverse fracture that may have comminution.
- Patient age also plays a role in fracture type and location. Pediatric patients most commonly sustain epiphyseal fractures at the phalanx base, whereas adult patients more commonly sustain transverse or oblique fractures of the phalanx shaft.

NATURAL HISTORY

- Minimally displaced fractures and stable fracture patterns have a high rate of union with minimal long-term loss of function.
- Displaced fractures and unstable fractures may lead to nonunion or malunion, resulting in loss of motion.

PATIENT HISTORY AND PHYSICAL FINDINGS

- The history should carefully document the mechanism of injury and time since injury. A higher-energy mechanism of injury may indicate greater surrounding soft tissue damage and the possibility of greater fracture instability. The time since injury is important, especially in pediatric patients, as delay in surgical intervention may preclude closed reduction if significant fracture healing occurs prior to intervention.
- A careful examination of the skin is important to rule out open fracture that would necessitate more urgent surgical treatment.
- The finger is often swollen and ecchymotic from the fracture.

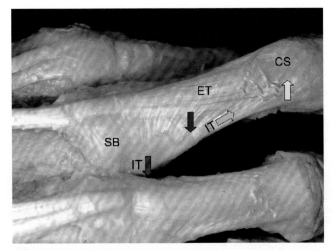

FIG 1 • Extra-articular proximal phalanx shaft fractures typically assume an apex volar angulation (*red arrow*). The lateral band (IT) insertion (*green arrow*) at the base of the proximal phalanx results in flexion of the proximal fragment (*blue arrow*) and the central slip (CS) insertion on the base of the middle phalanx pulls the distal fragment dorsally (*yellow arrow*). SB, sagittal band; ET, extensor tendon. (From Harman TW, Graham TJ, Uhl RL. Operative treatment of extra-articular phalangeal fractures. In Hunt TR, ed. *Operative Techniques in Hand, Wrist, and Forearm Surgery*. Philadelphia, PA: Lippincott Williams & Wilkins, 2011:287.)

- Rotational alignment of the finger should be evaluated by asking the patient to flex the digits. All four fingers should point in the same direction, toward the scaphoid tubercle.
  - If patients are unable to adequately flex the digits secondary to pain, the alignment of the fingernails can be compared to the contralateral hand with the fingers in full extension. Rotational malalignment is not well tolerated and is an indication for surgical intervention.
- Finger extension is carefully evaluated. Apex dorsal angulation of the fracture can result in relative lengthening of the extensor mechanism, resulting in an extensor lag at the proximal interphalangeal joint.

IMAGING

- Standard AP, lateral, and oblique radiographs are obtained.
- Advanced imaging with CT is rarely indicated. CT may be beneficial to evaluate articular congruity for condyle fractures and phalangeal base fractures.

DIFFERENTIAL DIAGNOSIS

- Proximal phalanx fracture
- Contusion
- Collateral ligament sprain/tear
- Arthritis
- Trigger finger
- Infection

NONOPERATIVE MANAGEMENT

- Nondisplaced and minimally displaced fractures without rotational malalignment may be treated nonoperatively with a cast or custom thermoplast splint.
- The risk of prolonged immobilization and resultant stiffness must be weighed against the risks of surgical intervention.

SURGICAL MANAGEMENT

- It cannot be overemphasized that the best surgical option is the least invasive option that provides fracture stability and the opportunity for early range of motion.

- Extensive exposure may result in permanent postoperative stiffness.
- Percutaneous techniques with near-anatomic alignment may be preferred to open treatment with anatomic alignment.
- Indications
  - Closed reduction and pinning
    - Acceptable alignment can be obtained by closed means.
    - Fracture is stable after pinning.
    - Of note, a limited incision to reduce the fracture, followed by percutaneous pinning, is also a treatment option
  - Open reduction with lag screws
    - Long oblique fracture with 2:1 ratio of fracture length:phalanx width
  - Open reduction with mini-fragment plate
    - Comminution
    - Transverse fracture or short oblique not amenable to lag screws or pinning

Preoperative Planning

- The surgeon should be prepared for both closed and open techniques.
- K-wires and mini-fragment screws and plates should be available.

Positioning

- The patient is placed in the supine position with the affected arm on a radiolucent hand table.
- Most surgical approaches are from the dorsum of the finger, and therefore the palm is placed down on the table.
- The surgeon sits in the axilla (if right handed) or at the head of the bed (if left handed) to allow the dominant hand to be used to place K-wires.

Approach

- For the techniques described in this chapter, the dorsal approach is used.
- Sharp dissection down to the extensor mechanism is performed to develop thick flaps that are not damaged by blunt dissection.

■ Open Reduction and Internal Fixation of Intra-articular Proximal Phalanx Condylar Fractures

- A midlateral incision is made on the side of the condylar fracture.
- Sharp dissection is carried out down to the extensor mechanism and thick flaps are raised.
- The interval between the central slip and lateral band is incised.
- The fracture site is identified and dorsal capsule incised to evaluate the articular surface.
- The collateral ligament is attached to the condyle and is the deforming force.
- The fracture is reduced under direct visualization.
  - This is accomplished by placing a 0.035-in. K-wire in the fragment and using it as a joystick to reduce the fracture. The K-wire can then sometimes be drilled across

the fracture site to temporarily stabilize the fracture. However, often the K-wire is at the wrong angle, and a second 0.035-in. K-wire is placed across the fracture site.
- Caution should be exercised when using tenaculum clamps or towel clips as the condyle fracture fragment is often very small and can be crushed by these larger clamps.
- I have found that gentle use of a hemostat to hold the fracture while the temporary K-wire is placed across the fracture site is useful and typically does not crush the condyle.
- Two or three (depending on the size of the condyle fragment) 1.2-mm mini-fragment screws are placed across the fracture (**TECH FIG 1**).
  - I do not recommend the use of standard lag screw technique for these fractures. I only drill the pilot hole and place a neutralization screw. The fracture fragment is small, and there is little room for error. Multiple passes

T E C H N I Q U E S

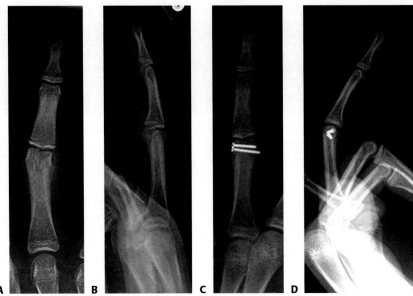

TECH FIG 1 • AP **(A)** and lateral **(B)** radiographs demonstrating an intra-articular condylar fracture of the proximal phalanx head. Postoperative AP **(C)** and lateral **(D)** radiographs demonstrate improved articular congruity after open reduction and internal fixation.

- with the drill can cause fragmentation of the fracture and results in fracture displacement.
- Anatomic reduction is confirmed on orthogonal radiographs.

- The wound is well irrigated and interval between the central slip and lateral bands closed with 4-0 Vicryl suture.
- The skin is closed using 4-0 nylon suture.

■ Closed Reduction and Pinning of Extra-articular Proximal Phalanx Shaft Fractures

- A closed reduction is performed and confirmed on orthogonal radiographs (**TECH FIG 2**).
- The MCP joint is flexed to 90 degrees.

- A 0.045-in. K-wire is taken freehand and placed at the midpoint of the metacarpal head in the AP plane and immediately medial or lateral.
  - In my experience, this starting point is more volar than expected.
- Using a combination of direct feel and fluoroscopy, the K-wire is passed medial or lateral to the metacarpal head and into contact with the base of the proximal phalanx.

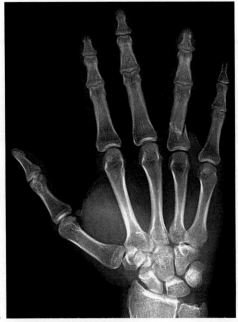
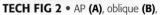
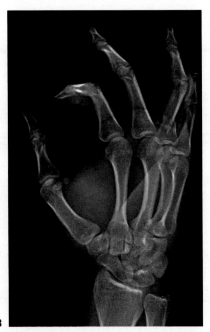

TECH FIG 2 • AP **(A)**, oblique **(B)**,

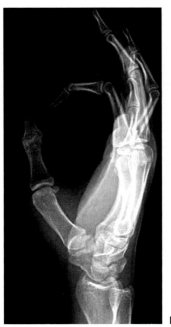
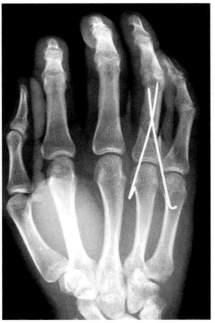
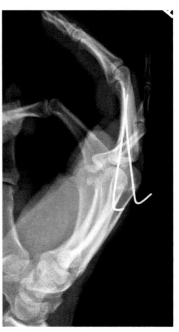

C   D   E

TECH FIG 2 (Continued) • and lateral **(C)** radiographs showing an extra-articular ring finger proximal phalanx shaft fracture with ulnar deviation and apex volar deformity. Postoperative AP **(D)** and lateral **(E)** radiographs showing improved alignment after closed reduction and percutaneous pinning.

- While holding the reduction, the K-wire is drilled into the phalanx base, across the fracture sire, and into the head of the proximal phalanx.
- Placement of the K-wire within the medullary canal (and not through the phalanx head into the PIP joint)

and maintenance of reduction is confirmed using fluoroscopy.
- This procedure is repeated to place a second 0.045-in. K-wire on the other side of the phalanx.
- The pins are bent and cut outside the skin for later removal.

■ Open Reduction and Internal Fixation of Extra-articular Proximal Phalanx Shaft Fractures With Lag Screws

- A longitudinal incision is made directly over the proximal phalanx. For more distal fractures, the incision is carried distally in a lazy S over the PIP joint, and for more proximal fractures, the incision is carried proximally in a lazy S over the MCP joint.
- Sharp dissection is carried out down to the extensor mechanism and thick flaps raised.
- Fracture exposure can be performed in two ways. I prefer to split the extensor mechanism longitudinally. I feel that this gives the best exposure of the fracture and allows the easiest screw placement. The problem with splitting the extensor tendon is postoperative extensor lag. Alternatively, the interval between the central extensor tendon and lateral bands can be developed.

- The fracture site is identified and fracture hematoma cleared.
- The fracture is provisionally reduced. For oblique fractures, this is often able to be accomplished with the use of a point-to-point tenaculum clamp or towel clamp.
  - Be careful to not overcompress with the clamp as this can cause iatrogenic fracture of the bone.
  - Check rotational alignment.
- A lag screw is then placed perpendicular to the fracture site. The pilot hole is drilled first, followed by the gliding hole. The countersink is then used as well (**TECH FIG 3**).
- An additional lag screw is placed perpendicular to the fracture site.
- Finally, a third screw is placed perpendicular to the other two screws.
- The extensor mechanism is closed with buried 4-0 Vicryl sutures.
- Close the skin with nylon sutures.
- Place the patient in splint with MCP flexed to 60 to 70 degrees, PIP and DIP fully extended.

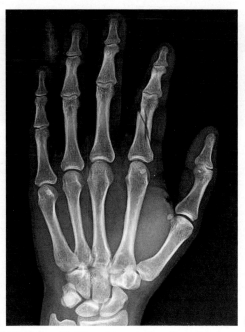 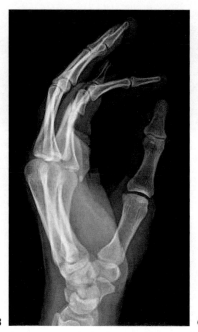 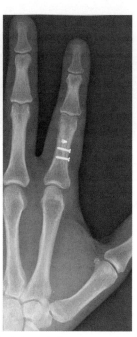

TECH FIG 3 • AP **(A)** and lateral **(B)** radiographs demonstrating an extra-articular fracture of the proximal phalanx shaft. Postoperative AP **(C)** radiograph demonstrates improved alignment after open reduction and internal fixation with a lag screws.

▪ Open Reduction and Internal Fixation of Extra-articular Proximal Phalanx Shaft Fractures With Mini-Fragment Plates

- The same approach is used as is described above for lag screw fixation.
- A 1.2 or 1.7-mm mini-fragment plate is chosen based on the size of the proximal phalanx.

- The smallest plate that will offer fracture stability is chosen and hardware prominence against the extensor mechanism may result in decreased range of motion.
- One screw is placed on each side of the fracture and rotational alignment evaluated (**TECH FIG 4A–D**).
- The remaining screws are then placed.
- The extensor mechanism is closed with buried 4-0 Vicryl sutures.
- The wound is closed using 4-0 nylon sutures.

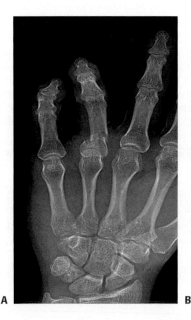 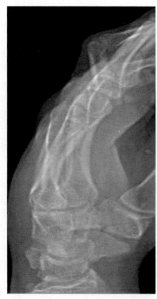

TECH FIG 4 • AP **(A)** and lateral **(B)** radiographs demonstrating an extra-articular fracture of the proximal phalanx base. Postoperative AP

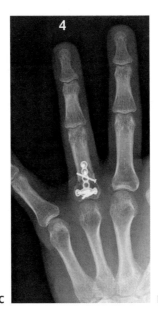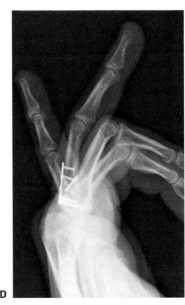

TECH FIG 4 (Continued) • **(C)** and lateral **(D)** radiographs demonstrate improved alignment after open reduction and internal fixation with a mini-fragment plate and screws.

C   D

PEARLS AND PITFALLS

Treatment	▪ Perform the least invasive procedure to achieve fracture stabilization.
Rehabilitation	▪ Start early ROM to decrease stiffness.
Starting point for K-wires	▪ The starting point for K-wires is more volar than expected.
Condylar fractures	▪ These fractures tend to have relatively little bone. Be careful to not overclamp these fractures as they can fall apart. Additionally, do not try to perform standard lag technique, just place neutralization screws.
Rotation	▪ Be sure to evaluate rotation before final hardware is placed and after all hardware is in place. Rotational alignment is critical.

POSTOPERATIVE CARE

- The patient is placed in a plaster splint with the MCP joints flexed to 70 degrees and PIP joints placed in full extension.
- If stable fixation has been achieved, the postoperative splint is removed at 7 to 10 days and the patient placed into a removable thermoplast splint with the MCP joints flexed to 70 degrees and the PIP joints left free to allow early ROM.
- If the fixation is of questionable stability, the patient is placed into a fiberglass cast that places the MCP joints to 70 degrees and PIP joints in full extension.
  - Pins are removed at 4 weeks and ROM initiated.
- At 6 weeks, all immobilization is discontinued and more aggressive ROM is started.

OUTCOMES

- Hornbach and Cohen[3] reported on 12 extra-articular proximal phalanx fractures treated with transarticular K-wire fixation.
  - Mean total active motion was 265 degrees and excellent results were obtained in 10 of 12 fractures.

- Faruqui et al.[4] reported on the outcomes of 50 isolated extra-articular proximal phalanx fractures that were treated with either transarticular or extra-articular cross-pinning.
  - The mean total active motion was 201 degrees in the transarticular group and 198 degrees in the extra-articular group.
  - The mean flexion loss at the PIP joint was 27 degrees.
  - Nearly 33% of patients in each group had an extensor lag greater than 15 degrees.
  - Secondary procedures were required in 6/25 patients in the transarticular group and 2/25 patients in the extra-articular group.
  - Hornbach and Cohen reported on 12 extra-articular proximal phalanx fractures treated with K-wire fixation at a mean follow-up of 20 months.

COMPLICATIONS

- Stiffness is a nearly universal complication after treatment of proximal phalanx fractures.
- Pin tract infections may occur when percutaneous pins are used.
- Malunion and nonunion may occur but are uncommon.

REFERENCES

1. Chung KC, Spilson SV. The frequency and epidemiology of hand and forearm fractures in the United States. *J Hand Surg [Am]*. 2001;26(5):908-915.
2. Gaston RG, Chadderdon C. Phalangeal fractures: displaced/nondisplaced. *Hand Clin*. 2012;28(3):395-401.
3. Hornbach EE, Cohen MS. Closed reduction and percutaneous pinning of fractures of the proximal phalanx. *J Hand Surg Br*. 2001;26(1):45-49.
4. Faruqui S, Stern PJ, Kiefhaber TR. Percutaneous pinning of fractures in the proximal third of the proximal phalanx: complications and outcomes. *J Hand Surg [Am]*. 2012;37(7):1342-1348.

Metacarpal Shaft Fractures

John R. Fowler and Thomas B. Hughes

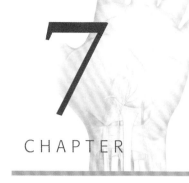

CHAPTER 7

DEFINITION

- A metacarpal head fracture is an intra-articular fracture of the metacarpal that is distal to the metacarpal neck.
- A boxer's fracture is a small finger metacarpal neck fracture.
- Metacarpal fractures constitute 30% of all fractures treated in the emergency department.
- Eighty-five percent of these fractures occur in males[1]

ANATOMY

- The metacarpals are concave volarly and articulate distally with the base of the proximal phalanx.
- The metacarpal base articulates with the distal carpal row.
  - The index and middle metacarpal bases articulate with the trapezoid and capitate. There is minimal motion at this articulation.[2]
  - The small and ring finger metacarpal bases articulate with the hamate. This articulation provides significant flexion and some rotation.[2]
- The deep intermetacarpal ligament connects the volar plates of each metacarpal, preventing significant shortening in the setting of fracture.[3]
- Tendon insertions and/or origins may contribute to fracture displacement.
  - FCR inserts on the volar base of the index metacarpal.
  - ECRL inserts on the dorsal base of the index metacarpal.
  - ECRB inserts on the dorsal base of the middle metacarpal.
  - ECU inserts on the dorsal base of the small metacarpal.
  - Interossei arise from the metacarpal shafts.

PATHOGENESIS

- Metacarpal neck fractures are the result of an axial load applied to a flexed MCP joint.
- The most common mechanism of injury is punching a hard object.[1]
- Metacarpal shaft fractures can result from axial load, torsion, and/or a direct blow.[3]
- The ring finger metacarpal has the narrowest shaft and therefore has a higher incidence of shaft fracture from a punching mechanism than do the other metacarpals.[1]
- Metacarpal base/CMC fracture dislocations are almost always the result of axial loading.

NATURAL HISTORY

- Pace et al.[4] compared 23 patients who underwent a closed reduction and casting for an isolated small finger metacarpal neck fracture with 43 patients who did not have a closed reduction.

- Despite improved angulation after reduction, at final follow-up, there was no difference in volar angulation between the two groups.
- Sletten and colleagues[5] randomized 85 patients with small finger metacarpal neck fractures that had more than 30 degrees of volar angulation to either nonoperative treatment or antegrade bouquet pinning. The authors found no difference in quickDASH, pain, satisfaction, range of motion, grip strength, or quality of life between the two groups. However, the operative group had a higher rate of complications and longer sick leave.
- Every 2 mm of metacarpal shortening results in 7 degrees of extensor lag.[6]

PATIENT HISTORY AND PHYSICAL FINDINGS

- The history often includes an axial load to the hand, usually with the fingers flexed.
- The history should include any history of open wounds or punching the mouth of another person to rule out "fight bite."
- "Fight bite" injuries require operative treatment to prevent deep infection.
- Special attention should be paid to the rotational alignment of the fingers with flexion.
  - All fingers should roughly point to the distal pole of the scaphoid.
  - Ensure that there is no scissoring.
  - Compare to the contralateral hand.
- The flexor tendons and collateral ligaments at each joint should be evaluated to ensure the absence of associated soft tissue injury.

IMAGING

- AP, oblique, and lateral radiographs of the hand should be obtained.
- Volar angulation should be measured on the true lateral view as the oblique view can overestimate true angulation.
- Consideration to CT scan can be given in cases of metacarpal base fractures to more accurately determine subluxation and for intra-articular metacarpal head fractures to more accurately determine the amount of articular step-off and displacement.

NONOPERATIVE MANAGEMENT

- Nonoperative treatment is appropriate for the vast majority of metacarpal neck and shaft fractures.

- Patients without rotational deformity and/or scissoring and without pseudoclawing are placed into a hand-based (neck fractures) or forearm-based (shaft fractures) ulnar gutter splint with the PIP joints left free for early motion
  - The splint is worn full-time for 4 weeks and then discontinued if the fracture site is no longer tender.
- Patients who are likely to be noncompliant with splint treatment are placed in short-arm ulnar gutter casts with the PIP joints left free.

SURGICAL MANAGEMENT

- Indications[3,7]
  - Metacarpal neck fractures with more than 10 to 15 degrees of volar angulation for the index and middle fingers and more than 40 degrees of volar angulation for the ring and small fingers
  - Metacarpal shaft fractures with more than 10 degrees of volar angulation for the index and middle fingers and more than 20 degrees of volar angulation for the ring and small fingers
  - Any rotational deformity or scissoring of the finger with flexion
  - Pseudoclawing
  - Multiple metacarpal fractures
  - Segmental bone loss
  - Open fractures

Preoperative Planning

- The surgeon should be prepared to perform multiple techniques depending on specific intraoperative findings.
  - Fractures that may seem treatable with percutaneous pinning are often deemed to require open reduction internal fixation if an acceptable closed reduction cannot be obtained or if intraoperative findings are more severe than previously thought.
- Consideration should be given to utilization of the technique that results in the least soft tissue disruption while still restoring alignment and stability.

Positioning

- The hand is placed on a radiolucent table
- A forearm tourniquet is used for local-sedation cases and upper arm tourniquet used for regional block/general cases

Approach

- Open approaches to the metacarpal are almost always dorsally based.
- Adjacent metacarpal fractures can be exposed through a single incision equidistant between the two bones.
- The periosteum is incised and can sometimes be closed over the fracture if lag screws or K-wires are used. This is not usually possible if mini-fragment plates are used.
- For intra-articular metacarpal fractures, the extensor mechanism is split longitudinally to access the articular surface and then closed after fixation is completed.

TECHNIQUES

■ Closed Reduction and Pinning of Metacarpal Neck Fractures

- The Jahss technique (**TECH FIG 1A**) is used to perform a closed reduction of the metacarpal neck.
- The reduction is confirmed on the lateral radiograph.

- While the reduction is held by the assistant, a 0.045-in. K-wire is placed into the metacarpal head, just ulnar to the extensor mechanism.
- The K-wire is then advanced across the fracture site and down the metacarpal shaft.

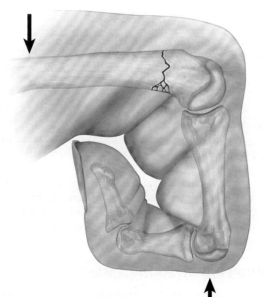

TECH FIG 1 • A. The Jahss technique. The metacarpophalangeal and proximal interphalangeal joints are flexed to 90 degrees and volar to dorsal force is placed on the proximal phalanx head. This reduces the volar angulation of the metacarpal neck fracture.

A

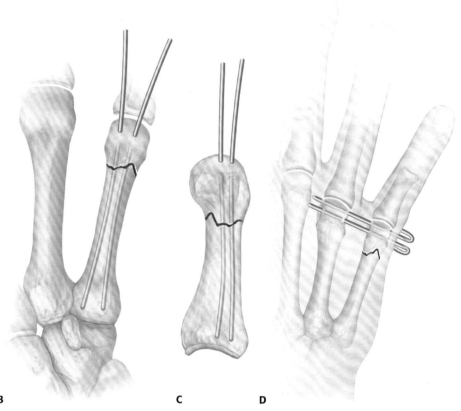

B   **C**   **D**

TECH FIG 1 (Continued) • **B,C.** AP and lateral depictions showing two K-wires placed longitudinally from the metacarpal head into the metacarpal shaft on either side of the extensor mechanism. **D.** Transverse pinning of a small finger metacarpal neck fracture to the ring finger metacarpal.

- A second 0.0450-in. K-wire is then placed into the metacarpal head, just radial to the extensor mechanism and advanced across the fracture site, into the metacarpal shaft (**TECH FIG 1B,C**).
- The reduction and intramedullary location of the K-wires are confirmed using orthogonal fluoroscopic views.

- Alternatively, for border digits, K-wires can be placed perpendicular to the metacarpal shaft and the fracture can be stabilized to the adjacent metacarpal (**TECH FIG 1D**).

■ Open Reduction and Internal Fixation of Metacarpal Neck or Shaft Fractures With Headless Compression Screws

- A 1-cm incision is made dorsally over the metacarpal head (**TECH FIG 2A**).
- The extensor tendon is split and dorsal arthrotomy performed (**TECH FIG 2B**).
- A 1.1-mm K-wire is placed into the metacarpal head and drilled retrograde to the level of the fracture (**TECH FIG 2C**).
  - The K-wire should be in the dorsal third of the metacarpal head on the lateral and not through the articular portion of the cartilage.
  - Consider using a longer K-wire so that you are able to pass the screw and not lose the K-wire into the metacarpal shaft.
- The fracture is then reduced and K-wire driven across the fracture site. Intramedullary location of the K-wire

and adequate reduction is confirmed on orthogonal fluoroscopic views.
- A cannulated headless compression screw is then placed over the K-wire (**TECH FIG 2D,E**).
  - We recommend a 3.0- to 3.5-mm screw with the exception of the ring finger because of the narrow diameter of its shaft. For the ring finger, we use a 2.0- or 2.5-mm screw.
    - Measure the width of the intramedullary canal as its isthmus prior to surgery to confirm that it is wide enough (at least 2 mm) to accept an implant.
  - The screw is inserted beneath the articular surface.
  - Attempt to center the screw on the fracture site to maximize compression, although this is difficult for metacarpal neck fractures given their proximity to the joint.
- The extensor split is closed with buried 4-0 Vicryl followed by 4-0 nylon for the skin.

TECHNIQUES

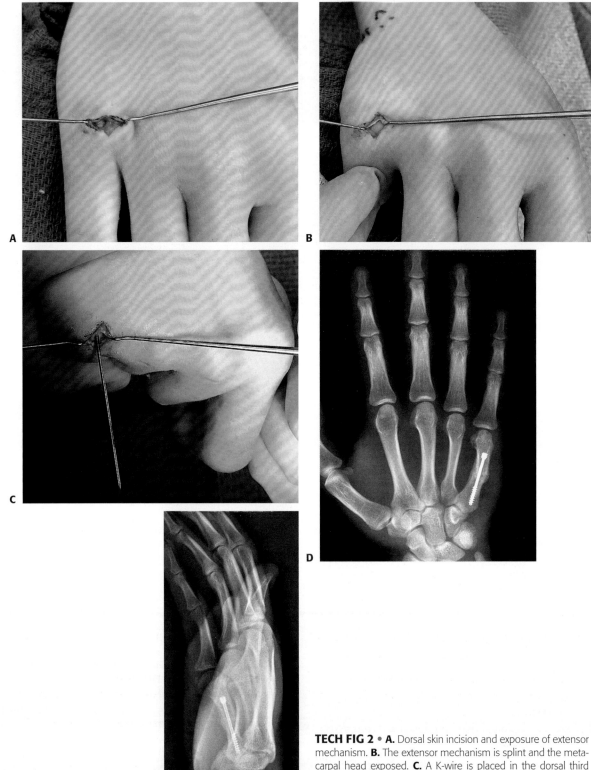

A

B

C

D

E

TECH FIG 2 • A. Dorsal skin incision and exposure of extensor mechanism. **B.** The extensor mechanism is splint and the metacarpal head exposed. **C.** A K-wire is placed in the dorsal third of the metacarpal head and driven retrograde across the fracture site after reduction has been performed. **D,E.** AP and lateral radiographs demonstrating a headless compression screw placed across the fracture site and within the metacarpal shaft.

Closed Reduction and Pinning of Metacarpal Shaft Fractures (Bouquet Technique)[8]

- A closed reduction is performed and confirmed on orthogonal radiographs. If an adequate closed reduction cannot be obtained, this technique is abandoned.
- A 2-cm longitudinal incision is made centered on the base of the metacarpal.
- Dissection is carried out down to bone, taking care to protect the extensor tendons.
- A small hole is made on the ulnar aspect of the metacarpal base (**TECH FIG 3A,B**), extra-articularly, taking care to not penetrate the radial cortex. This can be done using an awl or a small drill bit.

- Three round-tip 0.035-in. K-wires are gently bent (**TECH FIG 3C**).
- The fracture is reduced, and each K-wire is placed into the intramedullary canal and drilled across the fracture site and into the metacarpal head.
- The K-wires are placed in divergent directions to form a "bouquet" in the metacarpal head. It is often necessary to get the K-wires in the canal and across the fracture site, then use a needle driver to rotate the pins into divergent directions (**TECH FIG 3D,E**)
- Reduction is confirmed on fluoroscopy.
- The pins are cut outside the metacarpal base, taking care to leave enough K-wire protruding for easy removal.
- The skin is closed with nylon suture.

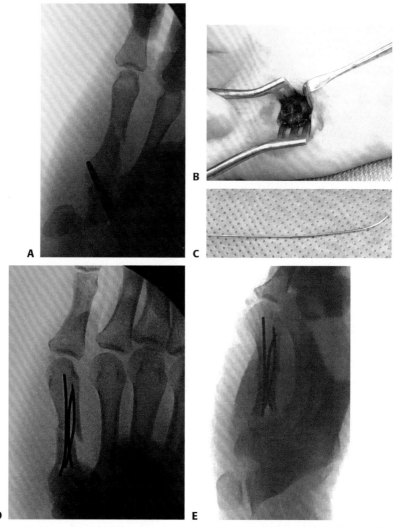

TECH FIG 3 • A. A radiolucent tool is used to locate the entry site for the pins, and the skin is marked with a marking pen. **B.** A 1- to 2-cm incision is made and dissection carried out down to bone. A 2.0-mm drill bit or curette is used to make a hole in the base of the metacarpal taking care to remain well extra-articular. **C.** The pins are bent with a gentle curve at the tip. **D,E.** Three pins are then placed into the intramedullary canal, and a needle driver is used to rotate them into divergent directions after being placed across the fracture site.

■ Open Reduction and Internal Fixation of Metacarpal Shaft Fractures With Lag Screws

- Open reduction and internal fixation with lag screws requires an oblique fracture line that is at least twice the width of the metacarpal shaft.
- For a single metacarpal fracture, the incision is placed directly over the metacarpal. For multiple adjacent fractures, the incision is placed midway between the metacarpals to allow access to both (**TECH FIG 4A**).
- Dissection is carried out bluntly down to the level of the extensor tendons (**TECH FIG 4B**).
- The tendon is retracted and periosteum incised over the metacarpal.
- The fracture is exposed and debrided (**TECH FIG 4C**).

- The fracture is provisionally reduced. For oblique fractures this can often be accomplished with the use of a point-to-point tenaculum clamp or towel clamp (**TECH FIG 4D**).
  - Care must be taken not to overcompress with the clamp, as this can cause iatrogenic fracture of the metacarpal.
  - Rotational alignment is checked (**TECH FIG 4E**).
- A lag screw is then placed perpendicular to the fracture site. The pilot hole is drilled first, followed by the gliding hole. The countersink is then used as well.
- An additional lag screw is placed perpendicular to the fracture site as well.
- Finally, a third screw is placed perpendicular to the other two screw. (**TECH FIG 4F**).
- Close periosteum over the fracture site if possible.
- Close skin with nylon sutures.
- Place the patient in splint with MCP flexed to 60 to 70 degrees, PIP and DIP fully extended.

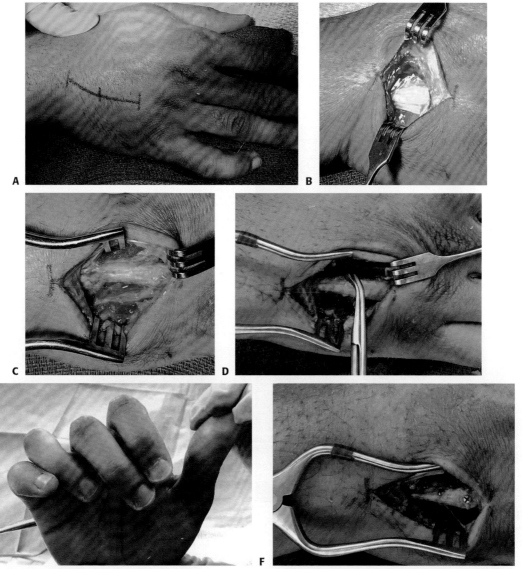

TECH FIG 4 • **A.** A longitudinal incision is made over the affected metacarpal shaft. **B.** Blunt dissection is carried out down to the extensor mechanism. **C.** The extensor mechanism is retracted and fracture site exposed. **D.** The fracture site is debrided of soft tissue and callus and provisionally reduced. **E.** Rotational alignment is confirmed prior to placing screws. **F.** Lag screws are placed and orthogonal radiographs obtained to confirm anatomic reduction.

Open Reduction and Internal Fixation of Metacarpal Shaft Fractures With Mini-Fragment Plates

- Open reduction internal fixation with mini-fragment plates and screws may be indicated for transverse fractures or fractures that cannot be adequately reduced and stabilized using percutaneous techniques (**TECH FIG 5A,B**)
- For a single metacarpal fracture, the incision is placed directly over the metacarpal (**TECH FIG 5C**). For multiple adjacent fractures, the incision is placed midway between the metacarpals to allow access to both.
- Dissection is carried out bluntly down to the level of the extensor tendons (**TECH FIG 5D**).
- The tendon is retracted and periosteum incised over the metacarpal.

- The fracture is exposed and debrided (**TECH FIG 5E**).
- The fracture is provisionally reduced (**TECH FIG 5F**).
  - Sometimes it is easier to fix the plate to one side of the fracture and then reduce the fracture to the plate. This is especially true of transverse fracture that are difficult to hold reduced using fracture clamps.
- Place one screw proximally and distally (**TECH FIG 5G**).
  - Check rotation of the finger (**TECH FIG 5H**) and radiographs.
  - If satisfied with alignment and rotation, fill remaining screw holes (**TECH FIG 5I–K**).
- Close periosteum over plate if possible.
- Close skin with nylon sutures.
- Place the patient in splint with MCP flexed to 60 to 70 degrees, PIP and DIP fully extended.

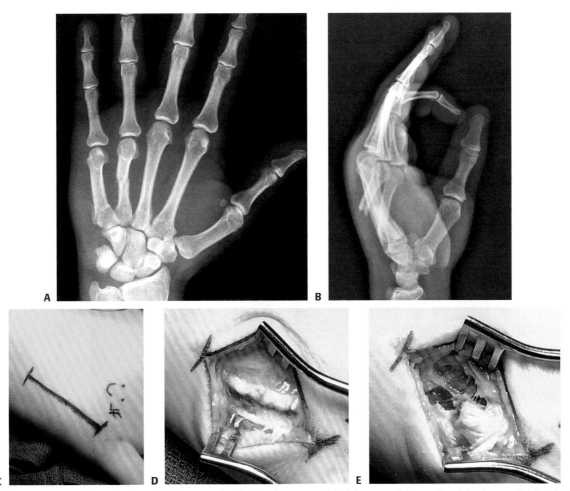

TECH FIG 5 • A,B. AP and lateral radiographs demonstrating displaced metacarpal shaft fractures of the small and ring fingers. **C.** A longitudinal incision is placed over the metacarpal shaft of the affected metacarpal. **D.** Blunt dissection is carried out down to the extensor tendon. **E.** The tendon is retracted and periosteum incised. The fracture is exposed and debrided.

TECHNIQUES

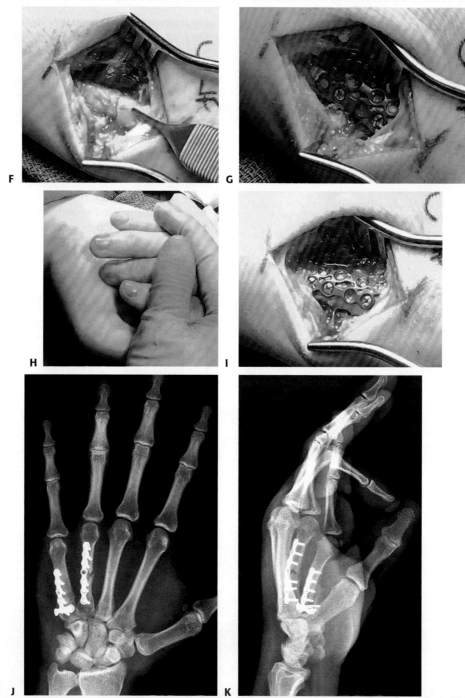

TECH FIG 5 (Continued) • **F.** The fracture is preliminarily reduced. **G.** The mini-fragment plate is affixed to the bone proximally and distally with one screw each. **H.** Rotational alignment is evaluated prior to placing the remaining screws. **I.** The remaining screws are placed and orthogonal radiographs scrutinized. **J,K.** Postoperative AP and lateral radiographs after plate fixation.

PEARLS AND PITFALLS

Indications	▪ Surgical treatment of metacarpal shaft fractures is indicated for rotational malalignment and/or volar flexion of more than 10 degrees for the index and middle fingers and more than 20 degrees for the ring and small fingers.
Rotation	▪ Once K-wires or screws have been placed, be sure to check rotation by flexing the fingers prior to definitive fixation and/or closure.
Open reduction and internal fixation with mini-fragment plates	▪ Do not waste time trying to achieve a perfect reduction before plate placement; sometimes it is easier to affix the plate to one side of the fracture and reduce the other side to the plate. Try to minimize soft tissue stripping.
Therapy	▪ If stable fixation, early ROM can be initiated at 10–14 d.

POSTOPERATIVE CARE

- Patients are immobilized in a nonremovable postoperative splint for the first 10 to 14 days. This splint flexes the MCP to 60 to 70 degrees and ideally leaves the PIP and DIP free for early motion.
- Sutures are removed at 10 to 14 days, and a forearm-based orthoplast splint is fabricated with the MCP joint in 60 to 70 degrees of flexion and PIP and DIP free for early motion.
- At 6 weeks, the splint is discontinued and therapy continued to regain full ROM.

OUTCOMES

- Ruchelsman et al.[7] reported on 20 patients at minimum 3-month follow-up who underwent limited-open retrograde headless screw fixation of metacarpal neck and shaft fractures. The union rate at 6 weeks was 100%, and all patients regained full composite fist by 3 months and extensor lag resolved by 3 weeks. Mean grip strength improved to 105% of the contralateral side.
- Doarn and colleagues[9] reviewed nine patients with nine metacarpal fractures treated with retrograde headless screw fixation at mean follow-up of 36 weeks. The union rate was 100% at a mean of 49 days, and mean return to work was 6 weeks. Mean grip strength returned to 95% of the uninjured hand.
- Kim and Kim[10] randomized 46 patients with metacarpal neck fractures to antegrade or retrograde intramedullary pinning. The authors found similar final radiographic alignment, but improved range of motion and DASH at 3 months in the antegrade pinning group.

COMPLICATIONS

- The complication rate depends greatly on the mechanism of injury and the amount of contamination in open injuries.
- Infection
  - The deep infection rate for closed metacarpal fractures treated operatively is 0.5% compared to 2% to 11% for operative treatment of open fractures.[11]
- Malrotation
  - Rotational deformity can significantly affect hand function.

- Malrotation of 5 degrees results in up to 1.5 cm of finger overlap with flexion.[11]
- Malunion
  - Volar angulation of the fracture or shortening can result in an extensor lag at the MCP joint.
    - For every 2 mm of shortening, there is 7 degrees of extensor lag.[6]
    - Due to natural hyperextension at the MCP joint, up to 6 mm of shortening may be acceptable in most patients.[11]
- The rate of nonunion approaches 6% in some series after ORIF.[12]

REFERENCES

1. Soong M, Got C, Katarincic J. Ring and little finger metacarpal fractures: mechanisms, locations, and radiographic parameters. *J Hand Surg [Am]*. 2010;35(8):1256-1259.
2. Kozin SH, Thoder JJ, Lieberman G. Operative treatment of metacarpal and phalangeal shaft fractures. *J Am Acad Orthop Surg*. 2000;8(2):111-121.
3. Diaz-Garcia R, Waljee JF. Current management of metacarpal fractures. *Hand Clin*. 2013;29(4):507-518.
4. Pace GI, Gendelberg D, Taylor KF. The Effect of closed reduction of small finger metacarpal neck fractures on the ultimate angular deformity. *J Hand Surg [Am]*. 2015;40(8):1582-1585.
5. Sletten IN, Hellund JC, Olsen B, et al. Conservative treatment has comparable outcome with bouquet pinning of little finger metacarpal neck fractures: a multicentre randomized controlled study of 85 patients. *J Hand Surg Eur Vol*. 2015;40(1):76-83.
6. Strauch RJ, Rosenwasser MP, Lunt JG. Metacarpal shaft fractures: the effect of shortening on the extensor tendon mechanism. *J Hand Surg [Am]*. 1998;23(3):519-523.
7. Ruchelsman DE, Puri S, Feinberg-Zadek N, et al. Clinical outcomes of limited-open retrograde intramedullary headless screw fixation of metacarpal fractures. *J Hand Surg [Am]*. 2014;39(12):2390-2395.
8. Foucher G. "Bouquet" osteosynthesis in metacarpal neck fractures: a series of 66 patients. *J Hand Surg [Am]*. 1995;20(3 Pt 2):S86-S90.
9. Doarn MC, Nydick JA, Williams BD, Garcia MJ. Retrograde headless intramedullary screw fixation for displaced fifth metacarpal neck and shaft fractures: short term results. *Hand (N Y)*. 2015;10(2):314-318.
10. Kim JK, Kim DJ. Antegrade intramedullary pinning versus retrograde intramedullary pinning for displaced fifth metacarpal neck fractures. *Clin Orthop Relat Res*. 2015;473(5):1747-1754.
11. Balaram AK, Bednar MS. Complications after the fractures of metacarpal and phalanges. *Hand Clin*. 2010;26(2):169-177.
12. Page SM, Stern PJ. Complications and range of motion following plate fixation of metacarpal and phalangeal fractures. *J Hand Surg [Am]*. 1998;23(5):827-832.

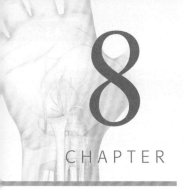

8

CHAPTER

Open Reduction for Carpometacarpal Joint Dislocation

John R. Fowler and Robert A. Kaufmann

DEFINITION

- Dislocation of the carpometacarpal (CMC) joint of the fingers may be simple (ligamentous disruption without fracture) or complex (associated with a fracture of the distal carpal row and/or metacarpal base).
- These injuries most commonly involve a dorsal direction of instability with subluxation or dislocation of the metacarpal base occurring relative to the carpal bones. Although rare, volar dislocations have been reported as well.

ANATOMY

- General
  - The index and middle finger CMC joints are more constrained than the small and ring finger CMC joints.
    - The index and long finger CMC joints have 11 and 7 degrees of flexion extension, respectively.[1]
    - The ring and small CMC joints have 20 and 44 degrees of flexion extension, respectively.[1]
  - This leads to increased incidence of small and ring finger CMC joint dislocations compared to index and middle CMC dislocations.
- Skeletal anatomy
  - The base of the index metacarpal is concave with radial and ulnar condyles that surround the trapezoid. The ulnar condyle also articulates with the long metacarpal and capitate, and the radial condyle has an articulation with the trapezium.[2]
  - The concave long metacarpal base articulates with the convex capitate and has a dorsoradial process that increases stability.[2]
  - The ring finger metacarpal base is locked by its articulations with the metacarpal bases of the middle and small finger and the hamate.[2]
  - The small finger metacarpal base has an ulnar slope and articulates with the hamate.[2]
  - Viegas et al.[3] classified the shape of the ring finger metacarpal base. The description is based on the number and positions of facets. The clinical relevance of this classification system is unclear.
- Ligamentous anatomy (**FIG 1**)
  - Conflicting descriptions exist in the literature with some authors reporting up to six dorsal and six volar ligaments to each CMC joint[4] and others reporting only one dorsal CMC ligament.[5]
  - Nakamura and colleagues[6] dissected 80 cadaver wrists and noted that the anatomy is different depending on which CMC is being studied.
    - The ring and small finger CMC joint have two distinct dorsal ligaments.

- The index and long finger CMC joints typically have three distinct dorsal ligaments.
- An intra-articular ligament exists between the long/ring finger metacarpal base and the capitate/hamate. This ligament resists dorsal dislocation even if the other volar and dorsal ligaments are cut.
  - Each CMC joint also has volar ligaments that resist dorsal dislocation.
    - The index and long CMC joints have two deep capsular ligaments that connect the metacarpal bases to the trapezium and two superficial ligaments that connect the metacarpal bases to the capitate.

PATHOGENESIS

- The most common mechanism of injury is punching a hard object with a closed fist.
  - Axial mechanical loading through a flexed MCP joint generates a rotational moment that causes a dorsally directed force on the metacarpal base.
- Yoshida and colleagues[7] found that capitate and hamate fractures were the most common fractures associated with ring and small finger CMC dislocations.

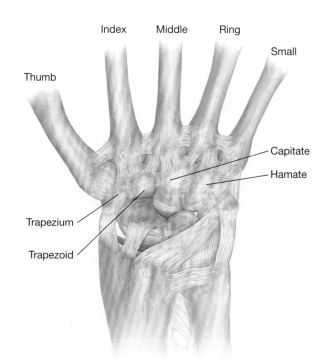

FIG 1 • Dorsal ligaments of the carpometacarpal joints.

- The ring and small finger CMC joints are more susceptible to injury than the index and long finger CMC joints due to increased mobility.[8]

NATURAL HISTORY

- Untreated CMC dislocations and fracture dislocations result in noticeable hand deformity, pain, limited range of motion, and decreased grip strength.[9]

PATIENT HISTORY AND PHYSICAL FINDINGS

- Most patients will present after punching a hard object with a closed fist. Other mechanisms can include an axial load on flexed metacarpals from a fall or motor vehicle accident.
- A thorough skin examination should be performed to rule out other injuries associated with punching, including "fight bite," which would require urgent surgical debridement.
  - Assessment of the soft tissues is focused on identifying skin disruption and extensor tendon damage.
- There is typically significant swelling, ecchymosis, and the inability to make a composite fist.
- Rotational malalignment is uncommon.

IMAGING

- Standard AP, lateral, and oblique radiographs are obtained (**FIG 2**).
- When a PA radiograph is taken in neutral, the normal CMC joints should have parallel articular surfaces, symmetric width between all CMC joint spaces (1–2 mm), and no overlapping joint surfaces.[10]
- Close attention must be paid to the lateral and oblique radiograph to evaluate for dorsal subluxation and/or dislocation of the metacarpal on the distal carpal row.
- On a true lateral radiograph the normal angle between the long axis of the index and small metacarpals should be

approximately 10 degrees. Angles near 40 degrees suggest dislocation.[11] Comparison to the contralateral side can be useful.
- An oblique radiograph with the forearm pronated 30 to 45 degrees from the PA will allow optimal visualization of the small and ring finger metacarpal base articulations with the distal carpal row.[11-13] Occasionally, a 15-degree pronation oblique is beneficial to fully assess the injury to the fourth and fifth CMC joints.[14]
- In unclear cases, consideration should be given to CT scan to further evaluate the CMC joint.[15]

DIFFERENTIAL DIAGNOSIS

- Metacarpal fracture
- Contusion
- CMC dislocation
- CMC fracture dislocation

NONOPERATIVE MANAGEMENT

- Nonoperative treatment may be considered if an adequate closed reduction can be obtained and remains stable. Close follow-up with weekly serial radiographs is recommended to ensure maintenance of the closed reduction.
- An ulnar gutter cast for fourth and fifth CMC injuries and a radial gutter cast for second and third CMC injuries are recommended. It is imperative that the cast prevent CMC subluxation through a dorsal mold. Keeping the MCP joint in no more than 40 to 50 degrees of flexion should prevent recurrence of dorsal subluxation at the CMC joints.

SURGICAL MANAGEMENT

Preoperative Planning

- The surgeon should be prepared to perform both closed and open reduction as needed to obtain a concentric reduction of the CMC joints.
- General or regional anesthesia is obtained.

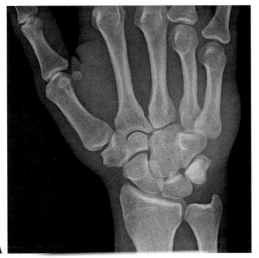
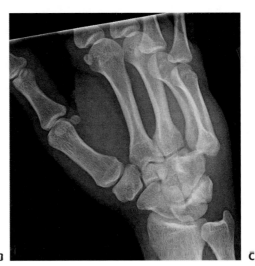
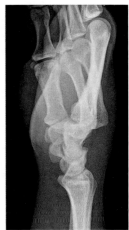

A   **B**   **C**

FIG 2 • PA **(A)**, oblique **(B)**, and lateral **(C)** radiographs demonstrating dorsal dislocation of the small and ring finger CMC joints.

- A drill and multiple K-wires should be available. A mini-fragment set is required to treat carpal fractures that may require open reduction and internal fixation.
- Intraoperative fluoroscopy is used to confirm adequate reduction and to direct K-wire placement.

Positioning

- The patient is placed in the supine position with the forearm pronated on a radiolucent table.
- The surgeon typically sits at the head of the bed to facilitate placement of K-wires.

Approach

- The approach to the CMC joint is dorsal and centered directly over the CMC joint. For multiple CMC dislocations, the incision can be placed between the two CMC joints.
- If all four CMC joints are dislocated and open reduction is required, a single incision can be placed over the middle finger metacarpal and thick flaps raised to visualize all four CMC joints.
- The dorsal ulnar and dorsal radial sensory nerves are fully visualized and freed up so that they can be gently retracted during the procedure.

■ Closed Reduction and Percutaneous Pinning

- A closed reduction is attempted with longitudinal traction on the affected metacarpal and dorsal to volar direct pressure on the metacarpal bases (**TECH FIG 1A,B**).
- The reduction is confirmed on AP, lateral, and oblique fluoroscopy images.
- While holding direct dorsal to volar pressure on the metacarpal bases, a 0.045-in. K-wire is drilled from the small finger metacarpal into the ring finger metacarpal, 1 to 2 cm distal to the CMC joint (**TECH FIG 1C**).
  - Familiarity with the location of the dorsal ulnar sensory nerve is imperative to avoid its injury. As a principle, avoiding the most dorsal ulnar region of the fifth metacarpal shaft will avoid injury to this nerve.

- If the ring finger metacarpal base is also involved, the K-wire is also drilled into the middle finger metacarpal shaft.
- A second 0.045-in. K-wire is placed in similar fashion, 1 to 2 cm distal to the first K-wire.
  - The second K-wire prevents rotation around the first K-wire.
- A third K-wire may be placed from the small finger metacarpal base into the hamate for added subluxation resistance.
- Fluoroscopy confirms maintained reduction of the CMC joints (**TECH FIG 1D–F**).
- The pins are cut below the skin.
- A well-padded volar splint is placed.

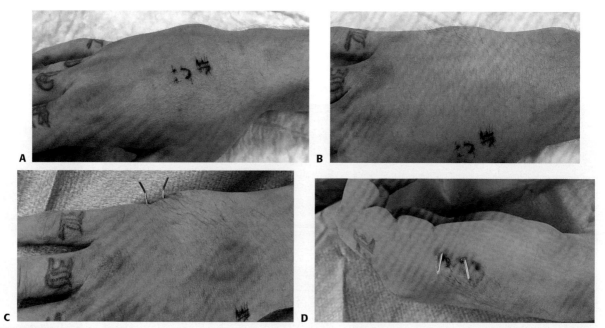

TECH FIG 1 • A. Photograph of the same injury in FIG 2 demonstrating the dorsal deformity associated with the dorsal dislocation of the metacarpal bases. **B.** Longitudinal traction is placed on the affected fingers and direct dorsal pressure is placed on the metacarpal base to reduced the dislocation. **C,D.** The pins in place after closed reduction and percutaneous pinning.

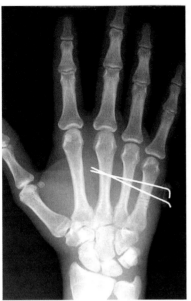
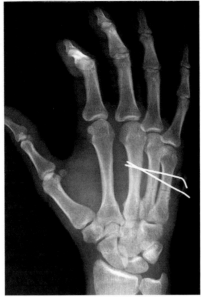
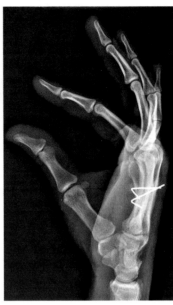

E   F   G

TECH FIG 1 (Continued) • **E–G.** AP, oblique, and lateral radiographs, respectively, showing placement of the percutaneous pins and reduction of the CMC bases (compare with FIG 2). Note that on the lateral view **(E)**, the metacarpals all line up and there is no dorsal subluxation of the small and ring finger metacarpal bases.

■ Open Reduction and Pinning With or Without Internal Fixation of Carpal Fractures

- A closed reduction is attempted with longitudinal traction on the affected metacarpal and dorsal to volar direct pressure on the metacarpal bases.
- If an adequate closed reduction cannot be maintained, an open reduction is performed.
- A longitudinal incision is made in between the small and ring finger metacarpal bases.
- Blunt dissection is carried out to the extensor tendons. The interval between the extensor digitorum communis to the ring finger and extensor digiti minimi is developed.
- The capsule over the CMC joints is incised longitudinally and sharply elevated radially and laterally to allow visualization of the joint.
  - Fibrosis and/or hematoma is cleared from the joint and a reduction performed.
- While holding direct dorsal to volar pressure on the metacarpal bases, a 0.045-in. K-wire is drilled from the small finger metacarpal into the ring finger metacarpal, 1 to 2 cm distal to the CMC joint.

- Similar to the closed reduction pinning algorithm, pins are placed into the middle finger metacarpal shaft when the ring CMC joint is also injured.
- If the ring finger metacarpal base is also involved, the K-wire is also drilled into the middle finger metacarpal shaft.
- A second 0.045-in. K-wire is placed in similar fashion, 1 to 2 cm distal to the first K-wire.
  - The second K-wire prevents rotation around the first K-wire.
- An additional K-wire may be placed from the small finger metacarpal base into the hamate for added stability.
- If there is a sizeable fracture of the dorsal lip of the hamate, this can be addressed using 1.2- or 1.5-mm mini-fragment screws (**TECH FIG 2**).
  - Ensure that the drill does not plunge through the volar cortex of the hamate given the close proximity of the ulnar nerve motor branch to the hook of the hamate.
- Fluoroscopy confirms maintained reduction of the CMC joints.
- The pins are cut below the skin.
- The CMC capsule is closed with absorbable suture. The skin is closed with 4-0 nylon.
- A well-padded ulnar gutter splint is placed.

T E C H N I Q U E S

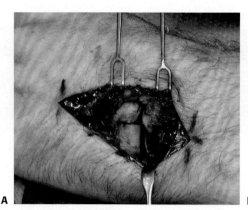 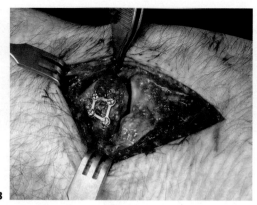

TECH FIG 2 • **A.** Fracture of the dorsal lip of the hamate. **B.** After internal fixation of the hamate with a mini-fragment plate. For small fragments, mini-fragment screws alone can be used.

PEARLS AND PITFALLS

Radiographs	■ Scrutinize the lateral and oblique radiographs to evaluate for dorsal subluxation/dislocation of the metacarpal base. Obtain a CT scan if necessary.
Preoperative workup	■ Have a low threshold to obtain a CT scan if necessary.
Fixation	■ At least two K-wires are needed to maintain joint alignment. Ensure that pins gain secure purchase in uninjured metacarpals in order to transmit forces away from zone of injury. Consider third pin directed obliquely from metacarpal into carpal bone to improve biomechanical rigidity of fixation.
K-wires	■ Bury K-wires under the skin for later removal at 10–12 wk. A longer period of fixation is required to allow healing of the dorsal ligaments.
Postoperative immobilization	■ Cast immobilization is recommended for nonoperatively treated injuries. ■ Immobilize unreliable postoperative patients in a cast after sutures are removed.

POSTOPERATIVE CARE

- Patients are placed in an ulnar gutter splint with the MCP joints free.
- Early finger motion is started to minimize stiffness.
- The postoperative splint is removed at 2 weeks and the patient is placed into either a removable thermoplast splint or a short-arm cast. This decision is based on the perceived reliability of the patient. Less reliable patients are placed into casts.
- Radiographs are obtained at 2, 6, and 10 weeks to ensure no further subluxation of the metacarpal base and to evaluate for healing of any carpal fractures that may have been present.
- Buried pins are typically removed in the operating room under sedation and local anesthetic at 10 to 12 weeks.

OUTCOMES

- Zhang et al.[9] reviewed 20 fracture dislocations of the small and ring finger CMC joints at mean follow-up of 1 year.
  - Mean Michigan Hand Questionnaire score was 98.
  - Patients obtained similar range of motion and grip strength to the contralateral hand.

- Patients treated without surgery had worse mean grip strength (31 kg vs 45 kg) and worse Michigan Hand Questionnaire score (72 vs 98).
- Gehrmann and colleagues[8] reported on 16 fracture dislocations of the small and ring finger CMC joints and 23 fracture dislocations of the small finger CMC joint treated with either closed reduction and pinning or open reduction and internal fixation at mean follow-up of 13 months.
  - Mean DASH score at final follow-up was 6.0 for small and ring finger dislocations and 7.2 for small finger dislocations.
  - Grip strength was 16% less than the uninjured side.
  - There were no cases of recurrent dislocation or subluxation.

COMPLICATIONS

- Post-traumatic arthritis may occur despite the surgeon's best effort. This is secondary to cartilage injury during the dislocation event.
- Finger stiffness is common secondary to swelling and pain.
- Recurrent dorsal subluxation/dislocation is uncommon but has been reported.

REFERENCES

1. El-Shennawy M, Nakamura K, Patterson RM, Viegas SF. Three-dimensional kinematic analysis of the second through fifth carpometacarpal joints. *J Hand Surg [Am]*. 2001;26(6):1030-1035.

2. Bushnell BD, Draeger RW, Crosby CG, Bynum DK. Management of intra-articular metacarpal base fractures of the second through fifth metacarpals. *J Hand Surg [Am]*. 2008;33(4):573-583.

3. Viegas SF, Crossley M, Marzke M, Wullstein K. The fourth carpometacarpal joint. *J Hand Surg [Am]*. 1991;16(3):525-533.

4. Gurland M. Carpometacarpal joint injuries of the fingers. *Hand Clin*. 1992;8(4):733-744.

5. Harwin SF, Fox JM, Sedlin ED. Volar dislocation of the bases of the second and third metacarpals: a case report. *J Bone Joint Surg Am*. 1975;57(6):849-851.

6. Nakamura K, Patterson RM, Viegas SF. The ligament and skeletal anatomy of the second through fifth carpometacarpal joints and adjacent structures. *J Hand Surg [Am]*. 2001;26(6):1016-1029.

7. Yoshida R, Shah MA, Patterson RM, et al. Anatomy and pathomechanics of ring and small finger carpometacarpal joint injuries. *J Hand Surg [Am]*. 2003;28(6):1035-1043.

8. Gehrmann SV, Kaufmann RA, Grassmann JP, et al. Fracture-dislocations of the carpometacarpal joints of the ring and little finger. *J Hand Surg Eur Vol*. 2015;40(1):84-87.

9. Zhang C, Wang H, Liang C, et al. The Effect of timing on the treatment and outcome of combined fourth and fifth carpometacarpal fracture dislocations. *J Hand Surg [Am]*. 2015;40(11):2169-2175, e2161.

10. Fisher MR, Rogers LF, Hendrix RW. Systematic approach to identifying fourth and fifth carpometacarpal joint dislocations. *AJR Am J Roentgenol*. 1983;140(2):319-324.

11. Parkinson RW, Paton RW. Carpometacarpal dislocation: an aid to diagnosis. *Injury*. 1992;23(3):187-188.

12. Liaw Y, Kalnins G, Kirsh G, Meakin I. Combined fourth and fifth metacarpal fracture and fifth carpometacarpal joint dislocation. *J Hand Surg Br*. 1995;20(2):249-252.

13. Cain JE Jr, Shepler TR, Wilson MR. Hamatometacarpal fracture-dislocation: classification and treatment. *J Hand Surg [Am]*. 1987;12(5 Pt 1):762-767.

14. Bora FW Jr, Didizian NH. The treatment of injuries to the carpometacarpal joint of the little finger. *J Bone Joint Surg Am*. 1974;56(7):1459-1463.

15. Pullen C, Richardson M, McCullough K, Jarvis R. Injuries to the ulnar carpometacarpal region: are they being underdiagnosed? *Aust N Z J Surg*. 1995;65(4):257-261.

9
CHAPTER

Reconstruction of Acute and Chronic Ulnar Collateral Ligament Injuries of the Thumb

John R. Fowler and Robert A. Kaufmann

DEFINITION

- An acute tear of the ulnar collateral ligament (UCL) is defined as an injury that is less than 12 weeks. Acute tears can often be repaired.
- A chronic tear is an injury that is older than 12 weeks. Chronically injured UCLs are often in need of reconstruction.
- The ligament integrity at the time of surgery is the primary determinant of whether a repair or a reconstruction may be performed. Chronic tears, especially in younger patients, can often still be repaired with excellent results. Acutely injured UCLs, particularly Stener lesions, may not be amenable to a repair and might benefit from a reconstruction effort.

ANATOMY

- The thumb UCL has proper and accessory components.
- The proper UCL is tight in 20 to 30 degrees of flexion.
  - The origin is from the metacarpal with the center of insertion 4.2 mm from the dorsum of the metacarpal and 5.3 mm proximal to the articular surface (**FIG 1**).
  - The insertion is on the proximal phalanx with a center of insertion 2.8 mm from the volar surface and 3.4 mm distal to the articular surface.[1]
- The accessory collateral ligament is tight in full extension.

- The accessory collateral ligament is volar to the proper and has an origin on the metacarpal and inserts into the volar plate and proximal phalanx base.
- The adductor pollicis longus inserts through its aponeurosis into the extensor hood over the metacarpophalangeal (MCP) joint.
- The dorsal capsule of the MCP joint acts as a secondary stabilizer in flexion.[2]
- The extensor pollicis longus, extensor pollicis brevis, and flexor pollicis longus provide dynamic joint stability.

PATHOGENESIS

- A forceful valgus stress to the thumb results in disruption of the UCL.
  - The ligament may tear and yet not retract substantially from its insertion into the proximal phalanx.
  - A "Stener lesion" is created when the stump of a completely ruptured UCL retracts proximally and then the adductor aponeurosis becomes interposed between the UCL and its insertion on the proximal phalanx[3] (**FIG 2**).
- Chronic repetitive valgus stress may result in UCL laxity. Antecedent trauma is likely the sentinel event that caused ligament damage, whose healing was interrupted through chronic reaggravation leading to laxity of the UCL complex.

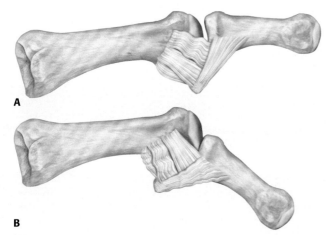

FIG 1 • The anatomy of the ulnar collateral ligament of the thumb metacarpophalangeal (MCP) joint. **A.** In extension, the accessory collateral ligament is taut. **B.** In flexion, the proper collateral ligament is taut.

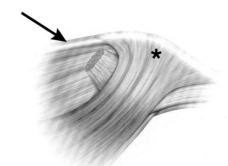

FIG 2 • A Stener lesion occurs when the stump of the ulnar collateral ligament (*arrow*) retracts and the adductor aponeurosis (*) becomes interposed between the ligament and its insertion on the proximal phalanx.

NATURAL HISTORY

- Acute tears of the UCL that do not heal with conservative treatment typically progress to chronic instability.
- Chronic instability results in weakness, pain, and degenerative changes that accompany joint laxity.

PATIENT HISTORY AND PHYSICAL FINDINGS

- Patients with acute injuries typically report a valgus load to the thumb. This may occur during athletic activities, from a fall or from a ski pole or strap.
- The mechanism of injury and chronicity of the injury should be documented.
- Physical examination
  - Inspection: Evaluate for swelling, ecchymosis, alignment.
  - Palpation: Palpate the insertion and origin sites of the RCL and UCL
    - Palpation of fullness over the metacarpal head may indicate the presence of a Stener lesion.
  - Provocative testing
    - Test the accessory collateral in full MCP extension.
    - Test the proper collateral in 20 to 30 degrees of flexion at the MCP joint: 30 degrees of deviation or more than 15 degrees compared to the contralateral side is diagnostic for a UCL tear.
    - Compare to the contralateral thumb.
    - Gross instability with the joint held in MCP extension heralds disruption of both the accessory and proper collateral ligaments and may obviate the need for MRI imaging.

IMAGING

- AP and lateral radiographs of the thumb should be obtained to determine if there is an avulsion fracture of the UCL and to rule out dislocation and/or concomitant fractures of the phalanx or metacarpal. Always review radiographs prior to provocative ligament stress testing to ensure that a nondisplaced avulsion fracture is not displaced through the examination effort.
- Stress radiographs of the thumb may be diagnostic for UCL tear.
- Advanced imaging including ultrasound or MRI may confirm the presence of a complete rupture of the UCL and/or Stener lesion.
  - Ultrasound has an accuracy of approximately 80% for detecting a complete tear of the thumb UCL.[4]
  - MRI has a sensitivity and specificity approaching 100% for complete tears.[5]

DIFFERENTIAL DIAGNOSIS

- Metacarpal or proximal phalanx fracture
- Contusion
- Ligament strain/sprain
- MCP dislocation
- MCP arthritis

NONOPERATIVE MANAGEMENT

- Indications for nonoperative treatment include incomplete or partial tears as well as nondisplaced avulsion fractures.
- Understanding when the injury occurred is important as acute injuries are better suited for nonoperative management.
- Nonoperative treatment consists of immobilizing the thumb MCP joint. A forearm-based thumb spica cast is effective regardless of patient compliance and is recommended, for a minimum of 6 weeks for an avulsion fracture and 8 weeks for a soft tissue injury.
- Patients can elect nonoperative treatment for complete tears; however, healing may be less reliable.
  - Landsman et al. reported that 85% of patients with an acute complete rupture of the thumb UCL and who were treated in a cast for 3 months reported no signs of pain or instability.[6]

SURGICAL MANAGEMENT

- Indications
  - Instability greater than 30 degrees with the thumb in 20 to 30 degrees of flexion represents injury to the proper collateral ligament.
  - Instability greater than 30 degrees with the thumb in extension represents injury to both the proper and the accessory collateral ligament.
  - Instability that is 15 degrees greater than the contralateral side
  - Palpation of a Stener lesion (retracted UCL ligament residing proximal to the adductor aponeurosis)
  - A bony avulsion with significant displacement that results in laxity to stress testing
  - Lack of a firm endpoint on examination

Preoperative Planning

- The surgeon should be prepared and comfortable to both repair or reconstruct the UCL.
  - Despite an acute tear, a midsubstance rupture may require reconstruction.
  - Some reported acute injuries actually represent a reaggravation of prior trauma making the UCL untenable for successful reattachment.
- Suture anchors and a drill should be available.
- Presence of the palmaris longus tendon should be established.

Positioning

- The patient is placed in the supine position with the arm on a radiolucent table.
- The surgeon typically sits in the axilla to allow the best visualization of the ulnar aspect of the thumb.

Approach

- The UCL is approached through either a straight or a curvilinear dorsal-ulnar incision.
- If a nonstraight incision is chosen, then the distal aspect should follow a gentle volar path to facilitate access to the insertion of the UCL on the proximal phalanx.

■ Acute Repair of the Ulnar Collateral Ligament[7]

Exposure

- The incision is centered over the MCP joint (**TECH FIG 1A**).
- Careful blunt dissection is carried out down to the extensor mechanism/adductor aponeurosis. The dorsal sensory nerves are identified and gently retracted (**TECH FIG 1B**).
- The adductor aponeurosis may be incised just off of the extensor pollicis longus or be removed as much as 5 mm. Preserving the distal portion of the adductor aponeurosis as it merges with the extensor pollicis longus facilitates later closure. Leaving the confluence of the adductor aponeurosis and the extensor pollicis longus intact allows for these structures to be closed in a distal to proximal manner essentially "pulling the zipper" in a retrograde manner (**TECH FIG 1C**).
- The aponeurosis is carefully dissected off of the underlying capsule. In chronic injuries, this step becomes more challenging but is often made easier if the adductor aponeurosis is identified in a location slightly more distal than the joint itself and dissected away from the capsule/UCL ligament complex.

- The capsule is then incised and the injured UCL identified (**TECH FIG 1D**). In most cases, the UCL is ruptured/avulsed from the proximal phalanx.
- The articular cartilage is inspected for degenerative changes, which, when present, represent a contraindication to UCL repair/reconstruction (**TECH FIG 1E**).

Suture Placement and Closure

- The proximal phalanx insertion site is debrided to ensure bleeding bone, and a suture anchor is placed at the center of the insertion site (**TECH FIG 2A,B**).
- The stump of the UCL tendon is trimmed back to healthy-appearing tissue and sutured to the bone using the sutures from the anchor. Additional 3.0 Vicryl sutures are placed between the UCL ligament and the periosteum/capsule that is just distal to the site of ligament insertion. One or two of these sutures can augment the biomechanical integrity of the repair (**TECH FIG 2C,D**).
- The adductor aponeurosis is closed using nonabsorbable suture in a retrograde manner (**TECH FIG 2E**).
- The skin is closed using 4-0 nylon sutures.

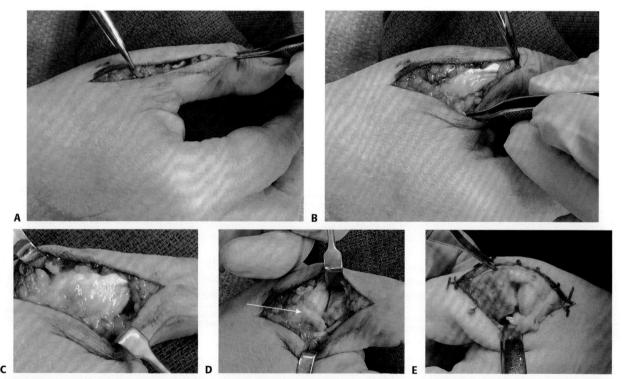

TECH FIG 1 • A. Planned incision for treatment of ulnar collateral ligament injuries. The curvilinear nature allows access to the insertion of the proper collateral ligament, which is along the volar edge of the proximal phalanx. **B.** The skin is incised and blunt dissection carried out down to the extensor mechanism. Sensory nerve branches may be crossing the incision in this location and must be identified and protected. **C.** The adductor aponeurosis is incised 5 mm from the extensor pollicis longus, leaving a cuff for later repair. **D.** The stump of the ulnar collateral ligament is identified (*arrow*). Most tears/avulsions occur off the proximal phalanx, but the surgeon must ensure that there is not a midsubstance or proximal rupture. **E.** The joint is inspected for signs of degenerative changes. Degenerative changes are a contraindication to repair and/or reconstruction.

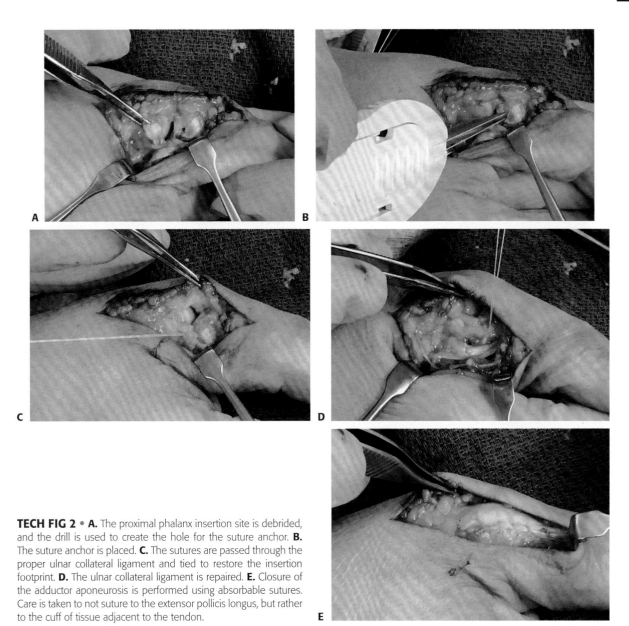

TECH FIG 2 • **A.** The proximal phalanx insertion site is debrided, and the drill is used to create the hole for the suture anchor. **B.** The suture anchor is placed. **C.** The sutures are passed through the proper ulnar collateral ligament and tied to restore the insertion footprint. **D.** The ulnar collateral ligament is repaired. **E.** Closure of the adductor aponeurosis is performed using absorbable sutures. Care is taken to not suture to the extensor pollicis longus, but rather to the cuff of tissue adjacent to the tendon.

■ Reconstruction of Chronic Tear Using Palmaris Autograft (Tunnel Technique)

Exposure

- The same incision is made for a repair or a reconstruction effort (**TECH FIG 3A**).
- Careful blunt dissection is carried out down to the extensor mechanism/adductor aponeurosis. Dorsal sensory nerves are identified and retracted (**TECH FIG 3B**).

- The adductor aponeurosis is incised just as it would be for a repair and carefully dissected off of the underlying capsule (**TECH FIG 3C**).
- The capsule is then incised and the unrepairable remnant of the ulnar collateral ligament is identified and excised (**TECH FIG 3D**).
- The articular cartilage is inspected for the presence of degenerative change. Significant damage is a contraindication to UCL repair/reconstruction.

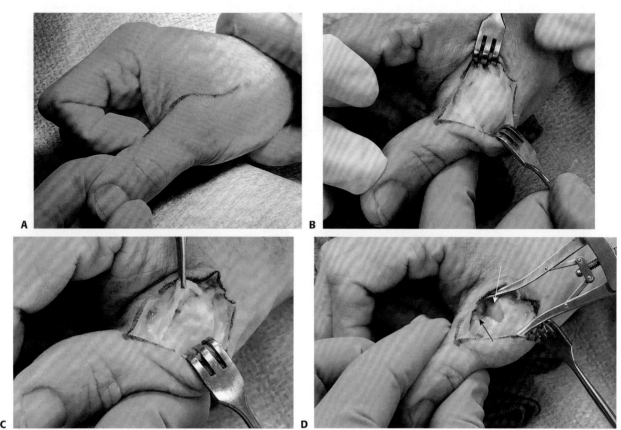

TECH FIG 3 • A. Planned curvilinear incision for ulnar collateral ligament reconstruction. **B.** Blunt dissection is carried out down to the level of the extensor mechanism and adductor aponeurosis. Care is taken to identify and protect sensory nerves. **C.** The adductor aponeurosis is incised and carefully elevated off the underlying capsule. A 5-mm cuff of tissue adjacent to the extensor tendons is left for later repair. **D.** In the case of a chronic collateral ligament tear, there is usually very little tendon identified. The origin (*white arrow*) and insertion (*black arrow*) of the proper ulnar collateral ligament are identified and debrided.

Palmaris Tendon Harvest

- A 1-cm longitudinal or transverse incision is made over the distal wrist crease (**TECH FIG 4A**).
- The palmaris longus is isolated and a Ragnell retractor placed under the tendon.
- Traction is placed on the palmaris longus and its course traced proximally.

- A longitudinal or transverse incision is made 10 cm proximal to the wrist crease.
- The palmaris longus is isolated here and transected. Blunt dissection is used to free connections between the underlying tissue.
- The palmaris is pulled through the distal wound and transected distally (**TECH FIG 4B**).

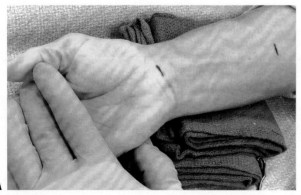
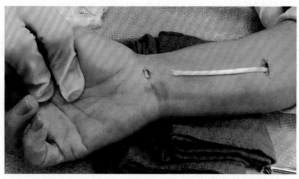

TECH FIG 4 • A. The palmaris longus tendon is palpated and skin incisions planned. **B.** The palmaris is identified distally and divided. It is then pulled out of the wound proximally and divided to obtain maximum length.

- The palmaris longus should be trimmed to no smaller than 2 to 3 mm in width.

Creating Bone Tunnels and Inserting the Tendon Graft

- A 2.0-mm drill bit is used to make a hole at the insertion of the proper collateral ligament on the proximal phalanx (**TECH FIG 5A**).
  - Recognize that the insertion is about 3 mm dorsal from the volar-most edge of the proximal phalanx and about 3 mm distal from the joint line.
- Leaving a generous bone bridge, a second hole is made dorsal to the first hole.
- Proximally, a single hole is made (using the same 2.0-mm drill bit) at the isometric point on the metacarpal head (at the origin of the proper collateral ligament).
- Two additional holes are made more proximal and dorsal to the hole at the proper collateral origin.
  - A curette may be used to both gently enlarge and connect the holes to allow for easier passage of the graft.

- A 4-0 nylon suture or Hewson suture passer is used to shuttle the palmaris autograft through the bone tunnels. The 4-0 nylon needle is secured by the needle driver at its tip and a loop created through which the graft is passed. The same technique can be used to efficiently pass the graft through all of the drill holes (**TECH FIG 5B**).
  - The palmaris is first passed through the tunnels in the proximal phalanx.
  - Both limbs are then passed through the isometric tunnel on the metacarpal head.
  - One limb is then passed through its respective tunnel on the dorsum of the metacarpal.
- The MCP joint is reduced and the tendon limbs tightened. The limbs are sutured to each other using a nonabsorbable 3-0 suture.
- The adductor aponeurosis is closed using absorbable suture (**TECH FIG 5C**).
- The skin is closed using 4-0 nylon horizontal mattress sutures.

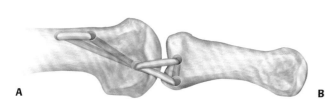

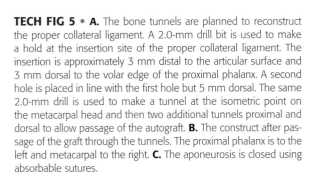

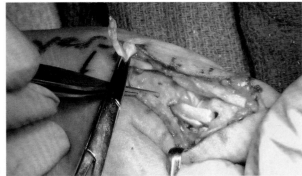

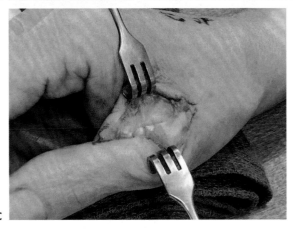

TECH FIG 5 • A. The bone tunnels are planned to reconstruct the proper collateral ligament. A 2.0-mm drill bit is used to make a hold at the insertion site of the proper collateral ligament. The insertion is approximately 3 mm distal to the articular surface and 3 mm dorsal to the volar edge of the proximal phalanx. A second hole is placed in line with the first hole but 5 mm dorsal. The same 2.0-mm drill is used to make a tunnel at the isometric point on the metacarpal head and then two additional tunnels proximal and dorsal to allow passage of the autograft. **B.** The construct after passage of the graft through the tunnels. The proximal phalanx is to the left and metacarpal to the right. **C.** The aponeurosis is closed using absorbable sutures.

Reconstruction of Chronic Tear Using Palmaris Autograft (Anchor Technique)

- The aforementioned surgical approach is followed, but instead of using bone tunnels, two anchors are employed
- A K-wire is placed into the center of the UCL origin on the metacarpal head (**TECH FIG 6A**).

- A 3.5-mm cannulated drill hole is placed over the K-wire to enlarge the hole.
- An Arthrex DX SwiveLock 3.5 mm × 8.5 mm forked tip anchor is used. The palmaris graft is placed over the fork, and the anchor is then seated into the bone. An Arthrex FiberTape suture can be incorporated with the repair for added strength (**TECH FIG 6B,C**).

- A K-wire is placed into the center of the UCL insertion on the proximal phalanx base. The center of the insertion is approximately 4 mm from the dorsum of the metacarpal and 5 mm proximal to the articular surface (**TECH FIG 6D**).
- A 3.5-mm cannulated drill hole is placed over the K-wire to enlarge the hole.
- The palmaris autograft is then placed over the forked tip on a second Arthrex DX SwiveLock anchor (**TECH FIG 6E**).

- It is important to leave a little bit of slack as the ligament will tighten as the anchor is seated into the bone.
- Prior to tightening the screw anchor, check stability and range of motion of the MCP joint.
- Once satisfied with the tension in the graft, range of motion, and stability, tighten the anchor.
- The free ends of the autograft are excised (**TECH FIG 6F**).
- The adductor aponeurosis is closed using nonabsorbable suture.
- The skin is closed in the usual manner.

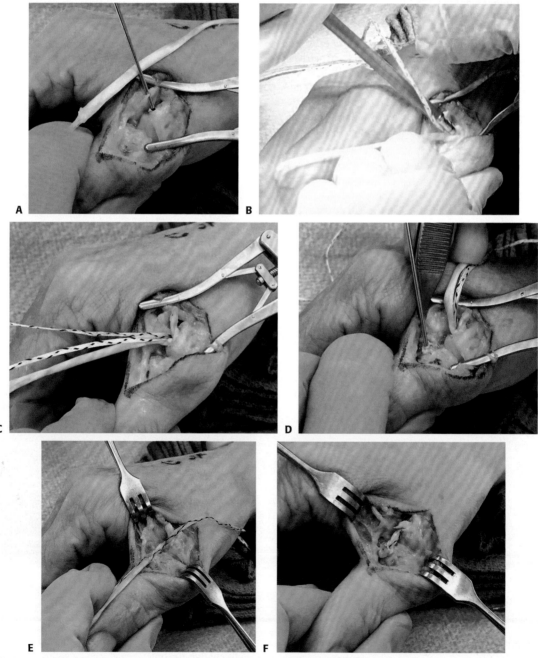

TECH FIG 6 • A. The guide wire is placed at the isometric point on the metacarpal head. **B.** The anchor is used to secure the graft and additional suture into the metacarpal head. **C.** After the graft and suture has been secured. **D.** The guide wire is placed into the insertion site on the proximal phalanx. **E.** The suture anchor is again used to secure the graft and suture down into the proximal phalanx. **F.** The construct after the extra tendon and suture has been removed.

PEARLS AND PITFALLS

Dorsal sensory nerve	▪ Carefully dissect and gently retract the dorsal sensory nerves.
Graft tension	▪ When repairing or reconstructing the UCL with bone tunnels, ligament tension may be maximized without overtightening the MCP joint as time-dependent soft tissue properties allow for dissipation of undue graft tension. Thumb stiffness is avoided as long as the MCP joint is flexed 30 degrees while being immobilized in the postoperative setting.
Adductor aponeurosis	▪ Leave the distal confluence of adductor aponeurosis with extensor pollicis longus tendon intact so that precise closure may be accomplished. Careful "teasing away" of aponeurosis from UCL/scar/capsule is important to ensure that the adductor aponeurosis maintains its biomechanical integrity when securely reattached to the extensor pollicis longus tendon.
Degenerative changes	▪ Degenerative changes are a contraindication to UCL repair and/or reconstruction. A fusion should be performed.
Placement of anchors/tunnels on proximal phalanx	▪ Remember that the insertion of the proper UCL is volar, only 3 mm dorsal to the volar edge of the proximal phalanx. Restoration of both proper and accessory collateral ligaments is ensured when bone tunnels are placed.

POSTOPERATIVE CARE

▪ A well-molded plaster thumb spica cast is placed. Care is taken to avoid any valgus force imparted to the MCP joint.

▪ The MCP joint is best held in 30 degrees of flexion status post repair or reconstruction effort. Due to "cam" appearance of metacarpal head, the ligament is tighter in flexion and may become unable to stretch out in patients who are immobilized and then heal in full extension.

▪ At the 2-week visit, the wound is inspected and patient placed in either a removable thermoplast splint or a short-arm thumb spica cast for an additional 4 weeks.

  ▪ Thumb IP joint and finger motion is encouraged.

OUTCOMES

▪ Operative treatment results in good to excellent results in over 90% of patients.

▪ Glickel et al. reported on 26 patients who underwent thumb UCL reconstruction using free tendon graft at an average of 3.9 years' follow-up.

  ▪ The authors reported excellent results in 20 patients, good results in 4 patients, and fair results in 2 patients.

  ▪ The operative thumb averaged a 10% increase in laxity compared to the nonoperative thumb and yet retained 80% of its arc of motion.

  ▪ Mild or intermittent pain with heavy use was reported in 8/26 thumbs; the remainder reported no pain.

COMPLICATIONS

▪ Thumb stiffness particularly when the MCP joint was immobilized in full extension.

▪ Persistent instability, which is more likely in a repair rather than a reconstruction effort.

▪ Injury to the radial sensory nerve during exposure and/or retraction.

▪ Fracture of the metacarpal and/or proximal phalanx when creating bone tunnels or during anchor placement.

▪ Degenerative changes of the MCP joint over time.

REFERENCES

1. Carlson MG, Warner KK, Meyers KN, et al. Anatomy of the thumb metacarpophalangeal ulnar and radial collateral ligaments. *J Hand Surg [Am]*. 2012;37(10):2021-2026.
2. Tsiouri C, Hayton MJ, Baratz M. Injury to the ulnar collateral ligament of the thumb. *Hand (N Y)*. 2009;4(1):12-18.
3. Tang P. Collateral ligament injuries of the thumb metacarpophalangeal joint. *J Am Acad Orthop Surg*. 2011;19(5):287-296.
4. Papandrea RF, Fowler T. Injury at the thumb UCL: is there a Stener lesion? *J Hand Surg [Am]*. 2008;33(10):1882-1884.
5. Hergan K, Mittler C, Oser W. Ulnar collateral ligament: differentiation of displaced and nondisplaced tears with US and MR imaging. *Radiology*. 1995;194(1):65-71.
6. Landsman JC, Seitz WH Jr, Froimson AI, et al. Splint immobilization of gamekeeper's thumb. *Orthopedics*. 1995;18(12):1161-1165.
7. Weiland AJ, Berner SH, Hotchkiss RN, et al. Repair of acute ulnar collateral ligament injuries of the thumb metacarpophalangeal joint with an intraosseous suture anchor. *J Hand Surg [Am]*. 1997;22(4):585-591.

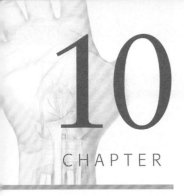

10 CHAPTER

Closed Reduction and Fixation of Bennett and Rolando Fractures

John R. Fowler and Thomas B. Hughes

DEFINITION

- A Bennett fracture (**FIG 1A**) is defined as an intra-articular base of the thumb metacarpal fracture consisting of a volar-ulnar fragment that is attached to the anterior oblique ligament.[1]
- A Rolando fracture (**FIG 1B**) is defined as a comminuted intra-articular metacarpal base fracture.[1] The fracture is often a T- or Y-type pattern.

ANATOMY

- The base of the thumb metacarpal has a saddlelike shape to accommodate its articulation with the trapezium. The articular surface is convex when viewed posterior to anterior and concave when viewed from lateral to medial.[2]
- The abductor pollicis longus inserts along the lateral edge of the metacarpal base.
- The anterior oblique ligament originates from the volar beak of the thumb metacarpal and inserts onto the trapezium (**FIG 2**).[2]
- The dorsal ligament complex is the strongest and thickest ligament complex around the thumb CMC joint. It consists of the dorsal radial and posterior oblique subligaments. If the dorsal ligament complex is disrupted, the joint is unstable even if the anterior oblique ligament is intact.[2]
- The intermetacarpal ligament runs transversely from the index metacarpal to the thumb metacarpal.

PATHOGENESIS

- Bennett fractures are caused by an axial load on the partially flexed thumb metacarpal.
- The anterior oblique ligament is attached to the volar-ulnar fragment and the trapezium (**FIG 3**). This holds the volar-ulnar fragment in place while the metacarpal base subluxates.
- The metacarpal base is displaced in a dorsal, radial, and proximal direction.
- Bennett fractures are classified using the Gedda classification (**FIG 4**).
- Rolando fractures are the result of an axial load on the thumb metacarpal that has a pilon effect on the articular surface.

NATURAL HISTORY

- As with other intra-articular fractures, articular congruity results in symptomatic arthritis at long-term follow-up.[3]
- Fractures that are not reduced result in chronic instability, pain, and decreased function.

PATIENT HISTORY AND PHYSICAL FINDINGS

- History should document the acuity of the injury, as chronic injuries may be less amenable to closed reduction.
- Patients typically describe a fall onto the thumb with axial loading. Alternatively, athletes may report a jamming-type

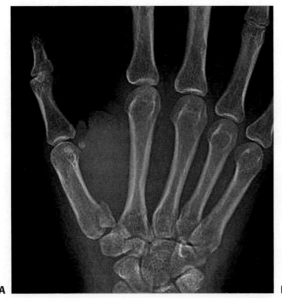

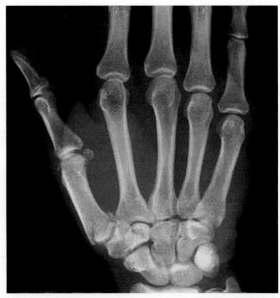

FIG 1 • PA radiographs demonstrating a Bennett fracture **(A)** vs a Rolando fracture **(B)**.

A   B

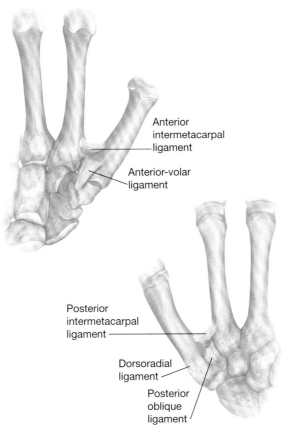

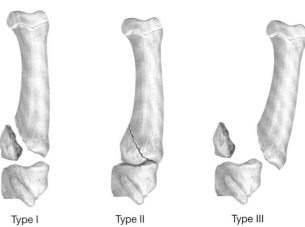

FIG 4 • The Gedda classification for Bennett fractures. Type I: large volar-ulnar fragment with subluxation of the thumb metacarpal. Type II: impaction of the articular surface without subluxation of the thumb metacarpal. Type III: avulsion of volar-ulnar metacarpal with dislocation of thumb metacarpal.

FIG 2 • Anatomy of the thumb carpometacarpal joint with special focus on the anterior oblique ligament and dorsal ligament complex.

injury from either a ball or contact with another player or the ground.
- There is often significant soft tissue swelling and ecchymosis around the thumb CMC joint.
- Evaluate the thumb MP collateral ligaments, the EPL, EPB, and FPL.
- Active and passive thumb motion is painful. There may be crepitus of the CMC joint.

IMAGING

- One must obtain at true AP (Robert's view) and true lateral radiograph (Bett's view) to assess the amount of articular incongruity.[1]
- A true AP is obtained by maximally pronating the forearm and placing the dorsum of the thumb on the cassette.
- A true lateral is obtained by pronating the forearm 20 degrees and placing the lateral border of the thumb on the cassette. The x-ray beam is angled 10 degrees distally.
- Computed tomography is not routinely needed for thumb metacarpal base fractures.

NONOPERATIVE MANAGEMENT

- Closed reduction and thumb spica casting is indicated for articular step-off of less than 1 mm.
- Because of comminution and articular incongruity, Rolando fracture is typically not treated nonoperatively.

SURGICAL MANAGEMENT

- Indications for surgery:
  - Articular step-off more than 1 mm[4]
  - Inability to reduce joint subluxation by closed reduction

Preoperative Planning

- The surgeon should be prepared to perform both closed reduction and open reduction as indicated by operative findings.
- Have mini-fragment plating system and K-wires available.

Positioning

- The patient is placed in the supine position with an upper arm tourniquet.
- The surgeon should sit at the axilla and assistant opposite.
- This allows the surgeon the ability to drill K-wires into the index metacarpal or trapeziometacarpal joint.

Approach

- Fractures that require open reduction and internal fixation are typically approached using the Wagner approach to gain access to the joint and fracture fragments.

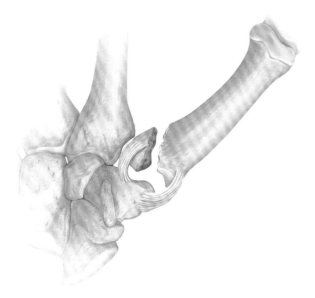

FIG 3 • The deforming forces in thumb metacarpal base fractures result in the characteristic radial displacement of the metacarpal shaft.

■ Closed Reduction and Pinning of Bennett and Rolando Fractures

- Longitudinal traction is placed on the thumb (**TECH FIG 1A**).
- The thumb is then abducted and pronated to reduce the fracture.
- Reduction is confirmed using fluoroscopy.
- A 0.045-in. K-wire is then drilled either into the trapezium or into the index metacarpal (**TECH FIG 1B–D**).

- A second K-wire is used if reduction to the index metacarpal is performed.
- Rolando fractures can also be treated with traction and pinning if alignment can be restored with traction. Pinning of individual fragments is typically not successful because there is often significant comminution.

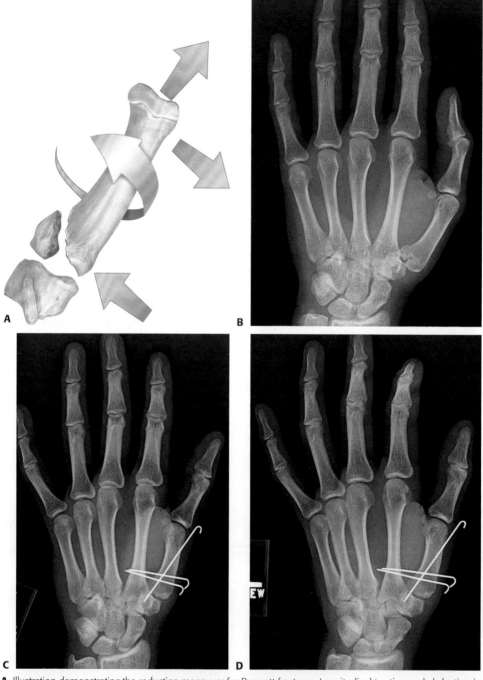

TECH FIG 1 • **A.** Illustration demonstrating the reduction maneuver for Bennett fractures. Longitudinal traction and abduction is performed. The surgeon's thumb places direct ulnar pressure on the base of the metacarpal, and the thumb is then pronated. **B.** PA radiograph demonstrating typical Bennett fracture. **C.** PA radiograph after pinning. **D.** Oblique radiograph after pinning.

Open Reduction and Internal Fixation of Bennett Fractures

- The Wagner approach is used.
  - The incision is made along the radial border of the thumb between the glabrous and nonglabrous skin.
  - Blunt dissection is performed down to the fascia overlying the thenar musculature. Branches of the palmar cutaneous branch of median nerve and branches of the dorsal radial sensory nerve are identified and carefully retracted.
  - The thenar muscles are elevated off of the metacarpal.
  - A longitudinal incision is made in the thumb CMC joint capsule.

- Do not strip the individual fragments of their soft tissue attachments.
- The fracture is reduced under direct visualization using ligamentotaxis and/or a fracture clamp and stabilized using K-wires or mini-fragment screws. We prefer to use 1.7-mm mini-fragment screws using a lag technique (**TECH FIG 2**).
  - A K-wire can be placed between the thumb metacarpal and index metacarpal to relieve compression stresses on the fracture site.
- Anatomic reduction of the joint surface is confirmed with direct visual inspection.
- The capsule is closed using nonabsorbable sutures and the skin is typically closed using interrupted nylon horizontal mattress sutures.

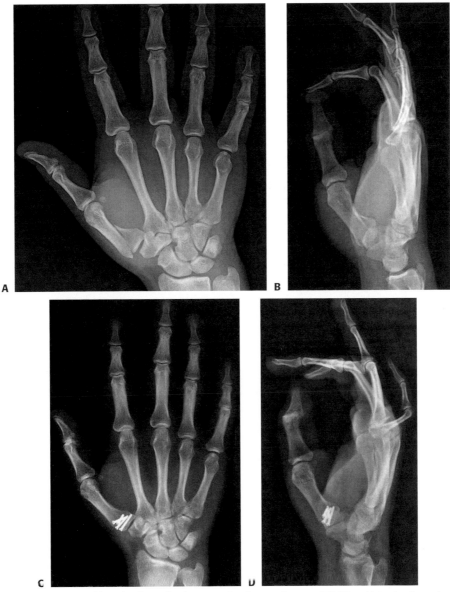

TECH FIG 2 • A,B. Preoperative PA and lateral radiographs demonstrating Bennett fracture. **C,D.** PA and lateral radiographs after open reduction and internal fixation with lag screws.

■ Open Reduction and Internal Fixation of Rolando Fractures

- The Wagner approach is used.
  - The exposure is similar to the approach above for Bennett fracture.
  - A longitudinal incision is made in the thumb CMC joint capsule.
  - Do not strip the individual fragments of their soft tissue attachments.

- The fracture is reduced under direct visualization using ligamentotaxis and/or a fracture clamp. A 1.7- or 2.3-mm mini-fragment plate can be contoured and used to stabilize the fracture fragments (**TECH FIG 3**).
  - A K-wire can be placed between the thumb metacarpal and index metacarpal to relieve compression stresses on the fracture site.
  - One or more additional K-wires may be necessary to capture additional fracture fragments or to pin the joint in distraction for stability.

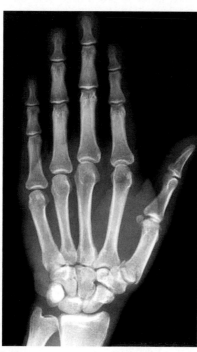
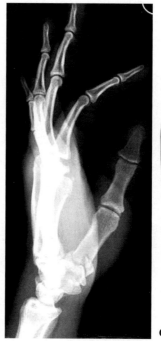
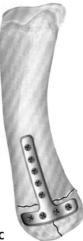

TECH FIG 3 • A,B. PA and lateral radiographs demonstrating a Rolando fracture. **C.** Illustration showing placement of a 2.3-mm mini-fragment T-plate to stabilize the intra-articular fragments.

PEARLS AND PITFALLS

Indications	■ Open reduction and internal fixation is indicated if there is more than 1 mm of articular step off after closed reduction.
Proper imaging	■ Obtain true AP and lateral radiographs to accurately assess articular step-off.
Hardware	■ Ensure that there are no intra-articular screws after ORIF.
Treatment	■ Perform the necessary procedure to restore articular congruity and reduce metacarpal subluxation.
Approach	■ Perform the Wagner approach to visualize the joint surface and directly visualize articular congruity.

POSTOPERATIVE CARE

- Patients are immobilized in a nonremovable thumb spica splint for 2 weeks.
- If closed reduction and pinning is performed, the patient is placed into a short-arm thumb spica cast for 2 weeks.

- The pin sites are examined at 4 weeks from surgery. If there is no erythema, the pins are left for another 2 weeks.
- If there is pin site irritation, the pins are removed and patient placed into thumb spica cast for another 2 weeks.

- If open reduction internal fixation was performed, the patient is placed in a thumb spica cast at the 2-week visit for 4 weeks.
- Hand therapy is started at 6 weeks to regain motion and strength.

OUTCOMES

- Middleton et al.[5] reported long-term outcomes of 62 patients who underwent closed reduction and pinning of Bennett fractures at mean follow-up of 11 years. Mean DASH was 3, and 94% of patients were satisfied with their outcome and none had undergone further surgery.
- Griffiths[6] followed 21 patients with Bennett fractures treated with closed reduction and casting and evaluated at mean 6.8 years after treatment. More than half of patients had lost reduction, but there was little correlation between lost reduction and functional disability or symptoms.
- Livesley[3] reported on 17 patients at a mean follow-up of 26 years and noted that all 17 had decreased motion and grip strength with radiographic evidence of arthritis and subluxation.

COMPLICATIONS

- Pin tract infections can occur if closed reduction and percutaneous pinning is performed.
- Post-traumatic arthritis with decreased motion and strength may develop despite treatment.
- Superficial sensory nerve injury may occur during open or percutaneous treatment.

REFERENCES

1. Carlsen BT, Moran SL. Thumb trauma: Bennett fractures, Rolando fractures, and ulnar collateral ligament injuries. *J Hand Surg [Am]*. 2009;34(5):945-952.
2. Edmunds JO. Current concepts of the anatomy of the thumb trapeziometacarpal joint. *J Hand Surg [Am]*. 2011;36(1):170-182.
3. Livesley PJ. The conservative management of Bennett's fracture-dislocation: a 26-year follow-up. *J Hand Surg Br*. 1990;15(3):291-294.
4. Liverneaux PA, Ichihara S, Hendriks S, et al. Fractures and dislocation of the base of the thumb metacarpal. *J Hand Surg Eur Vol*. 2015;40(1):42-50.
5. Middleton SD, McNiven N, Griffin EJ, et al. Long-term patient-reported outcomes following Bennett's fractures. *Bone Joint J*. 2015;97-B(7):1004-1006.
6. Griffiths JC. Bennett's fracture in childhood. *Br J Clin Pract*. 1966; 20(11):582-583.

Section III: Joints

11
CHAPTER

Volar Plate Arthroplasty of the Proximal Interphalangeal Joint

James T. W. Saunders and Amy M. Moore

DEFINITION

- Volar plate arthroplasty (VPA) of the proximal interphalangeal joint (PIP) involves the elevation and advancement of the volar plate in an attempt to resurface the fractured articular region of the middle phalanx and reduce dorsal subluxation of the PIP joint.

ANATOMY

- A combination of bony constraints, the volar plate and the collateral ligaments provide stability of the PIP joint (**FIG 1**).
  - The concave articular surface of the middle phalanx articulates with the convex condyles of the proximal phalanx, allowing the joint to function as a hinge.
  - The volar plate is a fibrocartilaginous structure that originates from the proximal phalanx via two strong checkrein ligaments. It inserts distally to the volar base of the middle phalanx. The volar plate resists PIP joint hyperextension.
  - The proper and accessory collateral ligaments are the primary restraints to radial- and ulnar-directed forces. The accessory collateral ligaments, situated volarly, attach to the lateral margin of the volar plate as it crosses the joint.

PATHOGENESIS

- The strong volar plate is frequently injured in dorsal PIP dislocations and/or hyperextension injuries of the PIP joint.
  - The most common injury is avulsion of the volar plate from the base of the middle phalanx due to the strength of checkrein ligaments and attachments to the accessory collateral ligaments.
  - The distal attachment often avulses a fragment of the base of the middle phalanx (**FIG 2**).
- Disruption of 40% to 50% of the volar articular surface of the base of the middle phalanx can lead to joint instability (ie, dorsal subluxation of the middle phalanx) requiring correction (**FIG 3**).[1]

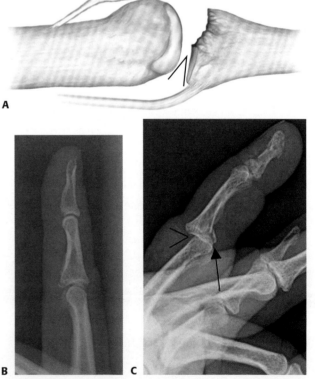

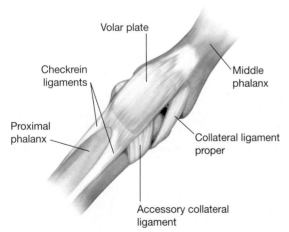

FIG 1 • Anatomy of proximal interphalangeal (PIP) joint. In this view of volar aspect of the joint, note the relationship between the volar plate and collateral ligaments. These structures create stability of the joint and are often injured with PIP joint dislocations.

FIG 2 • **A.** Illustration of volar plate avulsion with dorsal PIP dislocation. **B.** The middle phalanx subluxes dorsally, creating a V deformity of the dorsal joint. **C.** A volar bone fragment is commonly avulsed with the volar plate (*arrow*).

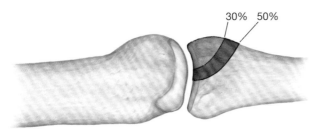

30% 50%

FIG 3 • Fracture stability. Fractures with 50% articular involvement are inherently unstable. Fractures with 30% to 50% involvement are tenuous and need to be evaluated closely for instability. Fractures of less than 30% tend to be stable.

NATURAL HISTORY

- Disruption of the volar plate with or without an associated base of middle phalanx fracture can lead to[2]:
  - Pain
  - Premature degenerative arthritis
  - Stiffness and loss of PIP joint motion
  - Persistent dorsal subluxation of the joint

PATIENT HISTORY AND PHYSICAL FINDINGS

- The most common cause of acute injury is an axial or dorsal load to the finger leading to a dorsal dislocation. The patients will often report that their finger was "jammed" or "dislocated."
- Patients most often reduce the joint themselves prior to presentation.
- On physical examination:
  - Patients have ecchymosis, edema, decreased range of motion, and tenderness located to the PIP joint.
  - Repeated dorsal dislocation on flexion of the PIP joint is characteristic of a volar plate disruption.

- Minimal resistance to hyperextension at the PIP joint is also suggestive of volar plate injury.
  - This is best tested under anesthetic block.
  - Always compare to noninjured digits.
- Acute or chronic development of a swan-neck deformity can suggest a volar plate injury.

IMAGING

- Appropriate preoperative radiographic imaging of the affected finger is important to assess bony injury. These include AP and lateral radiographs (**FIG 4A–C**).
- Radiographs in both flexion and extension allow the stability of the joint to be assessed when volar base of middle phalanx fractures exist.
- Preoperative live fluoroscopy is also useful to further assess stability of the joint in real time.
- Complex fractures can be evaluated with a high-resolution CT to evaluate bony fragment size and location (**FIG 4D**).
- In cases of acute or chronic instability without an underlying fracture, signs of arthritic damage or malalignment should be evaluated.

NONOPERATIVE MANAGEMENT

- Nonoperative management for PIP joint dislocations may be considered in those patients with stable injury patterns (less than 30% articular surface involvement).
- Stability may be confirmed with a lateral radiograph of the PIP joint.
- If mild subluxation of the PIP joint exists, the digit should be examined for adequate reduction with the joint blocked in 15 to 20 degrees of flexion using a dorsal blocking splint. If a dorsal blocking splint offers an adequate reduction, conservative treatment can be pursued with close follow-up. If more than 60 degrees of flexion is needed to maintain reduction, surgical intervention should be considered.

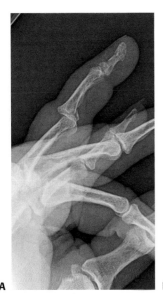
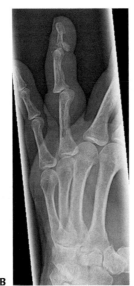
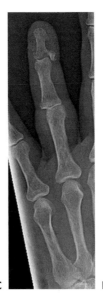
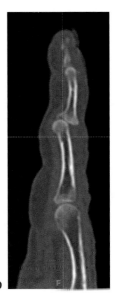

A   B   C   D

FIG 4 • **A–C.** Radiographs of the left ring finger demonstrate a fracture-dislocation of the PIP joint with dorsal subluxation. There is also a displaced intra-articular fracture of the distal phalanx. **D.** A CT scan of the affected digit can be obtained to evaluate the size and number of bony fragments involving the middle phalanx.

- Treatment options for stable PIP joints include dorsal blocking splint, buddy taping to a neighboring digit, and early motion. A figure-eight splint or silver ring splint may also be used.

SURGICAL MANAGEMENT

- For most PIP fracture-dislocations, joint reconstruction with a hemihamate arthroplasty (HHA) has largely replaced the use of VPA because of the HHA's ability to restore near-anatomic alignment of the joint. However, the HHA is technically demanding and has a steep learning curve. For inexperienced surgeons, the VPA is a reasonable conservative option.
- Indications:
  - Acute dorsal dislocation injury with gross instability
  - Acute fracture dislocation involving over 30% of the articular surface with subluxation of the middle phalanx.
  - Chronic dorsal subluxation with failed conservative management
  - Osteoarthritis of PIP joint[3]

Preoperative Planning

- Appropriate preoperative imaging is necessary to assess bony joint quality/deformity.
  - The dorsal cortex must be intact to perform VPA.
  - Articular surface of the proximal phalanx must also be intact.
- General, regional, or local anesthesia can be used.

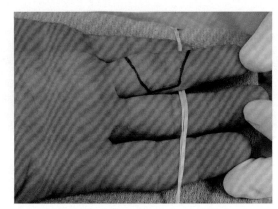

FIG 5 • Skin markings to access the volar aspect of the finger. A traditional Bruner incision is also acceptable.

Positioning

- Patient is placed in the supine position with the affected limb abducted on a radiolucent hand table.
- Tourniquet is placed on upper arm or forearm.
- A malleable lead/aluminum hand may be used to help retract the nonoperative digits.

Approach

- A volar approach through either a Chevron-shaped or Bruner-style incision is based over the PIP joint (**FIG 5**).

TECHNIQUES

■ Volar Plate Advancement for Base of Middle Phalanx Fractures

Exposure

- Exposure is planned from the A2 pulley to A4 pulley (**TECH FIG 1A**).
- A2 and A4 pulleys are preserved, but the flexor tendon sheath between them is incised and reflected.

- A Penrose drain can then be looped around the exposed flexor tendons to retract them, allowing visualization of the underlying volar plate (**TECH FIG 1B**).
- With the volar plate exposed, the fracture can be visualized by hyperextending the PIP joint.
- Incise and free the lateral margins of the volar plate from the accessory collateral ligaments with a Beaver or no. 15c blade.

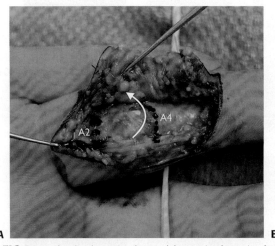
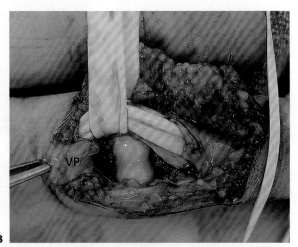

A   **B**

TECH FIG 1 • **A.** The distal margin of A2 and the proximal margin of A4 pulleys are identified (*purple dotted lines*), and the flexor tendon sheath is reflected laterally. The pulleys are maintained. **B.** The flexor tendons are reflected laterally and secured with a Penrose drain. The volar plate (VP) is incised and reflected proximally to expose the joint.

- The distal margin of the volar plate often maintains its attachments to the fracture fragment, which can be sharply excised if necessary.
- If not completely free, the volar plate is then divided transversely as distally as possible to maximize the length of the now proximally based flap.
  - This can be done by first placing a Freer elevator under the volar plate to identify the distal margin and then sliding a no. 15 blade under the volar plate to divide it.
  - It is important to obtain a volar plate flap as long and broad as possible.
- To further hyperextend or shotgun the joint (in cases of joint reconstruction), the collateral ligaments must be released from the middle phalanx at this point.

Preparation of the Middle Phalanx

- The middle phalanx is then prepared with a rongeur to make smooth the volar articular surface with careful maintenance of the dorsal articular surface and cortex (**TECH FIG 2A**).
- Two straight Keith needles are drilled through the middle phalanx base from volar to dorsal angling them slightly distally (**TECH FIG 2B**).
  - Each needle is started laterally at the volar margin of the cartilaginous surface and aimed toward the midline dorsally (toward the triangular ligament) to avoid injuring the lateral bands or central slip on the dorsal surface.
    - Flexing the DIP joint as the K-wires are driven will help prevent the DIP joint from being locked in extension if the extensor mechanism is caught with the pull-through suture.
  - In the situation of a middle phalanx fracture, the needles are started at the lateral margin of the remaining intact cartilaginous surface.

Passing and Setting the Suture

- A Prolene or stainless steel suture is passed in a grasping fashion around the fibrocartilaginous portion of the volar plate ending at the distal margin (**TECH FIG 3A**).
- After the needle is removed, the suture ends are fed through the holes in the Keith needles.
- The Keith needles are then manually pulled through the dorsal aspect of the finger using a needle driver.
  - If both needles can be brought out through the same hole in the triangular ligament, you can minimize the chance of injuring or entrapping the extensor mechanism.
- The suture is passed through a folded wad of petroleum-impregnated gauze for skin protection before being passed through a button.
- The suture tension is set temporarily over the button with the PIP joint extended to 0 degrees (**TECH FIG 3B,C**).
- Fluoroscopic images are taken to ensure an adequate reduction (**TECH FIG 3D,E**).
- It is important to observe congruent joint surfaces through a full range of motion on fluoroscopy.
- If hinging (gapping over the dorsal cortex) is still present, consider further advancement of the volar plate or releasing the dorsal joint capsule.
- Once satisfied with positioning, the sutures can be permanently secured over the button (**TECH FIG 3F**).
- The lateral margins of the volar plate are then sutured to the adjacent collateral ligament margins to restore three-dimensional stability.
- In the case of a base of middle phalanx fracture, an oblique Kirschner wire is placed to maintain 20 to 30 degrees of flexion and joint congruity.

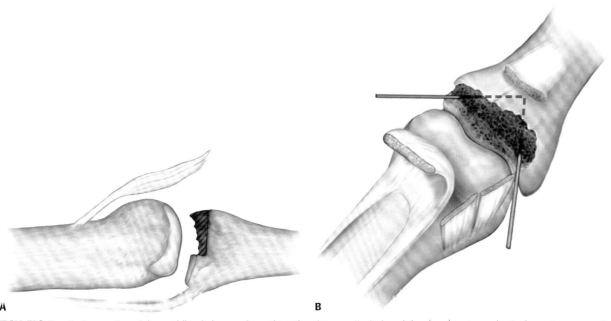

A   B

TECH FIG 2 • **A.** Preparation of the middle phalanx surface. The volar plate is reflected, and the dorsal cortex and articular surface are maintained. **B.** The *dotted lines* show the paths of the Keith needles for the pull-through technique. The needles are angled in a volar to dorsal direction toward the midline of the finger. They are also angled slightly in a proximal to distal direction to avoid injury to the central slip dorsally.

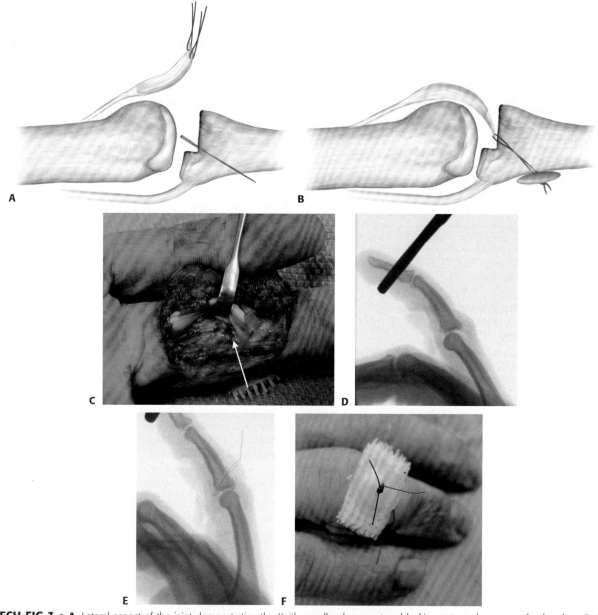

TECH FIG 3 • A. Lateral aspect of the joint demonstrating the Keith needle placement and locking suture placement of volar plate. **B.** The sutures are pulled through the middle phalanx and secured over a button. **C.** The volar plate is tensioned symmetrically (*white arrow*) to obtain joint congruity. **D.** Lateral radiograph demonstrates dorsal subluxation following a volar base of middle phalanx fracture. The middle phalanx is subluxed dorsally creating a dorsal V sign with overexaggeration of the dorsal joint space. Approximately 30% of the articular surface is involved in the fracture. **E.** Postreduction radiographs demonstrate restoration of joint congruity using a stainless steel wire with the volar plate arthroplasty. **F.** A petroleum-impregnated gauze strip is used to avoid injury to the underlying skin.

■ Correction of PIP Joint Instability Without a Middle Phalanx Fracture

- The procedure is similar to the volar plate arthroplasty for volar base of middle phalanx fractures with the following differences:
  - A postreduction K-wire can be replaced with a dorsal blocking splint if the reduction is maintained through a full arc of motion allowing for immediate mobilization of the PIP joint.
- Although the volar plate should still be separated from the collateral ligaments, the collateral ligaments do not need to be divided as the joint is not shotgunned open.

PEARLS AND PITFALLS

Fracture characterization	■ Patients with volar base of middle phalanx fractures need radiographs to assess the stability of the joint. ■ The dorsal cortex and articular surface must be intact. ■ The fracture pattern should be evaluated in flexion and extension preoperatively. ■ Volar plate arthroplasty is appropriate for volar base of middle phalanx fractures with greater than 40% of the articular surface involved.
Timing	■ Operative management within the acute time period avoids working against scar tissue.
Pull-through wire placement	■ Volar placement of the wire and angled distal to central slip is key to an adequate reduction. ■ Centralized dorsal placement of the wire will prevent entrapment of the extensor mechanism. ■ Symmetric tension setting of the volar plate will ensure adequate reduction.
Intraoperative fluoroscopy	■ Joint congruity throughout a full range of motion intraoperatively must be obtained and maintained.
Postoperative care	■ Initiate early guarded range of motion to prevent flexion contracture.

POSTOPERATIVE CARE

■ VPA for unstable volar base of middle phalanx fractures:
  ■ K-wire immobilization of the joint is maintained for 3 weeks.
  ■ DIP joint ROM is started immediately to promote tendon glide.
  ■ Active range of motion of the PIP joint is initiated 4 weeks following surgery.
  ■ Dynamic extension splinting is initiated if full extension has not been reached by 5 to 6 weeks following surgery.
  ■ The button and suture are removed 5 to 6 weeks following surgery.
  ■ Buddy taping is initiated once the dorsal blocking splint is discontinued at 6 weeks.
  ■ Return to sporting activities is permitted at 8 weeks as long as buddy taping is maintained.
■ VPA for nonfractured joints with restored congruency:
  ■ DIP and PIP range of motion is initiated the day after surgery with a dorsal blocking splint in place under the guidance of a hand therapist.
  ■ The button and suture are removed 5 to 6 weeks after surgery.
  ■ Buddy taping is initiated once the dorsal blocking splint is discontinued at 6 weeks.
  ■ Dynamic extension splinting is initiated if full extension has not been reached within 5 to 6 weeks after surgery.
  ■ Return to sporting activities is permitted at 8 weeks as long as buddy taping is maintained.

OUTCOMES

■ Reported outcomes vary greatly, but two long-term follow-up papers demonstrate maintenance of motion and stability of the reconstruction.
■ Eaton and Malerich in 1980 reviewed 24 patients over a 100-year period and noted the following[2]:
  ■ An average of 95 degrees of motion and a 6-degree flexion contracture if treated within 6 weeks from a fracture
  ■ An average of 78 degrees of motion and a 12-degree flexion contracture if treated after 6 weeks from the date of fracture

■ Dionysian and Eaton reported their VPA results of 17 patients with an average of 11.5 years' follow-up and found[4]:
  ■ Patients with VPA within 4 weeks of injury maintained total active ROM of 85 degrees.
  ■ Patients with VPA after 4 weeks of injury averaged 61 degrees of active ROM.

COMPLICATIONS

■ Complications are relatively uncommon with reports of patient satisfaction rates as high as 94%.[5]
■ Complications can include the following:
  ■ Redisplacement: Due to failure to achieve a stable reduction or suture failure
  ■ PIP joint angulation: Commonly due to a failure to recognize or manage an asymmetric fracture pattern
  ■ DIP joint stiffness: Failure to initiate early DIP motion or capturing the extensor mechanism in the pull-through suture can lead to stubborn DIP stiffness.
  ■ Flexion contracture: This is the most common complication and is due to splinting or stabilization in excessive PIP flexion or failure to initiate aggressive/hand therapist–supervised hand therapy at an appropriate interval.

REFERENCES

1. Calfee RP, Sommerkamp TG. Fracture-dislocation about the finger joints. *J Hand Surg [Am]*. 2009;34(6):1140-1147.
2. Eaton RG, Malerich MM. Volar plate arthroplasty of the proximal interphalangeal joint: a review of ten years' experience. *J Hand Surg [Am]*. 1980;5(3):260-268.
3. Burton RI, Campolattaro RM, Ronchetti PJ. Volar plate arthroplasty for osteoarthritis of the proximal interphalangeal joint: a preliminary report. *J Hand Surg [Am]*. 2002;27(6):1065-1072. doi: 10.1053/jhsu.2002.35871.
4. Dionysian E, Eaton RG. The long-term outcome of volar plate arthroplasty of the proximal interphalangeal joint. *J Hand Surg [Am]*. 2000;25(3):429-437.
5. Durham-Smith G, McCarten GM. Volar plate arthroplasty for closed proximal interphalangeal joint injuries. *J Hand Surg Br*. 1992;17(4):422-428.

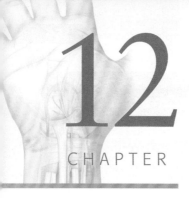

12

CHAPTER

Hemihamate Arthroplasty for the Proximal Interphalangeal Joint Fracture Dislocation

David Wei, Mark A. Vitale, and Amy M. Moore

DEFINITION

- Fracture dislocations of the proximal interphalangeal (PIP) joint are injuries in which the volar lip of the middle phalanx is fractured with accompanying instability of the middle phalanx on the proximal phalangeal head.
- The majority of PIP joint fracture dislocations are dorsal dislocations.
- PIP joint fracture dislocations are classified by their mechanical stability as well as the percentage of joint surface fractured and other radiographic parameters.[1]
- The most important radiographic determinant of stability is the percentage of the middle phalangeal articular surface that has been fractured:
  - Disruption of 30% or less of the articular surface is likely to be stable.
  - Thirty to thirty-five percent of articular surface involvement may be tenuous.
  - More than 50% of articular surface involvement is considered unstable.[1]
- Other radiographic signs of instability include the dorsal V sign and loss of continuity of the dorsal cortices of the proximal and middle phalanges.[2,3]
- Evaluation of mechanical stability is also important and can be tested by evaluating range of motion of the PIP joint using live fluoroscopic imaging or with radiographs in both full extension and full flexion (usually under a digital block). Injuries in which the PIP joint subluxates as the joint approaches extension are deemed unstable.
- Hemihamate arthroplasty, originally introduced by Hastings in 1999, is a method of reconstructing the damaged volar base of the middle phalanx by using the natural contour of the size-matched portion of the distal dorsal articular surface of the hamate.[4]

ANATOMY

- The bony anatomy of the PIP joint allows it to function as a hinge, permitting flexion and extension in the sagittal plane.
- The normal range of motion of the PIP joint is 0 to 120 degrees.
- Stability of the joint is conferred by a combination of bony constraints, the volar plate and the collateral ligaments (**FIG 1**).
  - The concave articular surface of the middle phalanx articulates with the convex condyles of the proximal phalanx. There is slight asymmetry between the proximal phalangeal condyles, which causes mild supination of the middle phalanx with flexion.[5]

- The volar plate is a fibrocartilaginous structure that is firmly attached distally to the volar base of the middle phalanx and which originates proximally from the proximal phalanx via two checkrein ligaments. The volar plate resists PIP joint hyperextension.
- The collateral ligaments are the primary restraints to radial- and ulnar-directed forces. They are composed of the proper and accessory collateral ligaments.
- Hemihamate arthroplasty takes advantage of the anatomy of the hamate (**FIG 2A**), which can replicate the volar proximal portion of the middle phalanx (**FIG 2B**), and cadaveric studies have demonstrated ideal suitability as an autologous graft.[6]
  - The distal surface of the hamate, which articulates with the base of the fourth and fifth metacarpals, contains a bicondylar facet that is separated by a central ridge.
  - The ridge closely replicates the bicondylar facet and central ridge of the proximal portion of the middle phalanx.
  - Though the contour of the hamate is more shallow than the contour of the middle phalanx (with the phalangeal radius of curvature ranging from 45% to 61% of the hamate) with proper orientation and tilting of the graft, a stable, congruent joint is achievable.[6]

PATHOGENESIS

- Two mechanisms of injury to the PIP joint have been described: avulsion and impaction shear.[7]
- Avulsion injuries occur when the PIP joint is hyperextended. The volar plate remains attached to the proximal phalanx, and the distal attachment avulses a fragment of the middle phalangeal volar lip (**FIG 3A**).

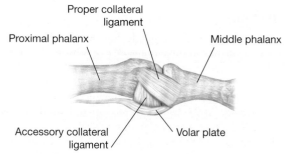

FIG 1 • Anatomy of the proximal interphalangeal (PIP) joint, including the proper (P) and accessory (A) collateral ligaments and the bony anatomy consisting of the convex condylar articular surface of the proximal phalanx (P1), which articulates with a concave articular surface of the middle phalanx (P2).

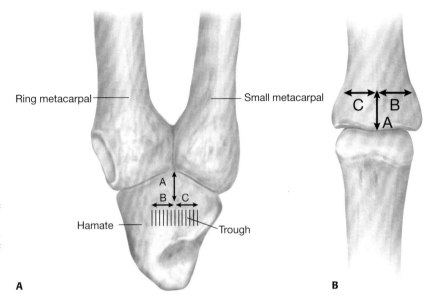

FIG 2 • The distal portion of the hamate bone of the carpometacarpal joint—which consists of a central ridge and bicondylar facet and articular cartilage distally, where it articulates with the articular cartilage of the fourth and fifth metacarpal bases **(A)**—is an ideal match in size, morphology, and dimensions to the volar proximal surface of the PIP joint of the digits **(B)**.

- Although avulsion fractures vary in size, there is typically no comminution.
- In impaction injuries, an axial load applied to the digit can drive the middle phalanx into the head of the proximal phalanx, creating a shear force through the middle phalangeal base. This creates a shear fracture of the volar lip.
- In this mechanism because the fractured base is impacted into the head of the proximal phalanx, the metaphyseal bone of the middle phalanx is often comminuted **(FIG 3B)**. When the volar fragment is sufficiently large, the buttressing effect of the volar margin of the middle phalanx and the restraint of the volar plate and collateral ligaments is lost, allowing the middle phalanx to displace dorsally.

NATURAL HISTORY

- The natural history of untreated dorsal PIP joint fracture dislocations is loss of motion, pain, and degenerative joint disease.[2]
- Even with adequate treatment, injury can result in chronic pain, stiffness, and swelling, as PIP joint injuries

are relatively unforgiving owing to the combination of bony injury, cartilage damage, soft tissue disruption, and scarring.[2,8]
- Traditional surgical options for unstable fracture dislocations of the PIP joint include external fixation, volar plate arthroplasty, and fracture fixation via percutaneous methods or open reduction and internal fixation.
  - When more than 50% of the volar aspect of the middle phalanx is injured, these traditional techniques lead to recurrent instability.[9]

PATIENT HISTORY AND PHYSICAL FINDINGS

- A patient's history will typically reveal a specific trauma in which the digit was "jammed" or "sprained"; the patient complaints of swelling, pain, and decreased range of motion.
- Physical examination should include a thorough examination of the skin. If surgery is needed and there is a compromised soft tissue envelope, percutaneous pinning or external fixation may be preferred to hemihamate arthroplasty.

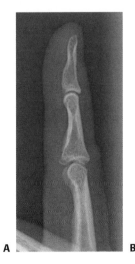
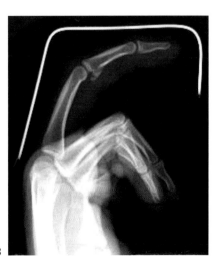

FIG 3 • **A.** Lateral radiograph of a middle finger demonstrating a small volar plate avulsion fracture without any evidence of PIP joint subluxation. **B.** Lateral radiograph of a ring finger demonstrating an impaction injury to the middle phalanx in which the base of the middle phalanx is driven into the head of the proximal phalanx resulting in comminution of the metaphyseal bone of the middle phalanx. This fracture was unstable and required closed reduction with a dorsal blocking splint and ultimately required surgical fixation.

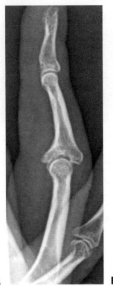 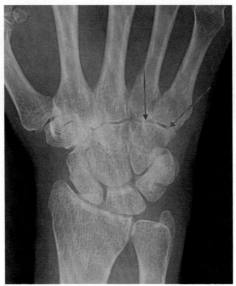 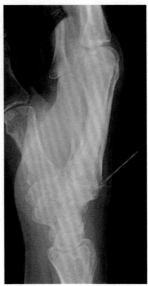 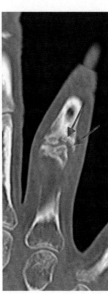

A   B   C   D

FIG 4 • A. Lateral radiograph demonstrating a patient with a 7-week-old dorsal PIP joint fracture dislocation with involvement of approximately 70% of the articular surface and an intact dorsal phalangeal base. **B,C.** PA and lateral radiographs demonstrating suitability of the ipsilateral hamate bone for a graft without evidence of fracture or degenerative joint disease. *Arrows* indicate location of harvest site. **D.** Coronal slice of a CT scan of the same patient revealing an ulnar-sided middle phalangeal defect with impaction causing ulnar deviation of the digit at the PIP joint (*arrows*). Fine slices via CT imaging allow for preoperative planning to determine how to contour the donor graft from the hamate.

- Physical examination should also include inspection for deformity, swelling, ecchymosis, malrotation, or angulation.
- Check for local tenderness to palpation of the PIP joint and assess the integrity of the flexor and extensor tendons.
- When imaging studies confirm dorsal dislocation, a gentle reduction should be attempted under local anesthetic.
- Once reduced, the joint should be inspected for passive and active stability.

IMAGING

- Basic radiographic imaging (including anteroposterior and lateral radiographs) of both the affected digit and the hand is necessary.
  - Lateral imaging of the PIP joint allows evaluation of the amount of articular surface that must be replaced (**FIG 4A**).
  - Wrist radiographs confirm that the hamate bone is intact and may serve as potential bone graft donor (**FIG 4B,C**).
  - In patients with prior injuries to the base of the ring or small finger carpometacarpal joints, the distal dorsal articular surface should be carefully inspected, and the contralateral hand should be considered for harvest of the hamate bone graft.
- In addition to radiographs, advanced imaging with a CT scan may be helpful in determining the three-dimensional nature of the middle phalanx defect.
  - Subtle radioulnar bony deficits, such as impaction and/or comminution may be visualized that are not apparent on radiographs (**FIG 4D**).

NONOPERATIVE MANAGEMENT

- Nonoperative management for PIP joint fracture dislocations may be considered in those patients with stable injury patterns (less than 30% articular surface involvement).

- Stability may be confirmed with a lateral radiograph of the PIP joint in full extension to ensure the absence of any dorsal subluxation.
- Treatment options include dorsal blocking splint, buddy taping to a neighboring digit, and early motion.
- For those PIP joint fracture dislocations that are unstable but reducible with PIP joint flexion of less than 30 degrees, nonsurgical management may be considered.
  - A dorsal blocking splint may be used to maintain reduction, and frequent radiographic follow-up is required to ensure the PIP joint remains congruent.
  - A figure-eight splint or silver ring splint may also be used.

SURGICAL MANAGEMENT

- Hemihamate arthroplasty is indicated for the treatment of unstable dorsal PIP joint fracture dislocations that are either acute or not amenable to ligamentotaxis or internal fixation, or subacute/chronic dislocations.
- Contraindications of this technique include any fractures involving the dorsal cortex, since the integrity of the dorsal cortex of the middle phalanx is necessary for hamate autograft fixation.
- Other considerations include those fractures with significant extension into the middle phalangeal shaft, as this can affect the positioning and recontouring of the articular surface.

Preoperative Planning

- Lateral radiographs of the PIP joint should be reviewed to estimate the size of the volar articular fragment that needs to be reconstructed.
- CT imaging may be useful in confirming the three-dimensional nature of the fractured volar rim and ensure

there is no dorsal cortical fracture or significant distal fracture extension along the volar cortex.

Positioning

- The patient is positioned supine on the operating table with the upper extremity on a radiolucent hand table.
- A malleable lead/aluminum hand may be used to help retract the nonoperative digits.
- The position of the surgeon should take into account the position of the fluoroscopic machine that most easily gives a perfect lateral radiograph of the PIP joint to be taken.

- One configuration is with the surgeon sitting at the head of the patient with the fluoroscopic C-arm coming from the end of the hand table in the horizontal position and the image intensifier closer to the surgeon. (See Pearls and Pitfalls, below.)

Approach

- A volar "shotgun" approach of the PIP joint is most commonly used and provides excellent exposure. Various skin flaps have been described to accomplish exposure of the volar aspect of the PIP joint.

■ Exposure

- We use a V-shaped Bruner incision, centered at the PIP joint flexion crease with the apex at the radial (the ulnar border could be used too), extending from the palmar digital crease to the DIP flexion crease.
- Raise skin flaps to expose the underlying flexor tendon sheath, and carefully identify both the radial and ulnar neurovascular bundles.
- Create an ulnar-based flap of the flexor tendon sheath by making transverse incisions distal to the A2 pulley and proximal to the A4 pulley, and also along the radial border.
  - Retraction of this flap ulnarly with a proximal and distal retraction suture helps to protect the neurovascular bundle just superficial to it.
- A Penrose drain can be used to retract the flexor tendons, exposing the underlying volar plate.
- Incise both radial and ulnar margins of the volar plate and elevate it from its distal attachment to the proximal phalanx to allow proximal retraction.
  - If the volar plate is still attached to the volar articular fragment, the fragment should be excised.
- Release both collateral ligaments off the proximal phalanx sharply, which may be done by using a knife at the level of the joint and cutting proximally along the

contour of the proximal phalangeal head so that the incised collateral ligaments can be redraped over the proximal phalanx to enhance healing.

- Now, the PIP joint may be fully hyperextended ("shotgunned") open, exposing the entirety of both articular surfaces (**TECH FIG 1**).

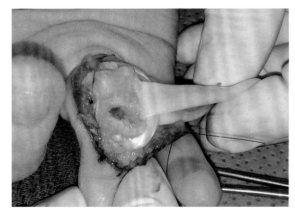

TECH FIG 1 • Shotgun exposure of the PIP joint of the ring finger with a PIP fracture dislocation exposing the head of the proximal phalanx and the fractured base of the middle phalanx. A small Penrose drain can be used to safely retract the flexor tendon system.

■ Middle Phalanx Preparation

- The base of the middle phalanx should be carefully inspected and correlated with preoperative radiographs and imaging.
- Use a rongeur or oscillating microsagittal saw on the middle phalanx to create a smooth articular interface to accept the hamate autograft.
  - A slow and careful approach during this step is recommended to avoid any excess removal of bone and to prevent fracture of the remaining dorsal bony cortex.
  - If possible, leaving a radial or ulnar bony articular lip may help to provide further stability of the hamate autograft.

- An ideal bone defect is one that begins at the articular surface and slopes toward the remaining intact volar cortex, which helps to cant the hamate graft and ultimately recreate the concave contour of the articular surface (**TECH FIG 2A**).
- The bone defect should be measured in preparation for hamate graft harvesting using either calipers or a small cut piece of a ruler.
- Dimensions that should be noted include the total width, the proximal to distal length, and finally the approximate amount of articular surface that must be recreated (**TECH FIG 2B,C**).

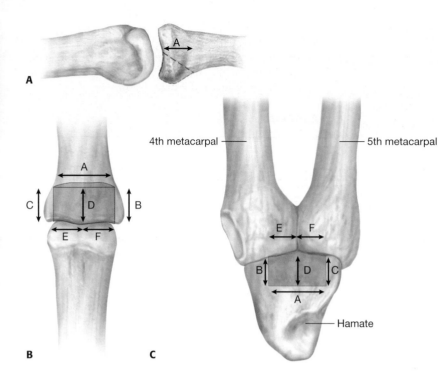

4th metacarpal — — 5th metacarpal

— Hamate

TECH FIG 2 • A. Illustration of the lateral PIP joint demonstrating the preferred bone defect to accept a hemihamate graft, with sloping at the articular surface toward the remaining intact volar cortex. **B,C.** Careful measurement of the dimensions of the missing volar phalangeal base with a caliper or ruler—including the total width, the proximal to distal length, and the amount of articular surface that must be reconstituted from the donor hamate graft—allows for a close match of the graft to its recipient site.

■ Hamate Autograft Harvest

- Identify the ring and small finger carpometacarpal joints using fluoroscopic guidance so the incision may be accurately positioned.
- Use either a transverse or longitudinal incision centered on the carpometacarpal joints.
- Retract and protect any cutaneous branches of the dorsal ulnar nerve as well as the extensor tendons to the ring and small fingers.
- Expose the CMC joints subperiosteally by incising the dorsal capsule longitudinally (**TECH FIG 3A**).
- Find the bony ridge between the ring and small finger CMC facets on the hamate. This will be used as the center of the graft.
- Using the previously measured dimensions of the PIP joint defect, mark the hamate using an indelible sterile marker, erring on the side of harvesting a slightly larger graft than necessary.
- Note that the central ridge on the hamate actually runs at an oblique angle from dorsal to volar. A previous cadaveric study has shown that the hamate has a central ridge and bicondylar facet with articular contours similar to the base of the middle phalanx.[6]
  - To ensure that the ridge remains central and in the correct orientation on the graft, make sure the hand is sufficiently pronated on the table before making any cuts (see Pearls and Pitfalls, below).
- With an oscillating saw or osteotome, make the sagittal and axial plane cuts first, remembering to take into

account the loss of bone that can be expected, depending on the thickness of the instrument used.

- Make the coronal plane cut last with a curved osteotome, as this is usually the most difficult cut to make and contributes directly to the concavity of the reconstructed articular surface. Two primary techniques can be used, antegrade or retrograde.
  - In the antegrade approach, a curved osteotome is used transversely along the proximal dorsal surface of the hamate and aimed into the ring and small finger CMC joint blindly. To ensure adequate thickness of the autograft using the antegrade approach, a small slice of bone is removed just proximal to the *axial* plane cut (**TECH FIG 3B**). This extra bone excision will provide room for the curved osteotome to obtain the correct depth of coronal plane cut (**TECH FIG 3C–E**).
  - In the retrograde approach,[10] the ring and small finger metacarpals are forcefully volarly subluxated to reveal the distal articular surface of the hamate, and the saw or osteotome is aimed volar and proximal to make a retrograde coronal cut.
  - Alternatively, a modification to this retrograde approach has been proposed[11] that exposes the distal articular surface of the hamate by resecting a portion of the ring and small finger metacarpal bases.
- Once excised, the hamate autograft can be further contoured and shaped to fit the recipient site with a fine rongeur.

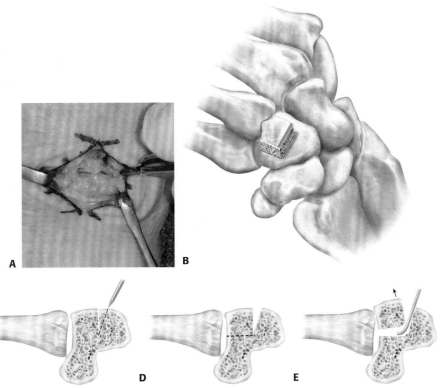

TECH FIG 3 • **A.** The donor site between the base of the fourth and fifth metacarpal and the dorsal aspect of the hamate can be exposed via either a longitudinal or transverse incision. The graft can be visualized after careful subperiosteal elevation. **B.** The coronal cut of the autograft harvest. To ensure adequate thickness of the autograft using the antegrade approach, a small slice of bone is removed just proximal to the axial plane cut (indicated in *pink*). **C–E.** This extra bone excision will provide room for the curved osteotome to obtain the correct depth of coronal plane cut.

■ Hamate Graft Fixation and Closure

- Provisionally fix the graft to the middle phalanx using a central 0.028-in. or 0.035-in. K-wire in a volar to dorsal direction (**TECH FIG 4A**).
- If the visual contour of the graft is satisfactory, use two 0.035-in. K-wires to secure both the radial or ulnar aspects of the graft to prevent any rotation (**TECH FIG 4B**).
- If 1.3-mm screws are used, there is no need to redrill, and the 0.035-in. K-wires may simply be replaced with screws.
- Depending on the size of the graft, a combination of two or three 1.0-, 1.3-, or 1.5-mm screws may be used (**TECH FIG 4C,D**).

- Visually verify the concavity of the articular surface, and fluoroscopically verify screw lengths and overall graft positioning. Ideally, screws will be bicortical such that no more than 1 thread length is visible beyond the dorsal cortex to avoid prominence of the screw tips dorsally (**TECH FIG 4E**).
  - Because of the discrepancy of cartilage thickness, a bony step-off visualized on fluoroscopy is not unusual despite visual confirmation of articular congruency; this may be ignored.
- If there is any prominence along the volar cortical surface, the graft may be contoured to match the volar cortex of the middle phalanx using a bur or a rongeur.
- Reattach the volar plate distally, and the flexor tendon sheath flap maybe placed underneath the flexor tendons as an additional layer.

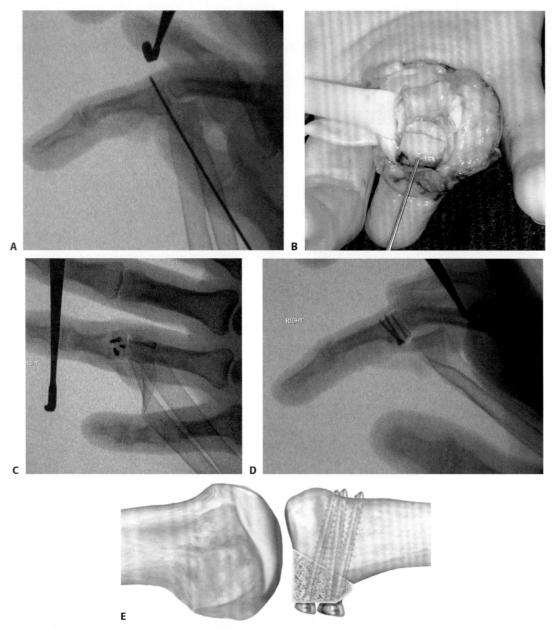

TECH FIG 4 • **A.** Provisional fixation of the hemihamate graft with a 0.035-in. K-wire. This K-wire hole can later be used for one of the screw holes if appropriately positioned. **B.** Using a shotgun approach, the surgeon can align the articular contour between the donor hemihamate graft and the remaining articular surface of the recipient dorsal phalangeal base. Because of slight mismatch in the width of the articular cartilage of the hemihamate graft and the phalangeal base, which may appear as a step-off on a radiograph or fluoroscopic image, it is more important to visually align the contour of the graft than it is to align the fluoroscopic contour of the underlying subchondral bone. **C.** AP intraoperative fluoroscopic view of final fixation of the hemihamate graft with one 1.0-mm and two 1.3-mm bicortical screws to form an inverted triangle demonstrates correction of preoperative ulnar deviation and good medial to lateral size match of the graft with the native middle phalanx. **D.** Lateral fluoroscopic view shows restoration of PIP joint stability. **E.** Screw fixation of the graft should ideally be bicortical but without more than one thread length of the screws beyond the dorsal cortex of the middle phalanx to avoid dorsal prominence.

PEARLS AND PITFALLS

Autograft contour	▪ Reconstructing the proper concavity of the articular surface of the base of the proximal phalanx is crucial. Cancellous autograft may be used distally to aid in tilting the graft to create a more concave articular surface.

Hamate autograft anatomy	▪ The central ridge separating the ring and small finger metacarpal facets on the hamate may not be purely perpendicular to the dorsal surface.
	 ▪ There are two methods to ensure graft harvest does not result in asymmetry:
	   ▫ Be sure to pronate the hand as much as possible such that the central ridge is as perpendicular to the floor as possible. This will help guide your cuts.
	   ▫ Fluoroscopy can help verify that the hamate ridge is indeed positioned perpendicular to the cut you make.
	 ▪ If you do an antegrade osteotomy, first use the saw to remove a very small section of hamate proximal to the graft so that you can harvest a deep enough graft with a curved osteotome when making your final cut in the coronal plane.

Hamate autograft coronal cut	▪ The last cut, or the coronal plane cut, of the hamate autograft is the cut that determines the amount of volar-dorsal articular surface harvested.
Radioulnar asymmetry	▪ A CT scan may be helpful in determining radioulnar asymmetry of the fracture fragment. When preparing the proximal phalanx, *keeping* this asymmetry can be helpful, as the hamate autograft may also be asymmetric.
Checking for passive motion	▪ After the proximal phalanx recipient site is prepared, make sure passive ROM of the reduced PIP joint is full. If necessary, an extensor tenolysis or joint contracture release should be performed. ▪ If this passive motion is not checked until after the autograft is secured, a joint contracture could lead to undue force on the graft and risk graft fixation failure.
C-arm fluoroscopy positioning	▪ Obtaining a lateral radiograph of the PIP joint is critical for evaluating the reconstructed joint bony anatomy. Using a C-arm from the end of the hand table in the horizontal position facilitates manipulation and imaging. ▪ The shoulder is abducted to 90 degrees, and the elbow is flexed at 90 degrees. With the XR beam horizontal to the floor, the forearm may be easily pronated and supinated until a perfect lateral of the PIP joint is obtained. ▪ If a lead hand is used, the other fingers may be fully extended and the shotgunned surgical finger flexed at the MP joint. ▪ Alternatively, an elastic bandage may be used to hold all the nonoperative fingers flexed in a fist with the shotgunned surgical finger extended at the MP joint.
Proximal phalanx preparation	▪ In order to reconstruct the concavity of the articular surface, it is important to prepare the proximal phalanx such that the graft will be tilted to recreate the cup shape of the volar lip. ▪ Creating a slope, rather than a right angle, from the articular surface down to the volar cortex will help with this.
Collateral ligaments	▪ The collateral ligament may be repaired to the volar plate for soft tissue coverage and a gliding surface over the bone graft for the flexor tendons.
Postoperative splinting	▪ A dorsal blocking splint may be used in about 20 degrees of PIP flexion as described in previous published reports, although they may be placed in closer to full extension if the reconstruction leads to a stable joint.
Graft disasters	▪ Should the graft that was obtained from the ipsilateral hamate be catastrophically contaminated or dropped, consider using the contralateral hamate.

POSTOPERATIVE CARE

▪ Authors have described various postoperative immobilization protocols including:
  ▫ Use of a 15-degree dorsal blocking splint to protect volar plate repair and avoid postoperative instability[8]
  ▫ Alternately, initial immobilization of the wrist and digit in extension for 3 or 4 days followed by a thermoplast extension splint to avoid a flexion contracture[11]
  ▫ We prefer to utilize a wrist-based (to protect the hamate graft harvest site) intrinsic-plus splint to include the affected finger and border digits for 1 week until sutures are removed. We then transition to a 15-degree dorsal blocking digital splint vs figure-eight splint initiating active wrist and digital range of motion under the supervision of a hand therapist 1 week after surgery with a home exercise program focusing on active range of motion techniques out of the splint.
▪ Protective splints are generally discontinued at 6 weeks, followed by initiation of passive range of motion.

▪ Full unprotected use for heavy lifting and sports is not allowed until bony union is verified by radiographs and clinical exam, which is anticipated at 3 to 4 months.

OUTCOMES

▪ A prior cadaveric study comparing the biomechanical characteristics of hemihamate arthroplasty vs volar plate arthroplasty found that although both techniques could adequately restore PIP joint stability, use of volar plate arthroplasty led to an increasing flexion contracture as the middle phalanx palmar base deficit increased.[12]
▪ Williams and coauthors followed 13 consecutive patients with unstable dorsal PIP fracture dislocations treated with hemihamate autograft for 16 months.[13] On average, 60% of the articular surface was involved on lateral radiographs. Average arc of motion of the PIP joint postoperatively was 85 degrees, VAS pain score was 1.3, grip strength averaged 80% of the contralateral side, and eleven patients were very satisfied with their function.

- Calfee et al. reported on a cohort of 33 patients with a combination of acute and chronic injuries with 4.5-year follow-up.[8] The average arc of postoperative PIP joint motion was 70 degrees, VAS score rating was 1.4, and grip strength averaged 95% of the contralateral grip strength. Outcomes were modestly better in injuries treated acutely (within 6 weeks of injury) compared to chronic injuries (injuries treated 6 weeks or later from injury).
- Afendras and coauthors reviewed the clinical outcomes of eight consecutive patients who underwent hemihamate arthroplasty at a minimum follow-up of 4 years.[14] The average arc of motion was 67 degrees at the PIP joint, and the VAS rating was 10 (on a 100-point scale), with 91% grip strength compared to the uninjured side.

COMPLICATIONS

- Williams and coauthors reported two patients with recurrent dorsal subluxation out of a total 13 consecutive patients.[13] The authors postulated the subluxation was due to failure of the volar plate repair and inadequate angulation of the graft such that the articular concave geometry was not sufficiently recreated.
- Others have suggested that adequate restoration of the middle phalangeal base provides sufficient osseous stability to prevent such subluxation and that extension block pinning and formal volar plate repair are rarely needed.[8,15]
- Two series with long-term follow-up found no instances of subluxation or dislocation.[8,14]
- One series reported intraoperative fracture of the dorsal cortex of the middle phalanx as a possible complication.[8]
- Flexor tendon pulley insufficiency is another reported complication if the critical A2 or A4 pulley systems that are repaired at the conclusion of the case become incompetent.[8]
- PIP joint flexion contracture has been reported and may potentially be avoided by adherence to a closely supervised postoperative hand therapy protocol.[8]
- Donor site pain in the wrist is an infrequent complication reported in 5% of cases,[15] and cadaveric studies have shown minimal evidence of instability of the fourth or fifth carpometacarpal joints following graft harvest.[6]
- Previous series have shown that radiographic signs of degenerative joint disease of the PIP joint have occurred in close to 50% of cases with long-term follow-up, but this has been observed in the absence of pain or other symptoms with no correlation between loss of joint space and functional outcomes.[8]

- In the patient series by Afendras, two of eight patients developed severe symptomatic arthritis, and two of eight developed mild degenerative changes.[14] The authors speculated that this may be due to nonanatomical mismatch of the joint surface and consequent abnormal load bearing, biologic failure of the graft, or chondral damage from the initial injury.

REFERENCES

1. Kiefhaber TR, Stern PI. Clinical perspective fracture dislocations of the proximal interphalangeal joint. *J Hand Surg [Am].* 1998;23A:368-380.
2. Mangelson JJ, Stern PJ, Abzug JM, et al. Complications following dislocations of the proximal interphalangeal joint. *Instr Course Lect.* 2014;63:123-130.
3. Light T. Buttress pinning techniques. *Orthop Rev.* 1981;10:49-55.
4. Hastings H, Carroll C. Treatment of closed articular fractures of the metacarpophalangeal and proximal interphalangeal joints. *Hand Clin.* 1988;4:503-527.
5. Leibovic SJ, Bowers WH. Anatomy of the proximal interphalangeal joint. *Hand Clin.* 1994;10:169-178.
6. Capo JT, Hastings H, Choung E, et al. Hemicondylar hamate replacement arthroplasty for proximal interphalangeal joint fracture dislocations: an assessment of graft suitability. *J Hand Surg [Am].* 2008;33:733-739.
7. Elfar J, Mann T. Fracture-dislocations of the proximal interphalangeal joint. *J Am Acad Orthop Surg.* 2013;21:88-98.
8. Calfee RP, Kiefhaber TR, Sommerkamp TG, Stern PJ. Hemi-hamate arthroplasty provides functional reconstruction of acute and chronic proximal interphalangeal fracture-dislocations. *J Hand Surg [Am].* 2009;34:1232-1241.
9. Deitch M, Kiefhaber TR, Comisar BR, Stern PJ. Dorsal fracture dislocations of the proximal interphalangeal joint: surgical complications and long-term results. *J Hand Surg [Am].* 1999;24:914-923.
10. Yang DS, Lee SK, Kim KJ, Choy WS. Modified hemihamate arthroplasty technique for treatment of acute proximal interphalangeal joint fracture-dislocations. *Ann Plast Surg.* 2014;72:411-416.
11. DeNoble PH, Record NC. A modification to simplify the harvest of a hemi-hamate autograft. *J Hand Surg [Am].* 2016;41:e99-e102.
12. Tyser AR, Tsai M, Parks BG, Means KR. Biomechanical characteristics of hemi-hamate reconstruction versus volar plate arthroplasty in the treatment of dorsal fracture dislocations of the proximal interphalangeal joint. *J Hand Surg [Am].* 2015;40:329-332.
13. Williams RMM, Kiefhaber TR, Sommerkamp TG, Stern PJ. Treatment of unstable dorsal proximal interphalangeal fracture/dislocations using a hemi-hamate autograft. *J Hand Surg [Am].* 2003;28:856-865.
14. Afendras G, Abramo A, Mrkonjic A, et al. Hemi-hamate osteochondral transplantation in proximal interphalangeal dorsal fracture dislocations: a minimum 4 year follow-up in eight patients. *J Hand Surg Eur Vol.* 2010;35:627-631.
15. McAuliffe JA. Hemi-hamate autograft for the treatment of unstable dorsal fracture dislocation of the proximal interphalangeal joint. *J Hand Surg [Am].* 2009;34:1890-1894.

Thumb Carpometacarpal Joint Fusion With Locking Plates

John M. Felder and Amy M. Moore

DEFINITION

- Arthritis of the thumb trapeziometacarpal (TMC) joint is common and leads to weakness, deformity, limitation of motion, and pain, particularly with pinch.
- Fusion of the TMC joint produces reliable relief of arthritic pain and a stable position of the thumb for pinch.
- Adequate postoperative thumb motion is maintained through movement at the thumb metacarpophalangeal (MCP) and scaphotrapezial joints.

ANATOMY

- The articular surface of the trapezium with the thumb metacarpal is saddle shaped, permitting a wide range of motion and palmar abduction (abduction perpendicular to the plane of the palm).
- The capsule of the TMC joint must be sufficiently lax to allow the wide range of motion of the thumb but contains key stout ligaments, such as the volar oblique and dorsoradial ligaments, that are critical for joint stability. Attenuation of these ligaments leads to joint incongruity and arthritis.

PATHOGENESIS

- In typical TMC joint osteoarthritis, progressive ligamentous laxity, intrinsic osseous instability, overuse patterns, and articular wear may all contribute to subluxation of the thumb metacarpal from the trapezium with resultant incongruous articulation, cartilage loss, and osteoarthritis.
- TMC joint arthritis may also result from prior fracture of the thumb metacarpal base or trapezium, typically in younger men.
- Fusion of the thumb TMC joint may also be desirable as an alternative to opponensplasty for positioning of the thumb in nerve palsies or brachial plexus injuries affecting thumb opposition.

PATIENT HISTORY AND PHYSICAL FINDINGS

- Any history of nontraumatic radial-sided hand pain, particularly pain localizing to the base of the thumb, may suggest TMC joint arthritis.
- Classically, this disease is most commonly encountered in postmenopausal women.
- Physical examination begins with inspection, which may show enlargement of the thumb TMC joint and prominence of the joint due to subluxation of the base of the metacarpal.

- In advanced disease, metacarpal adduction due to TMC joint subluxation may lead to compensatory hyperextension of the MCP joint, creating the so-called zigzag deformity.
- Maneuvers to elicit joint crepitus or tenderness at the joint include the grind test, palpation of the joint, and the thumb adduction or extension tests (and related tests),[1] which create sheer stress across the joint.
  - The CMC grind test is performed by applying an axially directed loading force to the thumb metacarpal and circumducting the thumb. Crepitus or reproduction of pain is considered a positive result.
  - For the adduction stress maneuver, the examiner is seated facing the patient. The patient places the affected hand on the examination table with the elbow flexed 90 degrees and the forearm in neutral rotation. The examiner places his or her ipsilateral hand such that the examiner's thumb rests dorsally over the head of the thumb metacarpal. The examiner's contralateral hand supports the ulnar side of the patient's hand to maintain the patient's wrist in neutral position to prevent ulnar deviation of the patient's wrist. The examiner firmly directs an adduction force downward onto the patient's metacarpal head until the patient's thumb metacarpal lies parallel to the midaxis of the index metacarpal or until a firm end point is reached. The re-creation of pain at the TMC joint is considered a positive test.
  - The thumb extension test is performed from the same starting position. The examiner places his or her ipsilateral thumb along the radial aspect of the distal thumb metacarpal, 5 to 10 mm proximal to the thumb MCP joint, and extends the thumb until the thumb metacarpal comes to lie in a plane parallel to the palm or until a firm end point is reached. Re-creation of pain at the TMC joint is considered a positive test.

IMAGING

- Standard PA, lateral, oblique, and Roberts view radiographs of the hand should be obtained. Roberts view of the thumb profiles the articular surface of the thumb TMC joint and provides optimal visualization of the thumb CMC joint. This view requires position of the forearm in maximal pronation with the dorsum of the thumb resting on the film cassette.

- Radiographic staging of thumb TMC joint arthritis[2] distinguishes between the following:
  - Stage I: Normal radiographs or TMC joint widening with symptomatic pain and laxity
  - Stage II: Mild joint space narrowing, osteophyte formation less than 2 mm
  - Stage III: Significant joint space narrowing or total loss of joint space, osteophyte formation more than 2 mm
  - Stage IV: Stage III also including scaphotrapeziotrapezoid (STT) joint arthritis
- Note that this staging system is useful for description of radiographic findings but is not used for prognosis or to guide treatment. Rather, clinical symptoms (eg, pain) direct treatment.

DIFFERENTIAL DIAGNOSIS

- First dorsal compartment (de Quervain) tenosynovitis
- Carpal tunnel syndrome
- Fracture
- STT joint arthritis
- Rheumatoid arthritis

NONOPERATIVE MANAGEMENT

- In the case of the TMC joint osteoarthritis, nonoperative management should always be attempted and consists of hand-based thumb spica splinting, nonsteroidal anti-inflammatory medications, and intra-articular steroid injections.
- In the case of nerve palsy requiring arthrodesis for thumb pinch stability, nonoperative management is not indicated and TMC joint fusion may be elected as a planned part of the reconstructive algorithm.[3]
- In either case, the patient's tolerance for joint fusion should be tested preoperatively with a period of immobilization of the TMC joint by rigid splinting before proceeding with arthrodesis.

SURGICAL MANAGEMENT

- Pain interfering with daily activities despite a period of nonoperative management and lack of ability to stabilize the thumb in space for opposition are indications for TMC joint fusion.
- For painful TMC joint osteoarthritis, resection and/or interposition arthroplasty is a reasonable alternative to fusion with similar outcomes.
  - Many authors favor TMC joint fusion for younger, higher-demand patients who require greater pinch strength and arthroplasty for older, less active patients.[4,5]
  - Because TMC joint arthroplasty with resection of the trapezium requires a prolonged period of postoperative splinting and therapy and may weaken the thumb for up to 6 months postoperatively, our preference is to perform TMC joint fusion for manual laborers who require a rapid return to work and hand strength.

Preoperative Planning

- Preoperatively, the patient must understand the implications of joint fusion on mobility; this is best demonstrated with a period of preoperative splinting.
- The thumb MCP joint should be assessed for stability prior to proceeding with TMC joint fusion. An unstable MCP joint will preclude stable pinch and, if arthrodesis of the MP joint is required for stability, this in combination with TMC arthrodesis may restrict thumb mobility so greatly as to interfere with thumb function.
- Radiographs should be assessed for osteopenia and be recognized when proceeding with the bony fixation required for arthrodesis. Disuse osteopenia is found with paralytic limbs.
- Radiographs should also be assessed for degenerative changes in adjacent joints such as the STT joint. Severe STT arthritis is a relative contraindication for CMC arthrodesis.[5]
- Surgery may be performed under general, local, or regional anesthesia. We prefer general anesthesia supplemented by local or regional blocks.
- Bone grafting is recommended for successful fusion; bone graft is taken from the distal radius or iliac crest in case of suboptimal contact between prepared bony surfaces.
- Fluoroscopy should be available.
- Power tools and a hand fixation set with locking plates should be requested for this case. We prefer the use of rigid locking plate fixation to traditional plates and K-wires in this procedure as often the bone is of poor quality. Locking plates provide inherent stability for bony fusion.

Positioning

- The patient is positioned supine on the operating room table, with the hand centered on a hand table.
- An upper arm tourniquet and exsanguination should be used for better visualization of neurovascular structures in the field, such as the radial artery and branches of the radial sensory nerve.

Approach

- A volar approach, a modified Wagner approach, or a dorsoradial approach to the TMC joint can be used.
- We prefer the dorsal approach, which requires identification and protection of the radial sensory nerve branches and radial artery but offers better visualization of the joint space and metacarpal, particularly if plate fixation is planned.

■ Dorsoradial Approach to Thumb TMC Joint Arthrodesis with Plate and Screw Fixation

Exposure

- A longitudinal incision is made from the midpoint of the dorsal surface of the thumb metacarpal to the proximal aspect of the radial styloid (**TECH FIG 1**).
- Superficial branches of the lateral antebrachial cutaneous (LABC) nerve and radial sensory nerve (RSN) are identified and protected (**TECH FIG 1B**).

- The abductor pollicis longus (APL) and extensor pollicis brevis (EPB) tendons are identified, and the interval between them is opened to create access to the joint (**TECH FIG 1C**).
- The radial artery is protected within the proximal field of dissection.
- The TMC joint capsule is identified in the depths between the APL and EPB tendons. At this point, it is useful to insert a Freer elevator at the presumed TMC joint space (**TECH FIG 1D**) and use fluoroscopy to verify correct position (**TECH FIG 1E**).

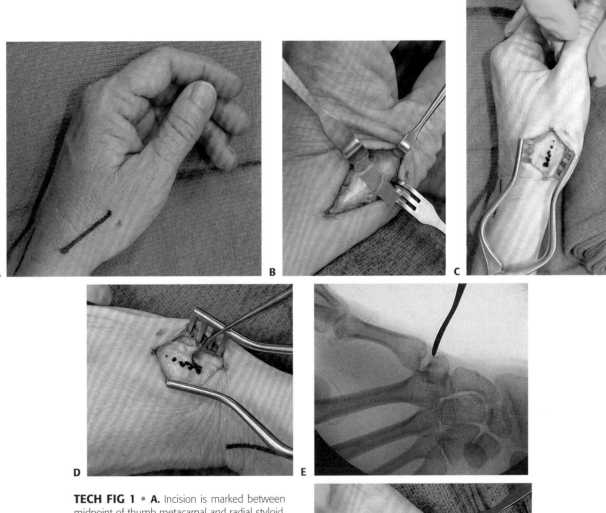

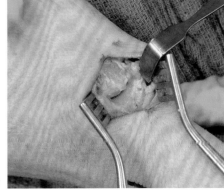

TECH FIG 1 • A. Incision is marked between midpoint of thumb metacarpal and radial styloid. **B.** The branches of the radial sensory and lateral antebrachial cutaneous nerves are identified and protected. **C.** The abductor pollicis longus and extensor pollicis brevis tendons are identified, and the interval between them is planned for exposure. **D.** A Freer elevator is used to identify the location of the TMC joint before making a capsular incision. **E.** Fluoroscopy confirms the correct location of the joint. **F.** The capsule of the TMC joint is incised, and capsular tissue is circumferentially elevated from the thumb metacarpal and trapezium.

- A longitudinal incision is made full thickness through the capsule to elevate the capsule from the metacarpal and the trapezium. An attempt should be made to preserve the edges of the capsule neatly for later closure (**TECH FIG 1F**).
  - Elevation of the capsule circumferentially from the metacarpal may cause detachment of the APL tendon insertion and it does not need to be reattached.

Fitting the Metacarpal Base to the Trapezium

- The thumb metacarpal base is delivered into the wound using two small Hohmann retractors.
- Using a rongeur or a slow-running bur, the metacarpal base is denuded of cartilage and subchondral bone, and the proximal medullary bone is fashioned into a ball or cone shape (**TECH FIG 2A,B**).

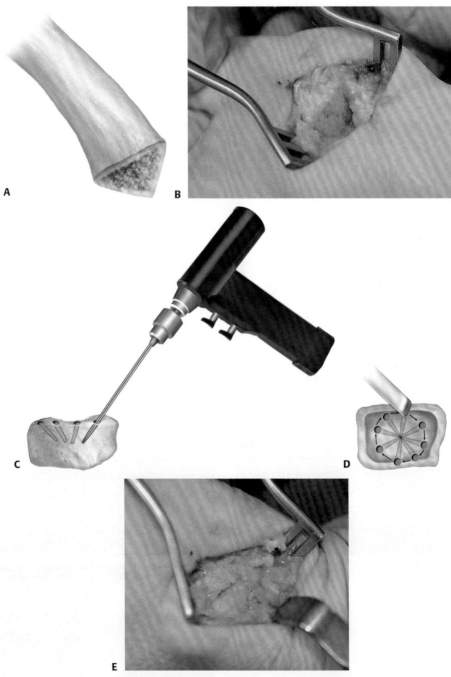

TECH FIG 2 • **A.** The metacarpal base is delivered into the wound, and a rongeur is used to fashion the medullary bone into a cone shape. **B.** Healthy cancellous bone is visualized. **C.** In preparing the trapezium surface, an option to allow for adequate bony contact is to use a K-wire to drill multiple holes into the trapezium at a 45-degree angle directed toward the center of the bone. **D.** A small osteotome is then used to excavate the central bone to allow the cone-shaped metacarpal base to fit into the trapezium. **E.** The metacarpal is fit onto the prepared surface of the trapezium.

- The articular surface of the trapezium is then removed and the medullary bone of the trapezium is fashioned into a cup shape to accommodate the cone of the metacarpal base. This can be done with a low-speed power bur or by using an awl.
  - Another option is to use a K-wire to drill multiple holes angled at 45 degrees toward the center of the trapezium (**TECH FIG 2C**). The holes are drilled sequentially at 2- to 3-mm intervals to create a circle, and the circumscribed cone-shaped fragment is then excavated with a small straight osteotome (**TECH FIG 2D**).[6]
  - Attention to detail is important when shaping the surface of the trapezium, as it may be a thin and degenerated bone with relatively little volume to allow for error. It is essential to be certain that the center of the "cone" has been denuded of cartilage or cortical bone and contains exposed medullary bone.
  - The metacarpal is fit onto the prepared surface of the trapezium (**TECH FIG 2E**).

Positioning the Thumb and Fixation

- At this point, attention is turned to proper positioning of the thumb. Ideal position is approximately 45 degrees from the coronal and sagittal planes of the hand. Slight pronation of the thumb tip may assist with pinch to the more ulnar digits.
  - Proper position is confirmed by seeing that the pulp of the thumb rests on the radial aspect of the index middle phalanx with the fingers in a relaxed, closed fist (**TECH FIG 3A**).
- Positioning should be secured using a K-wire for provisional fixation. This can initially be driven antegrade through the base of the thumb metacarpal toward the MCP joint and then reversed and driven retrograde to secure the base of the metacarpal to the trapezium.
- Once position is visually adequate, bony apposition is checked with fluoroscopy. Any areas of inadequate bony contact should be supplemented with cancellous bone autograft.
- Provisional K-wire fixation is maintained while placing a plate. Our preference is to use a locking 2.3-mm T-plate with the wings of the T placed over the trapezium and the long aspect of the plate extending onto the metacarpal shaft (**TECH FIG 3B**).
- Fluoroscopy should be used liberally to ensure that screws do not penetrate nearby joints (eg, STT) or the FPL tendon sheath. Once fixation is achieved, the K-wire is removed (**TECH FIG 3C,D**).

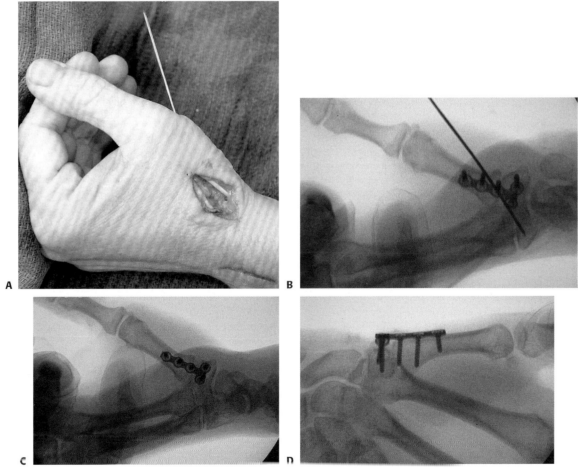

TECH FIG 3 • A. The thumb is positioned with it resting on the radial aspect of the index middle phalanx with fingers in gentle flexion. A K wire is used to secure the position prior to plate fixation. **B–D.** A locking T-plate is used to maintain the position of the thumb, and multiple fluoroscopic images are obtained to evaluate the plate position, the contact of the bony surfaces, and the length of the screws to avoid unwanted penetration into the STT joint or flexor pollicis longus.

- The capsule of the TMC joint should ideally be closed with buried suture.
- Supplement general anesthesia with local anesthetic injection before skin closure.

- The skin is closed with horizontal mattress sutures. Take care to avoid branches of the RSN during closure.
- The hand is dressed with short-arm thumb spica splint, leaving the IP joint free.

■ Dorsoradial Approach to Thumb TMC Joint Arthrodesis With K-Wire Fixation

- This procedure is identical to the above technique except that in place of a plate and screws, three 0.045-in. K-wires are used for fixation.
- This technique is most appropriate for patients with soft bone that will not accommodate a locking plate, such as patients with rheumatoid arthritis. We do not recommend use of K-wire fixation for fusion in patients with osteoarthritis.

- The first wire should follow the planned axis of bone fusion and may be driven using the antegrade (via the exposed TMC joint) followed by retrograde technique.
- The remaining two wires should be driven retrograde through the metacarpal into the trapezium at a divergence of 10 to 20 degrees from the axis of the first wire.
- Wires should not penetrate the STT joint.
- Pins are capped and left outside the skin for office removal at 6 to 8 weeks.
- Closure and dressings are as above.

PEARLS AND PITFALLS

Simulate fusion preoperatively	■ Place the patient in a hand-based thumb spica splint for several weeks preoperatively to ensure the patient understands what postoperative motion and hand function will be like.
Preparation of the bone	■ Careful preparation of the bone surfaces is essential for positioning and improved bony contact. This involves complete removal of articular cartilage and subchondral bone while maintaining the cup and cone formation of the joint.
Bone graft	■ Be prepared to harvest bone graft if needed to ensure excellent bony contact between fused surfaces. Our preference is to augment the fusion site with distal radius bone graft.
Nerve branches	■ Take great care to avoid damage to branches of the radial sensory nerve to prevent postoperative pain syndromes.
Position	■ Discuss positioning of the thumb preoperatively with the patient. Ideal position can be estimated by placing the thumb pulp over the index middle phalanx with the fingers resting in a flexed position.

POSTOPERATIVE CARE

- The short-arm thumb spica splint placed in the operating room is maintained for 2 weeks.
- Sutures are removed at 2 weeks, and the patient is placed into a short-arm thumb spica cast.
- If plate fixation is used, the cast is removed at 4 to 6 weeks postoperatively.
- If Kirschner wire fixation is used, the cast and pins are removed at 8 weeks.
- After cast removal, patients are given a custom-fabricated, removable forearm-based thumb spica splint leaving the interphalangeal joint free until definitive signs of bony healing are seen on x-ray.
  - Typically, bony healing on x-ray appears between 12 and 14 weeks (**FIG 1A–C**).
  - A CT scan can be performed to confirm union at 8 to 10 weeks (**FIG 1D**).
- Range of motion is initiated after cast removal with the help of a certified hand therapist (**FIG 1E,F**).

OUTCOMES

- Functional outcomes are typically excellent following thumb TMC joint arthrodesis. Clinically, it may be difficult to tell the difference between the thumb operated upon and the normal thumb.[6]
- Patients and surgeons should expect the operation to relieve the pain of arthritis, improve grip, and restore good stability to the thumb ray.[4]
- With proper positioning of the TMC joint in arthrodesis, compensatory motion of the MCP and STT joints typically allows patients to adduct the thumb to touch the base of the proximal phalanx of the index finger and to oppose the thumb to the tips of all fingers.[5]
- Thumb retropulsion and abduction from the plane of the palm will be decreased when compared with the unoperated side but are adequate to allow grasp around relatively large objects such as jar lids. Pinch strength is typically equal to the contralateral side.[7]

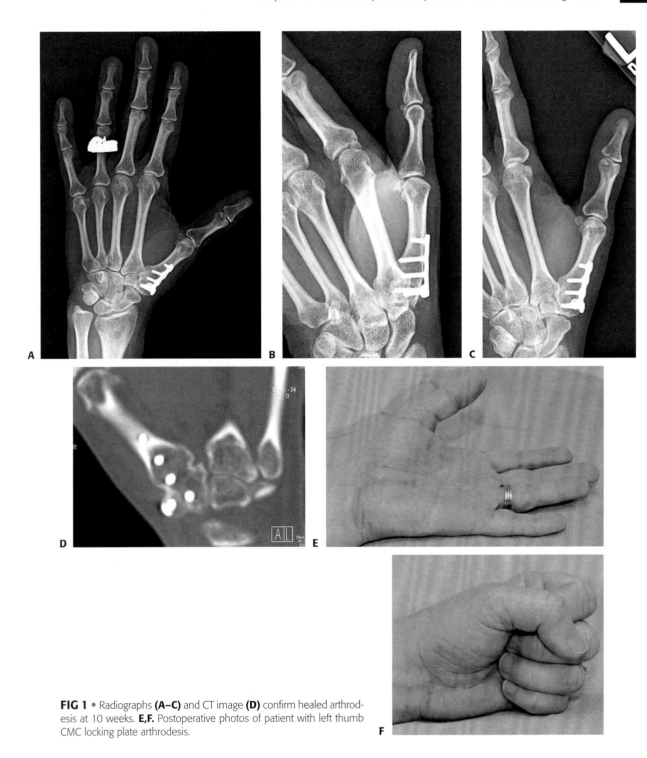

FIG 1 • Radiographs **(A–C)** and CT image **(D)** confirm healed arthrodesis at 10 weeks. **E,F.** Postoperative photos of patient with left thumb CMC locking plate arthrodesis.

COMPLICATIONS

- Nonunion is the most concerning complication and occurs at a reported rate of 13%.[8] Nonunion can be minimized by ensuring excellent apposition of cancellous bony surfaces, using bone graft and careful fixation technique. Careful attention to shaping of the cup and cone surfaces and avoiding the use of high-speed, heat-generating power saws may also help to prevent nonunion. Rigid stabilization with plate and screws may shorten casting time, but definitive increased overall union rate over K-wire fixation has not been shown.[5] Nonetheless, it is our preference to use locking plate fixation over K-wire fixation.

- Hardware-related pain or hardware prominence is a potential complication when using plate and screw fixation that may require return to the operating room.

- Hardware malposition (eg, within the STT joint) is a potential complication that is best avoided by intraoperative use of fluoroscopy in multiple planes.

- Radial nerve neuritis and complex regional pain syndrome are potential complications of this operation that are best avoided by careful identification and protection of nerve branches intraoperatively. However, the surgery should be approached with the knowledge that these complications may occur even despite careful surgical technique.
- Patients may complain of an inability to place the palm flat on a table or with difficulty in placing the hand in a pocket. These concerns are best addressed with thorough preoperative education and splinting.

REFERENCES

1. Gelberman RH, Boone S, Osei DA, et al. Trapeziometacarpal arthritis: a prospective clinical evaluation of the thumb adduction and extension provocative tests. *J Hand Surg [Am]*. 2015;40(7):1285-1291.
2. Eaton RG, Littler JW. Ligament reconstruction for the painful thumb carpometacarpal joint. *J Bone Joint Surg Am*. 1973;55(8):1655-1666.
3. Giuffre JL, Bishop AT, Spinner RJ, et al. Wrist, first carpometacarpal joint, and thumb interphalangeal joint arthrodesis in patients with brachial plexus injuries. *J Hand Surg Am*. 2012;37(12):2557-2563.e1.
4. Rizzo M. Thumb arthrodesis. *Tech Hand Up Extrem Surg*. 2006;10(1):43-46.
5. Goldfarb CA, Stern PJ. Indications and techniques for thumb carpometacarpal arthrodesis. *Tech Hand Upper Extrem Surg*. 2002;6(4):178-184.
6. Carroll RE, Hill NA. Arthrodesis of the carpo-metacarpal joint of the thumb. *J Bone Joint Surg Br*. 1973;55(2):292-294.
7. Stark HH, Moore JF, Ashworth CR, Boyes JH. Fusion of the first metacarpotrapezial joint for degenerative arthritis. *J Bone Joint Surg Am*. 1977;59(1):22-26.
8. Bamberger HB, Stern PJ, Kiefhaber TR, et al. Trapeziometacarpal joint arthrodesis: a functional evaluation. *J Hand Surg [Am]*. 1992;17A:606-611.

Section IV: Wrist Fractures and Carpal Instability
Arthroscopic Examination of the Wrist

Emily Krauss and Amy M. Moore

DEFINITION

- Wrist arthroscopy is a diagnostic and therapeutic tool to evaluate radiocarpal, intercarpal, and carpal pathology. Wrist arthroscopy has been described using both wet (fluid infiltrate) and dry techniques. Treatment applications include arthroscopic surgical procedures and arthroscopic-assisted open procedures.

ANATOMY

- Standard wrist arthroscopy portals are dorsal due to the relative lack of neurovascular structures (**FIG 1**).
- Portals to assess the radiocarpal joint are named relative to their location between extensor tendons. Volar portals, if used to assess the radiocarpal joint, are placed to avoid the major neurovascular bundles. The midcarpal joint can be assessed either by the dorsal midcarpal portals or by the volar radial midcarpal portal. The volar portals are used in select situations to evaluate the dorsal ligaments and are not standard portals for most situations.
- Standard diagnostic arthroscopy ports are described in Table 1.[1]
- Portals with special indications are listed in Table 2.[1]

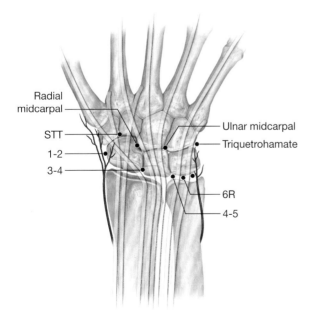

Radial midcarpal

STT

1-2

3-4

Ulnar midcarpal

Triquetrohamate

6R

4-5

FIG 1 • Dorsal wrist arthroscopy portals.

PATIENT HISTORY AND PHYSICAL FINDINGS

- Wrist arthroscopy is a diagnostic adjuvant to patient history and clinical examination.
- Patient evaluation is not complete without a thorough history of onset, aggravating and alleviating factors, history of trauma, occupational and repetitive motion history, and a complete history of interventions including injections, imaging, and surgical procedures.
- Physical examination should include an evaluation of wrist tenderness, tendinous pathology, carpal instability, distal radioulnar joint (DRUJ) pathology, and reproduction of symptoms with wrist loading. Details of a complete wrist physical examination are essential but beyond the scope of this chapter.

IMAGING

- Plain radiographs including posteroanterior, lateral, oblique, and clenched-fist views of the wrist may contribute to the differential diagnosis.
- A wrist arthrogram to test for triangular fibrocartilage complex (TFCC) tear can be unreliable in ulnar-sided wrist pain (sensitivity of 76%).[2]
- Wrist arthroscopy continues to be of value as a diagnostic tool in these cases. Arthroscopy is also useful in patients unable to obtain a 3T MRI or in patients suspicious for injury that could benefit from arthroscopic-assisted surgical intervention.

NONOPERATIVE MANAGEMENT

- Wrist arthroscopy is indicated as a diagnostic technique in patients with persistent wrist pain with no response to an appropriate trial of conservative management, including activity modification, splinting, nonsteroidal anti-inflammatories (NSAIDs), and cortisone injection.
- It may also be used as a diagnostic technique to stage the degree of injury (extent of ligament tear and articular wear) or pathology for further surgical planning.

SURGICAL MANAGEMENT

- Diagnostic indications:
  - Cartilage injuries
  - Chondromalacia
  - TFCC injury staging
  - Ligamentous instability (scapholunate interosseous ligament [SLIL] injury, lunotriquetral interosseous ligament [LTIL] injury)

Table 1 Standard Dorsal Wrist Arthroscopy Portals

Portal Name	Anatomic Landmarks	Purpose
1-2	Radial to EPL tendon at dorsum of snuff box	Inflow. Allows access to the radial styloid, scaphoid, lunate, and articular surface of the distal radius
3-4	Distal to Lister tubercle, between EPL and EDC tendons	Used as the main radiocarpal arthroscopic viewing portal
4-5	Distal to DRUJ. Follow ring finger metacarpal proximally, between EDC and EDM	Used as the main instrumentation portal for the radiocarpal joint; allows visualization of TFCC
6R	Radial (R) to ECU tendon	Instrumentation portal, visualize the TFCC and the ulnar wrist ligaments (ulnolunate, ulnotriquetral, and lunotriquetral)
6U	Ulnar (U) to ECU tendon	Outflow; allows access to dorsal rim of the TFCC or for instrumentation when debriding the volar LTIL
Radial midcarpal	In line with second metacarpal proximal to the capitate; identified by a depression between the capitate and scaphoid	Allows visualization of the scapholunate and lunotriquetral articulations, the STT joint, and the distal pole of the scaphoid
Ulnar midcarpal	In line with the 4th metacarpal, 1 cm distal to the 4-5 portal; identified by a depression at the lunotriquetral-capitate-hamate joint	Allows further visualization of the lunotriquetral articulation, distal lunate, and triquetral hamate articulation; used for instrumentation of the articulations

ECU, extensor carpi ulnaris; EDC, extensor digitorum communis; EDM, extensor digitorum minimi; EPL, extensor pollicis longus; DRUJ, distal radial ulnar joint; STT, scaphotrapeziotrapezoid joint; TFCC, triangular fibrocartilage complex.

- Wrist arthritis evaluation (intactness of lunate facet and midcarpal joint in salvage procedure surgical decision-making)
- Kienbock disease diagnostic staging (using 3-4 portal only to preserve vascular pedicle for a 4-5 extensor compartment artery vascularized bone graft)
- Treatment indications:
  - Ganglion excision
  - TFCC tear debridement or repair of foveal tears
  - Resection of radial styloid (radial styloidectomy in impingement)
- Ulnar styloid excision
- Proximal hamate excision (proximal arthritis in type II lunate)
- Chondroplasty
- Arthroscopic-assisted fracture reduction
  - Distal radius factures (comminuted or depressed articular fragments, evaluation of associated scapholunate ligament injuries)
  - Scaphoid fractures (using 4-5 portal for waist and proximal pole fractures)

Table 2 Special Indication Portals

Portal Name	Anatomic Landmarks	Purpose
Scaphotrapeziotrapezoid radial (STT-R)	In line with the index metacarpal just radial to the EPL at the level of the STT joint	Allows visualization and debridement of STT joint
Scaphotrapeziotrapezoid ulnar (STT-U)	In line with the index metacarpal just ulnar to the EPL at the level of the STT joint	Allows visualization and debridement of STT joint
Triquetrohamate	Ulnar to the ECU tendon at the level of the TH joint	Inflow/outflow. Allows visualization and debridement of the TH joint
Volar radial	Radial to the FCR tendon at the proximal wrist flexion crease, essentially through the floor of the FCR tendon sheath	Visualization of the DRCL and the volar aspect of the SLIL, visualization during DRUJ fracture reduction
Volar ulnar	Interval between flexor tendons and flexor carpi ulnaris and the ulnar neurovascular bundle	Visualization of the dorsal radioulnar ligament and volar aspect of the lunotriquetral ligament. Aids in repair or debridement of dorsal TFCC tears
Volar DRUJ port	Accessed through same skin incision of the volar ulnar portal, but the capsular entry is 5 mm to 1 cm proximal to the ulnocarpal capsular entry point	Volar aspect of DRUJ

ECU, extensor carpi ulnaris; EPL, extensor pollicis longus; DRCL, dorsal radial carpal ligament; DRUJ, distal radial ulnar joint; FCR, flexor carpi radialis; SLIL, scapholunate intercarpal ligament; STT, scaphotrapeziotrapezoid joint; TFCC, triangular fibrocartilage complex; TH, triquetrohamate.

- Septic wrist (complete irrigation through radiocarpal and midcarpal portals)
- Dorsal wrist capsular release
- Volar wrist capsular release (standard dorsal portals such as 3-4 and 6R; protect radioscaphocapitate ligament to prevent ulnar translation of carpus, and volar neurovascular structures and tendons can be at risk during release)
  - Contraindications:
    - Marked wrist swelling
    - Distortion of surface landmarks
    - Large capsular tears
    - Neurovascular compromise
    - Bleeding disorders
    - Infection
    - Specifically for dry wrist arthroscopy: using thermal probes, lasers, any heat-generating instrument

Preoperative Planning

- Equipment (**FIG 2A**)
  - 2.7-mm, 30-degree-angle scope with camera for the standard wrist arthroscopy and evaluation of the carpus
  - 1.9-mm, 30-degree-angle scope with camera for the DRUJ
  - Fiberoptic light source
  - Video monitor, printer for intraoperative photos, or digital system for direct video recording
  - Instrumentation:
    - 3-mm hook probe
    - Motorized shaver for debridement
    - Diathermy unit

- Ancillary equipment:
  - Motorized 2.9-mm bur for bony debridement or resection
  - Suture repair kits including TFCC repair kit or Tuohy needle for facilitating ligament repairs
- Equipment setup (**FIG 2B**)
  - Commercially available wrist arthroscopy traction tower
  - Above-elbow tourniquet
  - Shoulder holder
  - 5- to 10-lb sand bags or weights attached to arm sling for countertraction

Positioning

- The patient is positioned supine on the operating room table with the arm abducted at the shoulder and placed on an arm table.
- An above-elbow tourniquet is placed and the arm rested in a shoulder holder, with 5- to 10-lb weights attached to the arm sling (for countertraction).
- The arm is exsanguinated and the tourniquet insufflated prior to placing the fingers of the examination hand in the traction tower. Total traction force is generally 10 lb (4.5 kg).
- For use of dorsal arthroscopic examination portals, the surgeon sits at the patient's head facing the dorsum of the patient's wrist. For volar portals the surgeon sits over the patient's axilla (**FIG 3**).
- Ensure the arthroscopy camera is white-balanced and that the light source does not rest on the drape or the patient while turned on, as burns can occur.

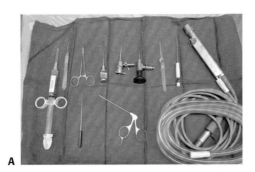

A

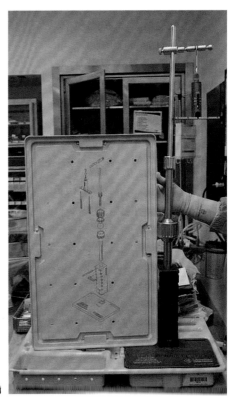

FIG 2 • **A.** Arthroscopy equipment. *Top row from left to right*: 22-gauge needle with 5-cc syringe of normal saline, 15 blade scalpel, mosquito or tenotomy scissors, blunt cannula, scope introducer port, 2.7-mm 30-degree arthroscopy, 18-gauge Jelco needle, small arthroscopy shaver, shaver apparatus. *Bottom row from left to right*: 3-mm probe, straight foreign-body grasper. **B.** Intraoperative ConMed Linvatec TractionTower Extremity Traction Device setup with diagram.

B

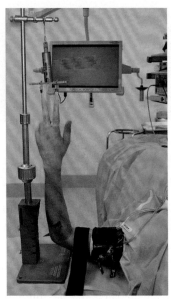

FIG 3 • Patient positioning for left wrist arthroscopy. Above elbow sterile tourniquet, countertraction above-elbow straps, traction device with 10 lb of traction. Surgeon sits at patient head for dorsal approach.

Approach

Classic "Wet" Wrist Arthroscopy

- A structured approach to wrist arthroscopy is important for efficiency and good visualization.
- Portals are established by palpating surface anatomic landmarks, prior to inserting a 22-gauge needle into the joint space. If inserting into the 3-4 portal first, the needle should be inserted 10 degrees palmar to account for the volar inclination of the radius.
- The joint is then injected with 5 cc of saline and subsequent aspiration to confirm position within the wrist joint.
- Vertical or transverse (within natural wrist creases) shallow incisions are made to avoid injury to dorsal sensory nerve branches, and a blunt mosquito or spreading tenotomy dissection is used to dissect the soft tissue down to the wrist capsule.

- The wrist capsule is then pierced (by holding the instrument like a dart) and a blunt trocar fitted with an inflow valve is inserted to introduce the scope cannula into the wrist.
- An 18-gauge angiocatheter can be placed in the 6U portal for sufficient outflow if wet technique performed.
- Structures that should be visualized in any standard arthroscopy include radius articular surface; the proximal scaphoid, lunate, and triquetrum; the SLIL both from radiocarpal and midcarpal; the LTIL both from radiocarpal and midcarpal; the radioscaphocapitate ligament; the ulnolunate (UL) ligament; the ulnotriquetral (UT) ligament; the articular disc of the TFCC; and the radial and peripheral TFCC attachments.
- Diagnostic wrist arthroscopy usually begins with the dorsal 3-4 portal to evaluate the volar ligaments. However, establishing dorsal portals first but beginning the examination using the volar radial portal to visualize the palmar SLIL and dorsal radiocarpal ligament (DRCL) can minimize iatrogenic trauma to the dorsal capsular structures and errors in diagnosis.
- A standard dorsal diagnostic arthroscopic examination uses primarily the 3-4 portal and combinations of the 4-5 portal and 6R to fully visualize the structures. From the 3-4 portal, visualization of the entire radiocarpal joint should be possible, using the 4-5 or 6R portals for probe insertion. 6U is primarily used for fluid outflow or for instrumentation for the palmar LTIL treatment.

Dry Wrist Arthroscopy

- Dry wrist arthroscopy is less commonly performed but has some theoretical advantages. However, with regard to safety with shaving or thermal procedures, we recommend the wet technique.
- Advantages:
  - Avoids fluid extravasation
  - Avoids risk of fluid-associated compartment syndrome
  - Less soft tissue swelling, capsular distention, possibly resulting in less postoperative pain
  - Larger portals and larger instruments
  - Larger portals facilitate more surgical procedures using arthroscopic technique (eg, partial wrist fusion).[3]

■ Diagnostic Arthroscopy

- Begin with the 3-4 portal distal to Lister tubercle between extensor pollicis longus (EPL) and extensor digitorum communis (EDC) tendons.
- After placement of a 22-gauge needle with a 10-degree volar tilt trajectory, inject and aspirate 5 cc of saline to confirm placement within the radiocarpal joint.
- Make a short superficial incision followed by blunt dissection using tenotomy scissors to the wrist capsule and bluntly puncture the dorsal wrist capsule. Gently insert the blunt trocar for the arthroscope (2.7-mm 30-degree angle).

- An 18-gauge angiocatheter can be inserted at the 6U portal for fluid drainage
- The 3-4 portal is a "workhorse" portal of wrist arthroscopy allowing a nearly panoramic examination of the radiocarpal joint.
- Throughout the arthroscopy, evaluation should include articular surfaces, synovitis, loose body identification and removal, and the integrity of wrist ligaments.

TECHNIQUES

■ Radial Structures

- Begin radially to examine the articular surfaces of the distal radius, proximal scaphoid, and proximal lunate. The dorsal aspect of the scaphoid is also visualized. Some features of the DRC joint capsule are also seen radially.
- The radioscaphocapitate (RSC) ligament is seen originating from the tip of the radial styloid and passing distally anterior to the proximal pole of the scaphoid.
- Identify the interligamentous sulcus separating the RSC and the long radiolunate (LRL) ligaments as a landmark for orientation (**TECH FIG 1**). The LRL arises from the palmar rim of the distal radius and passes anterior to the proximal pole of the scaphoid.
- The short radiolunate ligament (SRL) is just ulnar to the LRL, seen as an amorphous structure with surface blood vessels. The ligament passes vertically and integrates with the SL ligament in the proximal anterior third.
- The scapholunate ligament can then be seen covering the remaining proximal and distal aspects of the scapholunate joint and is fibrocartilaginous in this section. The ligament is frequently the same color and brightness as the articular surfaces and may be a concave or a convex bulge across the scapholunate joint. The SL ligament should be followed, by lowering the arthroscope parallel to the long axis of the forearm and turning the scope camera, as it courses dorsally to the reflected dorsal radiocarpal (DRC) ligament of the joint capsule. Note any signs of hemorrhage, synovitis, and attenuation (**TECH FIG 2**).
- Just ulnar to the SL ligament, the SRL ligament originates from the volar rim of the radius at the lunate fossa and forms the volar joint capsule, inserting on the proximal lunate. Ulnar and continuous with the SRL is the UL ligament. There may be a perceptible fold between the two ligaments.
- The DRC joint capsule may be visualized dorsally, generally after examination of the LT and TFCC. The DRC is normally generously lined with synovium in this region.
- Table 3 covers the 3-4 portal field of view.

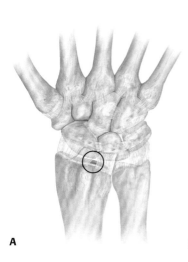 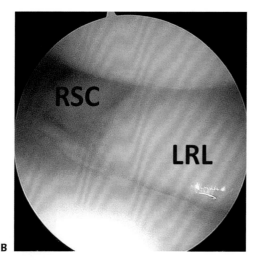

TECH FIG 1 • **A.** Diagram of a right wrist from dorsal approach, with 3-4 portal view marked. Note the radioscaphocapitate (*RSC*) ligament radially and the long radiolunate ligament (*LRL*) in the field of view. **B.** Radioscaphocapitate and long radiolunate ligaments as viewed intraoperatively from the 3-4 portal, scaphoid above.

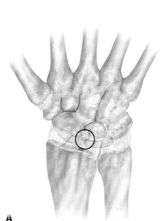 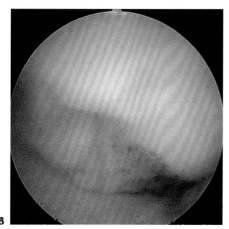 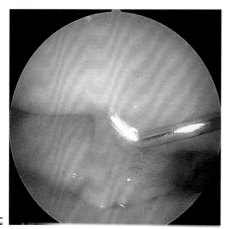

TECH FIG 2 • **A.** Diagram of right wrist, dorsal arthroscopy, indicating arthroscopic view of the scapholunate (SL) ligament from radiocarpal joint using the 3-4 portal. **B.** Intraoperative view of synovitis of the SL ligament from the radiocarpal joint. **C.** SL ligament probed by 3-mm probe from radiocarpal joint.

Table 3 3-4 Portal Field of View

Surface Anatomic Landmark: Distal to Lister tubercle, between EPL and EDC

Portal Field of View

Portal Name	Radial	Central	Volar	Dorsal/Distal	Ulnar
3-4 Portal	Scaphoid and lunate fossa, volar rim of radius	Proximal scaphoid and lunate, dorsal and membranous SLIL	RSC, RSL, LRL, ULL	Oblique views of DRCL insertion onto dorsal SLIL	TFCC radial insertion, central disk, ulnar attachment, PRUL, DRUL, PTO, PSR

Ulnar Structures

- A 4-5 portal can also be used to visualize the UL ligament and UT ligaments; however, in most patients, adequate examination can be accomplished by 3-4 portal plus a midcarpal arthroscopy.
- From the radiocarpal joint, immediately ulnar to the UL ligament is the UT ligament inserting on the volar edge of the triquetrum. The prestyloid recess can then be visualized at the junction between the UT and the palmar radioulnar (PRU) ligaments.

- Using the 4-5 portal, the pisotriquetral orifice can be visualized just anterior to the proximal articular surface of the triquetrum. Reposition the arthroscope to visualize the articular surface of the pisiform and the flexor carpi ulnaris (FCU) tendon passing through the orifice.
- Moving dorsally, the proximal region of the lunotriquetral ligament (LT) is localized by identifying the sulcus or concavity in the otherwise convex articular surfaces of the lunate and triquetrum (**TECH FIG 3**). Note any signs of hemorrhage, synovitis, or attenuation.
- Table 4 covers the 4-5 portal field of view.

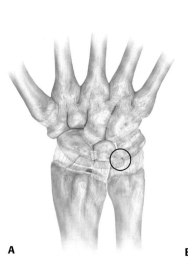

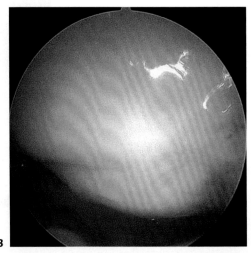

TECH FIG 3 • A. Diagram of right wrist, dorsal arthroscopy, indicating arthroscopic view of the lunotriquetral (LT) ligament from the radiocarpal joint using the 3-4 portal. **B.** Intraoperative view of the LT ligament from the radiocarpal joint.

Table 4 4-5 Portal Field of View

Surface Anatomic Landmark: Between EDC and EDM in Line with Ring Metacarpal, Slightly Proximal to the 3-4 Portal

Portal Field of View

Portal Name	Radial	Central	Volar	Dorsal/Distal	Ulnar
4-5 Portal	Lunate fossa, volar rim of radius	Proximal lunate, triquetrum, dorsal and membranous LTIL	RSL, LRL, ULL	Poorly seen	TFCC radial insertion, central disk, ulnar attachment, PRUL, DRUL, PTO, PSR

TFCC Evaluation

- From the 4-5 portal, the articular disc of the TFCC can be seen proximal, interposed between the dorsal radioulnar (DRU) and palmar radioulnar (PRU) ligaments. The articular disc is fibrocartilage and may be the same color and brightness at the articular surface of the lunate fossa (**TECH FIG 4A,B**).
- A 3-mm probe inserted from the 6R portal can be used to palpate the transition from the articular surface of the distal radius to the articular disc. The probe can be used to estimate the resting tension of the disc by pushing and releasing the probe pressure on the disc. Hypermobility of the articular disc is described as a trampoline sign (**TECH FIG 4C**).
- The dorsal radioulnar (DRU) and palmar radioulnar (PRU) ligaments should be identified as they converge toward their ulnar attachments.

- In patients with ulnar-sided wrist pain, it may be useful to use the volar ulnar portal to assess the palmar LTIL and dorsal radioulnar ligament and the region of the extensor carpi ulnaris subsheath. This portal also allows for assessment of the radial TFCC attachment.
- TFCC tears can be arthroscopically classified according to Palmer's classification to guide conservative, arthroscopic, or open treatment (**TECH FIG 5**).[4]
- TFCC repair can be accomplished using instrumentation introduced through the 6U portal, although some authors advise open repair, particularly at the ulnar styloid, to avoid injury to the dorsal cutaneous branch of the ulnar nerve at the 6U portal.
- Table 5 covers 6R portal fields of view.

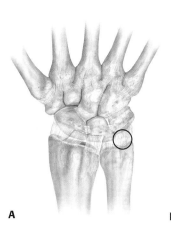 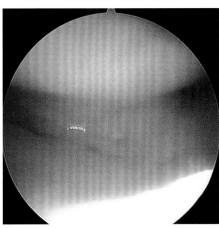 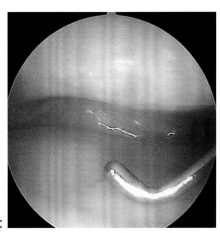

TECH FIG 4 • A. Diagram of right wrist, dorsal arthroscopy, indicating arthroscopic view of the triangular fibrocartilage complex (TFCC) using the 3-4 portal. **B.** Intraoperative view of the TFCC articular disc (*bottom*), fovea (*far center*), and lunate proximal articular surface above. **C.** Intraoperative arthroscopic view of a 3-mm probe, inserted through the 4-5 portal, testing an intact TFCC articular disc.

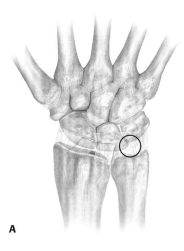 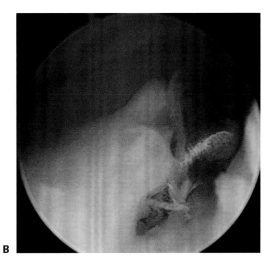

TECH FIG 5 • A. Radiograph demonstrating orientation of arthroscopic view. **B.** Intraoperative arthroscopic view of a 3-mm probe crossing a large peripheral Palmer class 1B TFCC tear.

TECHNIQUES

Table 5 6R Portal Field of View

Surface Anatomic Landmark: Radial Side of ECU Tendon

Portal Field of View

Portal Name	Radial	Central	Volar	Dorsal/Distal	Ulnar
6R Portal	Poorly seen	Proximal lunate, triquetrum, dorsal and membranous LTIL	ULL, ULT	Poorly seen	TFCC radial insertion, central disk, ulnar attachment, PRUL, DRUL, PTO, PSR

Midcarpal Arthroscopy

STT Joint

- Midcarpal examination can be performed from either the radial or ulnar midcarpal port or occasionally the scaphotrapeziotrapezoid joint (STT) port.
- When using the radial midcarpal portal, orientation can be quickly established by recognizing the concave surfaces of the proximal row articular surfaces and the dramatically convex articular surface of the head of the capitate and pole of the hamate (**TECH FIG 6**).
- Identify the cleft at the proximal extent of the capitohamate joint.
- Reorient the scope to direct it distally into the dorsal aspect of the midcarpal joint over the STT joint. This is accomplished by dropping the scope into a line tangential to the plane of the forearm.
- Rotation of the arthroscope in this region will visualize the STT joint and the curvature of the distal articular surface of the scaphoid. A cleft can be visualized between the trapezium and trapezoid and the radial aspect of the STT ligament along the lateral aspect of the STT joint.
- Moving the arthroscope proximally from the STT joint, the scaphocapitate (SC) articulation comes into view. The SC joint is a "tight" joint, and transverse fibers of the SC ligament are sometimes seen but not always due to difficulty positioning the arthroscope.

SL Joint

- As the arthroscope is continually drawn more proximally, the distal cleft of the SL joint is visualized. The SL joint should be visualized from at least two portals to change the orientation of view and prevent a false sense of a step-off.
- When visualizing the SL joint, take care to ensure that the arthroscope is not exerting pressure on either the scaphoid or lunate, forcing them out of alignment.
- The SL joint should be evaluated visually and by using a 3-mm probe according to the Geissler grading scale (**TECH FIG 7**).[5]
- Under normal conditions, it is difficult to pass an arthroscopic probe into the SL or LT joint and rotate it. When there is a SL ligament disruption, the scope can enter into the joint space; this is referred to as the "drive-through sign" (**TECH FIG 8**).
- From the midcarpal portals, the volar midcarpal joint capsule, with its generous synovial stratum, can be assessed, as well as the "space of Poirier" by palpating the volar capsule with the probe to detect a groove between the arcuate ligament (RSC and UC) and the lunate.

Ulnar Structures

- A complete assessment of the midcarpal joint includes the ulnar structures. Moving the scope ulnarly, the distal articular surface of the lunate can be inspected as well as the LT joint cleft (**TECH FIG 9**).

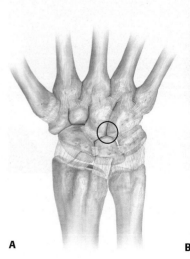 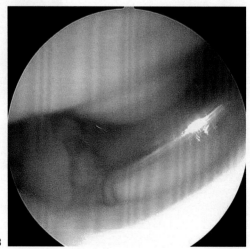

A **B**

TECH FIG 6 • A. Diagram of the right wrist, dorsal arthroscopy of the midcarpal joint from the radial midcarpal portal. **B.** Visualization of the capitohamate joint allows for orientation in the midcarpal joint.

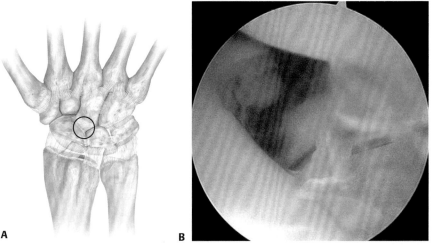

TECH FIG 7 • **A.** Diagram of right wrist, dorsal arthroscopy of the midcarpal joint, indicating arthroscopic field of view of the SL joint from the radial midcarpal portal. **B.** Hemorrhagic synovitis at the scaphocapitate joint.

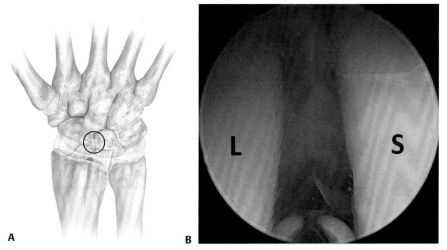

TECH FIG 8 • **A.** Diagram of the right wrist. **B.** "Drive-through sign" of the SL interval indicating a Geisler-type IV injury.

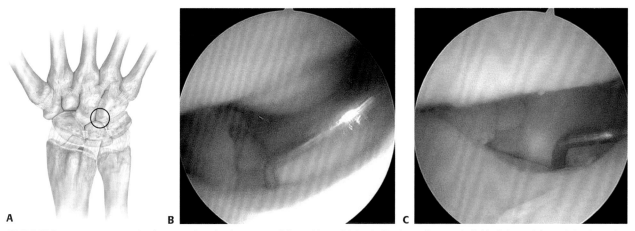

TECH FIG 9 • **A.** Diagram of right wrist, dorsal arthroscopy of the midcarpal joint, indicating arthroscopic field of view of the LT joint from the radial midcarpal portal. **B.** Intraoperative arthroscopic view of the capitate and hamate above, and (**C**) a 3-mm probe inserted through the ulnar midcarpal portal testing an intact LT joint.

Table 6 Radial Midcarpal Portal Field of View

Surface Anatomic Landmark: Radial Side of the Third Metacarpal Axis Proximal to the Capitate in a Soft Depression Between the Capitate and Scaphoid

Portal Field of View

Portal Name	Radial	Central	Volar	Dorsal/Distal	Ulnar
Midcarpal radial portal	STT joint, distal scaphoid pole	SLIL joint, distal scaphoid, distal lunate	Radial limb of arcuate ligament, ie, continuation of RSC ligament	Proximal capitate, CHIL, oblique views of proximal hamate	LTIL joint, partial triquetrum

- The LT can be palpated with a 3-mm probe and can also be graded using the Geissler grading scale.[5]
- Further ulnar movement can assess the palmar ligaments (ulnocapitate, triquetrocapitate, and triquetrohamate) after gently scraping the volar capsule synovial stratum.
- By dorsally rotating the scope at this position, the articular surfaces of the distal triquetrum (spiral shaped) and the proximal hamate (elliptical shape) can be inspected.

- Further ulnar movement of the scope will visualize a large joint recess and the "bare area" on the capitate neck and head and the pole of the hamate; however, due to excess synovial tissue, this view is often obscured.
- Tables 6 and 7 cover the radial and ulnar midcarpal portal fields of view, respectively.

Table 7 Ulnar Midcarpal Portal Field of View

Surface Anatomic Landmark: 1 cm Distal to the 4-5 Portal, Aligned with the Fourth Metacarpal, at the Lunotriquetral-Capitate-Hamate Joint

Portal Field of View

Portal Name	Radial	Central	Volar	Dorsal/Distal	Ulnar
Midcarpal ulnar portal	Distal articular surface of scaphoid	Distal lunate	Volar limb of arcuate ligament, ie, continuation of triquetrocapitolunate	Oblique views of proximal capitate, CHIL, proximal hamate	LTIL joint, triquetrum

PEARLS AND PITFALLS

Incisions	▪ Superficial longitudinal (or transverse) dermal incision followed by blunt dissection with a mosquito (or tenotomy dissection) to protect the extensor tendons and dorsal sensory nerve branches
Portal placement	▪ Reposition the trocar if not inserting easily, to avoid chondral injury. Always use the blunt trocar to enter into the joint.
Arthroscopy fluid	▪ Normal saline is injected to confirm placement of portals in the wrist, and arthroscopic examination can be performed either with or without fluid. However, use of heat-producing equipment should only be performed with arthroscopic fluid to avoid thermal injuries. We recommend the wet technique.
Inadequate views	▪ Synovitis, fractures, ligament tears, and tight wrist capsule may limit the field of view during wrist arthroscopy requiring use of more portals to adequately assess the wrist.
Traction	▪ Wrist traction often diminishes throughout the examination and should be readjusted to avoid inadvertent chondral injury from instruments.
Standardization	▪ A standard approach to wrist arthroscopy optimizes efficiency and ensures a thorough and complete examination of the wrist.
Dry Arthroscopy	
Preventing capsule collapse	▪ The valve of the sheath of the scope should be open at all times for air to circulate within the joint; otherwise, the capsule will collapse inward when using suction, obstructing the view.
Limited use of suction	▪ Open the suction only when needing to aspirate something, or debris may be stirred up that may stick to the tip of the scope.

PEARLS AND **PITFALLS** *(Continued)*

Avoiding splashes	▪ Avoid using the burs or osteotomes too close to the tip of the scope as minor splashes may block your vision. Minor splashes can be removed by gently rubbing the tip of the scope on the local soft tissue.
Clearing field with saline	▪ When a clear field is needed, a syringe with 5–10 mL of saline may be connected to the side valve of the scope and then aspirated with an arthroscopic shaver to get rid of blood and debris. The negative pressure exerted by the shaver will suck the saline into the joint without any pressure on the plunger and prevent extravasation.
Preventing suction clog	▪ Periodic saline aspiration from an external basin or by joint irrigation, and systematic joint flushing in some procedures (intercarpal arthrodesis, arthroscopic proximal carpectomy) during prolonged use of burs, which may cause heating of instrument and local burns

POSTOPERATIVE CARE

- Splinting:
  - Diagnostic: 4 to 7 days for comfort.
  - Arthroscopic reduction and scapholunate pinning: sugar-tong splint for 2 weeks, followed by short-arm cast for 8 weeks. Pins are removed at 10 weeks. Removable splint for 2 to 4 more weeks.
  - Open ligament repair with scapholunate pinning: sugar-tong splint for 2 weeks, followed by short-arm cast for 10 weeks. Pins are removed at 10 weeks. Removable splint for 2 to 4 more weeks.
  - TFCC debridement: volar resting splint for 2 weeks, and then begin range of motion exercises.
  - TFCC arthroscopic repair: sugar-tong splint for 2 weeks, followed by above-arm Munster cast for 4 weeks, followed by Munster splint until 45 degrees of nontender pronation and supination was achieved, and then volar resting wrist splint until full rotation achieved.
- Activity modification:
  - After splinting, gentle active range of motion of the wrist is encouraged. Gentle activities of daily living are resumed, but lifting is limited to less than 10 lb based on any repairs that have been performed.
  - Wrist capsule stiffness is a frequent complaint in post-arthroscopy patients, and patient education is critical regarding active range of motion and duration of expected stiffness.
  - Gradual strengthening should be encouraged, and involvement of certified hand therapists can optimize recovery.

OUTCOMES

- TFCC tear diagnosis.
  - A recent retrospective review of 908 patients with arthroscopic-confirmed TFCC tears illustrated only a 0.53 to 0.55 positive predictive value of clinical tests and a positive predictive value of MRI of 0.41 to 0.44 in diagnosing a TFCC tear. Arthroscopy is the standard for diagnosing and staging TFCC tears.[6]
- Scapholunate ligament treatment
  - In partial SL ligament tears, 85% treated by arthroscopic debridement have reported satisfactory improvement in symptoms. Only 67% with complete tear reported satisfactory outcomes with debridement alone.[7]
  - Arthroscopic reduction and K-wire pinning of SL instability is most beneficial in patients with instability for less than 3 months and a gap of 3 mm or less in the SL interval (83% symptomatic relief compared to 53% symptomatic relief if instability was present for longer, or a greater than 3-mm SL interval gap were present).[8]
- Lunotriquetral ligament treatment.
  - In a small series of LT ligament tears treated with arthroscopic debridement alone, 100% (six patients) with partial injury reported resolution of symptoms after debridement, and 78% (nine patients) with complete tear reported symptom resolution.[7]
- Wrist ganglion treatment
  - A systematic review of arthroscopically treatment volar wrist ganglions reported a recurrent rate of 0% to 20% (mean 6%) and a 7% complication rate. A higher complication rate was reported for arthroscopic treated of volar wrist ganglia in the midcarpal joint as the procedure is technically more difficult.[9]
- Fracture-reduction assistance
  - In case series of acute and nonunion scaphoid fractures, arthroscopy has been shown to aid in the assessment of fracture reduction.[10] In acute scaphoid fractures, one series illustrated median time to union of 62 days and average return to work 21 days after surgery.[10]
  - A randomized-control trial of arthroscopically vs fluoroscopically assisted reduction of intra-articular distal radius fractures treated with volar locking plate illustrated no statistical difference in radiographic or functional outcomes, including range of motion (ROM) and disabilities of the arm, shoulder, and hand (DASH) scores, between the two groups.[11]

COMPLICATIONS

- Most complications are related to injury of the dorsal cutaneous sensory nerve branches, particularly:
  - Superficial radial nerve in the 1-2 portal
  - Dorsal cutaneous branch of the ulnar nerve from the 6U portal
  - Palmar cutaneous branch of ulnar nerve from volar ulnar portal
  - Ulnar neurovascular bundle injury from over-retraction or poor portal placement
- Chondral injury from trochar insertion
- Venous bleeding
- Loss of wrist motion (particularly forearm supination)
- Fluid extravasation
- Infection
- Minor contact burns at the portals and dorsal skin by the full-radius resector and bur may occur in dry arthroscopy
- Meticulous technique is essential to reduce the above complications.

REFERENCES

1. Wolff JM, Dukas A, Pensak M. Advances in wrist arthroscopy. *J Am Acad Orthop Surg.* 2012;20:725-734.
2. Smith TO, Drew BT, Toma AP, Chojnoswki AJ. The diagnostic accuracy of X-ray arthrography for triangular fibrocartilaginous complex injury: a systematic review and meta-analysis. *J Hand Surg Eur.* 2012;37:879-887.
3. Jones CM, Grasu BL, Murphy MS. Dry wrist arthroscopy. *J Hand Surg [Am].* 2015;40:388-390.
4. Palmer AK. Triangular fibrocartilage complex lesions: a classification. *J Hand Surg Am.* 1989;14:594-606.
5. Geissler WB, Freeland AE, Savoie FH, et al. Intracarpal soft-tissue lesions associated with an intra-articular fracture of the distal end of the radius. *J Bone Joint Surg.* 1996;78:357-365.
6. Schmauss D, Pohlmann S, Lohmeyer JA, et al. Clinical tests and magnetic resonance imaging have limited diagnostic value for triangular fibrocartilaginous complex lesions. *Arch Orthop Trauma Surg.* 2016;136(6):873-880.
7. Weiss AP, Sachar K, Lowacki KA. Arthroscopic management of partial scapholunate and lunotriquetral injuries of the wrist. *J Hand Surg [Am].* 1997;22:344-349.
8. Whipple TL. The role of arthroscopy in the treatment of scapholunate instability. *Hand Clin.* 1995;11:37-40.
9. Fernandes CH, Miranda CD, dos Santos JB, Faloppa F. A systematic review of complications and recurrence rate of arthroscopic resection of volar wrist ganglion. *Hand Surg.* 2014;19:475-480.
10. Slutsky DJ, Trevare J. Use of arthroscopy for the treatment of scaphoid fractures. *Hand Clin.* 2014;30:91-103.
11. Yamazaki H, Uchiyama S, Komatsu M, et al. Arthroscopic assistance does not improve the functional or radiographic outcome of unstable intra-articular distal radial fractures treated with a volar locking plate. *Bone Joint J.* 2015;97B:957-962.

Ligament Reconstruction for Chronic Scapholunate Dissociation

Mark Morris and Kevin C. Chung

DEFINITION

- Scapholunate instability is the most common form of carpal instability.
- Injury to the scapholunate interosseous ligament (SLIL) and subsequent dorsal intercalated segmental instability (DISI) results in scapholunate advanced collapse (SLAC) if untreated.[1]
- Chronic tears generally require reconstruction rather than primary repair.
- Static vs dynamic instability[2]
  - Static instability: Any or all of the radiographic changes discussed below in the imaging section, seen on plain radiographs
  - Dynamic instability: Normal plain radiographs, but with stress radiographs, any or all radiographic changes are seen.
- Fixed vs reducible deformity
  - Fixed deformity: Static radiographic changes are not passively correctible.
  - Reducible deformity: Static radiographic changes are passively correctible.

ANATOMY

- The lunate, or the intercalated segment, is connected to the scaphoid via the scapholunate ligament and to the triquetrum via the lunotriquetral ligament.
- The scaphoid is inclined to flex, whereas the triquetrum is inclined to extend. Disruption in either ligamentous complex results in intercalated instability.
- The scapholunate ligament is a C-shaped structure that connects the dorsal, proximal, and volar surfaces of the scaphoid and lunate.[3] It has three portions (FIG 1):
  - Dorsal portion
    - 2 to 3 mm thick
    - Greatest rupture strength and is responsible for rotational and translational restraint
  - Proximal membranous portion
  - Volar portion
    - 1 mm thick

PATHOGENESIS

- SLIL disruption occurs when the wrist is forced into extension, supination, and ulnar deviation.[4]
- SLIL injuries range from sprains, partial tears, or complete tears
- The SLIL usually fails at the scaphoid bone-ligament interface.

NATURAL HISTORY

- With complete rupture of the SLIL, the scaphoid flexes and the lunate is now free to be pulled into extension either by the triquetrum[5] or because of its own natural tendency due to its shape.[6] This produces the DISI pattern.
- Left untreated, the DISI deformity results in abnormal radiocarpal contact.
- Flexion and hypermobility of the scaphoid leads to a predictable pattern of degenerative changes, resulting in SLAC wrist.
- SLAC was initially described in three stages but has been more recently described in five stages of degenerative changes:
  - Stage I: radioscaphoid
  - Stage II: scaphocapitate
  - Stage III: lunocapitate
  - Stage IV: triquetrohamate
  - Stage V: radiolunate

PATIENT HISTORY AND PHYSICAL FINDINGS

- Patients complain of radial-sided wrist pain exacerbated by loading activities, weak grip, swelling, and loss of wrist range of motion.
- Tenderness to palpation in the anatomic snuffbox or over the scapholunate interval, just distal to Lister tubercle
- Pain with extremes of wrist extension and radial deviation
- Diminished grip strength on examination
- Watson scaphoid shift test may be positive in scapholunate dissociation (FIG 2).[7]
  - The examiner places his or her thumb over the scaphoid tuberosity and the fingers over the dorsal radius. The other hand is used to move the wrist passively from ulnar to radial deviation. The scaphoid is extended with the wrist in ulnar deviation and flexed with the wrist in radial deviation. The examiner applies pressure on the scaphoid tuberosity while moving the wrist from ulnar to radial deviation. This prevents the scaphoid from flexing. If the SLIL is completely torn, the proximal pole subluxes dorsally out of the scaphoid fossa, inducing pain on the dorsoradial aspect of the wrist. When pressure is released, a clunk may occur. This indicates self-reduction of the scaphoid back into its normal position.
- Scapholunate ballottement test may also be positive.
  - The examiner holds the patient's scaphoid between the thumb and index finger. The thumb is placed over the tuberosity, and the index finger is placed over the proximal pole. The thumb and index fingers of other hand are used to hold the lunate. The examiner attempts to move the scaphoid and lunate in opposite directions.
  - This test is positive when it elicits pain.

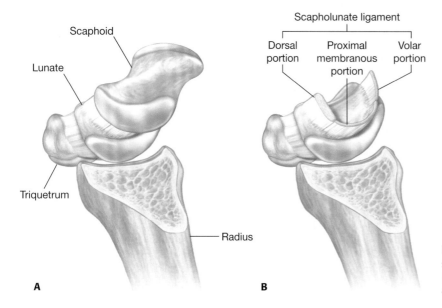

FIG 1 • The scapholunate ligament is a C-shaped structure that consists of a stronger dorsal portion (2–3 mm thick), a proximal membranous portion, and a volar ligamentous portion (1 mm thick).

IMAGING

- Radiographs may demonstrate the following findings suggestive of SLIL injury:
  - Terry Thomas sign: Scapholunate diastasis of more than 3 mm on standard PA radiographs (**FIG 3A**)[8]
  - Signet ring sign: The presence of a flexed scaphoid on standard PA radiographs produces a cortical hyperdensity that resembles a signet ring (see **FIG 3A**).[5]
  - Angular changes in the carpal bones
    - The normal scapholunate angle ranges from 30 to 60 degrees. An angle over 60 degrees is seen with SLIL injury (**FIG 3B**).
    - The normal capitolunate angle ranges from –15 to 15 degrees. An angle greater than 15 degrees is seen with SLIL injury.
    - The normal radiolunate angle ranges from –10 to 10 degrees. An angle greater than 10 degrees is seen with SLIL injury.
  - Quadrangular lunate: The lunate appears rectangular on standard PA radiographs as it moves into extension.
  - Disruption of Gilula lines as the relationship of the proximal carpal row is lost.
  - The presence of degenerative changes involving the radiocarpal or midcarpal joints is a contraindication for ligament reconstruction.

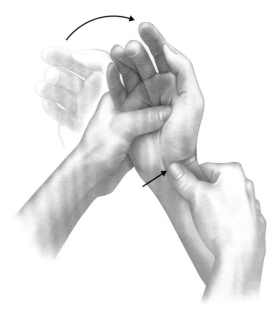

FIG 2 • Watson scaphoid shift test. The examiner uses his or her thumb to apply pressure over the scaphoid tuberosity while using the other hand to move the wrist from ulnar to radial deviation.

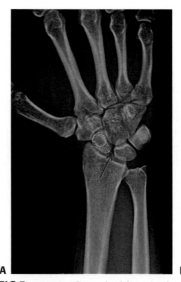
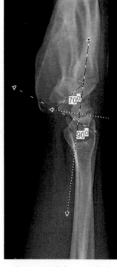

FIG 3 • **A.** PA radiograph of the wrist showing diastasis of the scapholunate interval (*arrow*). A signet ring sign can also be seen here (*circled*), which is produced when the scaphoid is flexed so the tubercle is superimposed on the waist of the scaphoid. **B.** The scapholunate angle is formed by the intersection of the scaphoid axis (a line drawn between the most palmar point of the distal pole and the most palmar point of the proximal pole) and the lunate axis (a line drawn perpendicular to a line drawn between the most distal palmar and dorsal points of the lunate). A scapholunate angle greater than 70 degrees indicates a DISI deformity.

- MRI can be performed to identify tears when radiographs are normal.
  - The sensitivity of a 3-T MRI ranges from 65% to 89% for complete scapholunate ligament tears. The sensitivity of MRA is reported to be 85% to 100%.
  - The sensitivity of both MRI and MRA is poor for partial ligament tears.[8]

DIFFERENTIAL DIAGNOSIS

- Partial SLIL tear
- Radiocarpal arthritis
- Scaphoid fracture
- Keinbock disease

NONOPERATIVE MANAGEMENT

- Nonoperative management of complete SLIL tear is unsuccessful and reliably results in radiocarpal and midcarpal degenerative changes.

SURGICAL MANAGEMENT

- Direct repair is rarely an option for a chronic SLIL tear.
- Capsulodesis is an option for dynamic scapholunate dissociation if secondary stabilizers are intact and there is no cartilage degeneration. Capsulodesis is not indicated in the case of static scapholunate dissociation.
- Ligament reconstruction

Preoperative Planning

- The surgeon can consider diagnostic wrist arthroscopy prior to ligament reconstruction. This will help to better characterize the articular surfaces of the carpal bones, as well as to better delineate the degree of ligament injury.

Positioning

- The patient is positioned supine on the operating table. The operative extremity is draped out on a hand table.
- We prefer to use regional anesthesia for this operation. General anesthesia can also be used.
- A tourniquet is applied.
- An examination under anesthesia is performed. A Watson shift test is done to feel for a clunk.

Approach

- Volar and dorsal incisions are made.
- The volar incisions are used to harvest the flexor carpi radialis (FCR) graft.
- The dorsal incision is used for most of the reconstruction.

■ Exposure

- Dorsal
  - An 8-cm longitudinal dorsal wrist incision is centered over Lister tubercle (**TECH FIG 1A**).
  - The extensor retinaculum over the third compartment is opened, and the extensor pollicis longus (EPL) is retracted radially.
  - The dorsal wrist capsule is opened through a longitudinal incision to expose the scapholunate interval (**TECH FIG 1B**).

- Volar
  - Three 1-cm incisions are made along the course of the flexor carpi radialis (FCR; **TECH FIG 1C**).
  - An oblique Wagner incision is made over the scaphoid tuberosity.
  - The radial sensory nerve is at risk with this incision and must be preserved.
- The scar tissue is excised between the scaphoid and lunate.

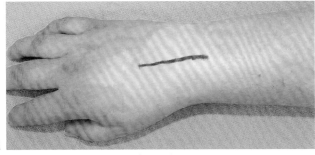

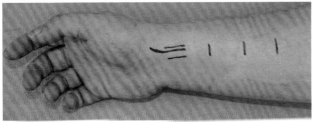

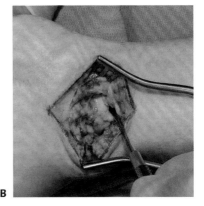

TECH FIG 1 • **A.** Dorsal wrist incision. **B.** The scapholunate interval is exposed. The Freer elevator in this image is in the scapholunate interval. **C.** Volar wrist incisions.

■ Reduction of Scaphoid and Lunate and Creation of a Bone Tunnel

- Two 0.062-inch K-wires are placed dorsally into the scaphoid and lunate. The K-wires are used as joysticks to aid in reduction (**TECH FIG 2**).
  - Threaded wires may provide better purchase of the scaphoid and lunate so joystick wires do not pull out.
- Wires must be drilled away from the anticipated tunnel for the planned ligament reconstruction.
- To correct the DISI deformity, the surgeon must extend the scaphoid and flex the lunate. Direct the scaphoid wire proximally and the lunate wire distally.
- To create a bone tunnel, a K-wire is passed from the scaphoid tuberosity to the dorsum of the scaphoid along its axis.
- A cannulated 2.7-mm drill is passed over the wire from the dorsum to the palmar side.

Harvesting and Passing a Strip of Distally Based FCR Tendon

- A distally based 3-mm-wide by 8- to 10-cm-long strip of FCR tendon is harvested from the radial aspect of the tendon (**TECH FIG 3**).

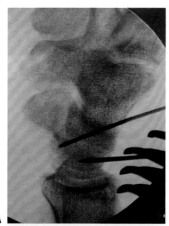

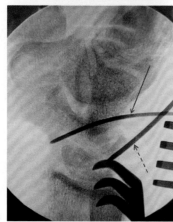

TECH FIG 2 • **A.** K-wires are used for reduction of the scaphoid and lunate. **B.** The scaphoid wire is directed proximally to extend the scaphoid (*solid arrow*), whereas the lunate wire is directed distally to flex the lunate (*dashed arrow*).

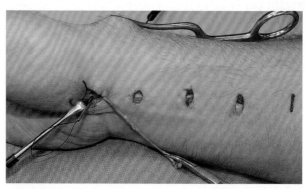

TECH FIG 3 • The distally based FCR tendon graft is harvested and passed though the scaphoid tunnel.

- The FCR tendon rotates 90 degrees within the sheath at the wrist. It is important to follow the fibers so the tendon is not inadvertently transected. Do not slide the scissors through the tendon fibers; cut along the fibers to maintain the integrity of the tendon.
- A grasping suture is placed at the cut end of the distally based FCR tendon and is then passed through the scaphoid tunnel from volar to dorsal.
- Forcing a wide strip of FCR through the scaphoid tunnel can fracture the scaphoid. It is better to harvest a narrow strip of FCR tendon.

Reduction of the Scapholunate Interval

- The scapholunate interval is reduced using the joystick K-wires. The K-wires can only correct the flexion-extension deformities of the scaphoid and lunate. A bone reduction clamp or towel clip is used to reduce the gap between the two bones.
- Reduction is maintained by passing new K-wires across the scapholunate and scaphocapitate joints.
- Confirm reduction of the scapholunate interval with fluoroscopy. Once this is done, the joystick K-wires can be removed.

Securing the FCR to the Lunate and Closure

- A bur is used to make a shallow trough on the dorsum of the lunate.
- The FCR tendon graft is secured to the midportion of the trough using a 1.8-mm bone anchor suture (**TECH FIG 4A**).
- The remaining portion of the tendon graft is passed through a slit in the distal portion of the dorsal radiotriquetral ligament and is sutured back to itself over the lunate (**TECH FIG 4B**).
- The dorsal capsule is first repaired using 3-0 Ethibond suture.
- The tourniquet is released and hemostasis is obtained.
- The EPL is transposed dorsal to the extensor retinaculum to avoid ischemic rupture that may occur due to postoperative swelling in the EPL sheath. The extensor retinaculum is also closed using 3-0 Ethibond suture.
- Skin is closed using 4-0 nylon suture.

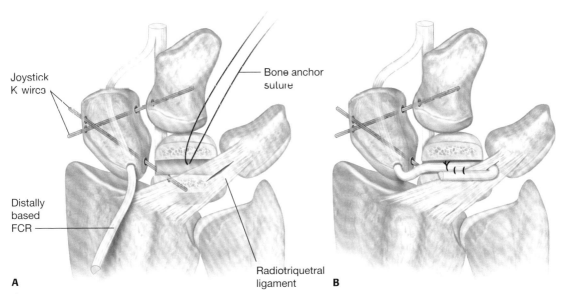

TECH FIG 4 • **A.** The FCR tendon is secured into the trough in the lunate using a 1.8-mm bone anchor suture. **B.** The remaining FCR tendon graft is sutured back over itself.

PEARLS AND PITFALLS

Technique	■ Some authors recommend a ligament-sparing capsulotomy to expose the scapholunate interval. To do so, the capsular incision is made in line with the fibers of the intercarpal and radiocarpal ligaments, and a trapezoid capsular flap is raised.
	■ The superficial radial nerve and palmar cutaneous branch of the median nerve are at risk with the volar portion of the surgery and should be identified and protected.
	■ The FCR tendon can be inadvertently transected as it rotates 90 degrees at the wrist. Be careful and follow the fibers rather than blindly sliding the scissors to harvest the graft.
	■ The scaphoid can be fractured if the surgeon attempts to force a wide graft through the tunnel. The tendon graft should be approximately 3 mm wide.
	■ K-wires are cut under the skin to avoid pin tract infection. The K-wires are removed in the operating room in 8 wk.
Therapy	■ In therapy, initial restriction of radial and ulnar deviation lessens the force on the SLIL ligament reconstruction.

POSTOPERATIVE CARE

- The patient is placed in a volar wrist splint postoperatively.
- The splint and operative dressings are taken down after 10 to 14 days, and the wound is examined. Sutures are removed at this time.
- The patient will remain splinted for 8 weeks.
- After 8 weeks of splinting, the patient is transitioned to a removable volar wrist splint for an additional 4 weeks. Gentle active wrist range of motion is started at this time. We do not send the patient to therapy because injudicious stressing of the wrist to get more motion will disrupt the reconstruction. Our goal is painless motion and whatever motion the patient can achieve is the suitable motion. This expectation must be presented to the patient before surgery; we inform the patient that there is no good wrist operation and all wrist operations trade pain relief for decreased wrist motion.

- Initial restriction of radial and ulnar deviation lessens the force on the ligament reconstruction.
- K-wires are removed 6 to 8 weeks after surgery.

OUTCOMES

- Most patients will have mild to no pain after initial recovery from surgery.[9–12]
- Most patients feel subjective improvement and would have the operation again.[9]
- Studies have shown a slight loss of wrist motion after surgery (**FIG 4**).
  - Total wrist motion averaged 85% of contralateral (uninjured) wrists in one study at an average of 10 years of follow-up.[11]
  - A more recent study of 20 patients with a mean follow-up of 24 months showed that wrist flexion was reduced by a mean of 19 degrees, and extension was decreased by a mean of 14 degrees.[12]

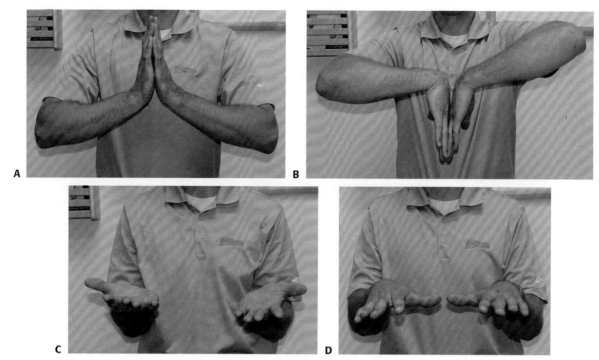

FIG 4 • Five-month postoperative clinical photographs after scapholunate ligament reconstruction with FCR tendon autograft. This patient demonstrates a minor loss of motion of the operative (**left**) wrist, as is to be expected. This loss of motion did not cause him any discomfort or disability. He was very satisfied with his outcome.

- Radial and ulnar wrist deviation has been shown to be 68% and 86% of contralateral wrists, respectively, in one study and equal to contralateral in another.[9,10]
- Grip strength has been shown to be 78% to 85% of contralateral (uninjured) strength after a modified Brunelli reconstruction.[10–12]
- Radiographic parameters improve after surgery. In one study, the average preoperative scapholunate gap was 5.1 mm, which was reduced to 2.4 mm at surgery and was 2.8 mm at final follow-up at an average of 10 years.[11] Scapholunate angle has been shown to improve to within normal limits immediately after surgery but may increase again after longer follow-up.[10–12]
- Most patients avoid degenerative changes of the wrist.[10–12]

COMPLICATIONS

- Damage to superficial radial nerve or the palmar cutaneous branch of the median nerve.
- Scar tenderness.[9]
- Complex regional pain syndrome.[9,10]
- SLAC wrist occurred in 1 out of 19 patients in one study with a mean of 37 months of follow-up,[10] 1 out of 8 in another study with a mean of 10 years of follow-up,[11] and 3 out of 20 in another study with a mean of 24 months of follow-up.[12]
  - Ligament reconstruction should not be performed in patients who already have degenerative changes on radiographs.

REFERENCES

1. Watson K, Ballet FL. The SLAC wrist: scapholunate advanced collapse pattern of degenerative arthritis. *J Hand Surg Am.* 1984;9:358-365.
2. Taleisnik J. Post-traumatic carpal instability. *Clin Orthop Relat Res.* 1980;149:73-82.
3. Berger RA. The gross and histologic anatomy of the scapholunate interosseous ligament. *J Hand Surg Am.* 1996;21A:170-178.
4. Mayfield JK, Johnson RP, Kilcoyne RK. Carpal dislocations: pathomechanics and progressive perilunar instability. *J Hand Surg Am.* 1980;5A:226-241.
5. Taleisnik J. Current concepts review. Carpal instability. *J Bone Joint Surg Am.* 1988;70:1262-1268.
6. Kaur JM. Functional anatomy of the wrist. *Clin Orthop Relat Res.* 1980;149:9-20.
7. Watson HK, Ashmead D, Makhlouf MV. Examination of the scaphoid. *J Hand Surg Am.* 1988;13(5):657-660.
8. Ramamurthy NK, Chojnowski AJ, Toms AP. Imaging in carpal instability. *J Hand Surg Eur.* 2016;41(1):22-34.
9. Van den Abbeele KLS, Loh YC, Stanley JK, Trail IA. Early results of a modified Brunelli procedure for scapholunate instability. *J Hand Surg Br.* 1998;23:258-261.
10. Chabas JF, Gay A, Valenti D, et al. Results of the modified Brunelli tenodesis for treatment of scapholunate instability: a retrospective study of 19 patients. *J Hand Surg Am.* 2008;33:1469-1477.
11. Nienstedt F. Treatment of static scapholunate instability with modified Brunelli tenodesis: results over 10 years. *J Hand Surg Am.* 2013;38A:887-892.
12. Elgammal A, Lukas B. Mid-term results of ligament tenodesis in treatment of scapholunate dissociation: a retrospective study of 20 patients. *J Hand Surg Br.* 2016;41E(1)56-63.

Lunotriquetral Ligament Reconstruction Using a Slip of the Extensor Carpi Ulnaris Tendon

Mark Morris and Kevin C. Chung

DEFINITION

- Isolated injury to the lunotriquetral (LT) ligament is less common than injury to the scapholunate (SL) ligament.
- LT ligament injury can be found in isolation or in combination with other injuries, such as in the case of a perilunate dislocation.
- The mechanism of LT ligament injury is debated but may be secondary to a dorsally applied force to a palmar-flexed wrist. Perilunate dislocation is thought to occur when the wrist is forced into hyperextension and ulnar deviation.[1]
- LT disruption can be the result of acute trauma or secondary to degenerative or inflammatory conditions.
- LT injury ranges from partial tears to complete dissociation. Partial tears or attenuation of the ligament are more common and result in dynamic instability, whereas complete dissociation leads to static collapse.
- Volar intercalated segment instability (VISI) occurs after complete disruption of the LT ligament, dorsal radiotriquetral ligament, and volar radiolunate ligament.
- VISI may occasionally be seen in uninjured wrists, in contrast to dorsal intercalated segment instability (DISI), which is always pathologic.

ANATOMY

- The LT ligament is C-shaped, consisting of dorsal, proximal membranous, and palmar portions (**FIG 1**). In contrast to the SL ligament where the dorsal portion is thickest and strongest, the palmar region of the LT ligament is the thickest and strongest portion.[2,3]
- Secondary stabilizers of the LT joint include the ulnocarpal (ulnolunate, ulnocapitate, and ulnotriquetral), midcarpal (triquetrohamate and triquetrocapitate), and dorsal carpal (dorsal intercarpal and radiotriquetral) ligaments (**FIG 2**).
- Complete tear of only the LT ligament will not result in VISI deformity because the secondary stabilizers maintain the lunate and triquetrum in position.
- The scaphoid has a tendency to flex, whereas the triquetrum has a tendency to extend. The lunate, or intercalated segment, is balanced by these two opposing forces.

PATHOGENESIS

- Isolated LT tear is thought to occur when a dorsally applied force is applied to a palmar-flexed wrist. This force causes the dorsal LT fibers to tear. The volar radiolunate ligaments remain intact and tether the proximal lunate on the volar side, leading to palmar flexion.

- Reverse perilunate injuries occur from falling on an outstretched hand with the wrist extended, pronated, and radially deviated. This mechanism can also result in an isolated LT tear, followed by lunocapitate dislocation, and then SL dissociation (**FIG 3A**).[4]
- Perilunate injuries occur when the wrist is forced into hyperextension and ulnar deviation. Mayfield describes four stages of perilunate injury (**FIG 3B**).[1] LT injuries occur in Mayfield III and IV perilunate injuries.
- Inflammatory arthritis or degenerative LT lesions may also lead to instability.

NATURAL HISTORY

- The natural history of LT injuries has not been clearly defined; however, they may lead to degenerative changes of the wrist.

PATIENT HISTORY AND PHYSICAL FINDINGS

- Patients present with ulnar-sided wrist pain.
- Patients may or may not report a history of trauma.
- Patients may have tenderness to palpation over the dorsal LT joint.

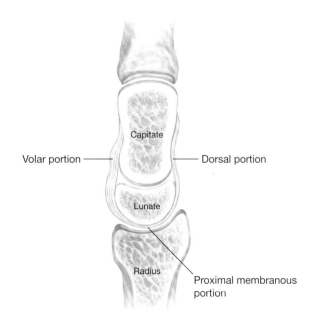

FIG 1 • The lunotriquetral ligament is C-shaped, consisting of palmar, dorsal, and proximal membranous portions. The palmar portion is the thickest and strongest portion of the ligament.

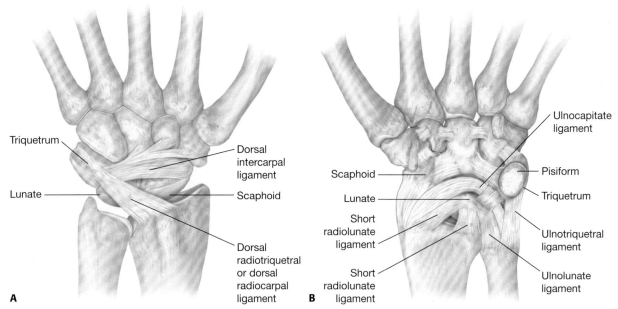

FIG 2 • A. Dorsal wrist ligaments. The important dorsal secondary stabilizers of the lunotriquetral joint are the dorsal intercarpal and dorsal radiotriquetral (also known as dorsal radiocarpal) ligaments. **B.** Volar wrist ligaments. The important volar secondary stabilizers of the lunotriquetral joint are the short and long radiolunate ligaments, the ulnolunate ligament, the ulnocapitate ligament, and the ulnotriquetral ligament.

- LT compression test: Radially directed pressure is applied over the triquetrum. This may elicit pain in patients with LT instability (**FIG 4A**).
- LT ballottement test: The lunate is stabilized with the thumb and index finger of one of the examiner's hands. The other hand is used to displace the triquetrum and pisiform dorsally and palmarly. Pain, crepitus, and joint laxity are seen in patients with LT instability (**FIG 4B**).
- Ulnar deviation with pronation and axial compression may elicit instability and a painful clunk.

- Limited range of wrist motion
- Diminished grip strength

IMAGING

- A PA radiograph may show a break in Gilula lines. There is often a step-off between the lunate and triquetrum.
- It is rare to see a gap in the LT interval on radiographs with LT injuries, in contrast to SL injuries where a gap is seen. Plain radiographs may be normal (**FIG 5**).

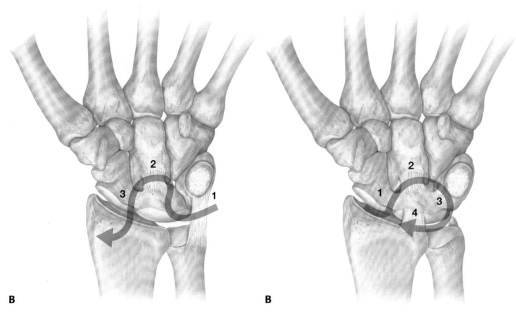

FIG 3 • A. Reverse perilunate injuries start on the ulnar side of the wrist starting with an isolated LT tear, followed by lunocapitate dislocation, and then scapholunate dissociation. **B.** Mayfield's four stages of perilunate injury. Stage 1: Disruption of scapholunate ligament or scaphoid fracture. Stage 2: Lunocapitate dislocation. Stage 3: Lunotriquetral dissociation or triquetrum fracture. Stage 4: Lunate dislocation.

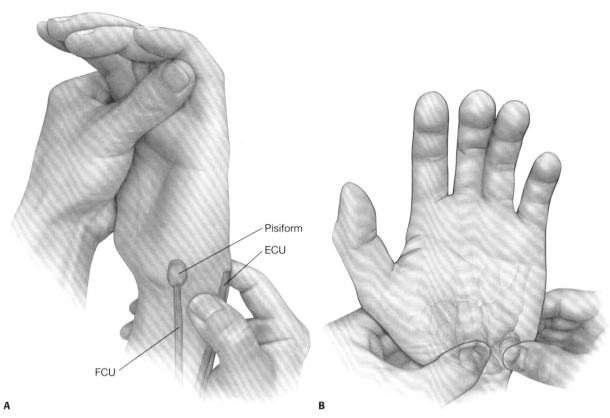

Pisiform
ECU
FCU

A   **B**

FIG 4 • **A.** Lunotriquetral compression test. The examiner applies radially directed pressure over the triquetrum. **B.** Lunotriquetral ballottement test. The lunate is stabilized with the thumb and index finger of one of the examiner's hands. The other hand is used to displace the triquetrum and pisiform dorsally and palmarly.

- A lateral radiograph may show a VISI deformity, marked by volar tilting of the lunate. This indicates injury to the LT injury along with injury to the dorsal radiotriquetral ligament (**FIG 6**).
  - The SL angle is less than 30 degrees with a VISI deformity.
  - The capitolunate angle increases to over 15 degrees with a VISI deformity.
- MRI is not reliable for imaging of LT ligament injuries.

DIFFERENTIAL DIAGNOSIS

- Ulnar impaction syndrome
- Distal radioulnar joint instability
- Extensor carpi ulnaris subluxation
- Triangular fibrocartilage complex injuries
- Pisotriquetral arthritis
- Hook of hamate fracture

FIG 5 • PA, oblique, and lateral radiographs of a patient with a lunotriquetral injury. There is no apparent widening of the lunotriquetral interval or VISI deformity seen here; however, a lunotriquetral ligament tear was found on wrist arthroscopy after the patient failed nonoperative management.

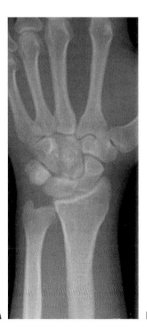
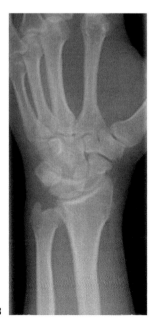
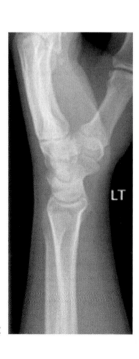

A   **B**   **C**

LT

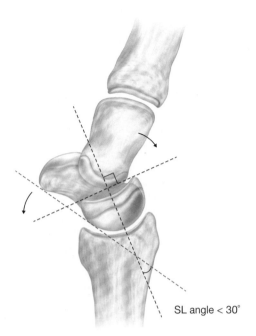

FIG 6 • The VISI deformity is marked by the lunate in a flexed position, which decreases the scapholunate angle and increases the capitolunate angle.

NONOPERATIVE MANAGEMENT

- The appropriate management of an acute LT injury is immobilization in a cast for 8 to 12 weeks. Patients who present with subacute or chronic LT injuries should also be treated first with immobilization, but the timing is less well-defined and can be determined by the patient's symptoms during immobilization.[5]
- Midcarpal injections with local anesthetic and corticosteroids may be a helpful adjunct to immobilization.

SURGICAL MANAGEMENT

- Surgical management is indicated in patients with symptomatic LT dissociation that is not relieved by nonoperative management.
- The goal of surgery is to restore stability to the proximal carpal row and to realign the lunocapitate axis.

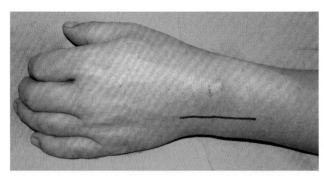

FIG 7 • A dorsal wrist incision is used, centered between the fourth and fifth compartments.

- Ligament reconstruction should be reserved for patients without arthritic changes.
- If degenerative changes are already present, the surgeon should consider arthrodesis or proximal row carpectomy.

Preoperative Planning

- The surgeon can consider diagnostic wrist arthroscopy prior to ligament reconstruction. This will help to better characterize the articular surfaces of the carpal bones, as well as to better delineate the degree of ligament injury.

Positioning

- The patient is positioned supine on the operating table. The operative extremity is draped out on a hand table.
- We prefer to use regional anesthesia for this operation. General anesthesia can also be used.
- A tourniquet is applied.
- An examination under anesthesia is performed to evaluate for a clunk. The distal radioulnar joint can be assessed under anesthesia as well.

Approach

- A 6-cm longitudinal incision is used, centered over the dorsal wrist between the fourth and fifth compartments (**FIG 7**).
- Alternatively, two incisions can be used—one incision over the dorsal wrist joint, and another proximally over the ECU tendon harvest site.

■ Exposure and Tendon Harvest

- A longitudinal skin incision is centered over the dorsal wrist, between the fourth and fifth compartments.
- The wrist capsule is incised longitudinally (**TECH FIG 1A,B**). The LT interval should now be visible (**TECH FIG 1C,D**).
- Excise scar tissue from between the lunate and triquetrum.
- The ECU tendon is identified in the proximal portion of the incision.

- A distally based slip of ECU tendon is harvested from the radial aspect of the tendon (**TECH FIG 1E,F**).
- The tendon graft should be 3 mm wide by 8 to 10 cm long.
- The strip of tendon graft is dissected to its insertion at the base of the small finger metacarpal.

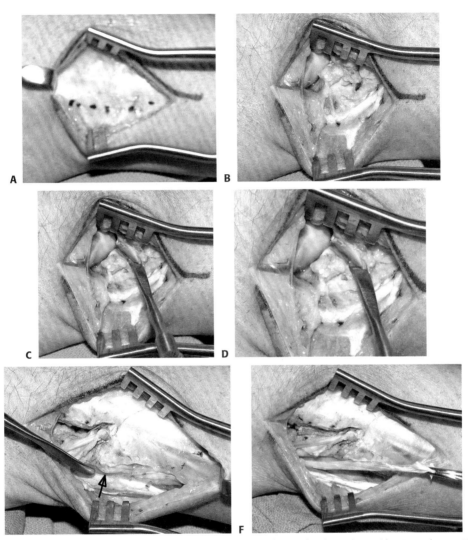

TECH FIG 1 • **A,B.** Longitudinal incision of the wrist capsule. **C,D.** The lunotriquetral interval is shown here with a Freer elevator. The lunotriquetral ligament here is ruptured. **E.** The intact ECU tendon (*arrow*). **F.** A 3-mm strip of distally based ECU tendon is harvested.

■ Reduction of the Lunate and Triquetrum and Creation of Bone Tunnels

- Two 0.062-in. Kirschner wires (K-wires) are inserted into the dorsal lunate and triquetrum to be used as joysticks for reduction (**TECH FIG 2A**). Be sure to keep the K-wires out of the way of the planned tunnels in each bone.
- To correct the VISI deformity, the lunate is extended by retracting the lunate K-wire proximally and the triquetrum is flexed by retracting the triquetral K-wire distally.

- To create the bone tunnels, a K-wire is placed in the triquetrum from the distal, dorsal, ulnar aspect toward the proximal, palmar, radial corner. Once acceptable placement is confirmed, a 2.5-mm cannulated drill is used to create a bone tunnel in the triquetrum over the K-wire (**TECH FIG 2B,C**).
- The lunate bone tunnel is then created in similar fashion by placing a K-wire from the distal, dorsal, and radial corner of the lunate to the proximal, palmar, and ulnar corner. A cannulated drill is again used over the K-wire to form the tunnel.
- The tunnels should converge at the volar margin of the LT joint and should remain extra-articular.

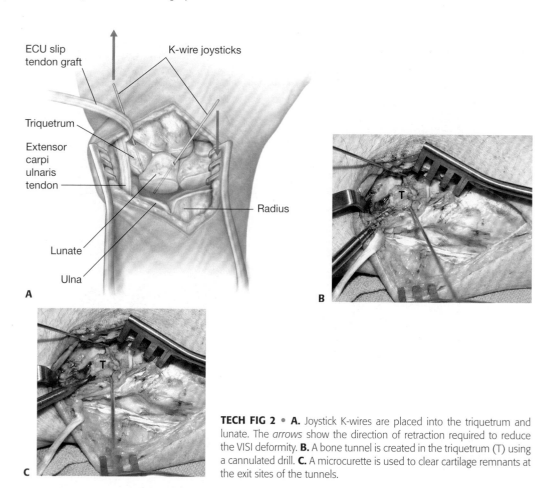

TECH FIG 2 • **A.** Joystick K-wires are placed into the triquetrum and lunate. The *arrows* show the direction of retraction required to reduce the VISI deformity. **B.** A bone tunnel is created in the triquetrum (T) using a cannulated drill. **C.** A microcurette is used to clear cartilage remnants at the exit sites of the tunnels.

■ Passing and Securing the ECU Tendon Graft

- The tendon is passed through the bone tunnels using a wire or suture. First pass the tendon from the dorsum of the triquetrum to the LT interval and then from the LT interval to the dorsum of the lunate (**TECH FIG 3A**).

- Alternatively, after passing the graft through the triquetrum, a small bone anchor can be used to secure the tendon graft to the lunate (**TECH FIG 3B,C**). The VISI deformity must be corrected with the joystick K-wires prior to fixation with an anchor.
- Next, the ECU graft is secured to itself over the remnant of the LT ligament.

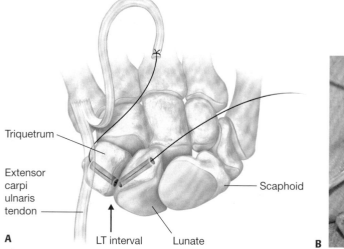

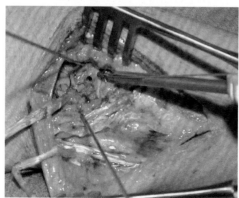

TECH FIG 3 • **A.** Bone tunnels are made through the triquetrum and lunate. A wire or suture (pictured) is used to feed the graft through the bone tunnels. **B,C.** A mini-Mitek anchor can be used to fix the graft to the lunate.

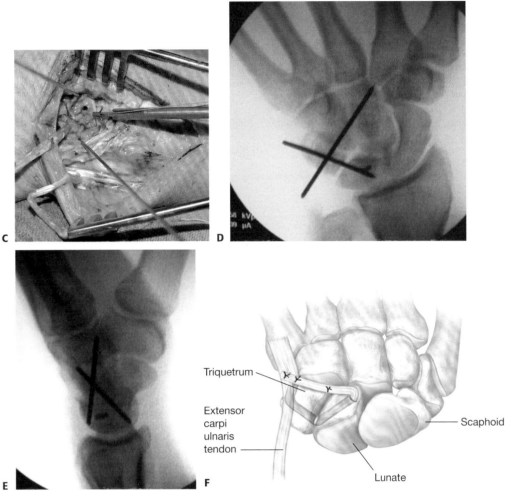

TECH FIG 3 (Continued) • **D,E.** One or two K-wires are inserted to hold the reduction of the lunotriquetral joint. Here, an additional wire was placed through the triquetrum into the hamate and capitellum. **F.** After passing the tendon graft through the triquetrum and lunate, the free end is sutured back to itself.

- First, the VISI deformity is corrected as described earlier with the joystick K-wires.
- The corrected position is held with a third K-wire passed through the triquetrum and lunate (**TECH FIG 3D,E**). The triquetrum should also be pinned to the capitate

to fixate the reduced construct; otherwise, the triquetrum may rotate around the single K-wire to lose the reduction.
- The end of the tendon graft is then sutured back to itself using 3-0 Ethibond sutures (**TECH FIG 3F**).

■ **Closure**

- The wrist capsule is closed tightly with 3-0 Ethibond suture.
- The extensor retinaculum over the fourth and fifth compartments is closed using 3-0 Ethibond suture.

- The joystick K-wires are removed at this time.
- The K-wire traversing the LT joint is left in place and is cut deep to the skin. This is done to avoid pin tract infections from a pin that will be left in place.

PEARLS AND PITFALLS

Technique	▪ Branches of the dorsal ulnar sensory nerve should be protected. The dorsal sensory branch of the ulnar nerve arises 8 cm proximal to the pisiform and passes dorsal to the FCU and pierces the fascia 5 cm proximal to the pisiform. It reaches the dorsal hand in close proximity to the ulnar styloid process.
	▪ The ECU tendon graft should not be more than 3 mm wide. If it is too wide, it will be difficult to pass through the drill holes in the lunate and triquetrum.
	▪ Joystick K-wires are used to correct the VISI deformity. The lunate wire is placed obliquely from a distal to proximal direction, and the triquetral wire is placed from an oblique proximal to distal direction. The VISI deformity is corrected by making both wires perpendicular to the axis of the forearm.
	▪ An alternative technique to drilling bone tunnels is to use a sharp curved awl. This is less traumatic and may help to avoid fracturing the carpal bones.
	▪ Ulnar shortening osteotomy may be performed at the same time as LT ligament reconstruction in a patient with concomitant ulnocarpal abutment.
Postoperative	▪ Pain is significantly improved in most patients after this procedure.
Therapy	▪ Do not be too aggressive with therapy or the repair can fail. Long-term satisfaction is high even though patients do typically lose some wrist range of motion.

POSTOPERATIVE CARE

- The patient is placed in a volar wrist splint immediately postoperatively.
- Incisions are examined and sutures are removed after 10 to 14 days.
- The patient is kept in a volar wrist splint for 8 weeks.
- K-wires are removed after 8 weeks.
- The patient can start gentle range of motion exercises after K-wires are removed. Wrist stiffness is common (**FIG 8**).

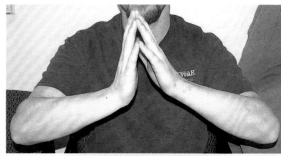

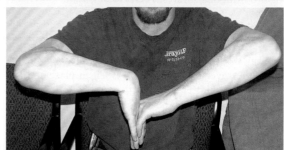

FIG 8 • Six-month follow-up after lunotriquetral ligament reconstruction. Although the patient lost some wrist range of motion, he was satisfied with his result.

OUTCOMES

- Shin et al.[6] demonstrated that patients who had LT ligament reconstruction had lower reoperation rates than did patients treated with direct repair or arthrodesis.
- Shahane et al.[7] studied 46 patients who underwent LT ligament reconstruction with ECU tendon. After a mean of 19 months of follow-up, 19 patients (41%) had excellent outcomes, 10 (22%) had good outcomes, 11 (24%) had satisfactory outcomes, and 6 (13%) had poor outcomes based on Mayo wrist scores. Forty of 46 patients said that they had substantially improved and would undergo the operation again.

COMPLICATIONS

- Injury to the dorsal branch of the ulnar nerve
- Pisotriquetral pain
- Reflex sympathetic dystrophy
- Residual instability

REFERENCES

1. Mayfield JK, Johnson RP, Kilcoyne RK. Carpal dislocations: pathomechanics and progressive perilunar instability. *J Hand Surg [Am]*. 1980;5(3):226-241.
2. Berger RA. The gross and histologic anatomy of the scapholunate interosseous ligament. *J Hand Surg [Am]*. 1996;21A:170-178.
3. Ritt MJ, Bishop AT, Berger RA, et al. Lunotriquetral ligament properties: a comparison of three anatomic subregions. *J Hand Surg [Am]*. 1998;23A:425-431.
4. Murray PM, Palmer CG, Shin AY. The mechanism of ulnar-sided perilunate instability of the wrist: a cadaveric study and 6 clinical cases. *J Hand Surg [Am]*. 2012;37(4):721-728.
5. Wagner ER, Elhassan BT, Rizzo M. Diagnosis and treatment of chronic lunotriquetral ligament injuries. *Hand Clin*. 2015;31:477-486.
6. Shin AY, Weinstein LP, Berger RA, Bishop AT. Treatment of isolated injuries of the lunotriquetral ligament in comparison of arthrodesis, ligament reconstruction, and ligament repair. *J Bone Joint Surg Br*. 2001;83:1023-1028.
7. Shahane SA, Trail IA, Takwale VJ, et al. Tenodesis of the extensor carpi ulnaris for chronic, post traumatic lunotriquetral instability. *J Bone Joint Surg Br*. 2005;87:1512-1515.

Fixation of Acute Scaphoid Fractures

Ketan Sharma, James T. W. Saunders, and Amy M. Moore

DEFINITION

- The scaphoid is the most commonly fractured bone of the carpus.
- *Acute* scaphoid fractures are defined as occurring within 3 to 4 weeks of the inciting event.
- *Displaced* scaphoid fractures are defined as exhibiting more than 1 mm displacement or more than 10 degrees angulation.
- Operative treatment of acute scaphoid fractures remains challenging due to the complex geometry and tenuous blood supply of the scaphoid itself.
- Herbert's system classifies fractures into four types[1]:
  - Type A—stable and acute
  - Type B—unstable and acute
  - Type C—delayed unions
  - Type D—established nonunion

ANATOMY

- The scaphoid spans the proximal and distal carpal rows, and serves as an important dynamic link between the two.
- The scaphoid articulates with the radius, lunate, capitate, trapezoid, and trapezium.

- These numerous articulations mean that over 80% of the surface area of the scaphoid is covered with cartilage and not periosteum.
- This characteristic limits both ligamentous structural integrity and vascular healing potential.
- This also means the scaphoid heals predominantly through primary bone healing (intramembranous ossification), which can result in a paucity of callus formation and weak early union.[2]
- The scaphoid bone is divided into three regions: the proximal pole, waist, and distal pole (or tubercle [**FIG 1**]).
- The proximal pole of the scaphoid articulates with the distal radius within the scaphoid fossa, and is coupled to the neighboring lunate within the proximal row via the strong scapholunate (SL) ligament.
  - This ligament prevents the scaphoid from falling into a flexed position, and is crucial for carpal stability.
- Vascular supply to the scaphoid is provided through two main branches of the radial artery (**FIG 2**).
  - The dorsal branch supplies 70% to 80% of the total vascularity, enters at the dorsal ridge distally, and supplies the entire proximal pole.

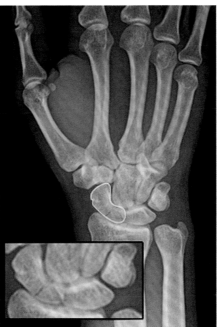 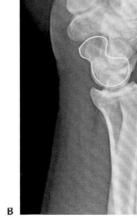

FIG 1 • **A.** PA **(B)** and lateral radiographs showing nondisplaced fracture of the scaphoid waist (scaphoid outlined in *yellow*; fracture magnified in inset in **A**). The scaphoid is divided into three regions (proximal pole, waist, distal pole) and serves as an important dynamic link between the proximal and distal carpal rows.

A   B

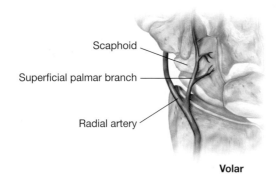

Scaphoid

Superficial palmar branch

Radial artery

Volar

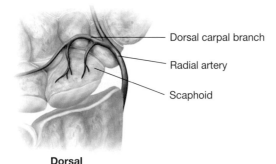

Dorsal carpal branch

Radial artery

Scaphoid

Dorsal

FIG 2 • The scaphoid is supplied by dorsal and volar branches of the radial artery, which predominantly distribute to the proximal and distal poles, respectively. This unique retrograde vasculature has important implications concerning healing of waist and proximal pole fractures.

- The volar branch supplies 20% to 30% of the total vascularity, enters through the tubercle, and supplies the distal pole and distal tuberosity predominantly.[3]
- The proximal pole receives the majority of its blood supply through retrograde intraosseous vascular flow from these arteries and is therefore susceptible to avascular necrosis (AVN) when this supply is disrupted by the fracture.

PATHOGENESIS

- The most common mechanism of injury of the scaphoid is a hyperextension of the wrist more than 95 degrees, coupled with an ulnar deviation.[4]
  - A volar tensile force leads to failure and propagation of a fracture through the body of the scaphoid to the dorsal surface where compression loading occurs.
  - Impingement on the dorsal rim of the distal radius during hyperextension may also contribute to waist fractures.
- Proximal pole scaphoid fractures likely occur from dorsal subluxation during forced hyperextension.
- Less commonly, hyperflexion and axial loads may also produce scaphoid fractures.

NATURAL HISTORY

- The natural history of scaphoid fractures remains integral to treatment strategy.
- Healing potential is fundamentally a function of fracture potential and available vascularity.
  - More proximal fractures have poorer blood supply, leading to decreased healing potential, which can produce nonunion or AVN.

- Fracture displacement disrupts the blood supply and decreases healing potential.
- Fractures displaced more than 1 mm or angulated more than 15 degrees have an increased risk of nonunion.
- Displaced or untreated scaphoid nonunions will predictably progress to dorsal intercalated segmental instability (DISI) type carpal instability, and eventually scaphoid nonunion advanced collapse (SNAC) arthrosis.
  - In patients with a nonunion, up to 97% will demonstrate arthritic change within 5 years of the injury.[5]
- Risk factors for scaphoid nonunion include delayed treatment, inadequate immobilization, proximal fractures, comminution, and concomitant carpal injuries.[6]

PATIENT HISTORY AND PHYSICAL FINDINGS

- Patients with acute or subacute scaphoid fractures typically present with a history of a high-energy fall or a wrist hyperextension–type injury.
- Patients present with radial-sided wrist pain, swelling, and loss of range of motion (ROM), most predominantly on dorsiflexion.
- Physical examination signs include the following:
  - Wrist edema over the dorsal/radial aspect of the wrist (occasionally accompanied by ecchymosis)
  - Pain on active or passive extension of the wrist localized to the dorsal/radial aspect
  - Focal pain on palpation within the anatomic snuffbox (space between the first and third extensor compartments at the level of the wrist). Always compare to the contralateral side as this is inherently a tender area.
  - Pain on palpation of the scaphoid tubercle volarly
  - Dorsal/radial wrist pain on resisted extension of the second digit
  - Decreased ROM of the wrist
  - Pain on axial loading of the wrist (scaphoid compression test)

IMAGING

- Radiographs should be obtained on any patient suspected of having a scaphoid fracture.
  - Dedicated scaphoid views should be achieved with the wrist in ulnar deviation, an oblique view, a PA view, a lateral view, and a clenched fist view (allows assessment of dynamic instability of the scapholunate ligament).
  - Approximately 25% of scaphoid fractures are not visible on initial radiographs, posing a diagnostic barrier.
  - Any patient with a high clinical probability of scaphoid injury but a negative plain film series either should be splinted for 10 to 12 days before obtaining repeat films or should undergo more sensitive additional imaging (CT or MRI).
- CT scans taken in the axis of the scaphoid offer additional information regarding the architecture or displacement and have utility in diagnosing acute fractures not seen on plain films. They are also useful in assessing for bony union or nonunion after treatment has been initiated (**FIG 3**).
- MRI is helpful in identifying occult fractures in the acute setting. The addition of gadolinium, as a contrast agent, can be used to assess the vascularity of the proximal pole if there are concerns of AVN.

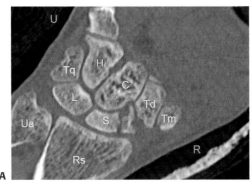 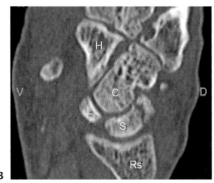

FIG 3 • A. Coronal and **(B)** sagittal CT slices showing a nondisplaced comminuted fracture of the scaphoid waist. Preoperative CT scans can provide additional diagnostic utility especially concerning degree of comminution, and postoperative scans can also allow for superior evaluation of malunion or nonunion. S, scaphoid; L, lunate; Rs, radius; Ua, ulna; C, capitate; H, hamate; Tq, triquetrum; Td, trapezoid; Tm, trapezium; R, radial; U, ulnar; V, volar; D, dorsal.

- A displaced/unstable scaphoid fracture is defined as:
  - Cortical displacement 1 mm or greater
  - More than 10 degrees of angular displacement
  - Comminution at the fracture site
  - Radiolunate angle of more than 15 degrees
  - Scapholunate angle of more than 60 degrees
  - Intrascaphoid angle of more than 35 degrees

DIFFERENTIAL DIAGNOSIS

- Wrist sprain
- Distal radius fracture
- Fracture of other carpal bones
- Ligamentous injury (most commonly, SL)
- Preiser disease (spontaneous AVN of the scaphoid)

NONOPERATIVE MANAGEMENT

- Nonoperative management, in the form of cast immobilization, is effective only in low-risk scaphoid fractures that meet all of the following criteria:
  - Acute fractures (less than 4 weeks old)
  - Nondisplaced
  - Favorable location (distal pole)
- Nondisplaced fractures of the scaphoid waist remain controversial regarding operative vs nonoperative treatment.
  - Nondisplaced waist fractures can be treated nonoperatively with immobilization for 10 to 12 weeks with close follow-up, with union rates as high as 90% in this scenario.[1]
  - Patients with a nondisplaced scaphoid waist fracture who wish to mobilize early (highly active persons, athletes, manual workers, or those in high-demand occupations) should undergo operative fixation.
- Nondisplaced and displaced fractures of the proximal pole should be surgically managed to minimize the risk of AVN.
- Splint or cast immobilization should immobilize at least the wrist and thumb CMC but does not need to include the entire thumb.[7] Above-elbow casting is not needed.
- Nondisplaced distal pole fractures have a high rate of union after cast immobilization for 6 to 8 weeks.
- Union, especially for conservatively treated scaphoid waist fractures, should be assessed with a CT scan to assess for bony bridging at approximately 8 to 10 weeks after the injury.

SURGICAL MANAGEMENT

- Surgical management is best for fractures that are unstable or displaced.
- An open approach is indicated for[8] the following:
  - Proximal pole fractures
  - A displaced, unstable fracture of the scaphoid waist
  - Associated carpal instability or perilunate instability
  - Associated distal radius fracture. Both fractures can be addressed at one operative time and will allow for early mobility.
- A percutaneous approach is indicated for the following:
  - Nondisplaced fractures of the scaphoid waist
  - A displaced fracture of the scaphoid waist
  - Proximal pole fractures
- Percutaneous fixation is technically difficult and has not been shown to have better outcomes. Thus, the authors advocate for an open approach to the scaphoid.
- Both percutaneous and open procedures can be performed from the volar or dorsal approach depending on fracture characteristics.
  - In general, fractures of the proximal pole are approached dorsally to allow for anterograde screw fixation and compression across the fracture. This approach maximizes the amount of screw threads distally.
  - Scaphoid fractures with associated carpal instability are also approached dorsally to allow for adequate exposure of the proximal carpal row. A K-wire can be placed in the lunate to assist reduction of the proximal scaphoid pole via its attachment through the scapholunate ligament. This assists obtaining and maintaining carpal realignment with scaphoid screw fixation.
  - Approaching scaphoid waist fractures, which have a tendency to flex volarly at the fracture site, from the dorsal approach makes reduction more challenging, as the wrist must be flexed to bring the axis of the scaphoid above the dorsal lip of the distal radius. In these cases, a volar approach can be used.

Preoperative Planning

- Imaging studies should be thoroughly reviewed to confirm fracture geometry.
- Required equipment includes
  - K-wires
  - Portable mini-fluoroscopy ("mini C-arm")

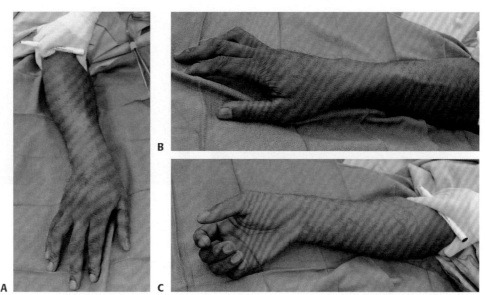

FIG 4 • A. The patient should be positioned supine, with the shoulder abducted to 90 degrees on an arm board. **B,C.** The forearm can then be supinated or pronated depending on the choice of a volar or dorsal approach, respectively.

- Cannulated headless compression screws, in which the differential thread pitch exerts compression across the fracture site[1]

Positioning

- Anesthesia should be general or regional.
- The patient should be positioned supine, with the shoulder of the affected upper extremity abducted to 90 degrees on an arm board (**FIG 4**).
- The fluoroscopy unit should be draped and readily available.
- A pneumatic tourniquet should be applied to the proximal upper arm.

- Intravenous antibiotic prophylaxis should be provided prior to tourniquet inflation.
- The upper extremity should be prepped and draped in the standard sterile fashion.
- The upper extremity should then be exsanguinated using an Esmarch bandage, and then the tourniquet should be inflated (to either 250 mm Hg or at least 100 more than systolic blood pressure).

Approach

- Scaphoid fractures can be approached from a volar or dorsal approach.

TECHNIQUES

■ Open Reduction and Internal Fixation of Scaphoid Fracture: Dorsal Approach

Exposure

- Make a longitudinal 3- to 4-cm-long incision in the dorsal forearm and hand starting at the ulnar aspect of the Lister tubercle and extending distally (**TECH FIG 1A**).
- Dissect through subcutaneous tissue; elevate skin flaps on either side above level of extensor retinaculum. Identify and protect any crossing radial sensory nerve branches.
- Incise the distal aspect of the extensor retinaculum over the third compartment. Identify the junction of the second and third dorsal compartments.

- Identify and retract EDC ulnarly and ECRB, ECRL, and EPL radially to expose the underlying radiocarpal capsule. The tendons can remain in their compartment but must be identified to avoid inadvertent transection during exposure of the capsule.
- Make a limited capsulotomy to expose the scaphoid. The scaphoid can be approached through a transverse limb just distal to dorsal radius (**TECH FIG 1B**). An inverted T incision can be extended if further exposure is needed.
- Elevate the capsular flap to expose the proximal pole of the scaphoid, the S-L ligament, and the underlying fracture. Be careful to avoid stripping the dorsal ridge vessels entering at scaphoid waist.
- Evacuate fracture hematoma.

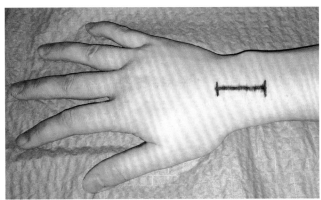
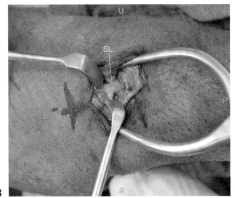

TECH FIG 1 • **A.** Longitudinal approximately 4-cm incision designed along the axis from the Lister tubercle to the long finger metacarpal. This incision is used for a dorsal approach to the scaphoid. **B.** Intraoperative photograph of the dorsal approach depicting scaphoid and intact scapholunate (SL) ligament. Note the position of the buried screw head as well. P, proximal; D, distal; U, ulnar; R, radial.

Fracture Reduction and Fixation

- Apply longitudinal traction on IF and LF to distract the carpus.
- If needed to assist in fracture reduction, insert 0.045-in. K-wires perpendicular into proximal and distal scaphoid fragments (**TECH FIG 2**).
- Reduce fracture; confirm by assessing congruity of radioscaphoid and scaphocapitate articulations.
- Once reduction is confirmed, temporarily fixate with derotational 0.045-in. K-wires. Drill first wire dorsoulnar

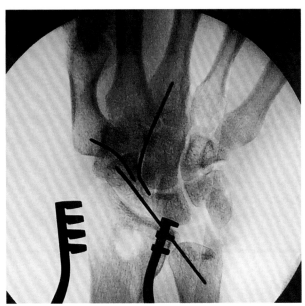

TECH FIG 2 • Inserting 0.045-in. K-wires into proximal and distal fragments to act as "joysticks" may significantly assist in fracture reduction. Also note the placement of a derotational 0.045-in. K-wire for temporary fixation, once the fracture is appropriately reduced. Importantly, this wire should be placed parallel to but not within the central axis of the scaphoid, to avoid interfering with screw placement.

to central axis of scaphoid, into the trapezium. Drill a second wire, if needed, volar and radial to central axis of scaphoid. Be careful to ensure that derotational wires will not interfere with screw placement and/or prevent compression within the central axis of the scaphoid (see **TECH FIG 2**).

Guidewire Placement

- Guidewire placement should originate at the membranous portion of the origin of the scapholunate ligament. For very proximal fractures, the starting point should be the mid-aspect of the membranous portion of the scapholunate ligament, to be as proximal as possible.
- Flex the wrist, and insert the guidewire down the central axis of the scaphoid. This should be in line with the thumb metacarpal.
- Confirm central axis placement via PA, lateral, and 30-degree pronated lateral radiographs.
- Advance the wire up to the scaphotrapezial joint without entering the joint itself.

Screw Insertion

- Determine screw length via the guidewire. With minimal displacement of the fracture, screw length should be 4 mm shorter than guidewire length to account for the cartilage thickness.
- Advance the guidewire into the trapezium.
- Use the cannulated drill to manually drill over the wire. Be careful to not overdrill the distal scaphoid, which could result in screw migration into the scaphotrapezial joint.
- Remove the drill and insert the screw along the central axis of the scaphoid.
- Remove the guidewire.
- Confirm screw position via radiographs (**TECH FIG 3**).
- Close the radiocarpal capsule and then the extensor retinaculum if completely released, then skin.

TECHNIQUES

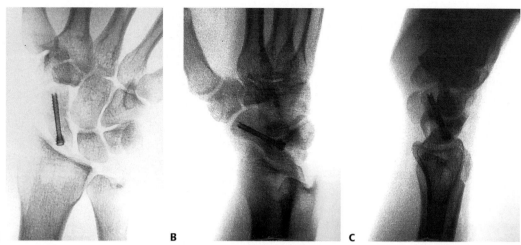

TECH FIG 3 • Final confirmation of appropriate screw position via PA **(A)**, lateral **(B)**, and 30-degree pronated lateral **(C)** radiographs. Note the screw positioning lies within the scaphoid cortex on all views, reducing the chance of undesired prominence.

■ Open Reduction and Internal Fixation of Scaphoid Fractures: Volar Approach

Exposure

- Palpate the tubercle of the scaphoid after radially deviating the wrist.
- Design a 3- to 4-cm incision centered over the palpated tubercle, extending proximally over the FCR tendon sheath and distally over the base of the thumb.
- Incise the FCR sheath and retract the tendon ulnarly, exposing underlying volar wrist capsule.
- Distally, divide thenar muscles over the distal scaphoid and trapezium.
- Incise the volar wrist capsule longitudinally, avoiding injury to the articular cartilage.
- Divide the radiolunate and radioscaphocapitate ligaments in the proximal field to visualize the proximal pole of the scaphoid.
- Use a Freer elevator to expose the scaphotrapezial joint. Limit dissection over the radial scaphoid to avoid injury to dorsal vessels.
- Evacuate fracture hematoma and irrigate.

Fracture Reduction and Fixation

- Apply longitudinal traction to the wrist and reduce the fracture. Consider using pointed reduction forceps or placing 0.045-in. K-wires into proximal and distal scaphoid fragments to assist in reduction.
- Place provisional 0.045-in. K-wire, starting from volar distal to dorsal proximal, for temporary fixation. Ensure the trajectory is not along the central axis of the scaphoid.
- To expose starting position for screw placement dorsally, resect small portion of proximal volar trapezium.
- Place central axis guidewire.
- Determine screw length via the guidewire. With minimal displacement of the fracture, screw length should be 4 mm shorter than guidewire length to account for the cartilage thickness.
- Advance the guidewire into the radius.
- Use the cannulated drill to manually drill over the wire.
- Insert the cannulated screw along the central axis; confirm via PA, lateral, and 30-degree pronated lateral radiographs.
- Repair radiolunate and radioscaphocapitate ligaments.
- Close the volar wrist capsule, then skin.

PEARLS AND PITFALLS

Preservation of scaphoid blood supply	▪ Avoid dissection on the dorsal ridge of the scaphoid. ▪ Limit dissection of capsule.
Guidewire positioning	▪ During dorsal approach, pronate and flex the wrist to ensure appropriate trajectory. ▪ During volar approach, resect small volar lip of trapezium to expose starting position in distal pole of scaphoid. ▪ Ensure the guidewire is placed along the central axis.
Screw position	▪ Assess screw length and prominence intraoperatively via 45-degree supination oblique and pronated oblique radiographs. ▪ Screw length should be 4 mm shorter than measured length. ▪ Stop drilling 2 mm short of the distal pole when using the dorsal approach. ▪ Place the screw in the central axis. ▪ Bury the headless compression screw beneath the cortical surface of the scaphoid to prevent screw prominence and cartilage erosion.
Small proximal pole fracture	▪ Consider a smaller screw such as Acutrak Mini to prevent proximal fragment comminution.
Unstable fracture reduction	▪ Place perpendicular joystick K-wires into proximal and distal fragments to aid in reduction. ▪ Stabilize fragments prior to screw insertion via derotational K-wires.

POSTOPERATIVE CARE

- Patients should be placed in a volar thumb spica splint.
- Patients should strictly elevate at home to reduce edema and pain.
- Frequent ROM exercises of the digits are crucial to prevent unwanted stiffness.
- At 2 weeks postoperatively, patients should return for suture removal and exchange to a removable forearm-based thumb spica splint. ROM exercises of the thumb are started at this point.
  - Fractures that involve the proximal pole, or fractures with significant comminution, should be immobilized for 6 to 10 weeks.
- Radiographs should be taken at the 2-, 6-, and 12-week postoperative time points to assess for fracture healing (**FIG 5**).
- CT scans can be considered to better assess for fracture union at 12 weeks or later if there are concerns about healing.

OUTCOMES

- Outcomes depend on type of treatment, timing of treatment, and location of screw placement.

- A recent systematic review concluded that internal fixation reduces the risk of nonunion compared with cast immobilization (1.7% vs 10%, respectively). However, the two treatments did not differ in terms of eventual postoperative pain, tenderness, long-term grip strength, ROM, functional outcome, and satisfaction, although internal fixation may produce quicker return to function and transiently improved ROM and grip strength.[9]
- Rigid internal fixation theoretically allows for earlier physical therapy, lesser time to union, improved ROM, and quicker functional recovery. This has been corroborated by studies that have showed high rates of union and good overall outcomes using open techniques[10] (**FIG 6**).
- Time to initiation of treatment highly influences union rates:
  - Scaphoid fractures treated before 4 weeks have a significantly higher union rate than do those treated after 4 weeks.[11]
  - Nondisplaced fractures casted within 3 weeks of injury have a 90% to 100% union rate,[12] whereas those casted between 6 weeks and 6 months from injury demonstrate a 90% union rate, but approximately twice as long duration to achieve a union.[13]
- Central screw placement exhibits more rapid progression to union, in cases of scaphoid nonunion.[14]

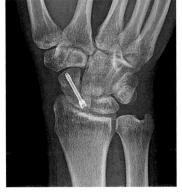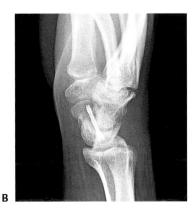

FIG 5 • **A:** PA and (**B**) lateral PA and lateral radiographs showing reduced, internally fixed, and united scaphoid waist fracture at roughly 3 months postoperatively.   **A**   **B**

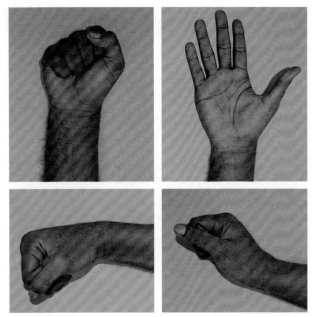

FIG 6 • Early outcome (at 12 weeks postoperatively) depicting intact grip and wrist flexion/extension.

COMPLICATIONS

- Screw prominence, erosion of the scaphotrapezial articulation, and erosion of the distal radius articular surface are possible if the screw length is not accurately estimated intraoperatively.
- Displaced waist and proximal pole fractures can lead to nonunion and potential AVN.
- Rare but potential other complications include wound infections, hypertrophic scarring, injury to sensory branch of radial nerve, and damage to scaphotrapezial articulation.

REFERENCES

1. Kang L. Operative treatment of acute scaphoid fractures. *Hand Surg.* 2015;20(2):210-214.
2. Ruby LK, Stinson J, Belsky MR. The natural history of scaphoid non-union: a review of fifty-five cases. *J Bone Joint Surg Am.* 1985;67A: 428-432.
3. Gelberman RH, Menon J. The vascularity of the scaphoid bone. *J Hand Surg [Am].* 1980;5:508-513.
4. Weber ER, Chao EY. An experimental approach to the mechanism of scaphoid waist fracture. *J Hand Surg [Am].* 1978;3:142-148.
5. Mack GR, Bosse MJ, Gelberman RH, et al. The natural history of scaphoid non-union. *J Bone Joint Surg Am.* 1984;66:504-509.
6. Lindstrom G, Nystrom A. Natural history of scaphoid non-union with special reference to "asymptomatic" cases. *J Hand Surg Br.* 1992;17:697-700.
7. Buijze GA, Goslings JC, Rhemrev SJ, et al. Cast immobilization with and without immobilization of the thumb for nondisplaced and minimally displaced scaphoid waist fractures: a multicenter, randomized, control trial. *J Hand Surg [Am].* 2014;39(4):621-627.
8. Leslie IJ, Dickson RA. The fractured carpal scaphoid: natural history and factors influencing outcome. *J Bone Joint Surg Br.* 1981;16B: 225-230.
9. Symes TH, Stothard J. A systematic review of the treatment of acute fractures of the scaphoid. *J Hand Surg Eur.* 2011;36E:802-810.
10. Bedi A, Jebson PJL, Hayden RJ, et al. Internal fixation of acute, non-displaced scaphoid waist fractures via a limited dorsal approach: an assessment of radiographic and functional outcomes. *J Hand Surg [Am].* 2007;32A:326-333.
11. Langhoff O, Andersen JL. Consequence of late immobilization of scaphoid fractures. *J Hand Surg Br.* 1998;13B:77-79.
12. Cooney WP, Dobyns JH, Linsheid RL. Nonunion of the scaphoid: analysis of the results from bone grafting. *J Hand Surg [Am].* 1980;5:434-445.
13. Mack GR, Wilckens JH, McPherson SA. Subacute scaphoid fractures: a closer look at closed treatment. *Am J Sports Med.* 1998;26:56-58.
14. Trumble TE, Clarke T, Kreder HJ. Non-union of the scaphoid: treatment with cannulated screws compared with treatment with Herbert screws. *J Bone Joint Surg Am.* 1996;67A:428-432.

Scaphoid Nonunion: Nonvascularized Bone Reconstruction

Matthew L. Iorio and Jason H. Ko

DEFINITION

- Scaphoid nonunion is defined as failure to heal within 6 months. The incidence of scaphoid nonunion is between 4% and 50%.
  - Nonunion may be evidenced by pain and tenderness at the anatomic snuffbox and scaphoid tubercle, and decreased wrist extension.
- Radiographs demonstrate a wide, sclerotic fracture cleft, potentially with cyst formation (**FIG 1**).
- Unstable nonunions demonstrate loss of the normal length and shape of the scaphoid, often with a dorsal intercalated segmental instability (DISI) deformity.
- When not corrected, carpal instability ensues, and a predictable pattern of degenerative changes known as scaphoid nonunion advanced collapse (SNAC) arthritis occurs.
- The preferred treatment for scaphoid nonunions is internal fixation with autologous bone grafting.
- Nonvascularized bone grafts have been the traditional treatment for scaphoid nonunion, although avascular necrosis (AVN) of the proximal pole is an indication for the use of vascularized bone grafts.

ANATOMY

- Seventy to 80% of the intraosseous vascularity comes from the dorsal scaphoid branches of the radial artery, entering through the dorsal ridge. These dorsal vessels enter the scaphoid waist in a retrograde direction, providing the single dominant intraosseous vessel to the proximal pole of the scaphoid.
- A minor volar contribution comes from radial artery or its superficial palmar branch, which gives off several volar scaphoid branches at the level of the radioscaphoid joint, entering the bone at its distal tubercle.
- Because of this unique vascular anatomy, the proximal pole of a fractured scaphoid is particularly prone to AVN, especially when the fragment is small.
- A nonunion through the scaphoid waist can lead to progressive flexion of the distal pole and extension of the proximal pole, leading to a "humpback deformity."
- Treatment and surgical approach will be influenced by whether or not a humpback deformity or DISI deformity is present.
- A proximal pole nonunion will not typically develop a humpback deformity; however, the risk of AVN is higher.

PATIENT HISTORY AND PHYSICAL FINDINGS

- Injury typically involves axial load across a hyperextended and radially deviated wrist.
- Tenderness can typically be found over the distal pole of the scaphoid volarly or along the proximal pole dorsally within the interval between the first and third extensor compartments.
- Ulnar-to-radial wrist deviation with pressure over the volar scaphoid pole may cause increased pain, as will active assist wrist flexion or extension or resisted pronation.

IMAGING

- Anteroposterior, oblique, and lateral radiographs of the scaphoid should be obtained.
  - Standard scaphoid view involves 30 degrees of wrist extension and 20 degrees of ulnar deviation.
  - Stress views with the fist tightly clenched may demonstrate dynamic instability of the scaphoid or nonunion site.
- Computed tomography (CT) with fine cuts may be beneficial in further characterizing the nonunion site, as well as associated humpback deformity, cyst formation, osteophytosis, and degenerative arthrosis.
  - Increased proximal pole sclerosis or density on imaging may indicate AVN, which, depending on the location of the nonunion, may limit both the ability to obtain viable bone margins as well as reliable fixation and osseous union.
- Magnetic resonance imaging can be used to assess for AVN of the scaphoid proximal pole.
- Evaluation of a potential degenerative posture or malunions of the scaphoid should be measured and documented as part of the initial evaluation. There is some debate as to which is superior in interobserver reliability, though they both

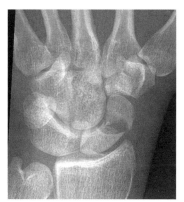

FIG 1 • Scaphoid waist nonunion characterized by a wide sclerotic fracture cleft with no evidence of bony healing.

function to evaluate deviations of scaphoid posture from a normative comparison in the setting of humpback deformity and collapse.

- A lateral intrascaphoid angle is obtained by drawing a line perpendicular to the proximal and distal articular surfaces.
  - A normal lateral intrascaphoid angle is 24 ± 5 degrees or less than 3 degrees.[1]
  - Increasing flexion results in a humpback deformity, with a lateral intrascaphoid angle greater than 35 degrees.
- The scaphoid height-to length ratio is evaluated on a lateral or sagittal image. A normal ratio is 0.60 ± 0.04.
  - For scaphoid length, a baseline is drawn along the volar scaphoid, and the length of the scaphoid is found from the most proximal to the most distal aspect.
  - For scaphoid height, the maximum height of the scaphoid was found on a line perpendicular to the baseline.

SURGICAL MANAGEMENT

- Nonvascularized bone graft reconstruction should be considered for the treatment of all scaphoid fracture nonunions that demonstrate no incidence of AVN of the proximal pole.
- Contraindications
  - Progressive pan-carpal arthrosis can follow prolonged scaphoid nonunions in a predictable pattern: SNAC wrist deformity.
  - The presence of radiocarpal or midcarpal sclerosis, with cyst formation, may indicate advanced disease with continued postoperative pain. In this instance, salvage procedures including proximal row carpectomy, limited intercarpal arthrodesis, or total wrist arthrodesis may be more reliable in regard to pain control.
  - Relative contraindications include the patient's suitability for surgery, smoking status, and understanding of the need for prolonged postoperative immobilization and use restrictions.

Positioning

- The patient is positioned supine on the operating room table with a well-padded tourniquet placed on the upper arm.
- General anesthesia or monitored anesthesia care (MAC) can be used, but supplementation with an infraclaviular or interscalene nerve block may markedly improve postoperative pain control.

Approach

- If a humpback deformity is present, a volar approach is used, which provides excellent exposure to the waist and distal pole of the scaphoid.
  - It also provides direct access to the extension osteotomy wedge for direct bone grafting and stabilization.
  - It may be possible that this exposure, by preserving the dorsal ridge vessel, may prevent iatrogenic devascularization of the scaphoid.
- If there is no humpback deformity, a dorsal or volar approach can be used, based on the location of the nonunion. Dorsal approaches are preferred for more proximal nonunions, and volar approaches are preferred for more distal nonunions.
- Either a volar or dorsal approach can be used with a waist nonunion without a humpback deformity.

■ Scaphoid Bone Grafting: Volar Approach

Exposure and Preparation of the Site

- Under tourniquet control and loupe magnification, a longitudinal incision is made in-line with the flexor carpi radialis (FCR) to the level of the proximal wrist crease, followed by a 60-degree angle at the volar junction of the glabrous skin. This will protect the radial artery and prevent a longitudinal scar across the flexor crease. This is also referred to as the Russe approach (**TECH FIG 1A–C**).
- The deep branch of the radial artery is visualized, and retracted radially.
- An intrasubstance longitudinal incision in the radioscaphocapitate (RSC) ligament can be created for exposure of the volar scaphoid. The incision and exposure should be at least distal to the scaphotrapezial joint, for preparation and visualization of screw placement.
- Following visualization of the scaphoid, 0.045-in. (or larger) K-wires may be placed proximal and distal to the fracture as "joysticks" to retract and see, and correct any humpback deformity that may be present (**TECH FIG 1D**).
- In the event of a malunion, an osteotomy can be performed; however, this should be done judiciously. We recommend only crossing 80% to 90% of the scaphoid waist with the osteotome to prevent penetration of the dorsal cortex and injury to the scaphocapitate joint or the dorsal ridge vessel.
- Disruption of the dorsal scaphoid can create an unstable fracture or make cancellous bone graft placement less secure.
- Following exposure, the nonunion site must be cleared of intervening fibrous material and necrotic bone, but viable cancellous bone should remain. A small dental pick or curette can be useful in this setting.

Obtaining Bone Graft

- If volar distal radius autograft is to be used, the pronator quadratus is incised and dissected subperiosteally to expose the volar cortex of the distal radius (**TECH FIG 2A**).
- The site of bone graft harvest should be confirmed with intraoperative fluoroscopy, being careful not to harvest graft too close to the radiocarpal joint.
- A structural corticocancellous bone graft can be obtained either with straight and curved osteotomes or with an oscillating saw.
  - If a saw is used, saline irrigation should be applied during the osteotomies to minimize thermal injury to the bone (**TECH FIG 2B,C**).
- Through the aforementioned cortical window, cancellous autograft can be harvested.
- For most scaphoid nonunions without AVN, distal radius autograft is sufficient.
  - However, iliac crest autograft is the traditional standard for scaphoid nonunion treatment. The anterosuperior iliac spine (ASIS) is palpated, and bone graft should be harvested 2 cm posterior to the ASIS.

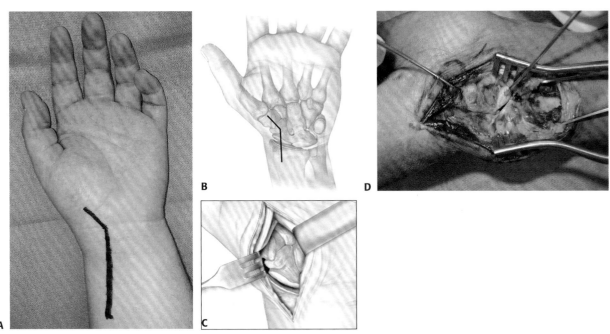

TECH FIG 1 • A–C. A volar Russe incision along the FCR tendon with an oblique extension over the scaphoid distal pole provides access to the volar scaphoid. **D.** Through this volar approach, 0.054-in. Kirschner wires used to joystick open the scaphoid fracture nonunion site, correcting the humpback deformity.

- The skin incision is made posterior to the ASIS, and dissection should proceed with monopolar cautery directly down to the iliac crest.
- Bicortical grafts from the inner table or outer table, or tricortical grafts, can be obtained, typically with an oscillating saw.

Stabilizing the Site

- The nonunion site can then be stabilized by either progressively packing either corticocancellous or cancellous graft into the site, effectively expanding the space and increasing the extension of the distal pole.
- K-wire joysticks can be used to provide an extension force through the fracture, and a longitudinal K-wire can be placed to provide a mechanical restraint to flexion.
  - In our experience, a combination of the two may work best, where the extension is corrected with the K-wires and stabilized longitudinally as best as possible and confirmed with fluoroscopy.
- This wire should be placed slightly off axis to avoid the ultimate trajectory of compression screw placement and directly capture the bone graft.
  - Alternatively, the wire can be placed slightly volar to the bone graft to prevent extrusion during compression.
- If a large cortical defect volarly is present in the extension wedge, a bone graft can be tailored to slightly overfill the space.
  - The longitudinal wire is then backed out just proximal to the fracture, the graft is press fit into the space, and the wire is readvanced (**TECH FIG 3**).

Scaphoid Fixation

- Osteosynthesis is then completed, most frequently with either K-wire or compression screw placement.

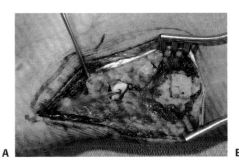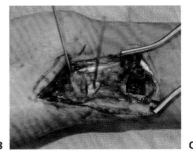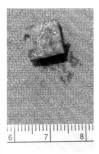

TECH FIG 2 • A. The pronator quadratus has been elevated subperiosteally off the volar surface of the distal radius. The purple markings are used to plan the osteotomies, which were confirmed with intraoperative fluoroscopy. **B,C.** A corticocancellous autograft is harvested from the volar distal radius. This type of graft can be used as a structural graft to correct a humpback deformity.

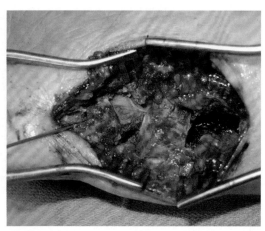

TECH FIG 3 • Corticocancellous autograft is press-fit into the scaphoid nonunion through a volar approach.

- For compression screw placement from the volar scaphoid, the guidewire can be advanced through either the trapeziometacarpal joint or scaphotrapezial joint, with similar outcomes.
  - In the scaphotrapezial approach, however, the volar beak or footplate of the trapezium should be first removed with a rongeur to prevent off-axis screw placement.

- The stabilizing K-wire should be left in place or repositioned if it is blocking the guidewire, to provide rotational control during drilling and compression.
- Following placement of the guidewire, the drill should be advanced with the aid of fluoroscopy to prevent penetration of the far cortex, as this may destabilize the distal screw and lead to screw loosening.
- Screw selection then is performed by drilling to the distal subchondral bone, measuring based off the guidewire, and selecting a screw length 4 to 6 mm shorter than the measured length to ensure that the screw is adequately buried in subchondral bone proximally, without distal extrusion.
  - Depending upon the manufacturer, there may be several screw widths to choose from, typically between 2 and 3 mm. This becomes relevant in either revising a prior attempt to heal an acute fracture with a compression screw or expectations in need for nonunion revision. That is, if the widest screw is chosen as the initial fixation and it fails, compression screw fixation may not be an option for salvage given the subsequent bone loss and instability. Therefore, initial fixation should be performed with a narrower screw, in case future revision with a wider screw can be performed (**TECH FIG 4**).

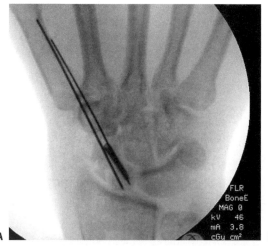
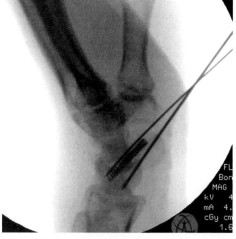

TECH FIG 4 • AP and lateral intraoperative fluoroscopic views of a headless compression screw to provide compression across the corticocancellous bone graft reconstruction. The radial K-wire in the AP view is used as a derotational pin, and the volar K-wire on the lateral view is used to further stabilize the small bone graft.

■ Scaphoid Bone Grafting: Dorsal Approach

Exposure and Preparation of the Site

- Under tourniquet control and loupe magnification, a longitudinal incision is made just ulnar to the Lister tubercle (**TECH FIG 5A**).
- A longitudinal cut or step-cut is made through the extensor retinaculum.
- The third dorsal compartment is released, and the EPL tendon is retracted radially.

- Subperiosteal dissection of the second and fourth dorsal compartments is performed to expose the dorsal distal radius.
- The posterior interosseous nerve (PIN) is located in the floor of the fourth compartment, and during the dorsal wrist approach, a PIN neurectomy can be performed to help minimize postoperative pain.
- A ligament-sparing capsulotomy or longitudinal capsulotomy is performed through the dorsal wrist capsule to expose the proximal scaphoid (**TECH FIG 5**).

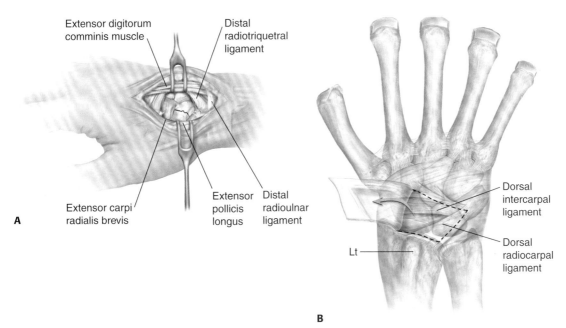

TECH FIG 5 • A. A dorsal longitudinal incision just ulnar to the Lister tubercle will give the surgeon access to both the scaphoid nonunion and the dorsal distal radius bone graft site. **B.** A ligament-sparing capsulotomy is performed parallel to the dorsal intercarpal (DIC) and dorsal radiocarpal (DRC) ligaments, along with a radial extension.

- The nonunion site is exposed and fibrous tissue removed until healthy-appearing cancellous bone is visualized both proximally and distally.
- Care is taken not to disrupt the scapholunate interosseous ligament during the procedure.

Scaphoid Fixation

- As described above, K-wires can be used as joysticks to gain control of the proximal and distal poles, and corticocancellous or cancellous autograft can be packed into the nonunion site.
- Fixation is achieved by headless compression screw, as described above. The derotational K-wire can be left in for temporary fixation.
- In proximal pole nonunions, if there is minimal bone proximally, screw fixation may not be possible, in which case, definitive fixation may be performed with K-wires.
- Allograft bone chips can be used to pack the bone graft donor site.

- With the volar approach, it is important to reapproximate the radioscaphocapitate ligament if it was cut during the procedure. This can be performed with 3-0 polyglactin suture.
- If volar distal radius bone graft was harvested, the pronator quadratus does not need to be repaired.

Closure

- The dorsal capsule is carefully closed with an absorbable suture, such as a 3-0 poliglecaprone-25 or polyglactin suture. The extensor retinaculum is closed with similar 3-0 suture, leaving the extensor pollicis longus tendon superficial to the retinaculum.
- Depending upon the volume of expected postoperative edema and skin quality, the skin is closed with either deep dermal stitches and a running subcuticular or horizontal mattress stitches with 4-0 nylon.
- The wrist is immobilized in a well-padded plaster short-arm spica splint.

PEARLS AND PITFALLS

Scaphoid preparation	▪ Degeneration of the radioscaphoid facet or post-traumatic arthrosis may predispose to ongoing pain and stiffness and should be considered a potential contraindication to scaphoid salvage techniques.
Distal radius bone graft harvest	▪ It is important to harvest bone graft 1 cm proximal to the radiocarpal joint to prevent injury.
PIN neurectomy	▪ During the dorsal wrist approach, the PIN can be identified in the floor of the fourth dorsal compartment and excised to help minimize postoperative pain.

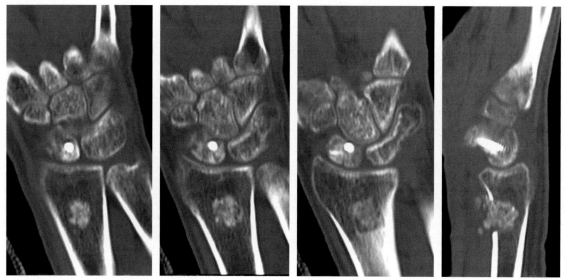

FIG 2 • CT scans obtained 6 weeks postoperatively after volar distal radius corticocancellous reconstruction of a scaphoid waist nonunion demonstrate healing across the proximal and distal autograft sites.

POSTOPERATIVE CARE

- The patient is placed in a well-padded thumb spica splint. At 2 weeks, the splint and stitches are removed and a thumb spica cast is applied.
- Casting is typically continued for a total of 10 to 12 weeks, with cast changes at 3- to 4-week intervals.
- X-rays should be obtained at each postoperative visit. CT scans can be obtained at the surgeon's discretion any time after 6 weeks postoperatively to determine extent of union (**FIG 2**).
- Exposed K-wires should be removed near 3 to 4 weeks to prevent pin site infections and possible bacterial colonization of the nonunion site. Buried wires can be removed in the office or operating room once union is verified.
- Osseous union is identified by bridging trabeculae on radiographs and absence of fracture site tenderness (**FIG 3**).

OUTCOMES

- In 1936, Matti described the original technique using an iliac crest corticocancellous bone strut as an inlay through a dorsal approach. Russe later offered a modified technique done via a volar approach to spare the blood supply and correct volar collapse. This technique demonstrated union rates ranging from 81% to 97%.[2]
- The Fisk-Fernandez technique employs a triangular or trapezoidal corticocancellous wedge from the iliac crest or distal radius that is placed as an intercalary structural graft to restore scaphoid length and correct carpal alignment. Such wedge-grafting techniques have demonstrated improved union rates when compared to Matti-Russe inlay grafting technique.[3–6]

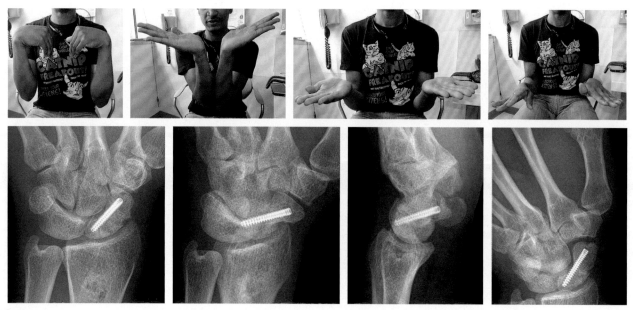

FIG 3 • Routine x-rays at 10 months postoperatively demonstrate complete healing of the scaphoid nonunion reconstruction, with pain-free range of motion.

- Sayegh and Strauch performed a systematic review comparing cancellous-only and corticocancellous grafts, reporting cancellous-only grafts provided a shorter interval to union, but corticocancellous grafts were associated with consistent deformity correction and improved Mayo wrist scores.[7]

COMPLICATIONS

- The most common complication is superficial wound or pin site infection, nerve irritation, and complex regional pain syndrome (1.25%).[8,9]

REFERENCES

1. Amadio PC, Berquist TH, Smith DK, et al. Scaphoid malunion. *J Hand Surg [Am]*. 1989;14(4):679-687.
2. Russe O. Fracture of the carpal navicular: diagnosis, non-operative treatment, and operative treatment. *J Bone Joint Surg Am*. 1960;42-A:759-768.
3. Fernandez DL. A technique for anterior wedge-shaped grafts for scaphoid nonunions with carpal instability. *J Hand Surg [Am]*. 1984;9(5):733-737.
4. Fernandez DL. Anterior bone grafting and conventional lag screw fixation to treat scaphoid nonunions. *J Hand Surg [Am]*. 1990;15(1):140-147.
5. Mulder JD. The results of 100 cases of pseudarthrosis in the scaphoid bone treated by the Matti-Russe operation. *J Bone Joint Surg Br*. 1968;50(1):110-115.
6. Stark A, Broström LA, Svartengren G. Scaphoid nonunion treated with the Matti-Russe technique. Long-term results. *Clin Orthop Relat Res*. 1987;(214):175-180.
7. Sayegh ET, Strauch RJ. Graft choice in the management of unstable scaphoid nonunion: a systematic review. *J Hand Surg [Am]*. 2014;39(8):1500-1506.e7.
8. Daly K, Gill P, Magnussen PA, Simonis RB. Established nonunion of the scaphoid treated by volar wedge grafting and Herbert screw fixation. *J Bone Joint Surg Br*. 1996;78(4):530-534.
9. Smith BS, Cooney WP. Revision of failed bone grafting for nonunion of the scaphoid. Treatment options and results. *Clin Orthop Relat Res*. 1996;(327):98-109.

19
CHAPTER

Scaphoid Fracture Nonunion: Vascularized Bone Reconstruction

Matthew L. Iorio and Jason H. Ko

DEFINITION

- Scaphoid fractures are among the most common upper extremity fractures, accounting for 70% of all carpal bone fractures.[1]
- Although most scaphoid fractures heal with nonoperative management, the tenuous blood supply of the scaphoid can lead to nonunion in 5% to 10% of cases even with appropriate treatment, and up to 55% of cases when there is displacement on initial injury (**FIG 1**).[2,3]
- The complications of scaphoid nonunion vary widely, from pain and decrease in function to carpal malalignment, progressive arthrosis, and eventual scaphoid nonunion advanced collapse (SNAC) (**FIG 2**).[3,4]
- To prevent such complications, surgical advances have been developed to treat scaphoid nonunions, including screw fixation, bone grafting, and, most recently, vascularized bone grafting.[5]
- Vascularized bone grafts (VBGs) have been shown to promote healing and realignment of recalcitrant scaphoid

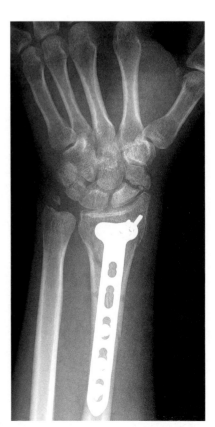

FIG 1 • Chronic scaphoid waist nonunion with tapered cortical edges.

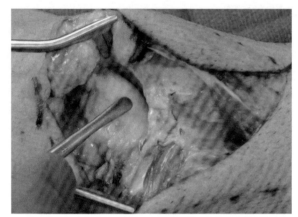

FIG 2 • Radiocarpal joint with avascular proximal scaphoid pole and cartilage fragmentation (Freer elevator).

nonunions in addition to re-establishing blood flow in cases with avascular necrosis (AVN).[6]

ANATOMY

- Seventy to 80% of the intraosseous vascularity comes from the dorsal scaphoid branches of the radial artery, entering through the dorsal ridge. These dorsal vessels enter the scaphoid waist in a retrograde direction, providing the single dominant intraosseous vessel to the proximal pole of the scaphoid.
- A minor volar contribution comes from the radial artery or its superficial palmar branch, which gives off several volar scaphoid branches at the level of the radioscaphoid joint, entering the bone at its distal tubercle.
- Because of this unique vascular anatomy, the proximal pole of a fractured scaphoid is particularly prone to AVN, especially when the fragment is small.
- Progressive collapse and flexion through the nonunion cause dorsal rotation of the lunate or subluxation of the midcarpal joint leading to a DISI deformity (dorsal intercalated segment instability).

PATIENT HISTORY

- Injury typically involves axial load across a hyperextended and radially deviated wrist.
- Tenderness can typically be found over the volar pole of the scaphoid or along the dorsal pole within the interval between the first and third extensor compartments.
- Ulnar-to-radial wrist deviation with pressure over the volar scaphoid pole may cause increased pain, as will active assist wrist flexion or extension or resisted pronation.

IMAGING

- Anteroposterior, oblique, and lateral radiographs of the scaphoid should be obtained.
- Standard scaphoid view involves 30 degrees of wrist extension and 20 degrees of ulnar deviation.
- Stress views with the fist tightly clenched may demonstrate dynamic instability of the scaphoid or nonunion site.
- Computed tomography (CT) with fine cuts may be beneficial in further characterizing the nonunion site, as well as associated collapse, cyst formation, osteophytosis, and degenerative arthrosis.
  - Increased proximal pole sclerosis or density on imaging may indicate AVN, which, depending on the location of the nonunion, may limit both the ability obtain viable bone margins as well as reliable fixation and osseous union.
- Magnetic resonance imaging can be used to assess for AVN of the scaphoid proximal pole.
- Evaluation of a potential degenerative posture or malunions of the scaphoid should be measured and documented as part of the initial evaluation. There is some debate as to which is superior in interobserver reliability, though they both function to evaluation deviations of scaphoid posture from a normative comparison in the setting of humpback deformity and collapse.
- A lateral intrascaphoid angle is obtained by drawing a line perpendicular to the proximal and distal articular surfaces.
  - A normal lateral intrascaphoid angle is 24 ± 5 degrees, or less than 3 degrees.
  - Increasing flexion results in a humpback deformity, with a lateral intrascaphoid angle greater than 35 degrees.
- The scaphoid height-to-length ratio is evaluated on a lateral or sagittal image. A normal ratio is 0.60 ± 0.04.
  - For scaphoid length, a baseline is drawn along the volar scaphoid, and the length of the scaphoid is found from the most proximal to the most distal aspect.
  - For scaphoid height, the maximum height of the scaphoid was found on a line perpendicular to the baseline.

SURGICAL MANAGEMENT

- Harvest of the osteocutaneous medial femoral condyle (MFC) microvascular flap provides simultaneous soft tissue and bone for reconstruction, ease of soft tissue recipient closure, and the ability to provide accurate postoperative monitoring of the microcirculation of the flap. Its routine use requires an understanding of the arterial variation of the descending geniculate arterial tree, as well as the blood supply to the overlying skin of the medial aspect of the knee.
- The free MFC corticoperiosteal flap has garnered increasing attention due to its many desirable attributes, including ease of dissection, surgical positioning facilitating a two-team approach, low donor-site morbidity, preservation of all major arteries to the distal extremity, variable size and shape for harvest and in-setting, and osteogenic potential.[7]

Contraindications

- Progressive pan-carpal arthrosis can follow prolonged scaphoid nonunions in a predictable pattern: SNAC wrist deformity.
- The presence of radiocarpal or midcarpal sclerosis, with cyst formation, may indicate advanced disease with continued postoperative pain. In this instance, salvage procedures, including proximal row carpectomy, limited intercarpal arthrodesis, or total wrist arthrodesis, may be more reliable for pain control.
- Relative contraindications include the patient's suitability for surgery, smoking status, and understanding of the need for prolonged postoperative immobilization and use restrictions.

Positioning

- The patient is placed supine on the operating room table, and a well-padded tourniquet is placed on the upper arm.
- General anesthesia or monitored anesthesia care (MAC) can be used, but supplementation with an infraclavicular or interscalene nerve block may markedly improve postoperative pain control.

■ Approach to Creation of the Bone Flap

- When there is no humpback deformity, a dorsally based vascularized bone flap from the distal radius, like the 4 + 5 extensor compartmental artery (ECA) flap or the 1,2-intercompartmental supraretinacular artery (1,2-ICSRA) flap, can be used to reconstruct a scaphoid nonunion.
- When a humpback deformity is present in the setting of AVN, however, a structural flap must be placed volarly, so a volar vascularized bone flap or a free MFC (or MFT) flap is required to properly correct the humpback deformity.

4 + 5 Extensor Compartmental Artery Vascularized Bone Flap

- The 4 + 5 ECA pedicle is based on retrograde flow between the anterior interosseous pedicle and the dorsal extensor compartmental arteries (**TECH FIG 1A,B**).

- Under tourniquet control, a standard dorsal approach to the wrist is used for exposure, incorporating prior incisions when appropriate.
- The dorsal radial sensory branches are identified and swept radially to protect them from iatrogenic injury.
- The third extensor compartment is opened and the tendon transposed.
- Retinacular flaps are elevated from the ulnar border of the Lister tubercle, moving radially and incorporating the retinaculum over the second dorsal compartment.
- Just distal to the radiocarpal joint and retinaculum, the fourth extensor compartment and tendons are mobilized from the dorsal capsule, preventing iatrogenic injury to the vascular pedicle.
- The tendons are then retracted ulnarly, exposing the anterior interosseous artery and neurovascular pedicle proximally and its distal anastomotic connections to the fourth and fifth extensor compartmental arteries.

TECHNIQUES

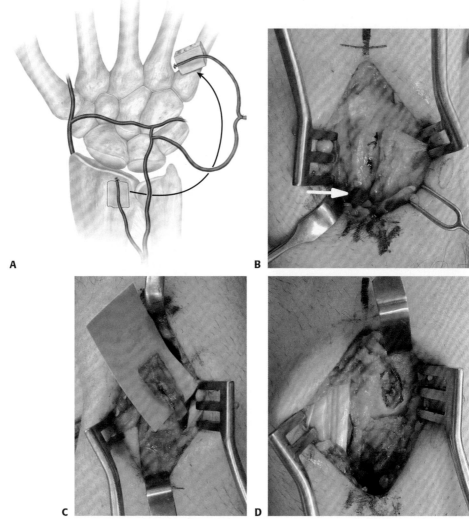

TECH FIG 1 • A. Illustration demonstrating the fourth and fifth extensor compartmental artery (4 + 5 ECA) flap and its axis of rotation. **B.** Fourth extensor compartment artery (*arrow*). **C.** Capsular vascularized bone graft distally based on the fourth extensor compartment artery. **D.** Placement of the distally based fourth ECA flap in the proximal pole of the scaphoid for avascular necrosis.

- Osteotomies are then designed with the vascular pedicle longitudinally centered and the distal transverse cut at least 1 cm proximal to the dorsal ridge of the radius.
- Distal to the site of osteotomy, the pedicle should be elevated with a sharp periosteal elevator or Freer.
- The proximal vessel is clipped, and the osteotomies are performed, taking great care to prevent disruption of the volar radial cortex.
- The flap is then reflected, with a wide cuff of capsular tissue around the retrograde ECA (**TECH FIG 1C,D**).
- The tourniquet can be released at this point to verify perfusion of the bone flap.

1,2-Intercompartmental Supraretinacular Artery Vascularized Bone Flap

- The 1,2-intercompartmental supraretinacular artery (1,2-ICSRA) is distally based from the dorsal continuation of the radial artery into the radiocarpal arch (**TECH FIG 2A**).

- Gentle exsanguination prior to tourniquet elevation can provide some continued turgor of the vascular pedicle, which can improve visibility and dissection.
- Prior dorsal longitudinal incisions can be incorporated when possible into a curvilinear dorsoradial longitudinal incision that follows the course of the EPL tendon (**TECH FIG 2B**).
- The dorsal radial sensory nerve should be identified in the interval next to the cephalic vein and carefully protected.
- Deep to this, the 1,2-ICSRA can be identified on the septum between the first and second extensor compartments, which are incised laterally to include a broad cuff of tissue including the accompanying venae comitantes (**TECH FIG 2C,D**).
- The vertical perforating nutrient branches of the pedicle enter the periosteum at an average of 15 mm proximal to the dorsal radiocarpal joint line.

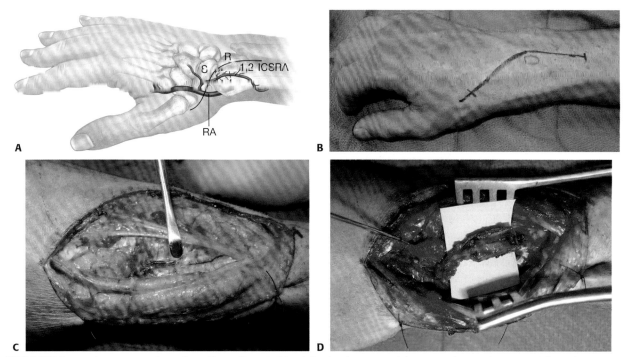

TECH FIG 2 • **A.** The 1,2-ICSRA bone flap with curvilinear incision following the course of the EPL tendon. **B.** The incision follows the course of the EPL tendon. **C.** 1,2-ICSRA vascular pedicle highlighted by the Ragnell retractor. **D.** The 1,2-ICSRA vascularized bone flap harvested.

- If desired, a dorsal radiocarpal capsulotomy can be performed to visualize the scaphoid nonunion.
- The proximal vessel is ligated with bipolar diathermy, and the flap is osteotomized with the vascular pedicle longitudinally centered.
- Prior to performing the distal osteotomy, a periosteal elevator should be used to elevate the periosteal sleeve and protect the distally based pedicle.

Superficial Palmar Branch of Radial Artery Vascularized Bone Flap

- The superficial palmar branch of the radial artery is a terminal transverse branch of the radial artery that arborizes on the distal cortex of the radius. The branch can be identified and preserved in the standard volar approach to the scaphoid, which may be useful especially in settings of humpback or flexion deformities that are typically approached from the volar wrist (**TECH FIG 3**).
- Following exsanguination and tourniquet control, a longitudinal incision in line with the flexor carpi radialis (FCR), with a lateral extension (approximately 45 degrees) at the wrist crease along the glabrous skin junction can be used for exposure.
- The superficial palmar branch is then identified in line with the FCR tendon, potentially originating 5 to 8 mm proximal to the radial styloid. It may be useful to identify the proximal radial artery and trace it distally to the take-off of the palmar vessel, thereby preventing inadvertent injury to the pedicle.
- The posterior sheath of the FCR tendon is then opened, and the volar wrist capsule is identified.
- A longitudinal incision in the radioscaphocapitate (RSC) ligament exposes the scaphoid and facilitates direct tendon repair at the time of closure.

- Following scaphoid preparation, the pronator quadratus is incised longitudinally and transversely to exposure the volar distal radius cortex.
- Care should be taken to harvest the graft at least 10 mm proximal to the volar rim to prevent disruption of the radioscaphoid facet.

Medial Femoral Condyle Microvascular Flap

- Flap dissection can be approached with or without the intent of harvesting a skin paddle, regardless of the variations in anatomy.

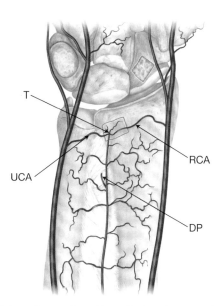

TECH FIG 3 • Volar vascularized bone flap based on the volar carpal artery.

- A Doppler signal can be routinely located over the apex of the medial condyle of the femur.
- A sweeping, curvilinear incision is created, starting at the Hunter canal and moving in distal and anterior directions to the midpoint between the medial border of the patella and the MFC, just anterior to the location of the Doppler signal (**TECH FIG 4A**).
- The incision then continues distal and posterior, stopping 2 to 3 cm below the joint line and just posterior to the midaxis of the leg.
- This skin incision is continued to the subfascial plane of the vastus medialis muscle, which allows the skin paddle to be rapidly elevated and retracted in a posterior direction as the vastus medialis is dissected in an anterior direction.
- The DGA can then be identified as the medial column of the femur is exposed. Dissecting subfascially ensures protection of all skin vessels that can branch off the distal DGA into the reflected skin.
- Through the fascial plane of the vastus medialis, the branching vessels emitting from the DGA can be identified, and the presence or absence of an SAB and/or DGA-CB is rapidly noted (**TECH FIG 4B,C**).
- Branches to the vastus medialis course in an anterior direction (penetrating the fascial plane) and are ligated.
- At this point, a decision is made regarding the approach for the skin paddle. This skin vessel is preferable because of the speed with which it can be dissected as well as the assurance that the skin and subcutaneous vasculature can be elevated anterior to the sartorius muscle and

adductor tendon, keeping the skin and bone segments in the same dissection interval (between the vastus medialis and sartorius muscles).
- If the SAB is selected as the means of supplying the skin segment, it requires a careful distal dissection to determine whether it is supported by skin branches that pass anterior to the sartorius muscle (45%) and in the same surgical interval as the bone component or posterior to the sartorius muscle (55%). If it does pass posterior, it will require a distal elevation of the skin segment and careful passage deep to the sartorius muscle to reunite it with the bone segment before completing the flap harvest.
- After determining the presence or absence of the DGA-CB and the SAB, we prioritize the DGA-CB because of its speed of dissection and ease of visualization.
- If the skin segment is quite large, or if initial dissection reveals that the SAB contributes to the skin perfusion while passing anteriorly to the sartorius muscle, both sources of skin perfusion (SAB and DGA-CB) can be harvested en bloc. Otherwise, the SAB is clamped, and the tourniquet is released. The Doppler signal over the apex of the MFC is again obtained.
- The initial sweeping incision allows many variations of oblique or longitudinally oriented ellipses to be designed, using the initial incision as the anterior border of the skin component, while capturing the Doppler signal for the benefit of postoperative monitoring.
  - Care is taken to harvest this in such a manner that primary closure is simply achieved.

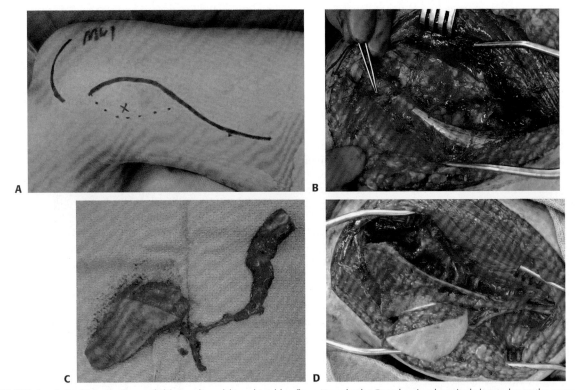

TECH FIG 4 • A. Markings for the medial femoral condyle and trochlea flaps. X marks the Doppler signal routinely located over the apex of the medial condyle of the femur. If a skin paddle is required, a sweeping, curvilinear incision is created at the midpoint between the medial border of the patella and the MFC. If no skin paddle is required, a longitudinal line just posterior to the medial femoral condyle can be used. **B.** In situ relationship of the medial femoral condyle bone flap and skin paddle based on the descending geniculate artery cutaneous branch (overlying sartorius tendon at the tip of the forceps). **C.** Free medial femoral trochlea flap based on the descending geniculate artery. Note the proximal origin of the saphenous artery branch, in this case from the descending geniculate artery, to provide irrigation for a skin paddle. **D.** Medial femoral condyle bone flap and skin paddle following osteotomy and elevation.

T E C H N I Q U E S

- The elevation of the posterior margin of the skin requires making note of the immediate proximity of the DGA-CB to the anterior surface of the adductor tendon.
  - This posterior incision should be carried down to the region posterior to the adductor tendon, giving wide berth to the DGA-CB.
- When deep and posterior to the adductor tendon, the scalpel is then used to approach the posterior aspect of the tendon and cautiously elevate the DGA-CB off the

adductor tendon while maintaining the adductor tendon integrity and preserving the critical DGA-CB.
  - This will enable the entire DGA and its periosteal branches to be preserved undisturbed on the surface of the cortical bone.
- The bone segment is dissected in the width, length, and depth required, and the flap is then harvested on the common DGA origin vessel (**TECH FIG 4D**).

■ Scaphoid Preparation and Fixation

- If cyst formation or bone loss is present without a humpback deformity, a longitudinal 1.1-mm K-wire can be placed radial to the longitudinal axis of the bone to preserve the alignment of the proximal and distal poles.
  - The wire should be placed through the proximal dorsal pole radial and volar to the longitudinal axis of the bone to avoid interference with the placement of a subsequent compression screw or visualization of the fracture.
  - The wire can be advanced anterograde and captured through the volar hand, bringing the proximal edge flush to cartilage cap to prevent injury to the scaphoid facet during manipulation.
  - The proximal and distal poles can then be distracted on the wire to facilitate visualization.
- Fluoroscopy is used to verify the nonunion site.
  - A no. 15 or beaver blade scalpel can be used to gently open the fracture site. Small curettes should be used to remove any intervening cystic or fibrous material (**TECH FIG 5A**).
  - If desired, a 0.8-mm K-wire can be used to sparingly trephinate the proximal and distal cancellous surfaces within the fracture, thereby increasing subsequent blood flow to the fracture site.
- The bone flap and nonunion site should be contoured using rongeurs or osteotomes. If an oscillating saw is used, the surgeon should be especially diligent about

water cooling the site and preventing heat-induced osteonecrosis (**TECH FIG 5B**).
- If a humpback deformity (flexion of the scaphoid through the nonunion site) is identified, a 1.1-mm K-wire should be placed in the proximal and distal poles to act as joysticks to correct the deformity prior to grafting and final fixation.
- If the nonunion site is expansive, the proximal and distal poles should be packed with cancellous autograft from the bone flap harvest site prior to insertion of the flap and definitive fixation.
- Osteosynthesis can be completed with a headless compression screw advanced from the proximal or distal pole, depending upon the orientation of the nonunion site.
  - Alternatively, K-wires may be used upon the surgeon's preference.
- The dorsal capsule is carefully closed with an absorbable suture, such as a 3-0 poliglecaprone-25 or polyglactin suture. The extensor retinaculum is closed with similar 3-0 suture, leaving the extensor pollicis longus superficial to the retinaculum.
- Depending upon the volume of expected postoperative edema and skin quality, the skin is closed with either deep dermal stitches and a running subcuticular or simply vertical mattress stitches with 4-0 nylon.
- The wrist is immobilized in a well-padded plaster short-arm spica splint.

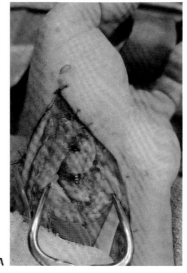 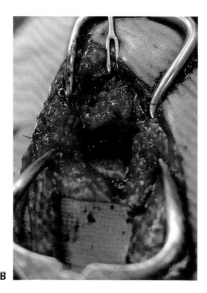

TECH FIG 5 • A. Scaphoid waist chronic fibrous nonunion with osteolysis. **B.** Preparation of the scaphoid prior to bone grafting, with resection of all fibrous and necrotic bone as visualized by bleeding tissue. Note restoration of the scaphoid distal pole extension from flexion ("humpback deformity") and the resultant bone void.

PEARLS AND PITFALLS

Scaphoid preparation	▪ Degeneration of the radioscaphoid facet or post-traumatic arthrosis may predispose to ongoing pain and stiffness and should be considered a potential contraindication to scaphoid salvage techniques.
	▪ A radial styloidectomy can be performed as an adjunctive technique in the setting of mild radioscaphoid arthrosis or to prevent impingement of the vascular pedicle to the bone flap (**FIG 3**).
	▪ A posterior interosseous neurectomy with distal transection, proximal crush, and transposition may be used during the initial exposure.
	▪ The adherent capsular tissue on the dorsal ridge of the scaphoid should be carefully preserved, as this may represent the blood supply to the scaphoid.
	▪ Following insertion of the bone flap, a 0.8-mm K-wire can be placed just dorsal to the flap to prevent migration or extrusion during application of a compression screw.
4 + 5 ECA; 1,2-ICSRA	▪ If prior dorsal capsulotomies have been made, the arterial pedicle may have been transected, rendering the 4 + 5 ECA vascularized bone flap unreliable.
	▪ Depending upon the width of the dorsal distal radius, the fourth or fifth ECA may be selected. However, great care should be utilized to prevent violation of the distal radioulnar joint or sigmoid notch when osteotomizing the fifth ECA-based bone flap as it is more ulnarly placed.
	▪ The 4 + 5 ECA bone flap must be osteotomized and elevated prior to full capsular exposure of the scaphoid; therefore, the surgeon should be aware of the potential dimensions of the flap based on preoperative imaging and design the osteotomies to be ample. In comparison, the 1,2-ICSRA should be identified and protected prior to the dorsal radiocarpal capsulotomy, but the bone flap does not need to be osteotomized and elevated prior to exposure of the scaphoid.
	▪ Osteotomies should be made at least 1 cm proximal to the radiocarpal joint to avoid penetration or disruption of the radiocarpal facets.
	▪ Undue traction or injury on the superficial dorsal radial sensory nerve may lead to increased or prolonged postoperative pain.
MFC	▪ Iatrogenic injury to the saphenous nerve should be avoided by careful identification to the neighboring saphenous artery branch and elevation of the nerve from the proposed skin paddle.
	▪ The skin component is usually elevated first, and attention is then turned to the bone segment. This is because posterior bone cuts will not be readily accessible until the skin paddle and the DGA-CB are reflected in an anterior direction.

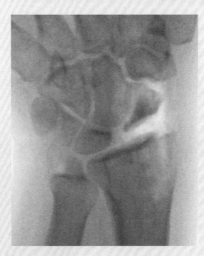

FIG 3 • Intraoperative image following resection of the radial styloid and proximal scaphoid pole with preservation of the scaphocapitate articulation.

POSTOPERATIVE CARE

▪ The patient is placed in a well-padded thumb spica splint. At 2 weeks, the splint and stitches are removed and a thumb spica cast is applied.

▪ Casting is typically continued for a total of 10 to 12 weeks, with cast changes at 3- to 4-week intervals.
▪ The authors advocate burying K-wires under the skin, since they are usually left in for 6 weeks. Buried wires can be removed in the office or operating room once union is

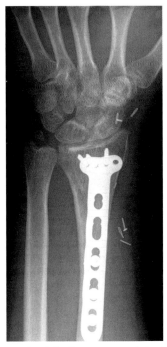

FIG 4 • Osseous union following MFC vascularized bone flap to the scaphoid waist. The dorsal branch of the radial artery at the wrist was used for inflow to the descending geniculate artery.

verified. Exposed K-wires should be removed near 3 to 4 weeks to prevent pin site infections and possible bacterial colonization of the nonunion site.

- X-rays should be obtained at each postoperative visit. CT scans can be obtained at the surgeon's discretion, but the authors recommend 10 to 18 weeks postoperatively to determine extent of union (**FIGS 4** to **6**).
- Osseous union is identified by bridging trabeculae on radiographs and absence of fracture site tenderness.

OUTCOMES

- Vascularized bone grafting of the scaphoid demonstrates union rates near 90%.[8]
- Across 6 studies (23.1%) involving 124 subjects following vascularized bone grafting to the scaphoid, preoperative pain was 5.20 and postoperative pain was 0.99 (on a 10-point scale), a 79.2% improvement. Two studies (7.69%) used Bach's criteria of pain and activity (BCPA) and Bach's criteria of pain activity limitation (BCPAL).[9] Across 34 patients, the BCPA improved from 4.32 preoperatively to 1.96 postoperatively, a 54.6% improvement; the BCPAL improved from 4.21 preoperatively to 1.77 postoperatively, a 57.9% improvement.
- Across all studies, regardless of metric, postoperative pain was improved at least 50% after vascularized bone grafting.

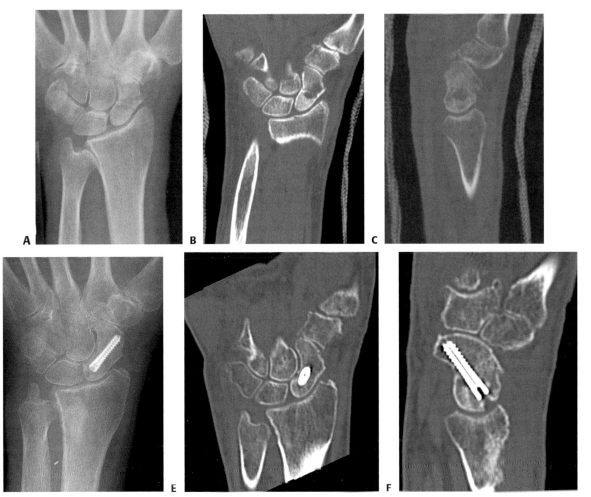

FIG 5 • **A–C.** Radiograph and CT scans showing chronic scaphoid nonunion, with cyst formation and osteolysis. **D–F.** Osseous union is seen following dorsal vascularized fourth + fifth extensor compartmental artery flap and compression screw.

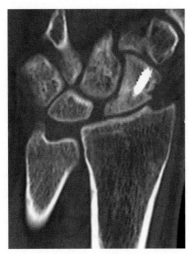

FIG 6 • Osseous union of the proximal scaphoid pole following medial femoral trochlea vascularized bone flap and compression screw.

- Previous studies have demonstrated that the ability to return to work and gainful employment have a significantly positive effect on the perceived health, physical function, and thus quality of life for individuals after injury.
- Vascularized bone grafting serves as a viable option to restore the normal anatomy of the radiocarpal joint and thus re-establish a patient's overall functionality.[6]

COMPLICATIONS

- The most common complication is superficial wound or pin site infection, nerve irritation, and complex regional pain syndrome (1.25%).
- Immediate postsurgical complications are typically only seen in microvascular cases with flap circulatory collapse.
- Errant osteotomies could potentially result in iatrogenic fracture of either the femur or distal radius.

REFERENCES

1. Dias JJ, Brenkel IJ, Finlay DB. Patterns of union in fractures of the waist of the scaphoid. *J Bone Joint Surg Br.* 1989;71(2):307-310.
2. Szabo RM, Manske D. Displaced fractures of the scaphoid. *Clin Orthop Relat Res.* 1988;230:30-38.
3. Mack GR, Bosse MJ, Gelberman RH, Yu E. The natural history of scaphoid non-union. *J Bone Joint Surg Am.* 1984;66(4):504-509.
4. Ruby LK, Leslie BM. Wrist arthritis associated with scaphoid non-union. *Hand Clin.* 1987;3(4):529-539.
5. Steinmann SP, Adams JE. Scaphoid fractures and nonunions: diagnosis and treatment. *J Orthop Sci.* 2006;11(4):424-431.
6. Shin AY, Bishop AT. Pedicled vascularized bone grafts for disorders of the carpus: scaphoid nonunion and Kienbock's disease. *J Am Acad Orthop Surg.* 2002;10(3):210-216.
7. Iorio ML, Masden DL, Higgins JP. The limits of medial femoral condyle corticoperiosteal flaps. *J Hand Surg [Am].* 2011;36(10):1592-1596.
8. Trumble TE, Clarke T, Kreder HJ. Non-union of the scaphoid: treatment with cannulated screws compared with treatment with Herbert screws. *J Bone Joint Surg Am.* 1996;78(12):1829-1837.
9. Bach AW, Almquist EE, Newman DM. Proximal row fusion as a solution for radiocarpal arthritis. *J Hand Surg [Am].* 1991;16(3):424-431.

Open Reduction and Fixation of Acute Perilunate Fracture Dislocation

CHAPTER 20

Grant M. Kleiber and Amy M. Moore

DEFINITION

- Perilunate dislocation refers to a pattern of ligamentous injuries and/or fractures involving the carpus. In a perilunate dislocation, the lunate remains in its anatomic position, and there is dorsal dislocation of the carpus in relation to the lunate.
- In a lunate dislocation, the lunate is volarly displaced outside of the lunate facet.
- Lesser arc injury refers to a purely ligamentous injury pattern.
- Greater arc injury implies at least one fracture in addition to the perilunate dislocation, the most common being the scaphoid and radial styloid.
- In the event of a greater arc injury, the injury pattern and the fractures are described using the nomenclature "trans-[fractured bone]" in addition to "perilunate dislocation." For example, a perilunate dislocation with a radial styloid and scaphoid fracture would be described as a "transradial styloid, trans-scaphoid perilunate dislocation."

ANATOMY

- The carpus is constrained by a network of dorsal and volar radiocarpal (extrinsic) and intercarpal (intrinsic) ligaments (**FIG 1**).

- The lunate is constrained by extrinsic ligaments on its volar surface only: the long radiolunate, short radiolunate, and ulnolunate ligaments.
- The lunate is constrained by intrinsic intercarpal ligaments on its radial and ulnar edges: the scapholunate and lunotriquetral ligaments.
- The scapholunate ligament is strongest at its dorsal aspect, whereas the lunotriquetral ligament is strongest at its volar aspect.
- The space of Poirier is an area of weakness in the volar wrist capsule, allowing the midcarpal joint to expand and contract during wrist motion. It is located between the radioscaphocapitate and the long radiolunate ligaments (see **FIG 1**).

PATHOGENESIS

- The biomechanical forces resulting in a perilunate dislocation are wrist hyperextension, ulnar deviation, and intercarpal supination.
- In a dorsal perilunate dislocation, there is rupture of the scapholunate and lunotriquetral ligaments, causing the carpus to dislocate dorsally off of the lunate.
- The lunate protrudes through the volar wrist capsule through the space of Poirier.

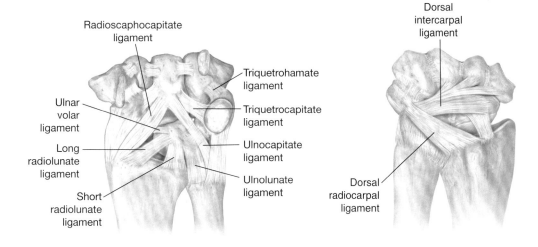

A   Volar   **B**   Dorsal

FIG 1 • **A:** The volar ligaments of the wrist include from radial to ulnar: radioscaphocapitate (RSC), long radiolunate (LRL), short radiolunate (SRL), ulnolunate (UL), and lunocapitate (UC), which overlies the ulnocapitate. Distally, the triquetrohamate and triquetrocapitate ligament stabilize the ulnar carpus (THC). The space of Poirier lies proximal to the arc between the radial and ulnar volar ligaments. **B:** The dorsal ligaments include the dorsal intercarpal ligament (DIC) and dorsal radiocarpal ligament (DRC).

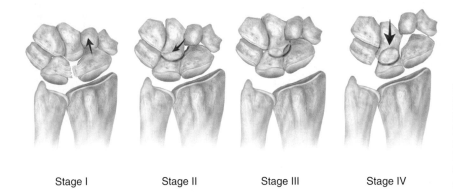

Stage I   Stage II   Stage III   Stage IV

FIG 2 • The Mayfield classification of perilunate injuries proposes a radial-to-ulnar progression of injury. In stage I, the scapholunate ligament is ruptured. Stage II is disruption of the capitolunate articulation. Stage III is disruption of the lunotriquetral ligament and dorsal dislocation of the carpus from the lunate. Stage IV is volar dislocation of the lunate out of the lunate fossa of the radius.

- The short radiolunate ligament typically remains intact in a perilunate dislocation, tethering the volar lunate to the volar lip of the radius.
- Mayfield classified perilunate dislocations as a progression of injury from radial to ulnar around the lunate[1] (**FIG 2**):
  - Stage I: Scapholunate disruption with rotation of scaphoid
  - Stage II: Capitolunate dissociation
  - Stage III: Lunotriquetral ligament rupture, dislocation of carpus dorsal to lunate
  - Stage IV: Lunate dislocation: lunate is dislocated volarly out of the lunate fossa.
- In a greater arc injury, there is transmission of force through the bony structures surrounding the lunate, resulting in at least one fracture in addition to the perilunate dislocation (**FIG 3**).

PATIENT HISTORY AND PHYSICAL FINDINGS

- Patients typically report a high-energy injury such as a fall from height or a motor vehicle collision.
- A full trauma workup should be initiated depending on the mechanism of injury.

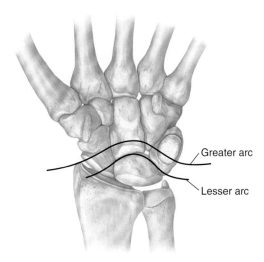

Greater arc

Lesser arc

FIG 3 • A lesser arc injury refers to a purely ligamentous pattern of injury, as described in the Mayfield classification. A greater arc injury describes the injury pattern traveling through at least one bony structure, such as the radial styloid, scaphoid, capitate, triquetrum, or ulnar styloid.

- Patients may present with acute carpal tunnel syndrome, with symptoms ranging from paresthesias to severe burning pain in their median-innervated digits.
- The examiner should perform a complete neurovascular examination of the hand including two-point discrimination to document sensory disturbance.
- The wrist is evaluated for edema, gross deformity, and tenderness.
  - Ecchymosis and edema over the volar wrist are often seen.

IMAGING

- Standard three-view wrist radiographs (PA, lateral, oblique) are sufficient for diagnosis in most cases.
- AP views demonstrate irregularity of the carpal rows, with a triangular lunate silhouette superimposed over other bones (**FIG 4A**).
- Lateral views shows the lunate tipped volarly relative to the remainder of the carpus in a "spilled teacup" sign (**FIG 4B**).
- In trans-scaphoid perilunate injuries, the displaced scaphoid proximal pole is seen attached to the lunate (**FIG 4C,D**).
- A CT scan may be helpful to identify and characterize carpal fractures in greater arc perilunate dislocations. Ideally, this study would be performed after reduction of the carpus.

DIFFERENTIAL DIAGNOSIS

- Scapholunate dissociation
- Scaphoid fracture
- Radiocarpal dislocation

NONOPERATIVE MANAGEMENT

- Closed reduction of the lunate should be attempted in all patients using the Tavernier maneuver (**FIG 5**).
- Conscious sedation is recommended for patient comfort and relaxation—facilitating reduction.
- The Tavernier maneuver:
  - The wrist is extended and the lunate is palpated volarly with the examiner's thumb.
  - Axial traction is placed on the patient's wrist, and gentle pressure is applied to the volar aspect of the lunate.
  - The wrist is then flexed forward while maintaining axial traction and volar pressure on the lunate. Successful reduction is often accompanied by a palpable "clunk."
  - Wrist radiographs are taken in traction to verify reduction, and a sugar tong splint is applied.
  - If reduction is unsuccessful, an open reduction should be performed in the operating room in an urgent manner.

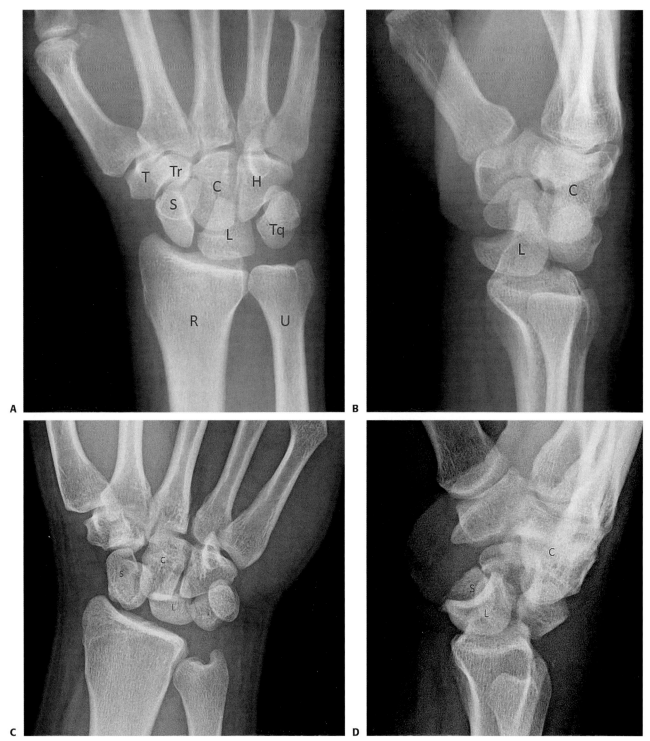

FIG 4 • A. AP radiograph of a perilunate dislocation demonstrates disruption of carpal rows and a triangle-shaped lunate (L) superimposed over the midcarpal joint. **B.** Lateral radiograph of a perilunate dislocation demonstrates dorsal translation of the carpus off the lunate, which is flexed forward. In this case, the lunate remains located within the lunate fossa of the radius. **C.** AP radiograph of a trans-scaphoid perilunate dislocation. The triangular shape of the lunate and disruption of the carpal arcs are demonstrated. **D.** Lateral radiograph demonstrates that in a trans-scaphoid perilunate dislocation the proximal pole of the scaphoid remains attached the lunate. The remainder of the carpus is dislocated dorsally. T, trapezium; Tr, trapezoid; C, capitate; H, hamate; S, scaphoid; Tq, triquetrum; R, radius; U, ulna.

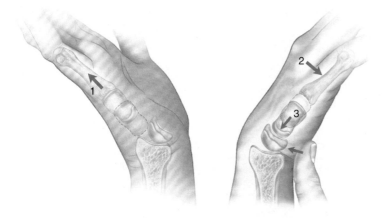

FIG 5 • The Tavernier's maneuver consists of (*1*) applying distal traction on the wrist while stabilizing the lunate with the opposite thumb. (*2*) The wrist is then extended and volar pressure is applied on the lunate to prevent dislocation into the carpal tunnel. (*3*) With traction and the lunate stabilized, the distal carpal row is reduced over the lunate into position with gentle wrist flexion.

SURGICAL MANAGEMENT

- If successful closed reduction is achieved, operative intervention and reconstruction can be performed several days later as a scheduled procedure but ideally within 1 week.
- Irreducible dislocations must be treated urgently to prevent median nerve impingement and devascularization of the lunate and displaced carpal bones.
- A surgical option for irreducible dislocations or for less experienced hand surgeons taking call is to take the patient to the operating room urgently for the volar approach to the carpus. An extended carpal tunnel release is performed to decompress the median nerve followed by open reduction of the carpus and repair of the volar lunotriquetral ligament and capsule. The dorsal approach can then later be performed by surgeons with expertise in the wrist.

Preoperative Planning

- As discussed previously, careful neurological exam should be performed including two-point discrimination to determine the baseline median nerve function.
- Any surgical equipment, such as hardware or suture anchors, should be available.
- A perilunate dislocation can be performed under regional or general anesthesia.

Positioning

- The patient is positioned supine with affected arm on a radiolucent hand table centered on the patient's axilla.
- A well-padded pneumatic tourniquet is placed on the upper arm.
- If an assistant is not available to assist with traction, end table traction with finger traps and 5 to 10 lb of weight will facilitate dissection and reduction during the procedure.

Approach

- A combined dorsal and volar approach is recommended for perilunate dislocations.
- Dorsal approach

- A 6- to 8-cm longitudinal incision centered over ulnar aspect of the Lister tubercle between the third and fourth extensor compartments provides good exposure. The radiocarpal and midcarpal joints are then exposed using a ligament-sparing capsulotomy, splitting the dorsal radiocarpal and dorsal intercarpal ligaments (**FIG 6**).[2]
- The dorsal approach is required in all patients for ligament repair and stabilization.
- Volar approach
  - A standard carpal tunnel release incision is extended across the wrist crease in a zigzag fashion for 2 to 3 cm.
  - The volar approach adds the benefit of open reduction of the lunate under direct visualization, volar lunotriquetral ligament repair, volar capsular repair, and median nerve decompression via the extended carpal tunnel release.

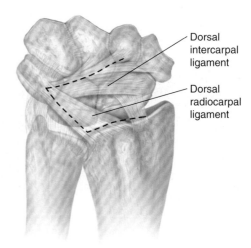

Dorsal intercarpal ligament

Dorsal radiocarpal ligament

Dorsal

FIG 6 • A dorsal ligament-sparing capsulotomy splits the dorsal radiocarpal (DRC) and dorsal intercarpal (DIC) ligaments, maintaining their fibers in continuity for added dorsal stabilization of the wrist with closure. (From Berger RA, Bishop AT. A fiber-splitting capsulotomy technique for dorsal exposure of the wrist. *Tech Hand Up Extrem Surg.* 1997;1:2-10.)

■ Lesser Arc Perilunate Dislocation

Volar Approach with Extended Carpal Tunnel Release and Open Reduction

- An extended carpal tunnel incision is made, crossing at least 2 to 3 cm proximal to the wrist crease.
- The transverse carpal ligament is divided along its ulnar aspect to avoid the median nerve, which may be displaced due to presence of the lunate within the carpal tunnel. As the carpal tunnel is released, blood is typically seen in this space.
- The antebrachial fascia is released proximally under direct vision, and the median nerve and flexor tendons are retracted radially.
- The lunate is visualized within the carpal tunnel, protruding from the volar wrist capsule and typically in a flexed position (**TECH FIG 1**). It is gently reduced into its anatomic position with axial traction on the wrist and gentle extension and pressure on the lunate.
- The volar lunotriquetral ligament is visualized and is repaired with nonabsorbable suture.
- The crescent-shaped tear in the volar wrist capsule is also repaired with nonabsorbable suture.

Dorsal Approach with Ligament Repair

Exposure

- The wrist is approached dorsally through a 6- to 8-cm incision centered on the ulnar aspect of the Lister tubercle via the third and fourth extensor compartments.
- Blunt dissection is carried over the extensor retinaculum to raise subcutaneous flaps radially and ulnarly. The radial sensory nerve and dorsal cutaneous branch of the ulnar nerve are identified and protected throughout the case.
- The extensor retinaculum is incised over the EPL tendon, which is transposed out of the retinaculum.
- The extensor retinaculum is then raised off of the fourth dorsal compartment and the second dorsal compartment, entering each through the open third compartment. Self-retaining retractors are placed, exposing the wrist capsule.
- A ligament-sparing capsulotomy is performed to enter the wrist joint, splitting the fibers of the dorsal radiocarpal ligament and the dorsal intercarpal ligament. A radially based capsular flap is raised by extending the proximal incision radially along the dorsal radius (**TECH FIG 2**).[2,3]
- The scaphoid, lunate, and triquetrum are visualized. Dorsal remnants of the scapholunate and lunotriquetral ligaments are identified. Typically, the ligaments are torn asymmetrically, with a larger piece on one side of the joint.

Reduction and Fixation

- Suture anchors are inserted in preparation for ligament repair. The anchor is inserted to the side of the joint with the smaller ligament fragment, so the sutures may be passed through the larger fragment.
  - Fluoroscopic imaging and direct visualization are used to ensure adequate placement of the anchors.
- The scaphoid is typically found to be flexed, and the lunate is extended. To correct the scapholunate angle, a 0.062-in. K-wire is inserted into the dorsum of the scaphoid and the lunate to act as a joystick.
- Using the K-wire joysticks, the scaphoid and lunate are aligned under lateral fluoroscopy to restore a scapholunate angle of 40 to 55 degrees (**TECH FIG 3A**). The K-wires can be provisionally secured together with a hemostat to hold this reduction.
  - Another option is to place a radiolunate K-wire to hold the reduced lunate in place and then the scaphoid can be reduced to the lunate using the K-wire joystick (**TECH FIG 3B**).
- The sutures attached to the anchors are now passed through the scapholunate and lunotriquetral ligaments and left untied until intercarpal pins are placed.
- Intercarpal pins are placed using 0.045-in. K-wires. Pins are placed to stabilize the scapholunate interval and the lunotriquetral interval.

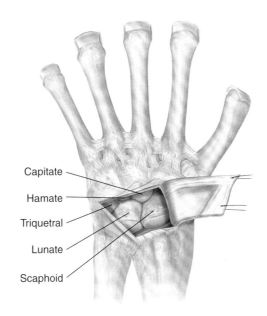

Capitate
Hamate
Triquetral
Lunate
Scaphoid

TECH FIG 2 • Using a ligament-sparing capsulotomy, a radially based capsular flap is raised to expose the carpus. (From Berger RA, Bishop AT. A fiber-splitting capsulotomy technique for dorsal exposure of the wrist. *Tech Hand Up Extrem Surg.* 1997;1:2-10.)

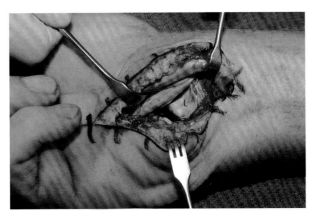

TECH FIG 1 • On volar approach to the wrist, the lunate (L) is seen protruding into the carpal tunnel through a crescent shaped rent in the volar wrist capsule.

- A scaphocapitate pin is placed to stabilize the scaphoid from flexing (**TECH FIG 3C**). Pins are buried beneath the skin to avoid pin-tract infection that invariably will occur when pins are left outside the skin for more than a few weeks.
- AP and lateral fluoroscopic radiographs are taken to ensure adequate reduction of the SL and LT interval, and a scapholunate angle of 40 to 55 degrees (**TECH FIG 3D**).

- If these films are satisfactory, the suture anchors are tied down.
- The wrist is irrigated copiously with normal saline to ensure no remaining osteochondral debris is present in the articular space.
- The capsulotomy, followed by the extensor retinaculum, is then closed with nonabsorbable sutures.

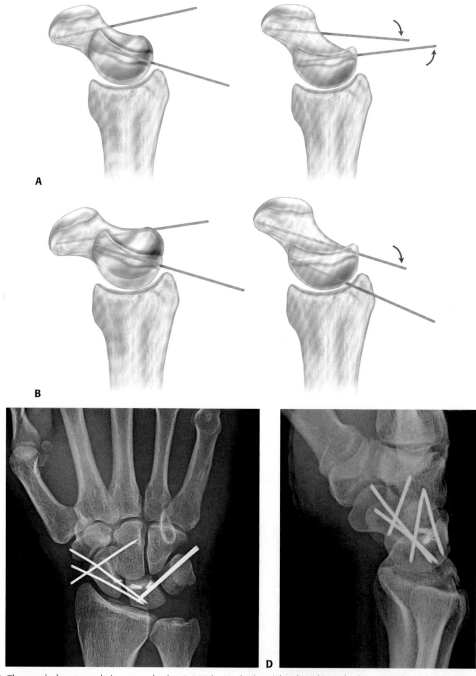

TECH FIG 3 • **A.** The scapholunate angle is restored using 0.062-in. K-wire joysticks placed into the lunate and scaphoid. These can be secured together with a hemostat to hold the reduction temporarily. **B.** Another option is to reduce the lunate and then place a radiolunate K-wire to stabilize the lunate. The scaphoid can then be reduced to the lunate to restore the scapholunate angle using a joystick. **C.** AP radiograph demonstrates that the carpus is stabilized with 0.045-in. K-wires after suture anchors have been place for reconstruction of the ligaments. Two K-wires are placed in the scapholunate and lunotriquetral intervals. A scaphocapitate (and/or a triquetrocapitate) K-wire can also be placed to stabilize the capitolunate joint if found to be unstable. **D.** Lateral view of carpus after K-wire stabilization and ligament repair demonstrates restoration of acceptable scapholunate angle.

■ Repair of Greater Arc Injury

Trans-scaphoid Perilunate Dislocation

- Greater arc injuries result in a fracture of an adjacent bone accompanying the perilunate dislocation. The scaphoid is the most common bone involved (**TECH FIG 4A,B**).
- The same volar and dorsal approaches are used as outlined above.
- The scapholunate ligament is most often intact in a trans-scaphoid perilunate dislocation (**TECH FIG 4C**), and the proximal pole of the scaphoid is displaced with the lunate (see **FIG 4D**).
- The scaphoid fracture is reduced under direct vision, aligning the cartilaginous surface of the scaphoid.
  - Joystick K-wires can be placed in the proximal and distal poles to aid in reduction and stabilization.

- The scaphoid is fixated with a dorsal cannulated compression screw using standard technique, with the caveat that the fracture will be less stable than typical scaphoid fractures.
- Use of distal radius bone graft is encouraged if significant comminution of the scaphoid is found. The graft can be easily taken from under the Lister tubercle in the same exposure.
- A guidewire is placed for a cannulated screw along the axis of the scaphoid, beginning proximally at the center of the membranous portion of the scapholunate ligament
- An antirotation parallel wire should be placed alongside the guidewire to stabilize the scaphoid fracture for overdrilling the guidewire.
  - Most cannulated screw systems have a parallel wire guide for placement of this wire. This step is highly recommended due to the instability of the fracture.

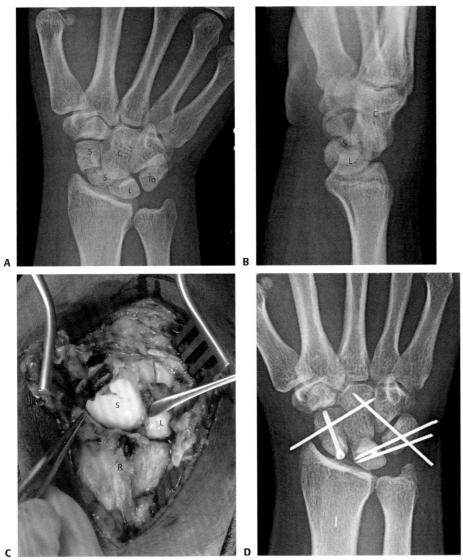

TECH FIG 4 • A. AP radiograph demonstrates a trans-scaphoid perilunate dislocation. In this greater arc injury, there is a scaphoid (S) waist fracture instead of a scapholunate ligament injury. **B.** The proximal pole of the scaphoid remains attached to the lunate (L) and flexes with it **C.** Image of right wrist demonstrates scaphoid fracture with intact scapholunate ligament (*). **D and E.** AP and lateral radiographs of open reduction and fixation of a trans-scaphoid perilunate injury with K-wire stabilization of the carpus and cannulated screw fixation of the scaphoid. C, capitate; R, radius Tq, triquetrum.

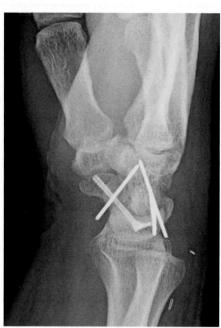

E

TECH FIG 4 (Continued)

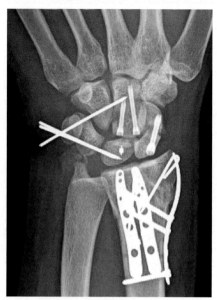

TECH FIG 5 • AP radiograph of a greater arc transradial styloid, trans-scaphoid, transcapitate perilunate dislocation. The distal radius fracture was treated with fragment-specific fixation, and cannulated screws were to repair the capitate and scaphoid fractures.

- The guidewire is measured and overdrilled, and an appropriately sized cannulated compression screw is placed over the wire.
- A scaphocapitate K-wire can be placed to further stabilize the lunocapitate joint as well as reinforce the scaphoid fixation if comminuted.
- The lunotriquetral ligament is repaired with suture anchors in the same manner described above, and the lunotriquetral interval is pinned with 0.045-in. K-wires (**TECH FIG 4D,E**).

Transradial Styloid, Trans-scaphoid, Transcapitate Perilunate Dislocation

- Greater arc injuries result in a fracture of an adjacent bone accompanying the perilunate dislocation. The scaphoid is the most common bone involved, and the technique for fixation of a trans-scaphoid perilunate is outlined above.
- Radial styloid fractures involving greater than one-third of the scaphoid fossa should be repaired to stabilize the volar ligamentous attachments.[4] This can be performed with cannulated screw fixation or a radial column pin plate. Anatomic alignment of the articular surface is critical.

- Transverse capitate fractures may be managed with cannulated compression screws, allowing the screws to be buried beneath the articular surface (**TECH FIG 5**).

Perilunate Dislocation Reconstruction with Posterior Interosseous Neurectomy

- The terminal branch of the posterior interosseous nerve (PIN) runs in the floor of the fourth dorsal compartment. It provides sensory innervation to the wrist joint.
- Perilunate dislocation and its subsequent reconstruction result in significant capsular trauma to the wrist joint. A PIN neurectomy should be strongly considered as an adjunctive procedure to decrease postoperative pain and improve long-term outcomes.
- The PIN can be consistently found 3 to 4 cm proximal and 1 cm ulnar to Lister tubercle, beneath the tendons of the fourth dorsal compartment.
- The nerve is carefully dissected free from the artery for a distance of 2 to 3 cm. The nerve is crushed proximally with a hemostat and distally 1 to 2 cm is resected. The proximal nerve is then cauterized.
- The proximal nerve end is transposed proximally along the course of the nerve, burying it beneath the forearm musculature to prevent symptomatic neuroma formation.

PEARLS AND PITFALLS

Irreducible perilunate dislocation	■ A closed reduction should be attempted in the emergency room under sedation. ■ If unable to reduce, open reduction should be performed in the operating room in an urgent fashion to decompress the median nerve and improve vascular supply to the displaced carpus.
Median nerve compression	■ Acute carpal tunnel syndrome commonly accompanies perilunate dislocation. These patients should be treated with urgent median nerve decompression and relocation of the lunate through a volar approach. ■ Carpal tunnel release should be performed in all patients due to trauma to the median nerve from the perilunate dislocation.
Technique: Ligament repairs	■ Suture anchors can be use to repair the scapholunate and/or lunotriquetral ligaments. ■ The anchors should be placed prior to the reduction and K-wire fixation of the interval to allow best visualization. ■ Once the interval is reduced and stabilized with K-wires, the sutures can be tied and secured.
Scapholunate angle	■ A normal scapholunate angle between 30 and 60 degrees should be restored, ideally between 40 to 55 degrees. ■ Place joystick K-wires into the scaphoid and lunate to extend the scaphoid and flex the lunate into an anatomic position (see **TECH FIG 3A**). ■ The lunate can also be stabilized with a temporary radiolunate pin (see **TECH FIG 3B**).
Posterior interosseous neurectomy	■ A PIN neurectomy should be strongly considered at the time of ligament repair to decrease postoperative pain. ■ The nerve is found in the floor of the fourth dorsal compartment.

POSTOPERATIVE CARE

■ The patient is placed in a sugar tong splint for 2 weeks, followed by 8 to 10 weeks of thumb spica cast immobilization.

■ K-wires are removed at 8 to 10 weeks. Burying pins beneath the skin results in fewer issues with pin-tract infections, but they may require removal in the OR.

■ Gentle range of motion exercises are begun after K-wire removal. Hand therapy is initiated to regain wrist motion.

■ A protective removable splint is worn between therapy sessions until pain and range of motion has stabilized. For greater arc injuries, the splint is worn until union is achieved.

OUTCOMES

■ Patients should expect decreased wrist range of motion, particularly flexion and extension, after this significant injury (**FIG 7**). Near-normal prono-supination is typically restored.
  ■ Total arc of motion for flexion/extension is reported from 57% to 83% of the contralateral side.[5–10]

■ A recent retrospective review of 65 cases reported that 85% of patients were able to return to their previous occupation.[5]

■ Despite adequate fixation and intervention, most patients (range 18%–92%) develop radiographic signs of radiocarpal and midcarpal arthrosis over time.[6,11]
  ■ In a study by Forli et al.,[6] 67% of their patients developed post-traumatic degenerative changes; however, they report that the arthrosis is well tolerated at an average follow-up of 13 years.

■ Proximal row carpectomy can be considered as a secondary salvage procedure in patients with avascular necrosis of the lunate or in delayed unrecognized perilunate dislocation.[12]

COMPLICATIONS

■ Multiple complications can result from the severe wrist trauma at the time of injury, as well as, from the operative procedure itself.

■ Complex regional pain syndrome has been reported to occur in up to 12% of patients.[5]

■ K-wire/pin-tract infections can occur.

■ Osteonecrosis of lunate or scaphoid has been reported at rate of about 8%.[5]

■ Carpal bone nonunion such as in trans-scaphoid perilunate dislocation is rare.[6,9]

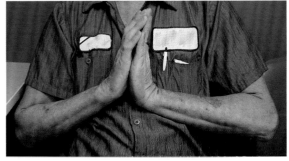
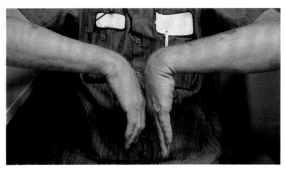

FIG 7 • At 6 months postoperatively, functional extension **(A)** and flexion **(B)** have been restored. However, range of motion is decreased compared to the uninjured hand.

REFERENCES

1. Mayfield JK, Johnson RP, Kilcoyne RK. Carpal dislocations: pathomechanics and progressive perilunar instability. *J Hand Surg [Am]*. 1980;5:226-241.
2. Berger RA, Bishop AT. A fiber-splitting capsulotomy technique for dorsal exposure of the wrist. *Tech Hand Up Extrem Surg*. 1997;1:2-10.
3. Berger RA, Bishop AT, Bettinger PC. New dorsal capsulotomy for the surgical exposure of the wrist. *Ann Plast Surg*. 1995;35:54-59.
4. Dumontier C, Meyer zu Reckendorf G, Sautet A, et al. Radiocarpal dislocations: classification and proposal for treatment: a review of twenty-seven cases. *J Bone Joint Surg Am*. 2001;83-A:212-218.
5. Israel D, Delclaux S, Andre A, et al. Peri-lunate dislocation and fracture-dislocation of the wrist: retrospective evaluation of 65 cases. *Orthop Tramatol Surg Res*. 2016;102:351-355.
6. Forli A, Courvoisier A, Wimsey S, Corcella D. Perilunate dislocations and transscaphoid perilunate fracture-dislocations: a retrospective study with minimum ten-year follow-up. *J Hand Surg [Am]*. 2010;35:62-68.
7. Sotereanos DG, Mitsionis GJ, Giannakopoulos PN, et al. Perilunate dislocation and fracture dislocation: a critical analysis of the volar-dorsal approach. *J Hand Surg [Am]*. 1997;22:49-56.
8. Trumble T, Verheyden J. Treatment of isolated perilunate and lunate dislocations with combined dorsal and volar approach and intraosseous cerclage wire. *J Hand Surg [Am]*. 2004;29:412-417.
9. Knoll VD, Allan C, Trumble TE. Trans-scaphoid perilunate fracture dislocations: results of screw fixation of the scaphoid and lunotriquetral repair with a dorsal approach. *J Hand Surg [Am]*. 2005;30:1145-1152.
10. Hildebrand KA, Ross DC, Patterson SD, et al. Dorsal perilunate dislocations and fracture-dislocations: questionnaire, clinical, and radiographic evaluation. *J Hand Surg [Am]*. 2000;25:1069-1079.
11. Herzberg G, Forissier D. Acute dorsal trans-scaphoid perilunate fracture-dislocations: medium-term results. *J Hand Surg Br*. 2002;27:498-502.
12. Rettig ME, Raskin KB. Long-term assessment of proximal row carpectomy for chronic perilunate dislocations. *J Hand Surg [Am]*. 1999;24:1231-1236.

Dorsal Capsulodesis for Scapholunate Stabilization With Extensor Carpi Radialis Longus Tenodesis

21

CHAPTER

Mark Morris and Kevin C. Chung

DEFINITION

- Scapholunate (SL) dissociation is the most common cause of carpal instability.
- SL dissociation can result in static or dynamic carpal instability.
  - Static instability: Radiographic changes are seen on standard wrist radiographs.
  - Dynamic instability: Standard radiographs are normal, but signs of instability are seen on stress radiographs.
- Partial SL interosseous ligament tears do not produce radiographic changes and often require arthroscopy for diagnosis.
- SL dissociation left untreated leads to dorsal intercalated instability (DISI) and eventually scapholunate advanced collapse (SLAC).[1]

ANATOMY, PATIENT HISTORY, AND PHYSICAL FINDINGS, IMAGING

- See Chapter 15 in the Hand section.

SURGICAL MANAGEMENT

- Dividing the SL interosseous ligament leads to altered radiocarpal kinematics and causes abnormal radiocarpal and ulnocarpal pressure distributions.[2,3]
- The radioscaphoid joint is normally congruent. However, when the scaphoid is subluxed because of SL instability, the load is shifted and abnormal contact points are created, leading to degenerative changes (**FIG 1**).[4]
- The goal of dorsal capsulodesis and extensor carpi radialis longus (ECRL) transfer is to maintain the extended position of the scaphoid in order to restore normal carpal alignment and avoid abnormal radiocarpal contact pressures that otherwise lead to pain and degenerative changes.
- Capsulodesis alone is contraindicated if there is static SL dissociation, whereas ECRL tendon transfer can be performed with static SL dissociation as long as reduction is possible in the operating room. Either procedure is contraindicated if radiocarpal or midcarpal degenerative changes are present.
- Capsulodesis is indicated for predynamic SL instability secondary to an isolated partial SL ligament tear (seen on arthroscopy) and for dynamic SL instability with intact secondary stabilizers and a technically repairable dorsal capsule.
- The main advantage of dorsal capsulodesis over tendon transfer is the technical ease of the procedure.
  - The disadvantage of dorsal capsulodesis is the predilection for attenuation of the repair over time and progressive carpal collapse.[5] Tendon transfer provides increased

strength of repair and the ability to maintain reduction of the scaphoid over time.

- Additionally, with a capsulodesis, the scaphoid is theoretically still unstable through much of the arc of wrist motion until it reaches the limit of flexion set by the capsulodesis. In contrast, a dynamic transfer should provide an extension force to the scaphoid throughout the entire range of wrist motion.[6]
- ECRL transfer to the scaphoid can be used as an alternative to capsulodesis for treatment of a partial SL ligament tear. ECRL transfer can be performed if the capsule is not technically repairable, which would obviously preclude capsulodesis.
- The ECRL tendon transfer was designed to re-establish a fluid scaphoid slider-crank motion and restore midcarpal kinematics without tethering the scaphoid or limiting wrist flexion.
  - A slider-crank mechanism converts linear motion to rotatory motion or vice versa, such as with a piston and crank shaft of an engine.
  - The slider-crank model of the wrist described by Linscheid et al.[7] explains wrist kinematics as a three-bar linkage

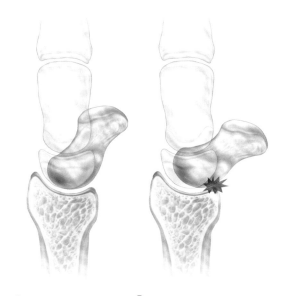

A **B**

FIG 1 • A. Normal orientation of the scaphoid and radius shows a congruent articulation between the scaphoid and the scaphoid facet of the radius. **B.** An area of abnormal loading of the radioscaphoid joint occurs when the scaphoid undergoes rotary subluxation. Disproportionate loading of the joint leads to degenerative changes.

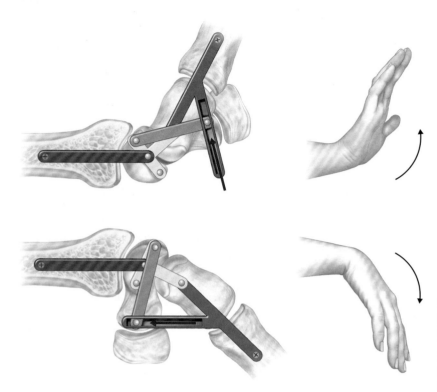

FIG 2 • The slider-crank model of the wrist joint posits a three-bar link between the radius, lunate, and capitate, with the scaphoid acting as the crank. The *red arrows* show the direction of force produced by the crank mechanism—a dorsally directed compressive force with extension of the wrist and a palmarly directed tensile force with flexion of the wrist.

composed of the radius, lunate, and capitate. The three bars are stabilized by the scaphoid, which acts as the crank. When the wrist is extended, the scaphoid "crank" causes dorsal rotation of the lunate by a dorsally directed compressive force. With flexion, the scaphoid causes flexion of the lunate via a palmarly directed tensile force (**FIG 2**).

- ECRL tendon transfer provides a consistent extension force to the scaphoid throughout the range of motion, as opposed to a dorsal capsulodesis, which acts merely as a checkrein to flexion of the scaphoid. By doing so, the scaphoid is able to influence the kinematics of the wrist throughout the arc of motion rather than just at the point limited by the checkrein.

Preoperative Planning

- Wrist arthroscopy has become the standard method of evaluation of interosseous ligament injuries. Geissler grading of ligament injuries as seen during arthroscopy is as follows[8]:
  - Grade 1: Attenuation/hemorrhage of interosseous ligament as seen from the radiocarpal joint. No incongruency of carpal alignment in the midcarpal space.
  - Grade 2: Attenuation/hemorrhage of interosseous ligament as seen from the radiocarpal joint. Incongruency/step-off as seen from the midcarpal space. A small gap may be seen between the carpal bones but smaller than the width of a probe.
  - Grade 3: Complete ligament tear seen from the radiocarpal joint. Incongruency/step-off of carpal alignment is seen from both the radiocarpal and midcarpal spaces. The probe can be passed through the gap between carpal bones.

- Grade 4: Complete ligament tear is seen from radiocarpal joint. Incongruency/step-off of carpal alignment is seen from both the radiocarpal and midcarpal spaces. Arthroscope (2.7 mm) can be passed through the gap in the carpal bones. Gross instability with manipulation.

Positioning

- The patient is positioned supine on the operating table. The operative arm is on a hand table.
- Regional or general anesthesia can be used.
- A tourniquet is applied.
- An examination under anesthesia is performed to check for instability.

Approach

- A dorsal approach to the wrist is utilized, centered over the Lister tubercle (**FIG 3**).
- The third dorsal compartment is identified but does not need to be opened in most cases.
- Dissection is performed between the second and fourth compartments to expose the scaphoid and lunate.

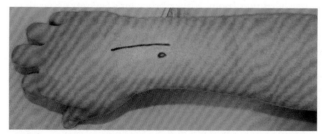

FIG 3 • A dorsal incision is centered over the Lister tubercle.

■ Dorsal Capsulodesis for Scapholunate Instability Using Suture Anchors

Exposure

- A 6-cm dorsal longitudinal incision is made, centered over the radiocarpal joint in line with the long finger metacarpal.
- Sharp dissection is carried down to the extensor retinaculum.
- Skin and subcutaneous tissue flaps are raised.
- The second and fourth compartments are elevated such that the tendons are maintained within the compartment.
- The wrist capsule is incised longitudinally to expose the scaphoid and lunate.
- The remaining dorsal SL ligament is assessed (**TECH FIG 1**).

Reduction

- Two 0.062-in. K-wires are placed into the dorsal scaphoid and lunate to act as joysticks for reduction.
- The scaphoid wire is retracted proximally to extend the scaphoid. The lunate wire is retracted distally to flex the lunate.
  - Fluoroscopy is used to evaluate the reduction.
- The assistant holds the scaphoid and lunate reduced using the joystick K-wires while the surgeon drills one K-wire percutaneously from the radial side of the wrist, through the scaphoid and lunate.

- A second K-wire is then drilled through the scaphoid into the capitate to prevent the scaphoid from rotating. This will hold the reduction.

Fixation

- A curette is used to debride the cortical bone from the distal dorsal scaphoid until cancellous bone is visible. This will provide a more favorable environment for healing the capsule to bone.
- Drill a hole using the Mitek anchor drill into the most distal part of the dorsal scaphoid. The drill hole should be placed adjacent to the scaphotrapezial joint, distal to the scaphoid axis of rotation. Place a 1.8-mm suture anchor (mini Mitek or similar) into the drill hole.
- Secure the dorsal capsule to the scaphoid by passing the suture from the anchor through the overlying capsule. Tie the suture securely to prevent the scaphoid from flexing.
- Final fixation is assessed fluoroscopically to confirm that the lunate is in neutral position and the carpal bones are aligned correctly (**TECH FIG 2**).
- The dorsal capsule is repaired using 3-0 Ethibond suture.

Closure

- The tourniquet is released and hemostasis is obtained.
- The extensor retinaculum is closed with 3-0 Ethibond suture.
- Skin is closed with a 4-0 Monocryl suture.

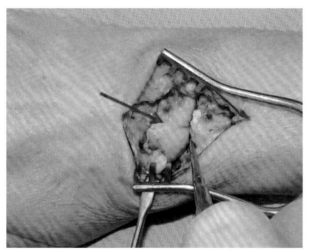

TECH FIG 1 • Exposure of the SL joint in this patient shows an intact dorsal SL ligament (*arrow*). This patient had normal wrist radiographs, and SL diastasis on wrist arthroscopy.

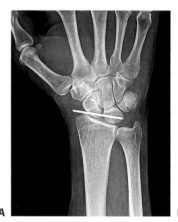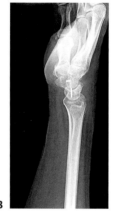

A   B

TECH FIG 2 • Postoperative AP and lateral radiographs show a suture anchor in the dorsal scaphoid and a K-wire traversing the SL joint.

■ Scapholunate Stabilization with Dynamic ECRL Tendon Transfer

Exposure and Reduction

- The skin incision is centered over the dorsal wrist joint between the third and fourth dorsal compartments and

extends from the Lister tubercle proximally to between the index and long finger metacarpal bases distally.
- Expose the ECRL and extensor carpi radialis brevis (ECRB) from the distal edge of the extensor retinaculum to their insertions on the index and long finger metacarpal bases, respectively.

- The extensor tendons are retracted ulnarly to expose the wrist capsule. The wrist capsule is incised longitudinally, just radial to the origin of the dorsal radiocarpal (DRC) ligament proximally and radial to the insertion of the dorsal intercarpal (DIC) ligament distally. This will expose the SL joint and the SL ligament tear.
- Reduce the scaphoid and lunate and pin in place, as described above in the capsulodesis section.

Tendon Transfer

- Prepare the ECRL tendon insertion site at the dorsal distal scaphoid (**TECH FIG 3A,B**).
- A trough is made the dorsal distal scaphoid in the same manner as described in the capsulodesis section, and one or two mini Mitek anchors are placed.
- Anchors can alternatively be placed after the tendon is harvested.
- To harvest the ECRL tendon, it is incised transversely from its insertion on the dorsal base of the second metacarpal (**TECH FIG 3C**).
- The tendon tension should be set to a length that will make it isotonic when docked into the scaphoid—the tendon transfer should provide equal tension to the scaphoid throughout the arc of wrist motion.
  - If the tendon is too short, tension will be too high with wrist flexion.
  - If the tendon is too long, tension will be too light with wrist extension.
- Any adhesions are released so the ECRL has full excursion.
- To secure the tendon transfer, extend the wrist and have the assistant retract the tendon distally to reach the scaphoid while the surgeon ties the tendon down tightly to the anchor. The tendon can otherwise retract during this step.

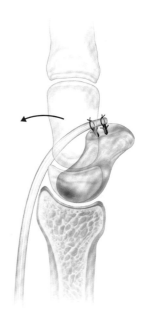

TECH FIG 4 • Two mini Mitek anchors secure the ECRL tendon graft, which pulls the scaphoid back into extension.

  - Use two mini Mitek anchors for more secure attachment (**TECH FIG 4**).

Closure

- The dorsal wrist capsule is closed with 3-0 Ethibond suture.
- The tourniquet is released and hemostasis is achieved prior to further closure.
- Skin is closed with a 4-0 Monocryl suture.

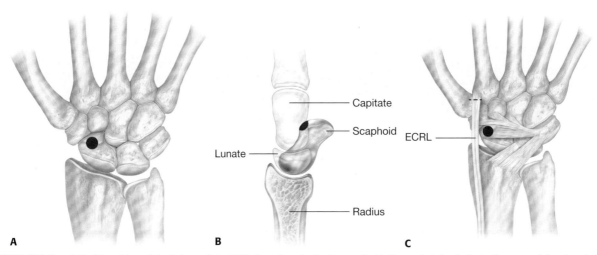

A   **B**   **C**

Capitate
Scaphoid
ECRL
Lunate
Radius

TECH FIG 3 • **A,B.** AP and lateral depictions of the ECRL insertion site in the scaphoid. The *red circles* indicate the area of the dorsal distal scaphoid to be curetted. **C.** The ECRL graft is harvested from the base of the second metacarpal. The *red circle* shows the location of the docking hole. The red line indicates where to transect the ECRL tendon from the insertion site on the index metacarpal base.

TECHNIQUES

PEARLS AND PITFALLS

Technique	■ When placing joystick K-wires, correction of the deformity will be easier if the scaphoid wire is directed proximally and the lunate wire is directed distally.
	■ When drilling a hole for a suture anchor, care must be taken to protect the vascular pedicle that inserts at the dorsal ridge of the scaphoid
	■ We recommend cutting K-wires under the skin to avoid pin tract infection. Infection is common when K-wires are left outside of the skin for more than 3 weeks.
Postoperative care	■ Wrist range of motion is expected to decrease by about 20%. Despite this, most patients have significant improvement in pain after this surgery.
Rehabilitation	■ Patients are instructed to avoid forceful axial loading of the wrist (especially activities like weight lifting or push-ups) for 6 months.

POSTOPERATIVE CARE

- Postoperatively, the patient is placed into a volar wrist splint for 8 weeks.
  - For capsulodesis, the wrist can be splinted in a neutral position.
  - After dynamic ECRL transfer or tenodesis, the wrist is splinted in 15 to 20 degrees of extension to prevent excessive tension at the ECRL insertion site.
- The wound is examined and sutures are removed (if nonabsorbable sutures are used) after 10 days.
- The K-wires are removed 6 to 8 weeks after the initial surgery.
- After 8 weeks of splinting, the patient is transitioned to a removable volar splint for an additional 4 weeks. Gentle active wrist range of motion can begin at this time.

OUTCOMES

- Dorsal capsulodesis
  - Gajendran et al.[9] studied 16 wrists in 15 patients who were treated with dorsal capsulodesis for chronic, flexible, static SL dissociation with follow-up of greater than 60 months (average 86 months). At final follow-up, average wrist flexion and extension were 50 and 55 degrees, respectively. Outcomes were also measured with disabilities of the arm, shoulder, and hand (DASH; average score 19), Short Form-12 (average score 78), and Mayo wrist score (average 78). Mayo scores were "excellent" in 38%, "good" in 19%, "fair" in 31%, and "poor" in 12% of patients. Grip strength was statistically unchanged from preoperative to final follow-up. Radiographs at final follow-up showed an average SL angle of 62 degrees, and an SL gap of 3.5 mm. Fifty percent of wrists (8/16) had evidence of arthritis on radiographs. Radiographic outcome did not correlate with subjective pain scores. The authors concluded that although dorsal capsulodesis did not prevent arthritic changes, patient satisfaction and functionality remained high after this surgery.
  - Megerle et al.[5] did a retrospective study of 59 patients who underwent dorsal capsulodesis, with a mean follow-up of 8.25 years (4.3–12 years). Although carpal alignment was significantly improved immediately postoperatively, results at long-term follow-up showed a return to preoperative alignment (mean SL angle 70 degrees at final follow-up). Eight patients required a salvage procedure at 2.33 years, and 10 patients had radiographic evidence

of arthritis at final follow-up. Mean DASH and Mayo wrist scores were 28 and 61, respectively. The authors concluded that although capsulodesis did not prevent degenerative changes, most patients had acceptable clinical outcomes at long-term follow-up.
- ECRL tenodesis: Bleuler et al.[10] studied 20 patients who were treated with dynamic ECRL tenodesis. All but one patient were satisfied with the functional outcome at short-term follow-up and would undergo the same surgery again if they had the choice. All patients were able to return to their former occupation between 1.5 and 4 months postoperatively.
- Combined ECRL tenodesis with dorsal capsulodesis: De Carli et al.[11] retrospectively reviewed 8 wrists in 8 patients who underwent combined ECRL tenodesis-capsulodesis for static SL dissociation with a minimum follow-up of 1 year (average 23 months). Average visual analog scale score (VAS: 0–10) postoperatively was 3. The mean DASH score was 13. Functional results were "excellent" in 2 cases and "good" in 6 cases. All patients lost some of their initial reduction on radiographs, but none had recurrence of carpal collapse.

COMPLICATIONS

- Infection
- Chronic regional pain syndrome
- Damage to the superficial radial nerve
- Loss of wrist range of motion
- Pin-tract infection
- Fracture

REFERENCES

1. Watson K, Ballet FL. The SLAC wrist: scapholunate advanced collapse pattern of degenerative arthritis. *J Hand Surg [Am]*. 1984;9:358-365.
2. Short WH, Werner FW, Green JK, Masaoka S. Biomechanical evaluation of the ligamentous stabilizers of the scaphoid and lunate. *J Hand Surg Am*. 2002;27A:991-1002.
3. Short WH, Werner FW, Fortino MD, et al. A dynamic biomechanical study of scapholunate ligament sectioning. *J Hand Surg Am*. 1995;20A:986-999.
4. Rajan PV, Day CS. Scapholunate interosseous ligament anatomy and biomechanics. *J Hand Surg Am*. 2015;40(8):1692-1702.
5. Megerle K, Bertel D, Germann G, et al. Long-term results of dorsal intercarpal ligament capsulodesis for the treatment of chronic scapholunate instability. *J Bone Joint Surg Br*. 2012;94B:1660-1665.
6. Bleuler P, Shafighi M, Donati OF, et al. Dynamic repair of scapholunate dissociation with dorsal extensor carpi radialis longus tenodesis. *J Hand Surg Am*. 2008;33A:281-284.

7. Linscheid RL, Dobyns JH, Beabout JW, Bryan RS. Traumatic instability of the wrist. Diagnosis, classification, and pathomechanics. *J Bone Joint Surg.* 1972;54(8):1612-1632.

8. Geissler WB. Arthroscopic management of scapholunate instability. *J Wrist Surg.* 2013;2(2):129-135.

9. Gajendran VK, Peterson B, Slater RR, Szabo RM. Long-term outcomes of dorsal intercarpal ligament capsulodesis for chronic scapholunate dissociation. *J Hand Surg Am.* 2007;32:1323-1333.

10. Bleuler P, Shafighi M, Donati OF, et al. Dynamic repair of scapholunate dissociation with dorsal extensor carpi radialis longus tenodesis. *J Hand Surg Am.* 2008;33A:281-284.

11. De Carli P, Donndorff A, Gallucci GL, et al. Chronic scapholunate dissociation: ligament reconstruction combining a new extensor carpi radialis longus tenodesis and a dorsal intercarpal ligament capsulodesis. *Tech Hand Up Extrem Surg.* 2011;15(1): 6-11.

Proximal Row Carpectomy

Patrick Reavey and Amy M. Moore

DEFINITION

- First described by Stamm,[1] proximal row carpectomy (PRC) is the removal of the scaphoid, lunate, and triquetrum, resulting in a neoradiocarpal articulation between the proximal capitate and the lunate fossa of the radius.
- PRC is one of the "motion-preserving" options for the treatment of degenerative carpal arthritis.

ANATOMY

- The proximal carpal row consists of the scaphoid, lunate, and triquetrum, and the distal carpal row includes the trapezium, trapezoid, capitate, and hamate (**FIG 1A**).
- Removal of the proximal carpal row converts a complex link joint to a simple hinge joint between the capitate and distal radius.
- Differences in the capitate and lunate morphology have been described as possible reasons for failure of PRC. However, biomechanical and clinical outcome studies have not demonstrated a significant relationship between carpal shape and failure.[2,3]
- The carpal bones are linked to the radius and ulna and to each other by a complex network of extrinsic and intrinsic ligaments.
  - The radioscaphocapitate (RSC) ligament extends from the radial styloid across the volar waist of the scaphoid to the capitate (**FIG 1B**).

- Identifying and preserving this ligament during PRC is crucial to prevent ulnar subluxation of the remaining carpus.

PATHOGENESIS

- A number of conditions can lead to painful radiocarpal arthritis.
  - Scapholunate advanced collapse (SLAC) and scaphoid nonunion advanced collapse (SNAC) occur secondary to chronic scapholunate (SL) ligament disruption and scaphoid fracture nonunion, respectively.
    - Both of these conditions result in progressive radiocarpal arthritis that starts between the radial styloid and scaphoid.
    - In later stages, these conditions can progress to a pancarpal arthritis and may involve the lunocapitate joint.
  - Kienbock disease is an idiopathic avascular necrosis of the lunate that can lead to varying degrees of intercarpal and radiocarpal arthritis.
- Treatment for each of these conditions varies based on the etiology and stage of disease at presentation. However, once significant arthritis has developed, conservative measures including splinting and steroid injections can minimize pain and improve function.

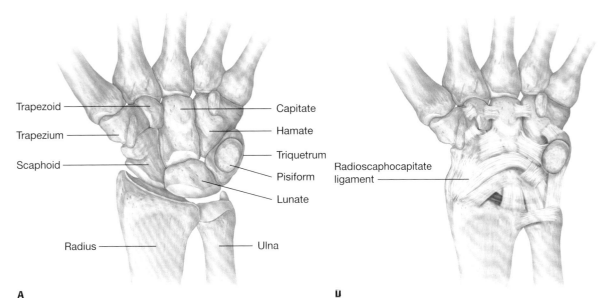

Trapezoid — Capitate
Trapezium — Hamate
Scaphoid — Triquetrum
— Pisiform
— Lunate
Radius — Ulna
Radioscaphocapitate ligament —

A   **B**

FIG 1 • **A.** Diagram of the carpus. **B.** Location of volar radioscaphocapitate ligament.

Table 1 Radiologic Staging Systems of Common Degenerative Wrist Arthritidis

Radiographic Stage	Kienboch's	SLAC	SNAC
1	No visible changes on x-ray, decreased vascularity on MRI	*Arthritis between scaphoid and radial styloid*	*Arthritis between scaphoid and radial styloid*
2	Sclerosis of lunate	*Arthritis between scaphoid and entire scaphoid facet of radius*	*Stage 1 + scaphocapitate arthritis*
3	A: lunate collapse, no scaphoid rotation B: lunate collapse, fixed scaphoid rotation	*Arthritis between capitate and lunate[a]*	*Periscaphoid arthritis*
4	*Degenerated adjacent intercarpal joints[a]*	Pancarpal arthritis	

Italics indicate stages appropriate for treatment with PRC.
[a]Lunocapitate arthritis is a contraindication to PRC, though capsular interposition or osteochondral resurfacing modifications may be performed in the presence of arthritis.
Kienbock, Lichtman classification; SLAC, Watson classification.

- PRC is usually reserved as a salvage operation for patients who have failed surgical treatment of earlier stages of the disease and have also failed trials of conservative management.[4,5] Table 1 covers staging of each condition and indications for PRC.
- PRC has also been described in the acute treatment of severe radiocarpal or carpal fracture dislocations[6] but is not recommended in the initial treatment of early SL dissociations.[7]

NATURAL HISTORY

- Carpal arthritis frequently presents with patients complaining of wrist pain, decreased range of motion and grip strength, and inability to perform daily activities without discomfort.
- Many patients will have a distant history of trauma or prior surgical procedures for an acute injury.

PATIENT HISTORY AND PHYSICAL FINDINGS

- Preoperative evaluation of a patient with wrist arthritis should include a detailed history, an assessment of functional limitations, measurement of wrist range of motion, and grip strength.
- History
  - A patient's occupation, age, and interests are key factors in determining if PRC is an appropriate procedure.
    - PRC is generally indicated in patients older than 40 who have low physical demands.
    - Younger patients and manual laborers have less ideal outcomes and higher failure rates after PRC.[3,8]
  - The operative records from prior surgeries should be obtained and the outcome of any trial of conservative therapy should be elicited.
  - Use of a patient-reported outcome measure (PROM) such as the Michigan Hand Questionnaire (MHQ), disability of the arm, shoulder, and hand (DASH), or Patient-reported Wrist Evaluation (PRWE) can be helpful in determining the patient's baseline functional disability and following postoperative outcomes.
- Physical examination
  - The skin is evaluated for scarring and/or previous incisions.
  - The wrist is evaluated for edema, gross deformity, and tenderness.
- Range of motion and grip strength
  - Active wrist flexion and extension as well as radial and ulnar deviation are measured with the forearm in neutral rotation.

- Total range of motion as well as the extent of each motion at which the patient experiences pain is determined.
- Grip strength is measured with a dynamometer.
- The bilateral wrist measurements are obtained and compared.
- Carpal examination
  - A detailed examination of the carpus is performed to elicit sites of discomfort to palpation and motion.
  - Evaluating for snuffbox tenderness, SL tenderness, and a Watson's is useful when determining the primary pathology leading to carpal arthritis but does not directly impact the decision to perform a PRC.
- Neurovascular examination
  - The examiner should perform a complete neurovascular examination of the hand.

IMAGING

- Standard three-view wrist radiographs (PA, lateral, oblique) are performed to evaluate for the extent of carpal arthritis.
- Specific evaluation of the lunocapitate joint on PA view is crucial to determining if PRC is an option for the patient because arthritic change at this joint precludes performing a PRC when a normal capitate is needed to articulate with the lunate fossa on the radius.
  - If there is any evidence of lunocapitate arthritis on x-ray, modifications of a PRC may be required (see below in techniques).
  - The patients should also be counseled that they may require conversion to an alternative procedure (ie, wrist fusion) intraoperatively.
- CT scan or MRI may be helpful in evaluating the pathologies that lead to carpal arthritis or the presence of synovitis in the intercarpal joints. However, they are not required prior to performing a PRC as the capitate can be visualized directly early in the procedure with options to perform alternative salvage procedures if necessary.

NONOPERATIVE MANAGEMENT

- Painful radiocarpal arthritis can initially be treated with splinting and/or steroid injections.

SURGICAL MANAGEMENT

- PRC is considered an appropriate salvage procedure if nonoperative measures fail or do not provide durable pain relief.
- Alternative salvage procedures include limited or total wrist arthrodesis.

Preoperative Planning

- As discussed above, evaluating the lunocapitate articulation helps in determining if a patient is a candidate for PRC.
- Mild arthritis of the proximal capitate may not be visualized on radiographs, so all patients should be counseled that they may require conversion to a limited wrist fusion intraoperatively.
- Any implants required for wrist fusion should be available in case they are needed.
- PRC can be performed under regional or general anesthesia.

Positioning

- The patient is positioned supine with the hand over a radioopaque hand table centered on the patient's axilla.
- A well-padded pneumatic tourniquet is placed on the upper arm.
- If an assistant is not available to assist with traction, endtable traction with finger traps and 5 to 10 lb of weight will facilitate dissection during the procedure.

Approach

- A dorsal radiocarpal approach between the third and fourth extensor compartments provides good exposure to inspect the radiolunate and lunocapitate articulations, remove the proximal carpal row, as well as to perform modifications to the PRC procedure or other salvage procedures.
  - A volar approach has also been described; however, this requires partial division and subsequent repair of the crucial RSC ligament.[9] This approach also limits options for alternative salvage procedures and is not recommended by the authors.
  - A PRC can be performed arthroscopically,[10,11] though this requires significant experience with these techniques and may not have long-term benefit to patients when compared to the standard procedure.[5]
- The key steps of a standard PRC are described below. Two modifications of PRC that can be performed in the setting of limited proximal capitate arthrosis are also described.

■ Standard Proximal Row Carpectomy

Exposure

- Exsanguinate the arm with Esmarch tourniquet and inflate the pneumatic tourniquet.
- Make a dorsal longitudinal incision approximately 8 cm in length over the carpus just ulnar to the Lister tubercle (**TECH FIG 1A**).
- Raise subcutaneous flaps ulnarly and radially just above the extensor retinaculum to protect sensory branches of the superficial radial and dorsal ulnar nerves.
- Identify the extensor pollicis longus (EPL) tendon proximal or distal to the retinaculum and divide the retinaculum sharply along the third dorsal compartment (**TECH FIG 1B**). Externalize and retract the EPL radially

so that the EPL does not rupture with swelling around the Lister tubercle after surgery.
- Raise the fourth compartment off the distal radius ulnarly in a subperiosteal fashion, with care not to injure the dorsal ligaments.
- Identify the extensor carpi radialis brevis (ECRB) tendon and place a Weitlaner to retract the ERCB and EPL tendons radially and the fourth dorsal compartment ulnarly.

Capsulotomy

- To enter the carpus, a longitudinal capsulotomy can be made in line with the division between the third and fourth dorsal compartments.
- However, designing an L-shaped capsulotomy provides good exposure for carpectomy and preserves the

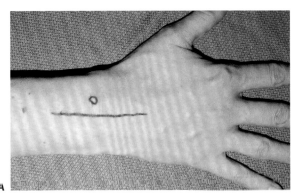
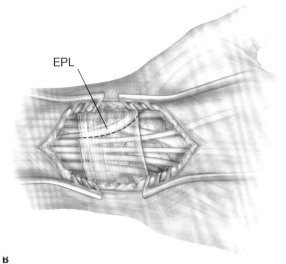

EPL

TECH FIG 1 • **A.** Incision for dorsal exposure of the carpus. *Circle marks* the Lister tubercle. **B.** Exposure of extensor retinaculum after raising subcutaneous flaps. The retinaculum is divided along the third compartment (*dashed line*).

TECHNIQUES

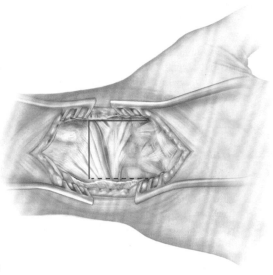
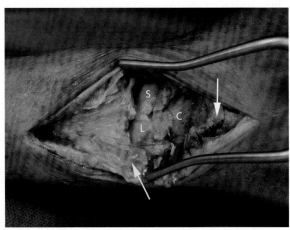

A   **B**

TECH FIG 2 • A. Markings for L-shaped capsulotomy (*solid line*). The *dashed line* indicates an incision to convert the capsulotomy into a distally based flap for capsular interposition. **B.** The capsular flap is raised and retracted to expose the carpus (*white arrow*). A portion of the dorsal cuff of capsule has been raised contiguous with the floor of the fourth compartment (*yellow arrow*). L, lunate; S, scaphoid; C, capitate.

dorsal capsule for use in an interposition flap if needed (see below).

- The longitudinal incision should be in line with the native position of the ECRB and connect to a capsular incision along the radiocarpal joint extending ulnarly.
- Leave a small cuff of capsule on the distal radius (**TECH FIG 2A**).
- Use a knife to raise the dorsal capsule off the carpal bones to completely expose the carpus (**TECH FIG 2B**).
- Once the carpus is exposed, inspect the lunate fossa of the radius and the proximal pole of the capitate for arthrosis.
  - If there is some arthrosis of the capitate, a modified PRC may be possible (see below).
  - In the setting of significant arthrosis, PRC should be aborted and the surgical plan changed to limited or complete wrist fusion.
- Once the decision is made to proceed with PRC, the proximal carpal bones are resected.

Bone Removal

- Place the patient's hand under traction with the help of an assistant or finger traps attached to weights off the end of the hand table. This aids in exposure and creates space between the carpal rows as well as the radius.
- Removal of the proximal row can be done in any order—scaphoid first or scaphoid last. However, there is more room for "error" during removal of the triquetrum, so surgeons with less experience may want to start with the triquetrum excision.
- The general steps to remove each bone is as follows:
  - First, divide any intact dorsal intrinsic ligaments to facilitate independent mobilization of each bone.
  - Use a penetrating towel clamp (or place small threaded Steinman pins or K-wires into the bones) to help manipulate each bone during dissection. Pins are especially useful in the setting of SNAC wrist to separately manipulate and dissect around the proximal and distal poles of the scaphoid.

- Use a Carroll elevator to bluntly begin the dissection around the volar aspect of each bone. A scraping sensation, as if dissecting subperiosteally, indicates the proper plane.
- Once enough of the attachments are released, the bone can be torqued to directly visualize the volar ligaments. At this point, sharp dissection with a knife can be used to release the ligaments directly off the bone.
- Piecemeal resection of the lunate and triquetrum (ie, with a rongeur or osteotome) is acceptable, but not advisable because it makes grasping and manipulating the bones difficult during final volar dissection. Thus, this technique is not recommended for the scaphoid.
- Key aspects of lunate excision:
  - It is crucial not to damage the cartilage on the proximal capitate and lunate fossa of the radius during lunate excision.
  - Hohmann retractors (or similar) should not be used around the lunate during dissection.
  - Consistent traction will provide space to ease dissection around the lunate.
  - Two wet 4 × 4 gauze can be tucked into the lunate fossa and around the proximal capitate to protect these cartilaginous surfaces during removal.
- Key aspects of scaphoid excision:
  - Slow and meticulous dissection along the volar waist of the scaphoid is imperative to preserve the RSC ligament.
  - Until each ligament is clearly visualized, all dissection along the scaphoid should be done bluntly.
  - Once the scaphoid has been removed, the intact RSC ligament should be visualized crossing from the radial styloid to the capitate (**TECH FIG 3**).

Completion and Closure

- After completing the carpectomy, fluoroscopy should be used to ensure complete resection. Small, retained portions of the distal scaphoid may not be symptomatic postoperatively,[5] but any other bone fragments should be removed.

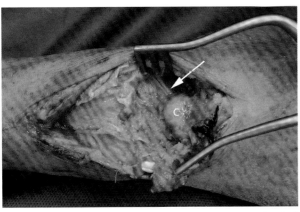

TECH FIG 3 • The proximal row has been resected. Note the thick radioscaphocapitate ligament in the volar capsule (*white arrow*). With forced ulnar translation, the capitate (*C*) does not migrate past the lunate fossa of the radius.

- Stress the carpus ulnarly to test the volar radiocarpal ligaments.
  - If the RSC ligament is adequately preserved, the capitate should not translate past the lunate fossa.
  - If the carpus does translate ulnarly, the RSC ligament was likely compromised and the pinning of the neoradiocarpal joint is recommended.
- Seat the capitate into the lunate fossa.
- Repair the dorsal capsulotomy with a 4-0 absorbable suture.
- Repair the extensor retinaculum with 4-0 suture leaving the EPL externalized, ie, transposed.
- Let down the tourniquet and check for hemostasis.
- A layered skin closure with a running subcuticular 4-0 suture (absorbable or non-absorbable) leaves a minimal scar.
- Patients are placed into a volar resting splint for postoperative comfort.

Proximal Row Carpectomy with Wrist Denervation

- Neurectomy of the posterior and anterior interosseous nerves may decrease postoperative pain and improve long-term outcomes.[8]
- Denervation can be completed at the beginning or end of the case.
- The tendons of the fourth dorsal compartment are isolated proximal to the extensor retinaculum and retracted ulnarly (**TECH FIG 4A**).
  - The posterior interosseous nerve and artery can be identified on the floor of the fourth dorsal compartment.

- The nerve is carefully dissected away from the artery, crushed proximally, and resected for a length of 1 to 2 cm. The proximal nerve end is then cauterized.
- The extensor tendons are then shifted radially and the interosseous membrane just proximal to the distal radioulnar joint is identified.
  - A 2- to 3-cm incision is made on the interosseous membrane and the anterior interosseous nerve and artery are identified just volar to the cut membrane (**TECH FIG 4B**).
  - The nerve is crushed proximally, and a 1- to 2-cm length of the nerve is resected with cauterization of the ends.
- After resection of the nerves, the procedure continues as described above.

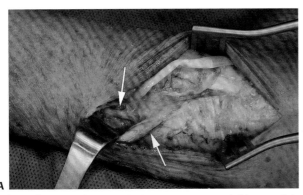
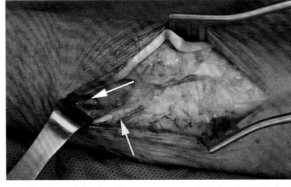

A   B

TECH FIG 4 • **A.** The posterior interosseous nerve (*white arrow*) is seen on the floor of the fourth compartment, which is retracted ulnarly (*yellow arrow*). **B.** A longitudinal incision has been made in the interosseous membrane (*circled*) and the anterior interosseous nerve is seen immediately below (*white arrow*). The fourth compartment remains retracted ulnarly (*yellow arrow*).

Proximal Row Carpectomy with Capsular Interposition

- The Salomon-Eaton modification of the PRC uses a dorsal capsular flap, which is interposed between the capitate and radius and can be performed in the setting of proximal capitate arthritis.[4,5,12]

- The procedure is performed the same as the standard PRC; however, it is required to perform the initial dorsal capsulotomy so that a distally based capsular flap can used (see **TECH FIG 2A**).
- After exposure of the capitate and presence of arthritis is confirmed, the proximal row is removed in the same manner as a standard PRC.

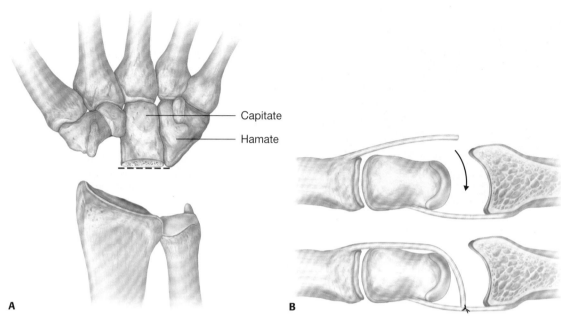

TECH FIG 5 • A. The proximal capitate is resected flush with the base of the hamate. **B.** The distally based dorsal capsular flap is sutured around the distal carpal bones to the volar capsule.

- In the traditional Salomon-Eaton procedure, the proximal capitate is then resected with a sagittal saw or osteotome to the level of the hamate (**TECH FIG 5A**). However, resection of the proximal capitate is not required for flap interposition and may result in deleterious injury to the remaining capitate and/or proximal hamate. The authors recommend leaving the capitate as is prior to flap interposition.
- The dorsal L-shaped capsulotomy is converted into a distally based rectangular flap by creating a longitudinal incision in the capsule on the ulnar aspect of the capitate.

- The dorsal flap is then sutured around the proximal capitate to the volar capsule with 4-0 nonabsorbable suture (**TECH FIG 5B**).
- A 0.062-in. K-wire is then inserted in a retrograde fashion from the capitate to the radius to secure it in the lunate fossa.
- As there is no dorsal capsule to close with this technique, closure begins with repair of the extensor retinaculum and proceeds in the standard fashion.

Proximal Row Carpectomy with Osteochondral Grafting

- This modification of PRC is indicated for resurfacing limited arthritis (less than 10 mm) of the proximal capitate.[13] The procedure uses an osteochondral graft harvested from one of the removed carpal bones that is placed into the proximal capitate articular surface.
- The procedure begins as in the standard PRC.
- Once the capitate is inspected and found to have a small area of cartilage loss (less than 10 mm), osteochondral grafting can be performed.

- The proximal row is removed as in the standard PRC; however, at least one of the bones must be removed en bloc to harvest the osteochondral graft.
- Once the proximal row is removed, the size of the cartilage defect in the capitate is determined and resected with a reamer for a depth of 10 mm.
- A harvesting dowel of matching diameter is then used to harvest a full-thickness osteochondral graft from one of the removed bones in an area of pristine cartilage, usually on the lunate or triquetrum.
- The graft is cut down to 10 mm in length and then gently impacted into the defect in the proximal capitate until the cartilage surface is flush.
- Closure proceeds in the same fashion for a standard PRC.

PEARLS AND PITFALLS

Patient selection	■ PRC has the longest durability in older patients (older than 40 years) with low physical demands.
Planning	■ Patients with evidence of lunocapitate arthritis on radiographs should not be offered PRC. ■ Designing the L-shaped capsulotomy in all patients reserves the dorsal capsule interposition flap as a bail out in cases with mild arthritis encountered intraoperatively.
Technique	■ Blunt dissection around the scaphoid is crucial to preserve the RSC ligament. ■ Failure to preserve this ligament may lead to poor alignment of the capitate and lunate fossa and early failure of the procedure.
Technique	■ Avoid damage to the proximal capitate and lunate fossa of the radius during removal of the proximal row.
Therapy	■ Early motion postoperatively allows for quicker return to of motion without any adverse outcomes.

POSTOPERATIVE CARE

■ Patients are seen in the office 2 weeks after surgery and the splint and sutures removed.

■ Standard radiographs of the wrist are obtained to confirm appropriate alignment of the radiocapitate articulation (**FIG 2**).

■ Patients in whom the RSC was protected and have maintained alignment can begin an early protected range of motion protocol.[14,15]

■ Strengthening of the wrist is reserved until 6 to 8 weeks postoperatively.

OUTCOMES

■ Postoperative pain from PRC generally takes 3 to 6 months to resolve.[3,4,16] However, once recovered, nearly all patients will note a significant decrease in their preoperative pain, and this continues to improve during the first postoperative year.

■ Patients can expect to regain between 50% and 85% of their contralateral wrist flexion-extension arc and 75% to 90% of grip strength relative to their contralateral side.[3–5,8,16,17]

  ■ Though the range of motion may be less than preoperatively, the decrease in patient's pain provides greater use of the hand, and most patients are extremely satisfied with the results of PRC.

■ Relative to alternative salvage procedures such as four-corner arthrodesis, PRC demonstrates better flexion and extension, though less radial deviation and grip strength.[12,18]

■ Long-term follow-up of PRC patients more than 10 years demonstrates a 10% to 15% failure rate with these patients requiring revision surgery for wrist arthrodesis.[3–5,8,16,17,19]

  ■ Younger patients (younger than 40 years of age) and manual laborers have a higher rate of failure,[3,5] though some authors report that 90% of high-demand patients are still able to function in their occupational capacity.[15,16,19]

  ■ All patients will end up with arthritis at the neoradiocarpal joint. However, most patients will still have good clinical outcomes that do not correlate with the degree of arthritis.[3–5,8,13,16,19]

■ Overall, the results of capsular interposition and osteochondral resurfacing during PRC are similar to those in standard PRC.[4,5,13]

COMPLICATIONS

■ The advantage of PRC is that it has a low complication rate and does not require bony union as in the alternative salvage wrist limited fusion procedures.

■ Improper selection of patients may lead to higher failure rates.

■ By far the most common complication of PRC is failure to preserve the RSC ligament during dissection. This requires prolonged immobilization postoperatively and leads to a higher likelihood of failure.

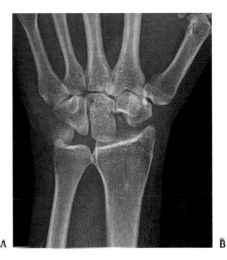 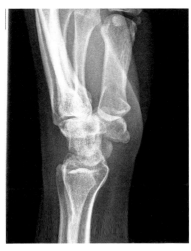

FIG 2 • Postoperative **(A)** PA and **(B)** lateral radiographs of a patient after proximal row carpectomy. Note the appropriate alignment of the capitate in the lunate fossa of the radius.

A   B

REFERENCES

1. Stamm TT. Excision of the proximal row of the carpus. *Proc R Soc Med.* 1944;38:74-75.
2. Tang P, Swart E, Konopka G, et al. Effect of capitate morphology on contact biomechanics after proximal row carpectomy. *J Hand Surg Am.* 2013;38A:1340-1345.
3. Wagner ER, Bravo D, Elhassan B, et al. Factors associated with improved outcomes following proximal row carpectomy: a long-term outcome study of 144 patients. *J Hand Surg Eur Vol.* 2016;41(5):484-491.
4. Balk ML, Imbriglia JE. Proximal row carpectomy: indications, surgical technique, and long-term results. *Oper Tech Orthop.* 2003;13(1):42-47.
5. Wall LB, Stern PJ. Proximal row carpectomy. *Hand Clin.* 2013; 29:68-78.
6. Della Santa DR, Sennwald GR, Mathys L, et al. Proximal row carpectomy in emergency. *Chir Main.* 2010;29:224-230.
7. Elfar JC, Stern PL. Proximal row carpectomy for scapholunate dissociation. *J Hand Surg Eur Vol.* 2011;36E(2):111-115.
8. Chim H, Moran SL. Long-term outcomes of proximal row carpectomy: a systematic review of the literature. *J Wrist Surg.* 2012;1:141-148.
9. Van Amerongen EA, Schuurman AH. Proximal row carpectomy: a volar approach. *Acta Orthop Belg.* 2008;74:451-455.
10. Culp RW, Talsania JS, Osterman AL. Arthroscopic proximal row carpectomy. *Tech Hand Up Extrem Surg.* 1997;1(2):16-19.
11. Weiss ND, Molina RA, Gwin S. Arthroscopic proximal row carpectomy. *J Hand Surg Am.* 2011;36A:577-582.
12. Salomon GD, Eaton RG. Proximal row carpectomy with partial capitate resection. *J Hand Surg Am.* 1996;21A:2-8.
13. Dang J, Nydick J, Polikandriotis JA, et al. Proximal row carpectomy with capitate osteochondral autograft transplantation. *Tech Hand Up Extrem Surg.* 2012;16:67-71.
14. Edouard P, Vernay D, Martin S, et al. Proximal row carpectomy: is early postoperative mobilization the right rehabilitation protocol? *Orthop Traumatol Surg Res.* 2010;96:513-520.
15. Jacobs B, Degreef I, De Smet, L. Proximal row carpectomy with or without postoperative immobilization. *J Hand Surg Eur Vol.* 2008;33E(6):768-770.
16. Green DP, Perreira AC, Longhofer LK. Proximal row carpectomy. *J Hand Surg Am.* 2015;40(8):1672-1676.
17. Richou J, Chuinard G, Moineau G, et al. Proximal row carpectomy: long-term results. *Chir Main.* 2010;29:10-15.
18. Bisneto ENF, Freitas MC, Leomil de Paula EJ, et al. Comparison between proximal row carpectomy and four-corner fusion for treating osteoarthrosis following carpal trauma: a prospective randomized study. *Clinics.* 2011;66(1):51-55.
19. Liu M, Zhou H, Yang Z, et al. Clinical evaluation of proximal row carpectomy revealed by follow-up for 10–29 years. *Int Orthop.* 2009;33:1315-1321.

Distal Radius Fractures

Shoshana W. Ambani and Kevin C. Chung

23
CHAPTER

DEFINITION

- Distal radius fractures encompass all fractures of the articular and distal metaphyseal components of the distal radius.
- They are the most common fracture of the human skeleton, with an annual incidence of over 640 000 cases in the United States.
- These fractures have a bimodal distribution, with peak occurrences in the 5- to 14-year-old and 75- to 84-year-old populations.
- Fractures of the distal radius distort the normal radiocarpal configuration, changing the biomechanical properties of the wrist joint.
- Nonanatomic alignment due to displaced fractures may lead to degenerative arthritis in the long term.

ANATOMY

- The distal radius has three concave articular surfaces: the scaphoid fossa, lunate fossa, and sigmoid notch (**FIGS 1** and **2A**).
- The dorsal aspect of the distal radius is convex and acts as a fulcrum for the extensor mechanism (**FIG 2B**).
  - The extensor pollicis longus tendon passes ulnar to the Lister tubercle, a dorsal landmark on the distal radius.

- Hand and forearm tendons and musculature are shown in **FIG 3**, and the extensor compartments of the wrist and anatomy of the dorsal wrist capsule are shown in **FIG 4**.
- Important anatomic considerations with regard to surgery of the distal radius are further delineated in the Techniques section of this chapter.

PATIENT HISTORY AND PHYSICAL FINDINGS

- Patients typically present with tenderness, swelling, and deformity of the wrist after a fall. Such a fall leads to compressive loading on the extended wrist.
  - The term FOOSH, which stands for "fall on outstretched hand," is a commonly used acronym describing this mechanism.
- Often, the wrist is described as having a "dinner fork deformity" upon examination (**FIG 5**).
- It is important to perform a comprehensive hand and wrist examination while paying particular attention to any median nerve symptoms that would indicate the presence of acute carpal tunnel syndrome.

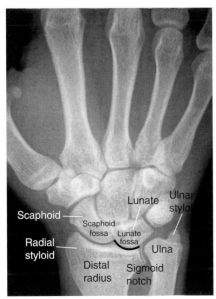

FIG 1 • The distal radius.

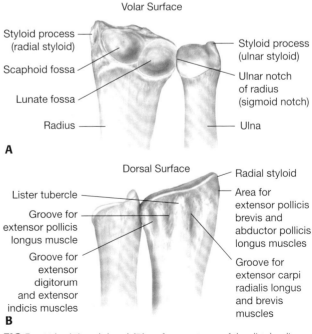

FIG 2 • Volar **(A)** and dorsal **(B)** surface anatomy of the distal radius.

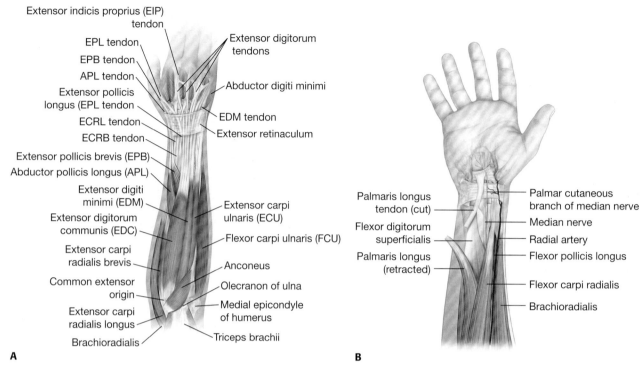

FIG 3 • Tendons and muscles of the dorsal forearm and hand **(A)** and the distal volar forearm and wrist **(B)**.

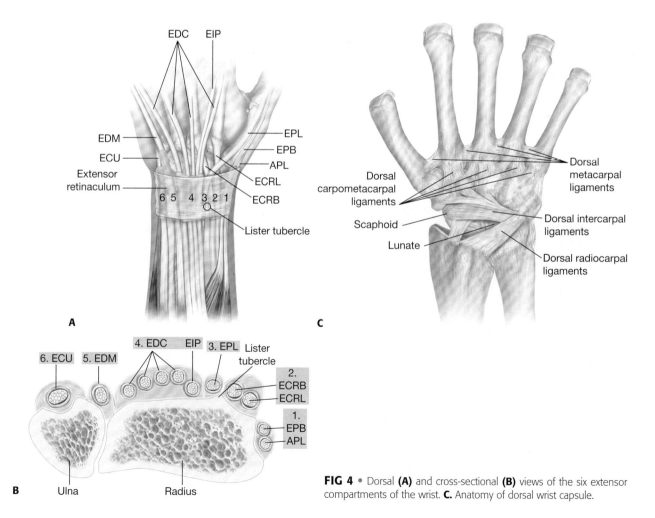

FIG 4 • Dorsal **(A)** and cross-sectional **(B)** views of the six extensor compartments of the wrist. **C.** Anatomy of dorsal wrist capsule.

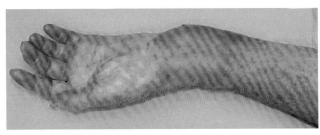

FIG 5 • Dinner fork deformity.

- Any open injuries should be noted and require urgent debridement.
- The distal ulna should be examined for dorsal prominence or instability, which may be indicative of a concomitant distal ulna fracture or a tear of the triangular fibrocartilaginous complex (TFCC) ligament.
- The elbow should be examined for tenderness at the radial head and collateral ligaments. Tenderness in this location may be indicative of a radial head fracture, elbow dislocation, or other elbow-related injury requiring attention.

IMAGING

- Standard imaging for all wrist injuries include posteroanterior (PA), oblique, and lateral radiographs.
  - On PA view, the distal radius has an average slope of 22 degrees in the radial-to-ulnar plane (radial inclination), with a radial height of about 10 to 12 mm (**FIG 6A**). The congruity of the distal radius articulation with the ulna at the sigmoid notch, as well as the radiocarpal joint itself, must be assessed.
  - On lateral view, the distal radius tilts about 12 degrees in the dorsal-to-volar plane (volar tilt) (**FIG 6B**).

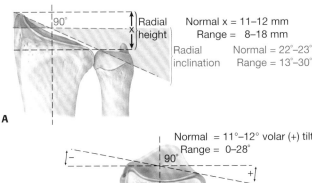

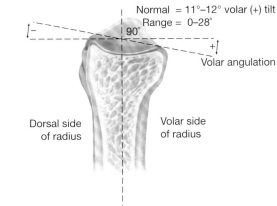

FIG 6 • **A.** Distal radius radial length and radial angulation. **B.** Distal radius volar tilt.

- If significant intra-articular comminution is present, a computed tomography (CT) scan may provide more information on the location and displacement of fracture fragments to aid in preoperative planning.

DIFFERENTIAL DIAGNOSIS

- Distal radius fractures can be differentiated from other wrist injuries, including the following, by careful examination and review of imaging.
  - Wrist sprain or contusion
  - Radiocarpal dislocation
  - Carpal bone fracture or dislocation, including fractures of the scaphoid
  - Carpal ligament injury, including injury to the scapholunate ligament
  - Fracture of the distal ulna or ulnar styloid
  - Distal radioulnar joint (DRUJ) injury
  - Degenerative arthritis
  - Inflammatory arthritis
  - Septic arthritis
  - Crystalloid arthropathy
- It is important to rule out other concomitant injuries, such as an acute median neuropathy.

CLASSIFICATION SYSTEMS AND EPONYMS

- Once diagnosed, distal radius fractures should be classified as open or closed, displaced or nondisplaced, and extra-articular or intra-articular. The structural elements and angles should be further described for clarity of the fracture pattern.
- Several classification systems exist for distal radius fractures, including the Muller AO, Frykman, Melone, Rayhack, Mayo Clinic, and universal classification systems. Given the plethora of independent classification systems, their use may complicate communication about fracture patterns. It is preferable to describe the fracture pattern directly.
- Eponyms were traditionally used to describe particular distal radius fractures but now only have historical significance. Common eponyms and nicknames include the following (**FIG 7**):
  - A Colles fracture is an extra-articular distal radius fracture featuring an apex volar deformity with dorsal comminution.
  - A Smith fracture, or "reverse" Colles fracture, is an extra-articular distal radius fracture with an apex dorsal configuration.
  - A die-punch fracture is an intra-articular depression fracture of the lunate fossa of the distal radius, resulting from a direct load transmitted through the lunate.
  - A Barton fracture is an intra-articular shear fracture of the distal radius, involving a fracture dislocation of the radiocarpal joint, either volarly or dorsally.
  - A Hutchinson fracture, or "chauffeur's fracture," is an isolated intra-articular fracture of the radial styloid. Chauffeurs often sustained injuries from manual crank starters that backfired.

INITIAL MANAGEMENT

- The goal of treating distal radius fractures is to achieve anatomic reduction, thereby maintaining wrist biomechanics.
- Initial management of any distal radius fracture requires closed reduction and immobilization.

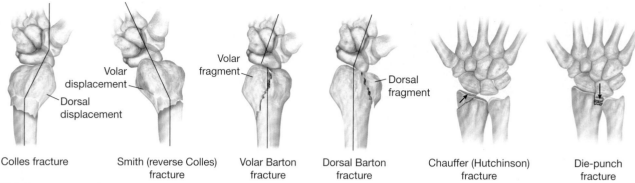

Colles fracture

Smith (reverse Colles) fracture

Volar Barton fracture

Dorsal Barton fracture

Chauffer (Hutchinson) fracture

Die-punch fracture

FIG 7 • Eponyms and nicknames for distal radius fractures.

- This can be done with the use of a "hematoma block," in which local anesthetic such as 1% lidocaine is injected dorsally into the fracture site. In addition, providing the patient with a benzodiazepine can help with muscle relaxation, thus minimizing deforming forces.
- The chance of success can be improved further with the use of continuous intravenous sedation, which provides better muscle relaxation than does a single benzodiazepine dose.
- The patient's index and middle fingers are then placed in finger traps suspended from an IV pole, with the shoulder abducted 90 degrees and elbow flexed at 90 degrees (**FIG 8A**). Weights are applied to the patient's elbow for traction (usually 5 to 15 lb), thereby distracting the fracture site.
- If necessary, a maneuver recreating the injury mechanism to disimpact the fracture site can be performed, followed by a reduction maneuver (**FIG 8B**).
- Notably, with simple distraction and sedation, the fracture often autoreduces without significant manipulation.
- A mini C-arm is employed to determine the adequacy of closed reduction in real time.
- Once reduction is achieved, with the patient still in finger traps, a sugar-tong splint is applied to stabilize the fracture site by preventing wrist flexion-extension and supination-pronation.
- Postreduction films are imperative.

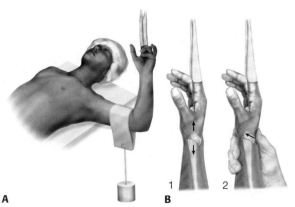

FIG 8 • **A.** General setup for closed reduction of a distal radius fracture. **B.** Reduction maneuver for dorsal displaced distal radius fractures. First, the wrist joint is placed in traction. Then, the physician's thumb is used to push the distal fragment volarly into alignment.

- If closed reduction is successful, strict immobilization over the next 6 to 8 weeks can lead to adequate fracture healing, obviating the need for surgery.
- An unstable fracture will not be maintained in a splint, however, and surgery should be considered pending patient circumstances.

NONOPERATIVE MANAGEMENT

- Nonoperative management consists of splinting or casting of stable fracture patterns. These are typically nondisplaced or minimally displaced fractures, or fractures that are well reduced.
- The patient's age, medical comorbidities, and functional level should be considered in determining whether or not to pursue nonoperative management vs surgical intervention.
- Patients being treated nonoperatively should be monitored with weekly radiographs for loss of reduction.
  - A volar tilt of 0 to 11 degrees dorsal tilt, radial shortening of 5 mm, and articular incongruity of 1 mm can be tolerated.
- Typically, the patient can be switched to a short-arm cast at 2 to 3 weeks for the remainder of the healing period.
- Early range of motion (ROM) of nonimmobilized joints is essential to prevent contracture. The cast should not extend past the metacarpophalangeal joints to allow finger ROM.

SURGICAL MANAGEMENT

- The goal of treatment is to restore anatomical alignment, thereby maintaining normal wrist biomechanics and decreasing the risk of developing degenerative arthritis.
- Indications for surgery include but are not limited to
  - Articular incongruity more than 1 to 2 mm
  - Radial shortening more than 5 mm
  - Dorsal tilt more than 10 to 20 degrees
  - Extensive comminution
  - Open fractures

Preoperative Planning

- Patient comorbidities must be assessed.
- Healthy patients are often given a regional block with intravenous sedation by the anesthesia team.
- Imaging should be thoroughly reviewed to develop a concrete operative plan.
- If the patient presents with median nerve symptoms, a concomitant carpal tunnel release should be considered.

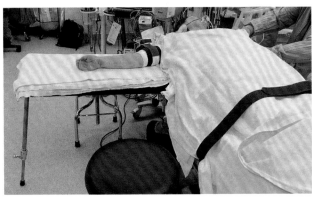

FIG 9 • Hand table setup.

Positioning

- Procedures on the distal radius are done on a hand table, with the surgeon seated (**FIG 9**).
- The patient is positioned supine on the operating bed as near to the hand table as possible.
- A tourniquet is placed on the upper arm.

Approach

- Surgical options for the treatment of distal radius fractures include percutaneous Kirschner wire (K-wire) fixation, external fixation, volar plate fixation, dorsal plate fixation, and dorsal bridge plate fixation.
- Percutaneous pinning with K-wires is indicated for unstable, displaced extra-articular distal radius fractures, simple intra-articular distal radius fractures, and displaced distal radius fractures in children and adolescents.
- External fixation uses ligamentotaxis to reduce and stabilize fracture fragments. Indications include unstable, irreducible extra-articular fractures, displaced intra-articular fractures that can be reduced in a closed or percutaneous fashion, and

highly comminuted fractures that are openly reduced and fixed with plates or pins but require further carpal unloading to promote healing. External fixation can be used as an adjunct to other fixation techniques should further stabilization be required.

- Volar-locking plate fixation is indicated for unstable, displaced extra-articular fractures, displaced intra-articular fractures, and volar shearing fractures. The introduction of volar-locking plating techniques has revolutionized the treatment of distal radius fractures by allowing early return of activity and by avoiding the problems of dorsal plating.
- Dorsal plating can be difficult in the presence of dorsal comminution and is associated with a higher rate of postoperative extensor tendon injury, adhesion, or rupture. Dorsal plate fixation is generally reserved for dorsal shear fractures or lunate facet fractures involving the dorsal cortex.
- Dorsal bridge plate fixation is designated for highly comminuted, intra-articular distal radius fractures, including those associated with significant metaphyseal and diaphyseal comminution, in particular subsets of patients:
  - Polytrauma patients with impaired ability to conduct activities of daily living
  - Patients who refuse external fixation for psychological or aesthetic concerns
  - Patients with extensive tendon injuries that will require multiple procedures followed by soft tissue and bony healing over an extended period of time
  - Patients with severe osteoporosis
    - For patients with osteoporosis and severe comminution of the distal radius, the bridging plate serves as an internal distractor that permits healing of the comminuted bone while giving the patient the latitude for self-care, with the bridging plate stabilizing the wrist.
    - At 2 to 6 months, when the distal radius has healed, the plate is removed and the patient can initiate wrist motion to regain mobility.

▪ Percutaneous Pinning

Equipment

- A tourniquet is not usually needed, although some surgeons advocate for its use to minimize soft tissue swelling during the procedure, thereby allowing improved palpation of bony landmarks.
- The pins are typically 0.062 in. K-wires, which are driven into bone using a power hand drill (**TECH FIG 1**).
- An intraoperative C-arm is required to assess fracture configuration and pin placement throughout the procedure.

Procedure

- We prefer the intrafocal Kapandji technique for percutaneous pinning of distal radius fractures, particularly if the bone is osteopenic and brittle.
- A K-wire is introduced dorsally into the fracture site as a lever to restore volar tilt (**TECH FIG 2A,B**)

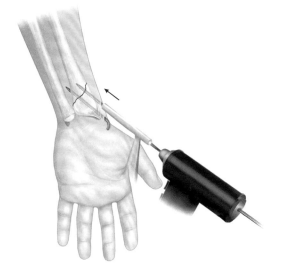

TECH FIG 1 • A power hand drill is used to insert K-wires

TECHNIQUES

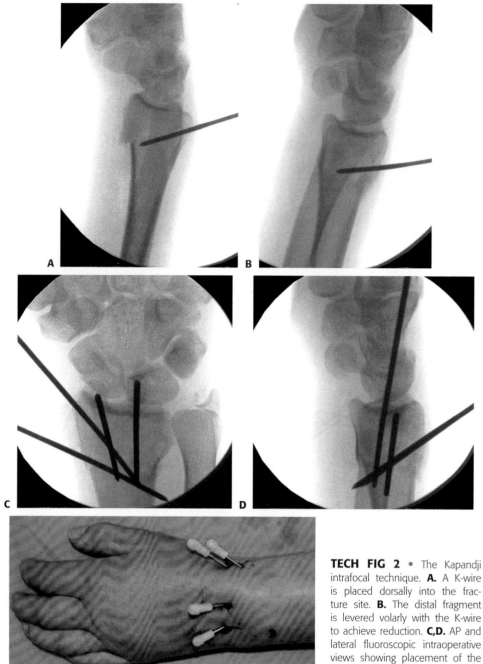

TECH FIG 2 • The Kapandji intrafocal technique. **A.** A K-wire is placed dorsally into the fracture site. **B.** The distal fragment is levered volarly with the K-wire to achieve reduction. **C,D.** AP and lateral fluoroscopic intraoperative views showing placement of the pins. **E.** K-wire pins in place.

- Once fracture reduction is achieved, one or two more K-wires are driven into the intact volar cortex at the same level, thereby buttressing the reduction. In a similar manner, the fracture can be levered radially to restore radial inclination.
- This is followed by placement of an additional buttressing K-wire.
- Once the fracture is stabilized by this buttressing technique, traditional pinning from the radial styloid and

from the dorsoulnar aspect of the radius through the fracture fragments can proceed (**TECH FIG 2C–E**).

Postoperative Care

- Patients are seen 2 weeks postoperatively in clinic for splint takedown, dressing change, and suture removal.
- A removable volar splint is applied.
- Gentle finger, wrist, and elbow ROM is allowed at this time.

- Serial x-rays are obtained at clinic visits to ensure stable bony alignment.
- In adults, K-wires are removed in the office at 5 to 6 weeks.
  - In pediatric patients, K-wires can be removed as early as 4 weeks, depending on radiographic and clinical signs of healing.

- Pin-track infection can lead to early removal of the pin, and if the infection is not treated or recognized, deep osteomyelitis can cause devastating problems.
  - Patients must be taught to clean the pin site meticulously twice a day with hydrogen peroxide on a cotton-tip applicator and then to seal the pin entry site with bacitracin ointment.

■ External Fixation

Equipment

- A variety of external fixator systems for treatment of distal radius fractures exist through different manufacturers. The surgeon must select an external fixator, and the instruction manual must be studied prior to use in the operating room.
- A tourniquet is useful to help maintain hemostasis during the procedure, particularly if done in conjunction with internal fixation.
- A C-arm is required intraoperatively to assess fracture configuration and pin placement.

Pertinent Anatomy

- The external fixator is placed parallel to the dorsoradial surface of the wrist, using pins at the proximal and distal ends.
  - The distal pins are placed in the second metacarpal.
  - The proximal pins are placed in the radial shaft, approximately 10 cm or one hand's breadth proximal to the radial styloid. This is the location of the abductor pollicis longus (APL) and extensor pollicis brevis (EPB) muscles as they traverse the radial shaft.
- One must have a solid understanding of the dorsal hand and forearm tendons and musculature (see **FIG 3A**) and the extensor compartments of the wrist (see **FIG 4A**).

Fracture Reduction

- The forearm is pronated on the hand table.
- The fracture is first reduced under fluoroscopic guidance.
- Percutaneous 0.062 in. K-wires may be placed dorsally as well as through the radial styloid to help maintain the reduction (**TECH FIG 3**).

Pin and External Fixation Frame Placement

- A 2-cm longitudinal incision is made dorsoradially just proximal to the APL and EPB tendons, about a hand's breadth proximal to the radial styloid.
  - Care is taken to visualize and protect the superficial radial nerve in this area.
- The first pin of the external fixator is inserted into the radial shaft in the deep interval between the extensor carpi radialis longus (ECRL) and extensor carp radialis brevis (ECRB) tendons.
- Then a 2-cm longitudinal incision along the dorsoradial aspect of the second metacarpal is made, taking care to retract and protect the extensor tendons and first dorsal interosseous muscle.
  - The second pin is placed through this incision.
- The external fixation frame is then slid into place over these initial two pins and tightened.
  - Using the open slots on the frame, the positions of the remaining two pins are marked, one in the metacarpal and one in the radial shaft.
  - These pins are then inserted at these locations (**TECH FIG 4A**).

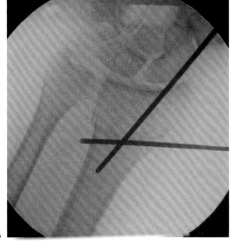
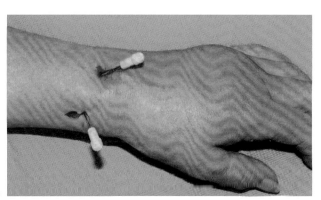

TECH FIG 3 • **A.** Fluoroscopy shows fracture reduction with K-wire pins in place. **B.** Pins in place through small wrist incisions.

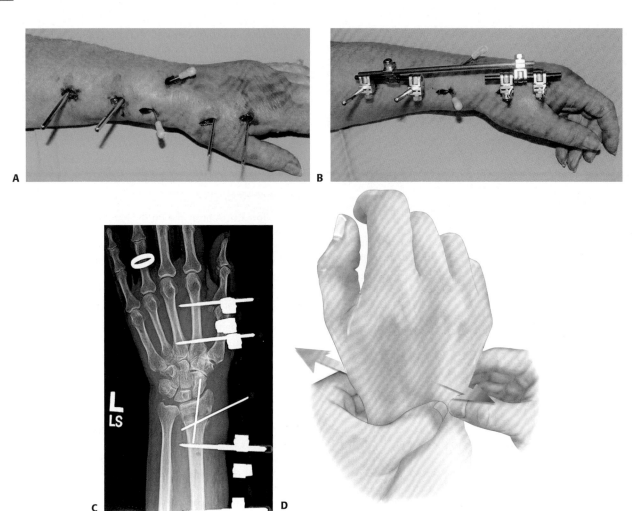

TECH FIG 4 • **A.** External fixator pin placement. **B.** Final placement of external fixator. **C.** Postoperative radiograph. **D.** Testing DRUJ instability.

- The external fixator frame is then further tightened to stabilize the reduction (**TECH FIG 4B,C**).
- At this point, all fingers should have passive flexion and extension, and the wrist should not be placed in excessive flexion or ulnar deviation.
- The DRUJ is also assessed for stability (**TECH FIG 4D**).
  - With the elbow flexed at 90 degrees on the hand table, displacement in the dorsal-palmar direction is tested in neutral position, supination, pronation, and radial deviation. Radial deviation should stabilize the DRUJ unless there is a disruption of the triangular fibrocartilaginous complex (TFCC).
  - DRUJ instability is defined as more than 8 mm of ulnar translation relative to the radius in the dorsal-palmar direction.
  - If unstable, the distal ulna is reduced and pinned to the radius.
- If a large ulnar styloid fracture is noted, this can be fixed with a K-wire.

Completion and Closure

- Simple, interrupted 4-0 nylon sutures are used to close the skin incisions, taking care to avoid injuring the branches of the superficial radial nerve.

- Nonadherent dressings are applied to the pin sites.
- A thick layer of gauze is used to push the skin down from being tented on the pins.
- A volar splint is applied for additional support.

Postoperative Care

- The splint and dressings are removed 7 to 10 days postoperatively to evaluate the pin sites and skin incisions. Sutures are removed.
- Finger ROM is encouraged.
- Nonadherent dressings are applied to the pin sites for the first 3 weeks. If there is drainage, half-strength peroxide is used on a cotton-tipped applicator to clean the sites daily.
- If percutaneous K-wires were placed to stabilize the reduction, they can be removed in the office after 3 to 4 weeks while the external fixator is left in place.
- The patient can shower with the external fixator in place once all sutures and percutaneous K-wires are removed and incisions are dry.
- The external fixator is removed in the office after 4 to 6 weeks once the fracture has healed on clinical and radiographic examination.

■ Volar Plating

Equipment

- A tourniquet is used for this procedure.
- Bipolar cautery is useful for coagulating crossing vessels during exposure.
- A number of volar-locking plate systems exist. The surgeon must select a plating system and review the instruction manual thoroughly prior to use in the operating room. Particular attention must be paid to the distal locking screw trajectory for proper plate placement.
- The C-arm is required intraoperatively to assess fracture configuration and hardware placement throughout the procedure.

Pertinent Anatomy

- The surgical interval is between the flexor carpi radialis (FCR) tendon and the radial artery and brachioradialis (BR) tendon (see **FIG 3B**).
- The median nerve lies in the plane between the flexor digitorum superficialis (FDS) and flexor digitorum profundus (FDP) muscle bellies in the forearm before emerging between FDS and flexor pollicis longus (FPL) more distally, entering the carpal tunnel at the wrist crease just deep to palmaris longus (PL).
- The palmar cutaneous branch of the median nerve arises 5 cm proximal to the wrist crease, between the PL and FCR. Notably, PL is absent in about 15% of the population.
- The FPL muscle overlies the pronator quadratus (PQ) and must be swept from radial to ulnar to expose PQ surgically.

- The PQ muscle is divided along its radial border and elevated to expose the bony surface of the distal radius and the associated fracture.
- The BR inserts into the distal radius and is often released during the procedure to decrease the deforming forces on the distal fragment, aiding fracture reduction.

Exposure

- The forearm is supinated on the hand table.
- A 6- to 8-cm incision is made at the radial aspect of the volar forearm between the FCR and the radial artery, ending just short of the wrist crease. If more distal exposure is required, the incision can be extended with a V-shaped zigzag (**TECH FIG 5A**).
- The FCR tendon sheath is entered, and the dissection proceeds along its radial aspect, to avoid the palmar cutaneous branch of the median nerve that is ulnar to the FCR, through the posterior sheath to expose the FPL muscle belly.
- The FPL is then swept ulnarly, exposing the PQ (**TECH FIG 5B**). The radial artery is also identified and retracted radially.
- An L-shaped incision is made through the PQ, releasing it radially and distally from the radius (**TECH FIG 5C**).
    - The PQ is elevated to expose the fracture site (**TECH FIG 5D**).
- The BR tendon can also be released at this point to further expose the distal fragment, which is usually displaced dorsally.

Fracture Reduction and Plate Fixation

- Next, fracture reduction is performed and may be provisionally held with K-wires.

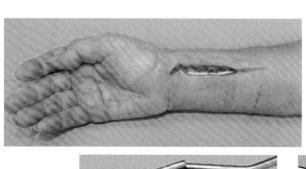
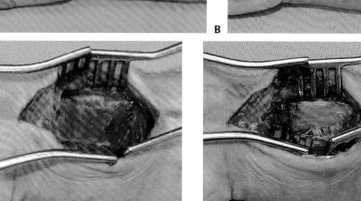

TECH FIG 5 • **A.** Skin incision with FCR exposed. **B.** The PQ is exposed. **C.** The PQ is cut radially and distally in an L shape. **D.** The distal radius is exposed.

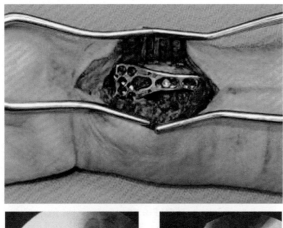

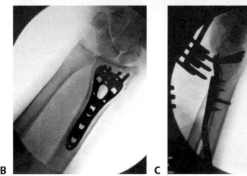

TECH FIG 6 • A. Volar plate placement. **B,C.** Intraoperative fluoroscopic images confirm appropriate plate placement.

- The volar plate is selected and placed centrally and distally on the radial shaft to capture the distal fragment.
- A screw is centrally placed through the elliptical plate hole into the radial shaft.
  - Although sizes can differ based on plating system, typically, a 2.0-mm drill bit is used, allowing for insertion of a 2.7-mm screw.
- Plate placement is then evaluated with C-arm fluoroscopy.
  - By loosening the shaft screw, the plate can be shifted proximally or distally as needed.
  - Once proper plate placement is achieved, the shaft screw is retightened. A second shaft screw is then inserted.
- With the wrist flexed, the distal screws are then placed, typically with a 1.8-mm drill bit and 2.4-mm screws.
  - Locking screws can be used if the fracture is already properly reduced.
  - However, if some separation exists between the distal fragment and the plate, a nonlocking screw can be placed initially to draw the bone to the plate.

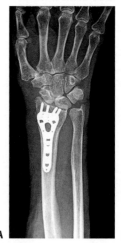
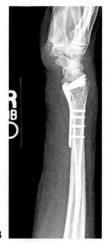

TECH FIG 8 • A,B. AP and lateral postoperative radiographs.

- Once the distal fragment is properly stabilized with a sufficient number of screws, the initial nonlocking screw can be exchanged for a locking screw, if desired (**TECH FIG 6A**).
- At this point, the provisional K-wires can be removed or left in place for 3 weeks if additional support is deemed necessary.
- Fluoroscopy is used to confirm appropriate plate placement (**TECH FIG 6B**).

Completion and Closure

- If the BR was released, it can be reattached with a step-cut lengthening maneuver.
- The PQ is then brought back over the plate and is sutured to the BR fascia using 3-0 Vicryl suture (**TECH FIG 7A**).
- The wound is closed with 3-0 Vicryl suture for the deep dermal layer, followed by a running subcuticular 3-0 Monocryl for the skin (**TECH FIG 7B**).
- A short-arm volar splint is placed for additional support, leaving the fingers free for ROM.

Postoperative Care

- Aggressive finger ROM is initiated immediately after surgery to decrease edema and avoid stiffness.
- The patient is evaluated in the clinic 10 to 14 days after surgery with repeat radiographs (**TECH FIG 8**), at which time gentle wrist ROM is initiated.

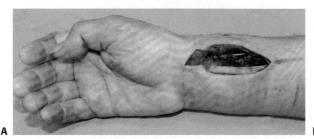
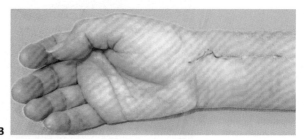

TECH FIG 7 • A. The PQ is reattached, covering most of the plate. **B.** Skin closure.

▪ Dorsal Plate Fixation

Equipment

- A tourniquet is used for this procedure.
- A dorsal T- or L-shaped plate of an appropriate length must be selected. This plate is typically a 2.4-mm low-profile plate.
- A C-arm is used intraoperatively to evaluate fracture configuration and assess hardware placement.

Pertinent Anatomy

- The extensor retinaculum divides the extensor tendons into six dorsal compartments and serves to prevent tendon bowstringing (see **FIG 4A,B**).
- The ECRL/ECRB tendons lie in the second extensor compartment.
  - Care must be taken in this area to avoid injury to the radial sensory nerve and dorsal radial artery.
- The extensor pollicis longus (EPL) tendon lies in the third extensor compartment, passing in a groove ulnar to Lister tubercle.
  - It must be released and mobilized to expose the dorsal distal radius.
- The extensor indicis proprius (EIP) and extensor digitorum communis (EDC) tendons lie in the fourth extensor compartment.
  - They are elevated subperiosteally, thereby minimizing tendon contact with dorsally placed hardware.
  - The fourth extensor compartment also contains the terminal branch of the posterior interosseous nerve (PIN), which traverses the floor along its radial aspect and can be sacrificed without clinical import.
- The distal radius articulates with the scaphoid and lunate via two hyaline-covered concave facets.
- The two most important ligaments associated with the dorsal wrist capsule are the dorsal radiocarpal (DRC/radiotriquetral) and dorsal intercarpal (DIC/scaphotriquetral) ligaments (see **FIG 4C**).

Exposure

- A 6- to 8-cm longitudinal incision on the dorsal wrist is made in line with the third metacarpal, just ulnar to Lister tubercle between the third and fourth extensor compartments (**TECH FIG 9**).

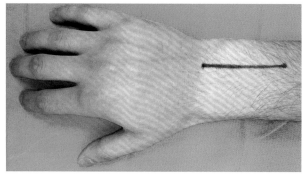

TECH FIG 9 • Planned incision on wrist.

- Care is taken to preserve the branches of the superficial radial nerve.
- Full-thickness flaps are raised to expose the extensor retinaculum.
- The third compartment is longitudinally incised, exposing the EPL tendon.
- The EPL tendon is released from its groove, and the retinaculum is divided between the septa of the third and fourth compartments.
- A periosteal elevator is used to elevate the fourth compartment in the subperiosteal plane to expose the bony surface.
- A longitudinal capsulotomy may be required to expose the articular surface, which is performed by releasing the dorsal capsular insertions from the distal nonarticular lunate.
- Once the fracture site and articular surface are exposed, Lister tubercle should be removed with a rongeur to allow the plate to sit flush on the dorsal cortex.

Fracture Reduction and Plate Fixation

- Fracture reduction is then accomplished with provisional K-wire fixation.
- A T-shaped plate is selected and contoured.
- Fluoroscopy is used to adjust the position of the plate proximally or distally as needed.
- Articular congruity is confirmed with fluoroscopy.
- The screws are applied sequentially to finalize plate (**TECH FIG 10**).
- Once the fracture is stabilized, the DRUJ is assessed for instability.
  - If deemed unstable, the DRUJ should be pinned percutaneously with the forearm in supination.

Completion and Closure

- The dorsal capsule and extensor retinaculum are closed with 3-0 and 2-0 nonabsorbable suture, respectively.
- The EPL tendon should remain in its new position superficial to the retinaculum.
- The skin is closed with simple interrupted 3-0 nylon suture.
- A volar splint leaving the thumb and fingers free is applied for postoperative comfort.

Postoperative Care

- The splint is removed at the first postoperative visit in 7 to 10 days, and active and passive finger ROM exercises are initiated.
- A removable short-arm volar splint is applied in neutral position, to be removed 5 to 7 times daily for wrist ROM exercises.
- A compression garment is applied for postoperative edema control.
- The splint can be weaned at 4 weeks to allow for activities of daily living.
- Once fracture healing has completed at about 6 to 8 weeks (**TECH FIG 11**), the splint is permanently discontinued.
  - However, if DRUJ instability was addressed in the procedure, the postoperative immobilization period is extended.

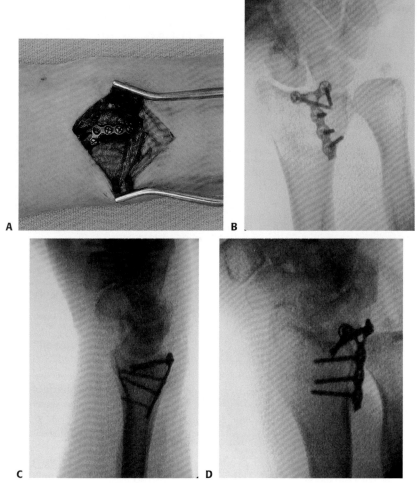

TECH FIG 10 • A. In situ plate placement. **B–D.** AP, lateral, and close-up lateral fluoroscopic views, respectively, showing final plate placement.

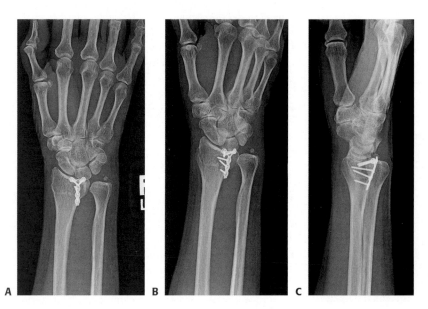

TECH FIG 11 • A–C. AP, oblique, and lateral postoperative radiographs.

■ Dorsal Bridge Plate Fixation

Equipment

- A tourniquet is used for this procedure.
- A distal radius bridge plate of an appropriate length must be selected. This plate is typically a 2.4-mm combination plate with smooth, beveled edges.
  - If such a plate is not available, a 2.7- or 3.5-mm limited contact dynamic compression plate (LC-DCP) can be used.
- A C-arm is used intraoperatively to help plan surgical incisions, evaluate fracture configuration, and assess hardware placement.

Pertinent Anatomy

- Dorsal bridge plate fixation is designated for highly comminuted, intra-articular distal radius fracture (**TECH FIG 12**).
- When placed, the bridge plate passes superficial to the joint capsule and periosteum within the second extensor compartment.
- The extensor tendons overlying the index finger metacarpal must be retracted to facilitate distal fixation of the bridge plate.
- The proximal portion of the bridge place is placed along the dorsoradial aspect of the radial shaft, adjacent to the BR.

Site Preparation and Exposure

- Fluoroscopy is used to mark the location of the proximal extent of the plate over the radial shaft, which should allow the placement of three screws at least 4 cm proximal to the fracture site.
  - The distal end of the plate should overlie the third or second metacarpal, no farther than the metacarpal neck.
  - These landmarks should guide incision placement.
- Two or three small longitudinal incisions are made dorsally to facilitate exposure (**TECH FIG 13A**).
  - A 4-cm incision is made over the dorsal midshaft of the index finger metacarpal. The extensor tendons are identified and retracted (**TECH FIG 13B**).
  - A second 4- to 6-cm incision is made dorsoradially overlying the radial shaft, just proximal to the EPB and APL muscles. The ECRL and ECRB tendons are identified and the radial shaft is exposed, allowing for placement of three screws at least 3 to 4 cm proximal to the fracture.

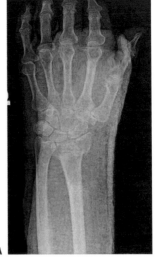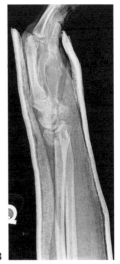

TECH FIG 12 • A,B. PA and lateral radiographs showing comminuted intra-articular distal radius fracture.

- A third separate 3-cm incision over Lister tubercle may also be made if an articular reduction or metaphyseal bone grafting is needed. The EPL tendon is mobilized to facilitate exposure and reduction.

Placement of the Plate

- Metzenbaum scissors are inserted, proximal to distal, along the floor of the second extensor compartment to create a tunnel, ensuring that the periosteum and joint capsule remain deep to the tunnel.
- The plate is then passed from the distal incision to the proximal incision (**TECH FIG 14A**), staying deep to the index finger extensor tendons.
- Manual traction of the wrist is used to obtain provisional reduction of the fracture, restoring radial length and inclination.
- Under fluoroscopy, the plate is aligned centrally over the index metacarpal and radial shaft.
- A bicortical screw is placed in the penultimate hole at the midline of the metacarpal shaft.
- While traction is reapplied under fluoroscopy to confirm fracture and plate alignment, the proximal end of the plate is clamped to the radial shaft using serrated bone-holding clamps.

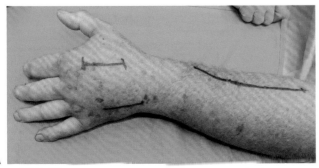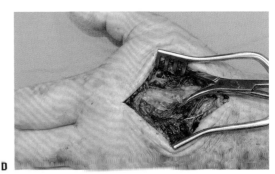

TECH FIG 13 • A. Planned incisions. **B.** Incision over index finger metacarpal.

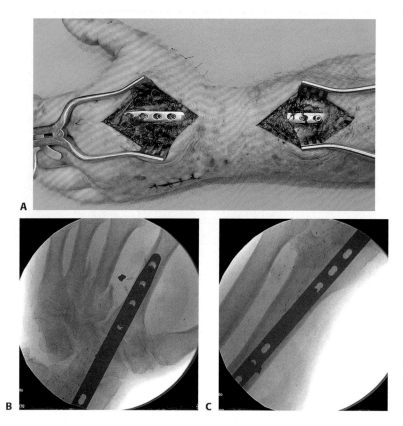

TECH FIG 14 • A. Dorsal plate placement. Intraoperative fluoroscopic images showing fixation at the second metacarpal **(B)** and at the radial shaft **(C)**.

- Fluoroscopy and clinical assessment are necessary to ensure restoration of radial length, radial inclination, and volar tilt, as well as absence of rotational abnormalities.
  - Supination and pronation of the forearm should be assessed to confirm full ROM.
- When plate position is deemed appropriate, three bicortical screws are placed proximally in the radial shaft, securing the plate.
  - Two additional bicortical screws are applied to the metacarpal, for a total of three distal points of fixation.
- Fluoroscopy is used to check plate placement (**TECH FIG 14B,C**).

Additional Fracture Reduction and Fixation

- Once the dorsal bridge plate is in place, any diaphyseal fragments amenable to lag screw fixation can be fixated to the radial shaft.
- If any further reduction of the articular surface is required, the third incision (explained above) can be used to release the EPL tendon and pass the plate.
- A dental pick can be used to reduce the articular incongruity.
- If possible, a 2.7-mm cortical screw is inserted through the plate directly under the lunate fossa as a buttress against subchondral collapse.
- Grafting with bone or allograft can also be performed to achieve subchondral and metaphyseal support of the articular reduction.

- K-wires (0.045 or 0.062 in.) can also be placed percutaneously to hold small articular fragments in reduction.

Completion and Closure

- Incisions are typically closed with 3-0 Vicryl sutures for the deep dermal layer, followed by a subcuticular running 3-0 Monocryl for the skin.
- A bulky dressing and volar wrist splint are applied for additional support, leaving fingers free for immediate active and passive ROM exercises.

Postoperative Care

- Active and passive digital ROM exercises are encouraged throughout the healing process.
- The first postoperative visit with radiographic films is at 7 to 10 days (**TECH FIG 15**), at which time a compression garment is applied to control edema, and a thermoplastic short-arm splint is provided.
- If K-wires were placed, they can be removed at 6 weeks.
- Patients may use the operated extremity for activities of daily living.
- Finger ROM, pronation, and supination are encouraged.
- Patients should not lift more than 5 lb. As long as restrictions are maintained, patients may return to work.
- Hardware removal can be scheduled at about 8 to 12 weeks after surgery, once bony healing has been achieved.
- Finger and wrist ROM exercises are initiated immediately after plate removal.

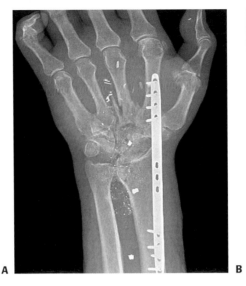
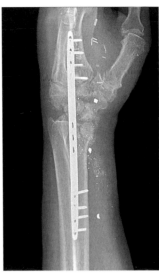

TECH FIG 15 • A,B. PA and lateral postoperative radiographs of dorsal bridge plate in place.

PEARLS AND PITFALLS

PERCUTANEOUS PINNING	
General K-wire technique	▪ Avoid multiple K-wire passes to prevent further fragmentation of fracture pieces, particularly in osteopenic bone.
Percutaneous pinning technique	▪ For pin placement, the authors prefer using a small longitudinal incision over the radial styloid to avoid skewering branches of the superficial radial sensory nerve and the extensor tendons. ▪ If the pins are placed percutaneously, caution is advised, as nerves and tendons can be easily damaged.
Adjunctive external fixation	▪ Consider concomitant external fixation in patients greater than 55 y of age and in younger patients if both the dorsal and volar cortices are comminuted.
Over-reduction	▪ Avoid over-reducing the fracture fragment, as excessive volar flexion can displace the fragment volarly.
Pediatric distal radius fractures	▪ Often, pediatric fractures can be reduced and stabilized with a single K-wire.
EXTERNAL FIXATION	
Alignment of external fixator	▪ The external fixator should be aligned at about 45 degrees dorsally from the radial midlateral axis. ▪ This dorsoradial position for external fixator placement should allow for full thumb ROM, particularly thumb retropulsion, with the fixator in place. ▪ Postoperative radiographs can also be obtained without obstruction by the fixator in this position.
General pin placement	▪ Pins should be bicortical and stable prior to external fixator frame placement. ▪ If the bone is weak and osteopenic, the proximal metacarpal pin may be placed through the second metacarpal base into the third metacarpal base for further stability. However, if the metacarpal pins are placed too deep, the motor branch of the ulnar nerve may be injured. ▪ When the proximal pins are placed between the ECRL and ECRB tendons into the radial shaft, the ECRL tendon acts as a protective barrier between the superficial radial nerve and the pins.
Percutaneous approach	▪ If the external fixator pins are placed percutaneously, whether in the radial shaft or in the second metacarpal, the superficial radial nerve can inadvertently be injured. ▪ The authors prefer using small incisions for direct visualization and protection of the nerve branches.
External fixator frame placement	▪ Avoid overdistraction of the frame, as this may lead to wrist stiffness or limited finger ROM. ▪ If the external fixator is placed in excessive flexion and ulnar deviation, carpal tunnel symptoms may occur. ▪ External fixators can be used to supplement the fixation of highly comminuted distal radius fractures with percutaneous pins or internal plating. External fixation serves to off-load the carpus during the healing process.

(Continued)

PEARLS AND PITFALLS (*Continued*)

VOLAR PLATING

Exposure	■ Avoid soft tissue stripping too far distally on the radius, as inadvertent release of the volar carpal ligaments will result in carpal instability. ■ Mobilizing the radial artery and ligating its ulnar-crossing branches will help to minimize bleeding and permit better exposure of the BR for release. ■ Avoid dissection ulnar to the FCR tendon, as the palmar cutaneous branch of the median nerve can be injured.
Release of the BR tendon	■ Not always necessary ■ Can be useful in fracture reduction ■ Dissection must proceed entirely on bone to avoid damage to the tendons of the first extensor compartment. ■ At the end of the procedure, the BR can be reattached using a step-cut lengthening maneuver.
Fracture reduction	■ A Freer elevator can be used to lever the distal fragment into place. It must be inserted through the fracture site into the dorsal cortex for complete disimpaction of the distal fragment to permit proper reduction. ■ Flexing the hand and wrist can promote reduction. ■ A large towel bump under the hand and distal fragment may be useful in the reduction maneuver. ■ Avoid over-reduction of the fracture, which can lead to volar displacement.
Intraoperative imaging	■ The C-arm is used to assess plate and screw placement. ■ The AP view confirms proper radioulnar placement of the plate. ■ The lateral view confirms proper proximal-distal placement of the plate. ■ A fossa lateral view, which is taken by holding the forearm at 22 degrees from the plane of the hand table, allows visualization of the radiocarpal joint space to ensure no screw penetration.
Screw placement	■ Avoid placing screws that are too long, as they may cause attritional extensor tendon rupture. The distal locking pegs or screws must be about 2 mm short of reaching the dorsal cortex. ■ Avoid screw penetration into the radiocarpal joint and DRUJ. ■ The distal screws are designed for subchondral support (distal row) and for dorsal fixation (proximal row) of the distal fragment.
Reattachment of the PQ	■ Often cannot be fully reattached due to plate prominence ■ Partial closure allows for some soft tissue coverage of the plate. ■ Avoid inadvertent suturing of the first extensor compartment tendons. ■ Some surgeons do not suture the PQ back into place at all.
Volar plate removal	■ Approximately 15%–20% of volar plates are eventually removed. ■ Reasons for removal of hardware included tenosynovitis, tendon rupture, pain, and prominent or intra-articular hardware.

DORSAL PLATING

Exposure	■ Full-thickness flaps are elevated, including skin, subcutaneous tissue, and superficial fascia. These flaps will contain and protect the dorsal sensory branches of the ulnar and radial nerves. ■ Elevating the fourth compartment in the subperiosteal plane minimizes plate contact with the extensor tendons. ■ Small incisions for provisional K-wire placement in the area of the radial sensory nerve are recommended to avoid damaging the nerve branches.
Dorsal capsulotomy	■ Can be performed to address fractures involving the articular surface. ■ Involves a longitudinal incision that detaches the dorsal capsular insertions from the distal nonarticular lunate. ■ The intercarpal ligaments must be protected. ■ Avoid entering the DRUJ. Radioulnar instability can result if the dorsal radioulnar ligament is divided.
Lister tubercle	■ The EPL tendon passes in a groove just ulnar to the Lister tubercle. ■ Lister tubercle is removed with rongeurs such that the plate can sit flush with the dorsal cortex and be less prominent.
Bone grafting	■ Cancellous bone grafting of metaphyseal defects can help support an articular reduction.
Screw placement	■ Avoid placing screws that are too long, as this can lead to irritation of volar structures.

DORSAL BRIDGE PLATE FIXATION

Incisions	■ Fluoroscopy is used to guide placement of incisions. ■ By holding the distal end of the plate at the index metacarpal neck-shaft junction, the proximal extent of the plate can be marked over the radial shaft. One must ensure that 3 screws can be placed at least 3 to 4 cm proximal to the fracture. ■ A third incision over the Lister tubercle can be made for articular reduction and metaphyseal bone grafting, if necessary.

PEARLS AND PITFALLS (*Continued*)

Dorsal bridge plate placement	■ The plate is placed along the floor of the second extensor compartment, deep to the index finger extensors and wrist extensors and superficial to the periosteum. ■ The plate should not extend distal to the index metacarpal neck. ■ The distal screw must be in the midline of the index metacarpal shaft to avoid rotary displacement of the fracture. ■ Applying traction with the forearm in 45–60 degrees of supination before applying the serrated clamp is helpful to avoid pronation of the distal fragment.
Overdistraction	■ Defined as a radiocarpal gap greater than 5 mm. ■ Can lead to loss of finger ROM secondary to extrinsic extensor tightness ■ Can lead to development of complex regional pain syndrome (CPRS).
Articular reduction and bone grafting	■ Failure to reduce articular fragments can lead to symptomatic radiocarpal arthrosis. ■ If an articular reduction is performed, bone grafting provides subchondral and metaphyseal support of the reduction. ■ Contraindications to bone grafting: 　■ Open fractures with gross contamination 　■ Soft tissue defects precluding primary wound closure
DRUJ instability	■ Defined as greater than 8 mm of palmar to dorsal translation of the ulna relative to the radius ■ Should be suspected in cases with large ulnar styloid fractures or displaced ulnar head fractures ■ After bridge plate placement, the DRUJ should be assessed for instability. ■ If DRUJ instability is detected, the forearm should be immobilized in supination for 3–4 wk.
Bridge plate removal	■ Plate removal can be electively scheduled at 8–12 wk after the initial surgery. ■ The plate should stay in place until radiographic osseous healing has occurred. Bridging callous should be seen in both the sagittal and coronal planes. ■ Bony healing may be difficult to visualize with a thick 3.5-mm plate in place. ■ Early removal of the plate can lead to fracture collapse. ■ Late removal of the plate may lead to extensor tendon attrition and rupture or permanent wrist stiffness.

OUTCOMES

■ Excellent long-term outcomes have been reported for all techniques when used in the appropriate patients.[1] Indeed, patient selection is critical.
　■ Over the past decade, however, internal fixation has become increasingly popular due to perceived early functional benefits.
■ Of the internal fixation options, volar plates are favored over dorsal plates due to fewer tendon-related complications.
■ With regard to external vs internal fixation, studies have shown no significant differences in grip strength, wrist ROM, radiographic alignment, and pain.
■ Still, the existing literature is heterogeneous with respect to reported outcomes for the treatment of distal radius fractures. As such, a unified approach has been recently proposed to integrate performance, patient-reported outcomes, pain, complications, and radiographs.[2]
■ For the elderly population, management of distal radius fractures has traditionally been dominated by closed reduction and immobilization.
　■ Nonoperative management was found to achieve satisfactory functional outcomes despite the presence of fracture malalignment.
　■ However, today's elderly population is more active than prior generations, which may indicate the need for more accurate fracture fixation for maintaining function. A multicenter prospective study to further investigate outcomes in this population is currently under way.

COMPLICATIONS

■ The overall complication rate after fixation of distal radius fractures has been reported to be as high as 30%.[3]
■ Pin-track or superficial infections associated with external fixation are the most common type of postoperative infection following distal radius fixation, with an overall incidence of 25%.
　■ *Staphylococcus aureus* is the most commonly isolated microbe.
　■ Nearly all reported infections resolve with oral antibiotics, with or without pin removal.
　■ Internal fixation of distal radius fractures, whether volar or dorsal, has lower infection rates, only up to 3%.
　■ Open fractures of the distal radius, regardless of fixation method, are associated with a higher rate of infection of 44%.
■ Clinically relevant extensor tendon injury or rupture is uncommon for both percutaneous pinning and external fixation, less than 1%. The use of small incisions to facilitate direct visualization and protection of important structures during pin placement is generally advocated.
　■ EPL rupture is, however, a well-documented complication of volar plating, with an incidence of 2% to 9%. It is typically caused by drill bit penetration or prominent dorsal screw tips. EPL rupture can also occur with nonoperative treatment. It is believed that the EPL near the Lister tubercle has poor intrinsic vascularity, and when combined with nutritional interference from hematoma, delayed EPL rupture ensues. Should EPL rupture occur, reconstruction can be performed with tendon grafting or an EIP tendon transfer.

- Extensor tenosynovitis may also occur with prominent dorsal screw tips from volar plating, with an incidence of up to 14%. This is addressed with hardware removal. In particular, dorsal plating is associated with an unacceptably high rate of extensor tendon complications, ranging from 19% to 48%. The advent of ultra–low profile plates appears to have decreased the incidence of such complications.
- Flexor tendon injury is less common than extensor tendon injury following fixation of distal radius fractures and is mostly associated with volar plating.
  - The FPL is the most frequently ruptured flexor tendon.
  - Flexor tenosynovitis may occur and may be treated with implant removal.
  - Some surgeons advocate repair of the PQ as a protective layer between volar hardware and flexor tendons.
- Carpal tunnel syndrome, or median neuropathy, can occur acutely, subacutely, or in a delayed fashion after distal radius fractures regardless of treatment method, operative or nonoperative, with an overall incidence of 8.5%.
  - Some surgeons advocate carpal tunnel release in all distal radius fractures undergoing fixation, whereas others limit this to patients with pre-existing or acute signs of median neuropathy.
- Superficial radial nerve (SRN) injury is most common with percutaneous pinning and external fixation, with an incidence of 4% to 13%. Using small skin incisions to facilitate direct visualization and preservation of the nerve branches during pin placement reduces this risk.
- Complex regional pain syndrome has been associated with distal radius fractures treated both operatively and nonoperatively, with rates ranging from 3% to 25%.
  - It is characterized by unexplained pain, swelling, vasomotor instability, and joint stiffness.
  - Type I (previously known as reflex sympathetic dystrophy) occurs secondary to a noxious event. Type II (also known as causalgia) is caused by direct peripheral nerve injury.

- The use of vitamin C for CPRS prophylaxis is controversial, but many still advocate it given its low side effect profile.
- Loss of reduction can occur following all forms of distal radius fixation and is most commonly seen with percutaneous pinning, followed by external fixation and subsequently internal plating.
  - Internal fixation with plates seems to maintain radiographic parameters better than other fixation methods.
  - Reoperation is performed in up to 80% of cases in which loss of reduction is discovered.
  - In particular, lunate facet fractures are prone to loss of reduction.
  - Some surgeons advocate other fixation methods as an adjunct to plating, such as pins, wires, sutures, or mini-screws.
- Nonunion after distal radius fixation is rare, with an incidence of less than 1%.
  - If nonunion is experienced, revision is indicated with plate fixation and autogenous bone grafting.
- Approximately 65% of patients with intra-articular distal radius fractures go on to develop radiographic evidence of radiocarpal arthritis, regardless of treatment modality.
  - Radiographic evidence of radiocarpal arthritis does not seem to correlate with patient symptoms or functional impairment, however, and functional outcomes seem to be no different from population norms.

REFERENCES

1. Horst TA, Jupiter JB. Stabilisation of distal radius fractures: lessons learned and future directions. *Injury.* 2016;47(2):313-319.
2. Waljee JF, Ladd A, MacDermid JC, et al. A unified approach to outcomes assessment for distal radius fractures. *J Hand Surg [Am].* 2016;41:565-573.
3. Lee DS, Weikert DR. Complications of distal radius fixation. *Orthop Clin North Am.* 2016;47(2):415-424.

Section VI: Rheumatoid Arthritis

Rheumatoid Arthritis of the Hand and Wrist

24

CHAPTER

Shoshana W. Ambani and Kevin C. Chung

DEFINITION

- Rheumatoid arthritis (RA) is a systemic autoimmune disease characterized by synovial inflammation, which results in progressive joint and soft tissue destruction that leads to deformity and disability.

PATHOGENESIS

- RA is an idiopathic disease affecting about 0.5% to 1.0% of the adult population, with both genetic and environmental factors, which are not fully understood.
  - For example, there is a three- to fourfold higher frequency in women compared to men. In addition, patients with the human leukocyte antigen-antigen D related (HLA-DR) allele have a 4 to 5 increased relative risk of RA.[1]
- Environmental links have also been made, particularly to smoking, caffeine, silica, and some infectious diseases.
- On a cellular level, autoreactive T cells and inflammatory cytokines have been found to play a critical role in the pathogenesis of RA.[2,3]
  - Tumor necrosis factor (TNF) and interleukin-6 (IL-6), for example, promote inflammatory cell accumulation, production of matrix metalloproteinases, and osteoclast activation, which ultimately results in the destruction of cartilage and bone.

DIAGNOSIS

- The diagnosis of RA is clinical, based on criteria developed by the American College of Rheumatology (ACR, previously the American Rheumatism Association) in 1987 to distinguish RA from other rheumatic diseases (Table 1).[4]
- In general, the diagnosis is made by recognizing a pattern of sign and symptoms, including a history of prolonged morning stiffness that may improve with activity, polyarthralgias, joint swelling, and fatigue.
- Blood work can help exclude the mimics of RA.
  - Anti–cyclic citrullinated peptide (anti-CCP) antibodies have been shown to be more than 90% specific for RA.[3-5]
  - Rheumatoid factor (RF), though not necessary to confirm the diagnosis of RA, is associated with more severe joint disease and extra-articular manifestations.
- Examination findings suggestive of RA include symmetrical polyarthritis and rheumatoid nodules.
- Arthrocentesis may be helpful in excluding septic arthritis.
- Radiographs may be obtained, revealing periarticular osteopenia, joint space loss, and erosions.
- In 2010, the ACR/European League Against Rheumatism (EULAR) developed further criteria for diagnosis in an effort to help identify patients who would benefit from disease-modifying antirheumatic drugs (DMARDS) early on before the irreversible effects of RA take place (Table 2).[6]

DIFFERENTIAL DIAGNOSIS

- Viral polyarthritis
- Systemic rheumatic diseases (eg, systemic lupus erythematosus, Sjogren syndrome, dermatomyositis, mixed connective tissue disease)
- Palindromic rheumatism
- Hypermobility syndrome and fibromyalgia
- Reactive arthritis and arthritis of inflammatory bowel disease
- Psoriatic arthritis

Table 1 1987 ACR Criteria for Rheumatoid Arthritis[a]

1. Morning stiffness
   - Located in and around joints
   - Duration ≥1 h before maximal improvement

2. Arthritis of ≥3 joint areas
   - At least 3 joints simultaneously have had soft tissue swelling or fluid, witnessed by a physician
   - May involve 4 possible joints: PIP, MCP, wrist, elbow, knee, ankle, and MTP joints

3. Arthritis of hand joints
   - At least 1 area with soft tissue swelling or fluid (wrist, MCP, or PIP joint)

4. Symmetrical arthritis
   - Simultaneous involvement of same joints on both sides of body
   - Bilateral involvement of PIPs, MCPs, or MTPs, without absolute symmetry, is acceptable

5. Rheumatoid nodules
   - Subcutaneous nodules over bony prominences, extensor surfaces, or in juxta-articular regions, observed by a physician

6. Serum rheumatoid factor
   - Demonstration of abnormal amounts of serum rheumatoid factor by any method for which the result has been positive in less than 5% of normal control subjects

7. Radiographic changes
   - Includes erosions or unequivocal bony decalcification localized to the involved joints
   - Osteoarthritic changes alone do not qualify

PIP, proximal interphalangeal; MCP, metacarpophalangeal; MTP, metatarsophalangeal.

[a]A patient is diagnosed with rheumatoid arthritis if at least 4 of the 7 criteria are met. Criteria 1 to 4 must have been present for at least 6 weeks.

From Arnett FC, Edworthy SM, Bloch DA, et al. The American Rheumatism Association 1987 revised criteria for the classification of rheumatoid arthritis. *Arthritis Rheum.* 1988;31(3):315-324.

Table 2 2010 ACR/EULAR Classification Criteria for Rheumatoid Arthritis

Classification Criteria	Score
• Add scores of categories A–D. • A score of ≥6/10 is required for diagnosis of RA.	
A. Joint involvement (any swollen or tender joint on examination, excluding DIPJ, first CMCJ, and 1st MTPJ)	
• 1 large joint	0
• 2–10 large joints	1
• 1–3 small joints (with or without large joint involvement)	2
• 4–10 small joints (with or without large joint involvement)	3
• Greater than 10 joints	5
Note: "Large" joints refer to shoulders, elbows, hips, knees, and ankles; "small" joints refer to MCPJ, PIPJ, 2nd–5th MTPJ, thumb IPJ, and wrists.	
B. Serology (at least 1 test result is needed for classification)	
• Negative RF *and* negative ACPA	0
• Low-positive RF *or* high-positive ACPA	2
• High-positive RF *or* high-positive ACPA	3
C. Acute-phase reactants (at least 1 result is needed for classification)	
• Normal CRP *and* normal ESR	0
• Abnormal CRP *or* abnormal ESR	1
D. Duration of symptoms	
• <6 weeks	0
• ≥6 weeks	1

CMCJ, carpometacarpal joint; DIPJ, distal interphalangeal joint; IPJ, interphalangeal joint; MCPJ, metacarpophalangeal joint; MTPJ, metatarsophalangeal joint; RF, rheumatoid factor; ACPA, anti–citrullinated protein antibody; CRP, C-reactive protein; ESR, erythrocyte sedimentation rate.
From Aletaha D, Neogi T, Silman AJ, et al. 2010 Rheumatoid arthritis classification criteria: an American College of Rheumatology/European League Against Rheumatism collaborative initiative. *Arthritis Rheum.* 2010;62(9):2569-2581.

- Polymyalgia rheumatic
- Crystalline arthritis (eg, gout, pseudogout)
- Infectious arthritis
- Osteoarthritis
- Paraneoplastic disease
- Multicentric reticulohistiocytosis

- Sarcoid arthropathy
- Fibroblastic rheumatism

IMAGING

- When evaluating the upper extremities, PA, oblique, and lateral radiographs of the hands should be obtained to assess the condition of the proximal interphalangeal joints (PIPJ) and metacarpophalangeal joints (MCPJ).
- Radiographs of the wrist will further serve to evaluate the distal radioulnar joint (DRUJ), midcarpal joint, and radiocarpal joint.
- Characteristic findings of RA include periarticular osteopenia, joint space loss, and marginal joint erosions (**FIG 1**). Often, these changes are not seen in early disease.
- MRI can be useful in detecting RA before radiographic changes can be detected. MRI can also identify bone marrow edema and synovial hypertrophy, which predict the development of erosive disease.

PATIENT HISTORY AND PHYSICAL FINDINGS

- Patients typically present between the third and sixth decades of life. Symptoms begin insidiously and grow over weeks to months. Patients complain of fatigue, malaise, generalized stiffness, and generalized arthralgias or myalgias.
  - In a small subset (10%–15%) of patients, the onset of RA is sudden, with fever, polyarthritis, lymphadenopathy, and splenomegaly developing over days to weeks.
- Inflammation of the synovial tissues (synovitis) develops gradually and often symmetrically in the hands, wrists, knees, and feet. Synovial hypertrophy (pannus) ultimately results in the destruction of ligaments, tendons, cartilage, and bone. Examination of affected joints reveals swelling, tenderness, warmth, and painful motion.
  - In the upper extremity, RA tends to affect the MCPJ, PIPJ, and wrists earlier and more frequently than it does other joints in the body. This is in part due to their high synovium-to-joint surface area ratio.
  - The distal interphalangeal joints (DIPJ) are typically spared from RA.

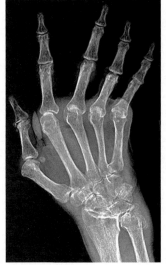 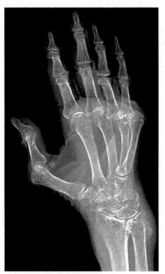 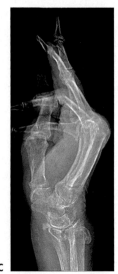

A **B** **C**

FIG 1 • Radiographs of rheumatoid hand and wrist showing periarticular osteopenia, joint space loss, and marginal joint erosions. **A.** AP view. **B.** Oblique view. **C.** Lateral view.

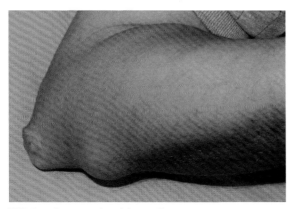

FIG 2 • Rheumatoid nodule on elbow.

- Patients may also present with rheumatoid nodules, vasculitis, pericarditis, pleural effusion, interstitial pulmonary disease, peripheral neuropathy, and keratoconjunctivitis sicca.
  - Rheumatoid nodules tend to develop on extensor surfaces or areas of contact pressure, such as the olecranon process at the elbow (**FIG 2**).
  - RA also affects the synovial lining of tendons, which can result in carpal tunnel syndrome, tendon rupture, tendonitis, and trigger digits.

Key Findings

- Wrist (carpus)
  - Midcarpal extension
  - Ulnar translocation of the carpus
  - DRUJ instability
  - Caput ulna (ulnar head dorsal dislocation, ECU subluxation, carpal supination)
  - Extensor tendon rupture, Vaughn-Jackson syndrome
  - Flexor pollicis longus (FPL) rupture (Mannerfelt lesion)
  - Carpal tunnel syndrome
- Hand
  - MCPJ and PIPJ arthritic changes
  - MCPJ volar subluxation and ulnar deviation
  - Sparing of the DIPJ

- Swan-neck deformity
- Boutonniere deformity

Wrist Joint

- Arthritic radiographic changes are initially noted at the scaphoid waist, the ulnar styloid, and the DRUJ and progress into the radiocarpal and midcarpal joints.
  - In later stages, severe erosion of the volar lip of the distal radius leads to lunate malposition (proximal migration, volar translation, volar angulation) and compensatory midcarpal extension.
- Three patterns of end-stage carpal arthritis can be encountered, depending on the degree of bony destruction and ligamentous instability.
  - First, wrist ankylosis (bony joint fusion) can occur, sometimes in acceptable alignment.
  - Second, the wrist can be arthritic but stable over time with limited ligamentous destruction.
  - Third, the wrist is unstable, characterized by progressive misalignment, whether ligamentous or bony in etiology.

Carpal Ligaments

- Normal carpal ligament anatomy is shown in **FIG 3A,B**.
- In RA, synovitis attenuates the radioscaphocapitate (RCC) ligament and the scapholunate (SL) ligament, causing ulnar translocation of the carpus.
- At the DRUJ, the triangular fibrocartilage complex (TFCC), including the dorsal and palmar radioulnar ligaments, is also destroyed by synovitis, leading to DRUJ instability and eventual dorsal dislocation of the ulnar head. The extensor carpi ulnaris (ECU) sheath is also destroyed, resulting in volar ECU subluxation and contributing to the supinated and radially deviated posture of the wrist (**FIG 3C**).
- The term *caput ulna* refers to the combination of dorsal ulnar head dislocation, volar ECU subluxation, and carpal supination (**FIG 3D,E**).

Tendons at the Wrist

- Synovitis develops within the extensor tendon compartments on the dorsal aspect of the wrist (**FIG 4**).

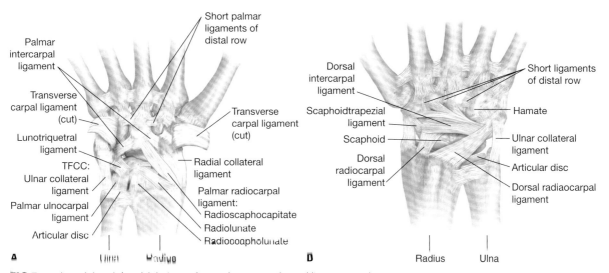

FIG 3 • Palmer (**A**) and dorsal (**B**) views of normal anatomy of carpal ligaments and TFCC.

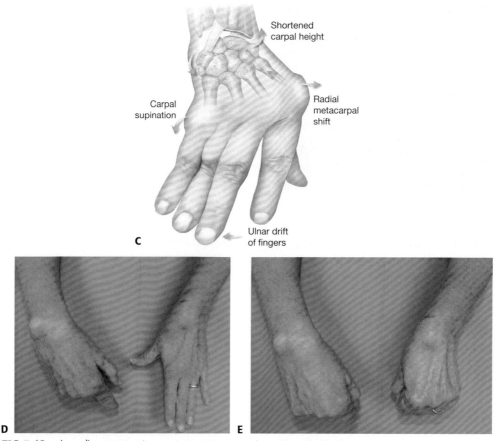

FIG 3 (Continued) • **C.** Wrist changes in RA. **D,E.** Caput ulna of the right hand.

- Pannus can be seen bulging proximally and distally from underneath the extensor retinaculum, taking on an hourglass appearance.
- Tendon rupture in RA results from direct pannus invasion and/or attritional wear over eroded bony edges.
  - In regions where the tendon is covered by tenosynovium (eg, extensor retinaculum, carpal tunnel, and digital flexor sheaths), tendons may be directly invaded by synovial pannus.

- In regions where tendon is closely related to joints (eg, the DRUJ, radiocarpal joint, and PIP joints), underlying proliferative synovitis may cause pressure ischemia leading to tendon rupture.
- Attritional rupture frequently involves the extensor digiti minimi (EDM) at the ulnar head, the extensor pollicis longus (EPL) at the Lister tubercle, and the FPL in the carpal tunnel, which is caused by a flexed, eroded scaphoid. An attritional FPL rupture is termed a *Mannerfelt lesion*.

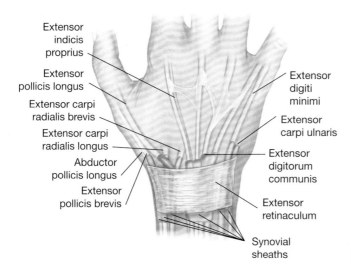

Extensor indicis proprius
Extensor pollicis longus
Extensor carpi radialis brevis
Extensor carpi radialis longus
Abductor pollicis longus
Extensor pollicis brevis

Extensor digiti minimi
Extensor carpi ulnaris
Extensor digitorum communis
Extensor retinaculum

Synovial sheaths

FIG 4 • Extensor tendons of the hand and wrist.

Table 3 Examining the Tendons of the Hand

Tendon	Examination Maneuver	Interpretation and Pearls
Extensor pollicis longus (EPL)	• With the patient's palm flat on a table, ask the patient to lift the thumb off the table.	If able to lift the thumb off the table (retropulsion), EPL is intact.
Extensor indicis proprius (EIP)	• Test independent extension of the index finger with the remaining fingers held in flexion.	It is important to test the integrity of EIP, as it is a common donor in tendon transfer procedures.
Extensor digitorum communis (EDC)	• With the finger passively placed in extension, ask the patient to maintain the finger in extension. If unable to maintain finger extension, there is either a tendon rupture or nerve palsy. • Next, test the *tendodesis effect* by passively flexing the patient's wrist and looking for concomitant finger extension. If the finger does not extend, tendon rupture is the diagnosis, as the tenodesis effect is preserved in nerve palsy.	• One must differentiate extensor tendon rupture from (1) ulnar subluxation of the extensor tendon over the head of the metacarpal and (2) posterior interosseous nerve (PIN) palsy secondary to elbow synovitis. • Patients with rupture of the EDC to one finger may still be able to extend that finger due to the juncturae connecting it to the adjacent fingers. • Usually, the finger cannot be extended if more than one EDC is ruptured.
Extensor digiti minimi (EDM)	Test independent extension of the small finger with the other fingers flexed.	• Patients may still be able to extend the small finger while extending the remaining fingers through an intact EDC or the juncturae connecting it to the ring finger.
Flexor pollicis longus (FPL)	Holding the thumb MCPJ in extension, ask the patient to flex the thumb IP joint.	• Intact thumb IP flexion indicates an intact FPL tendon.
Flexor digitorum superficialis (FDS)	FDS is checked for each finger by holding the patient's other fingers in extension and allowing the patient to actively flex the finger in question.	• If FDS is intact, the finger will bend at the PIPJ. • It is important to test the integrity of FDS to the ring and long fingers, as they are commonly used in tendon transfer procedures.
Flexor digitorum profundus (FDP)	FDP is checked for each finger by holding the PIPJ straight and asking the patient to flex the DIPJ.	• If FDP is intact, the finger will bend at the DIPJ.

- The most frequently ruptured tendons are the EDM, followed by the extensor digitorum communis (EDC) tendons of the small, ring, long, and index fingers; the EPL; the FPL; and, least commonly, the flexor digitorum superficialis (FDS) and profundus (FDP) tendons.
- Extensor tendon ruptures often progress from ulnar to radial, eventually affecting all digits, referred to as *Vaughn-Jackson syndrome*. Tendon ruptures occur suddenly, may not be painful, and must be differentiated from volar subluxation of the MCPJ, radial nerve palsy, and extensor tendon subluxation at the MCPJ. Flexor tendon ruptures occur less often.
- A thorough tendon examination (Table 3) is warranted to determine reconstructive options after tendon rupture (Table 4).

Table 4 Tendon Transfer Options for Rheumatoid Attritional Ruptures

Physical Findings	Ruptured Tendon(s)	Reconstructive Options
Lack of small finger extension	• EDM at ulnar head	• End-to-side repair of EDM to ring finger EDC
Lack of small and ring finger extension	• EDM at ulnar head • EDC to small finger • EDC to ring finger	• EIP transfer to EDM and ring finger EDC
Lack of small, ring, and long finger extension	• EDM at ulnar head • EDC to small finger • EDC to ring finger • EDC to long finger	• EIP transfer to EDM and ring finger EDC • End-to-side repair of long finger EDC to index finger EDC
Lack of small, ring, long, and index finger extension	• EDM at ulnar head • EDC to small finger • EDC to ring finger • EDC to long finger • EDC to index finger • EIP	• Long finger FDS to index and long finger EDC • Ring finger FDS to ring finger EDC and small finger EDC/EDM (whichever tendon is more robust)

Lack of thumb extension (retropulsion)	• EPL at Lister tubercle	• Preferred: EIP transfer to EPL
		• Alternatives:
		  ◦ ECRL to EPL
		  ◦ FDM to EPL

(Continued)

Table 4 Tendon Transfer Options for Rheumatoid Attritional Ruptures (*Continued*)

Physical Findings	Ruptured Tendon(s)	Reconstructive Options
Lack of thumb, index, long, ring, and small finger extension	• EDM at ulnar head • EDC to small finger • EDC to ring finger • EDC to long finger • EDC to index finger • EIP • EPL at Lister tubercle	• Long finger FDS transfer to EPL and index finger EDC • Ring finger FDS transfer to long and ring finger EDC and small finger EDC/EDM (whichever tendon is more robust)

Lack of thumb IPJ flexion	• FPL in carpal tunnel	• Preferred: BR transfer to FPL
		• Alternatives:
		  ◦ ECRL transfer to FPL
		  ◦ Long finger FDS transfer to FPL
		  ◦ Thumb IPJ fusion

Lack of independent PIPJ flexion (of any finger)	• FDS (any finger)	• PIPJ synovectomy (to prevent FDP rupture)
Lack of DIPJ flexion (of any finger)	• FDP (any finger)	• Preferred: DIPJ arthrodesis • Alternative: DIPJ tenodesis
Inability to flex PIPJ and DIPJ (of any finger)	• FDS and FDP (any finger)	• Staged flexor tendon reconstruction

BR, brachioradialis; DIPJ, distal interphalangeal joint; ECRL, extensor carpi radialis longus; EDC, extensor digitorum communis; EDM, extensor digiti minimi; EIP, extensor indicis proprius; EPL, extensor pollicis longus; FDP, flexor digitorum profundus; FDS, flexor digitorum superficialis; FPL, flexor pollicis longus; IPJ, interphalangeal joint; PIPJ, proximal interphalangeal joint.

Carpal Tunnel Syndrome

■ Within the carpal tunnel, synovial pannus and tenosynovitis can proliferate to the point of median nerve compression, causing carpal tunnel syndrome.

■ Synovitis between the scaphoid and lunate can cause SL ligament rupture and scaphoid collapse with its distal pole protruding into the carpal tunnel.

Joints of the Hand

■ In RA patients, the MCPJs and PIPJs are primarily affected, with relative sparing of the DIPJs. Radiographs reveal joint space narrowing from cartilage degradation and marginal bony erosions from pannus invasion. Joint capsules and collateral ligaments are stretched and invaded by pannus as well, leading to joint instability and deformity.

■ The radial and ulnar sagittal bands stabilize the extensor tendon over the dorsal midline of the MCP joint (**FIG 5A,B**). When the radial sagittal band is attenuated, the extensor tendon subluxes ulnarly, leading to ulnar deviation of the finger (**FIG 5C**). The MCPJs in RA patients are typically characterized by volar subluxation and ulnar deviation (**FIG 5D,E**). The MCPJ is a condylar joint, allowing for flexion, extension, radial deviation, and ulnar deviation. The extensor tendon is stabilized over the dorsal midline of the MCPJ by the radial and ulnar sagittal bands. The sagittal bands are connected to the volar plate. Because the lateral bands pass volar to the MCPJ and dorsal to the PIPJ, intrinsic muscle contraction through the lateral bands results in MCPJ flexion and PIPJ extension.

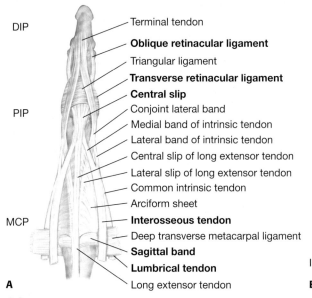

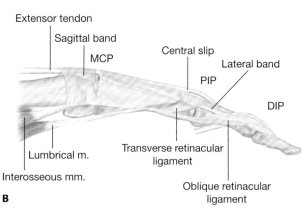

FIG 5 • **A,B.** AP and lateral views of normal anatomy of extensor tendons of the finger.

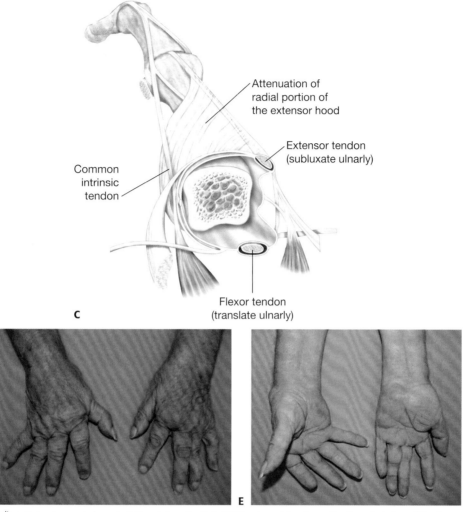

Attenuation of
radial portion of
the extensor hood

Extensor tendon
(subluxate ulnarly)

Common
intrinsic
tendon

Flexor tendon
(translate ulnarly)

C

D

E

FIG 5 (Continued) • **C.** Anatomy of ulnar deviation deformity. **D,E.** MCPJ volar subluxation with ulnar deviation of the fingers.

- In RA patients, ulnar deviation at the MCPJ is due to three things:
  - Erosion of the dorsoradial aspect of the joint capsule
  - The radially deviated wrist position causing an ulnar approach of the extensor tendons
  - Attenuation of the radial sagittal bands leading to ulnar subluxation of the extensor tendons

Swan-Neck Finger Deformity

- The swan-neck finger deformity (**FIG 6**) is characterized by PIPJ hyperextension with DIPJ flexion.
- This deformity is functionally debilitating due to loss of PIPJ flexion, which impedes pinching and grasping.
- Swan-neck deformities can result from pathology at the MCPJ, PIPJ, or DIPJ (Table 5).

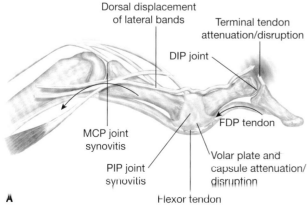

Dorsal displacement
of lateral bands

Terminal tendon
attenuation/disruption

DIP joint

MCP joint
synovitis

FDP tendon

PIP joint
synovitis

Volar plate and
capsule attenuation/
disruption

Flexor tendon

A

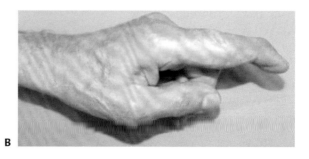

B

FIG 6 • **A,B.** Swan-neck deformity.

Table 5 Three Mechanisms Resulting in the Swan-Neck Deformity

Originating Joint	Mechanism of Swan-Neck Deformity
DIPJ	• Initially, the terminal tendon attenuates or erodes, resulting in a mallet finger. • This leads to increased extension at the PIPJ through the central slip, which is accentuated by MCP flexion. • Further attenuation of the PIP volar plate from synovitis leads to PIPJ hyperextension.
PIPJ	• Initially, the synovial pannus stretches and erodes the volar plate and capsule, allowing for PIPJ hyperextension. • The lateral bands slide dorsally, leading to extra slack in the extensor mechanism. • Slack in the extensor mechanism, combined with tightening of the flexor digitorum profundus (FDP) tendon, leads to DIPJ flexion.
MCPJ	• The volarly subluxed MCPJ posture leads to excessive pull through the extensor mechanism. • When the lateral bands migrate dorsally, the resulting tendon imbalance leads to PIPJ hyperextension and DIPJ flexion.

Boutonniere Finger Deformity

- Boutonniere deformities are less common than swan-neck deformities. They are also less debilitating given that PIPJ flexion, and thus, pinch and grasp are preserved.
- The pathology of boutonniere deformities always starts at the PIPJ, where disruption of the central slip at the base of the middle phalanx occurs. The dorsal capsule, transverse retinacular ligament, and triangular ligament also attenuate. As such, the lateral bands sublux to a position volar to the axis of the PIPJ, flexing the PIPJ.
- Hyperextension at the DIPJ occurs because the lateral bands continue to pull distally on the extensor mechanism at the terminal tendon (**FIG 7**).

Thumb Deformity (Types I to V)

- The boutonniere deformity (type I) is the most common thumb deformity in RA patients, characterized by MCPJ flexion, interphalangeal (IP) hyperextension, and radial abduction of metacarpal (**FIG 8**).
  - Synovial pannus at the MCPJ erodes dorsally, causing eventual rupture of the extensor pollicis brevis (EPB) tendon insertion and displacing the EPL ulnarly and volarly. This leads to MCPJ flexion and volar subluxation. IP joint hyperextension occurs secondarily and is exacerbated in patients with FPL rupture.
- A type II thumb deformity in RA is less common, characterized by thumb MCPJ flexion and IP extension in the setting of carpometacarpal joint (CMCJ) dislocation or subluxation.
- The swan-neck deformity (type III) is the second most common deformity of the thumb, with MCPJ hyperextension, IP flexion, and a metacarpal adduction contracture (**FIG 9**).
  - The volar beak ligament attenuates at the CMCJ, leading to CMCJ subluxation or dislocation and metacarpal adduction. MCPJ hyperextension occurs secondarily as the thumb compensates for the adducted metacarpal and is exacerbated by volar plate attenuation or erosion from pannus invasion.
- The type IV thumb deformity is termed the gamekeeper deformity, which develops secondary to synovial pannus destruction of the ulnar collateral ligament at the MCPJ.
- The type V thumb deformity is similar to the swan-neck deformity, with MCPJ hyperextension and IP flexion, but without the metacarpal adduction contracture.

Trigger Finger

- Trigger fingers in RA patients have a mechanism that is distinct from nonrheumatoid trigger fingers, occurring secondary to synovitis or small rheumatoid nodules in the flexor tendon.
- If the nodule is proximal to the A1 pulley, it can present similarly to a nonrheumatoid trigger digit, with locking in flexion or extension. However, a nodule just distal to the A2 pulley can result in locking in extension

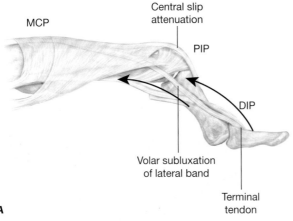

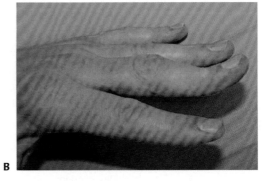

FIG 7 • A,B. Boutonniere deformity.

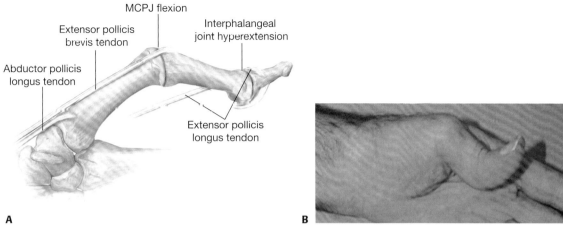

FIG 8 • A,B. Thumb boutonniere deformity.

or triggering during flexion. Also, multiple nodules or diffuse tenosynovitis can lead to loss of flexion and extension altogether.

- Treatment for trigger fingers in patients with RA involves flexor tendon synovectomy through windows in the flexor tendon sheath, along with excision of the rheumatoid nodule, if present.
  - The A1 pulley should not be completely released, as doing so would redirect the pull of the flexor tendon and contribute to ulnar deviation.

NONOPERATIVE MANAGEMENT

- The mainstay of RA treatment is medical, particularly with disease-modifying antirheumatic drugs (DMARDs): glucocorticoids, methotrexate (MTX), conventional DMARDs, and biologic DMARDs.[7] These medications prevent or reduce joint destruction, maintain or improve function, and can improve other aspects of the patient's general health. The goal of medical management in RA is not only clinical remission but also to prevent joint destruction with early medical intervention.[6]

- Oral glucocorticoids suppress inflammation and preserve joint structure. Glucocorticoids can also be injected into actively inflamed joints for pain relief.

- MTX, a folic acid antagonist, is often considered the first-line therapy for RA treatment, as it has been shown to decrease radiographic progression of the disease. MTX is potentially hepatotoxic, and the patient's liver enzymes should be checked at regular intervals. Since MTX is renally cleared, patients with chronic renal insufficiency should not be treated with MTX.

- Conventional DMARDS include hydroxychloroquine, sulfasalazine, and leflunomide, which are mild

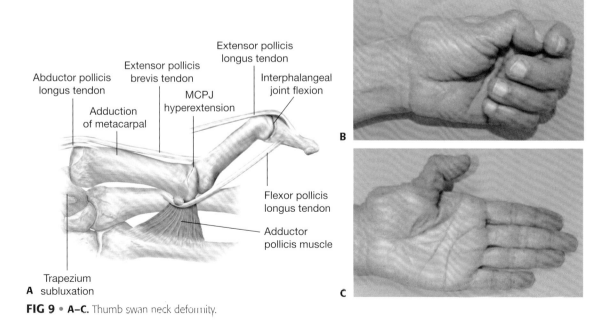

FIG 9 • A–C. Thumb swan neck deformity.

anti-inflammatory agents. These can be used single agents in mild RA or in combination with MTX or other agents.

- Biologic DMARDs include anti-TNF agents, such as etanercept, infliximab, and adalimumab. These are often used as second-line therapy for RA and can be added to MTX or other ongoing therapies. Anti-TNF agents are highly immunosuppressive and must be discontinued if an infection is encountered. Other biologic agents include abatacept and rituximab, which are safe when combined with MTX, and can be used if anti-TNF therapy has failed.

- Nonsteroidal anti-inflammatory drugs (NSAIDs) and other analgesics can be used in combination with DMARDs in the symptomatic treatment of pain in RA patients, but they do not have any significant impact on disease progression or function and should not be used as the primary or sole therapy in RA patients.

- Patients with RA should also be monitored for osteopenia and osteoporosis, which are common comorbid conditions in RA and can be accelerated with glucocorticoid therapy.

- Patients should also participate in physical and occupational therapy to maintain joint mobility and function, improve strength and endurance, and enhance cardiovascular fitness.

- Patients should be educated on the safe use of assistive devices, joint protection, and rest.

SURGICAL MANAGEMENT

- Although excellent clinical and radiographic results in patients with mild deformities or tenosynovitis have been obtained since the introduction of DMARDs, patients who develop severe joint deformities, tendon ruptures, and recalcitrant tenosynovitis will require surgical intervention.
  - The management of rheumatoid hand problems requires an integrated approach involving both the rheumatologist and the hand surgeon. Once medical management is optimized, the patient can be considered for surgery in an effort to provide pain relief, improve function, prevent disease progression, and improve appearance.

- Common surgeries for the rheumatoid hand include tendon reconstruction, correction of swan-neck deformities, correction of boutonniere deformities, and silicone arthroplasty of the MCP joints.

- Tendon transfers are indicated if there is rupture of the long digital flexor or extensor tendons. A thorough tendon examination (**FIG 10**; see Table 3) is critical in determining the appropriate reconstructive options (see Table 4).

- Although the typical swan-neck deformity involves a flexion contracture of the MCPJ, hyperextension of the PIPJ, and dorsally displaced lateral bands (see **FIG 6**), treatment is based on the flexibility of the PIPJ and condition of the joint cartilage. One must test active and passive PIPJ motion with the MCPJ in extension and flexion in order to evaluate intrinsic muscle involvement.
  - The Nalebuff classification[8] is useful for surgical decision-making (Table 6).

- Flexor tendon adhesions are suspected if PIPJ active motion is not nearly equal to its passive motion. On the other hand, if the PIPJ remains flexible regardless of MCPJ position (type I), a PIPJ extension-blocking splint may be enough to correct the deformity. If PIPJ flexion is restricted with MCPJ extension and radial deviation, ulnar intrinsic muscle tightness is present.

- Reconstructive surgery can be performed for a boutonniere deformity provided that the PIPJ has full passive extension. The Nalebuff classification of boutonniere deformities (see Table 6) classifies this as stage I or II. However, if a severe fixed flexion contracture exists, or if articular destruction is present (stage III), arthrodesis or arthroplasty of the PIPJ is recommended.

- In RA patients, silicone metacarpophalangeal joint arthroplasty (SMPA) is indicated to treat MCPJ contracture, subluxation, or dislocation. However, SMPA is not indicated in patients with other rheumatic conditions such as lupus, in which soft tissue laxity is present without the underlying joint destruction. In such patients, joint replacement would inevitably lead to joint dislocation due to the absence of healthy supporting ligaments.

- In RA patients with no evidence of MCP joint subluxation or arthritis, soft tissue reconstruction for correction of ulnar deviation finger deformities can be performed using the crossed intrinsic tendon transfer. The ulnar deviation deformity must be passively correctable. As such, this procedure is also useful in patients with lupus who do not have any underlying joint destruction.

Preoperative Planning

- Preoperative evaluation of RA patients is critical in reducing surgery-related morbidity and mortality.

- Many surgeons advocate that all RA patients should be seen in the preoperative anesthesia clinic due to a high incidence of comorbid conditions.

- A thorough evaluation with an electrocardiogram, complete blood count and differential, metabolic panel, chest radiograph, and cervical spine radiographs should be obtained.

- From a cardiac standpoint, RA can be associated with pericardial effusion, constrictive pericarditis, or conduction blocks, thereby impacting cardiac function. In addition, RA patients are at increased risk of coronary artery disease.

- Pulmonary involvement may include rheumatoid nodules, pleural effusions, or interstitial lung disease.

- Long-standing RA can be associated with Felty syndrome (splenomegaly, neutropenia, and secondary thrombocytopenia).

- Cervical spine flexion-extension radiographs are imperative as atlantoaxial instability is common in RA patients, placing patients at risk for spinal cord injury with routine procedures such as endotracheal intubation.
  - Patients with cervical instability should undergo fiberoptic intubation.
  - RA may also involve the cricoarytenoid and the temporomandibular joints, which can further complicate airway management.

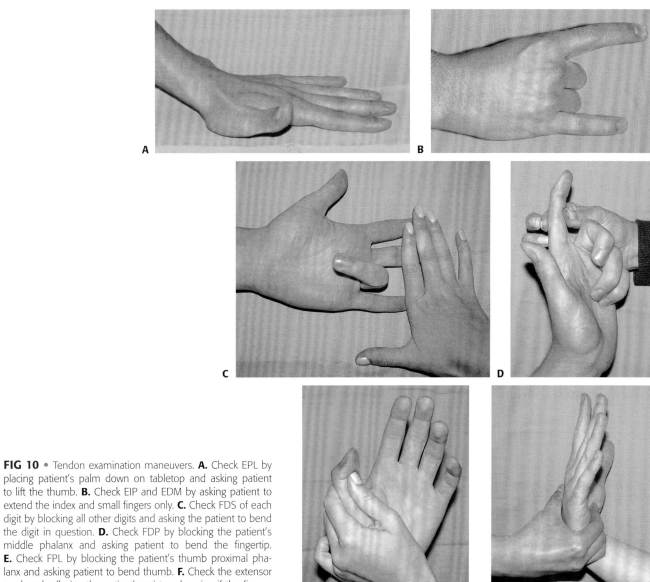

FIG 10 • Tendon examination maneuvers. **A.** Check EPL by placing patient's palm down on tabletop and asking patient to lift the thumb. **B.** Check EIP and EDM by asking patient to extend the index and small fingers only. **C.** Check FDS of each digit by blocking all other digits and asking the patient to bend the digit in question. **D.** Check FDP by blocking the patient's middle phalanx and asking patient to bend the fingertip. **E.** Check FPL by blocking the patient's thumb proximal phalanx and asking patient to bend thumb. **F.** Check the extensor tendons by flexing the patient's wrist and seeing if the fingers extend (the tenodesis effect).

Table 6 The Nalebuff Classification for Swan-Neck Deformities and Surgical Options

Type	Description	Surgical Goals/Options
I	PIPJ is flexible in all positions of the MCPJ	Must limit PIPJ hyperextension (splint, dermodesis, FDS tenodesis) and restore DIPJ extension (tenodermodesis, fusion)
II	PIPJ flexion is limited in certain MCPJ positions	Intrinsic release and/or MCPJ arthroplasty, in addition to procedures required for type I deformities
III	PIPJ flexion is limited irrespective of MCPJ positions	Restore PIPJ flexion by manipulation, lateral band mobilization, and lengthening of central slip
IV	PIPJ joints are stiff, with poor radio- graphic appearance	Arthrodesis of PIPJ is preferred, but implant arthroplasty may be considered

DIPJ, distal interphalangeal joint; FDS, flexor digitorium superficialis; PIPJ, proximal interphalangeal joint; MCPJ, metacarpophalangeal joint.

- Perioperative medication management should be discussed with the patient's rheumatologist. In general, corticosteroids can be continued, but patients may require a stress dose at the time of surgery.
  - MTX and other conventional DMARDs can generally be continued.
  - Biological DMARDs, on the other hand, are typically discontinued for 2 to 4 weeks before and after surgery. Again, discussion with the patient's rheumatologist is imperative.

Positioning

- Patients are positioned supine with the upper extremity abducted on a hand table.
- Care is taken to provide the appropriate neck support.
- A tourniquet is placed on the upper arm.

■ Tendon Transfers for Tendon Ruptures

Imaging and Planning

- Radiographs of the wrist to evaluate the DRUJ, midcarpal joint, and radiocarpal joint should be obtained.
  - Should these joints be involved, they must be addressed at the time of tendon reconstruction to prevent progressive deformity and rerupture of the reconstructed tendons.
- If tendon rupture is diagnosed, surgical reconstruction is indicated to restore function. Because the ruptured tendon ends are of poor quality, direct repair is usually not possible. Furthermore, myostatic contraction eventually leads to loss of the proximal end of the ruptured tendon, preventing the use of tendon grafts. Tendon transfer is the preferred reconstructive option.
- Depending on the number of ruptured tendons, surgery may involve a simple end-to-side repair to an intact adjacent tendon, or it may require transfer of a new motor-tendon unit (Table 5). It is also important to address the cause of tendon rupture at the time of tendon reconstruction to prevent rerupture.
  - If synovitis is the cause, a synovectomy must also be performed.
  - If joint instability or bony erosion is the cause, a procedure to address this should be performed as well.

Tendon Transfers for Extensor Tendon Ruptures

- After tourniquet inflation, a 6-cm longitudinal incision is made over the dorsal wrist in line with the long finger.
- Skin flaps are raised to expose the extensor retinaculum.
- The retinaculum is incised and elevated using a stair-step design (**TECH FIG 1A**).
  - The stair-step incision effectively lengthens the retinaculum to permit closure over the reconstructed tendons in the presence of swelling.
  - Also, if there is eroded bone exposed at the radiocarpal joint, half of the retinaculum can be used as a protective layer between bone and tendon, while the other half is closed over the tendons.
- Next, the septa between the second and sixth extensor compartments are divided, bringing the tendons together, typically revealing hypertophic synovial tissue encasing the tendons (**TECH FIG 1B**).
- Synovectomy is then sharply performed. Tendons that are invaded by synovial tissue are also completely excised (**TECH FIG 1C**).
- Tendon reconstruction then proceeds based on the tendons involved (see Table 4). All tendon junctures are secured with nonabsorbable braided suture (**TECH FIG 1D**).
- If EPL is to be addressed, a separate incision is made at the level of the thumb metacarpal, to identify the distal EPL tendon (**TECH FIG 1E**).
- The EIP tendon is often weaved into the EPL tendon (**TECH FIG 1F**), thereby restoring EPL function (thumb retropulsion).
- If three or more extensor tendons are ruptured, the FDS is used for the transfer.

- The FDS tendon is identified through a transverse incision in the distal palm and divided. The proximal end of the tendon is retrieved via a separate longitudinal incision in the distal volar forearm and passed in a subcutaneous tunnel radially in order to reach the extensor tendons on the wrist dorsum.
- A single FDS tendon can be transferred to up to three extensor tendons. If more than three extensor tendons are ruptured, however, transfer of both the ring and long finger FDS tendons should be considered.
- Once all tendons are addressed, the dorsal wrist capsule is closed using braided sutures. If the capsule is lax, it can be imbricated with these sutures.
- The forearm is placed in supination, and the capsule over the distal ulna is closed tightly with 3-0 braided sutures in a horizontal mattress fashion.
- Next, the extensor tendons are re-examined for laxity.
  - If lax, the extensor tendons can be tightened with horizontal mattress braided sutures.
  - Tension is set with all fingers in fully extended posture, as some postoperative stretching is anticipated.
- The extensor retinaculum is then repaired. If needed, the distal half can be used to augment the wrist capsular repair, placing it underneath the extensor tendons, and the proximal half is sutured over the tendons, recreating the pulley (**TECH FIG 1G**).
- The tourniquet is then released, hemostasis is achieved, and the skin is closed with 4-0 nylon simple interrupted sutures.
- Fingers are immobilized in fully extended position for 4 weeks, and then active range-of-motion (ROM) exercises are initiated.

Reconstruction of Ruptured Flexor Tendons

Grafting for FPL Rupture

- For the treatment of an FPL rupture caused by attritional wear against an eroded scaphoid (Mannerfelt lesion), exposure of the tendon is performed at the palm-wrist junction, and initially, a flexor tenolysis is performed.
- The osteophyte is then removed with a rongeur, and the capsule is closed to provide a smooth gliding surface.
- If the proximal and distal ends of the ruptured FPL tendon can be found within the palm-wrist incision, a small bridge graft from the palmaris longus (PL) is used in a Pulvertaft weave with 3-0 nonabsorbable braided horizontal mattress sutures (**TECH FIG 2**).
  - As an alternative, a strip of the FCR can be used instead of the PL.

Tendon Transfer for FPL Rupture

- If grafting within the palm or wrist is not possible, a tendon transfer is required. Here, the long finger FDS tendon transfer for FPL reconstruction is described.
  - A zigzag incision is made in the palm and the long finger FDS tendon is identified (**TECH FIG 3A**).
  - The long finger FDS is divided and brought into the palmar wound (**TECH FIG 3B,C**).
  - Through a Bruner incision on the thumb, the flexor tendon sheath is sharply opened and divided transversely, leaving enough tendon distally for suturing.

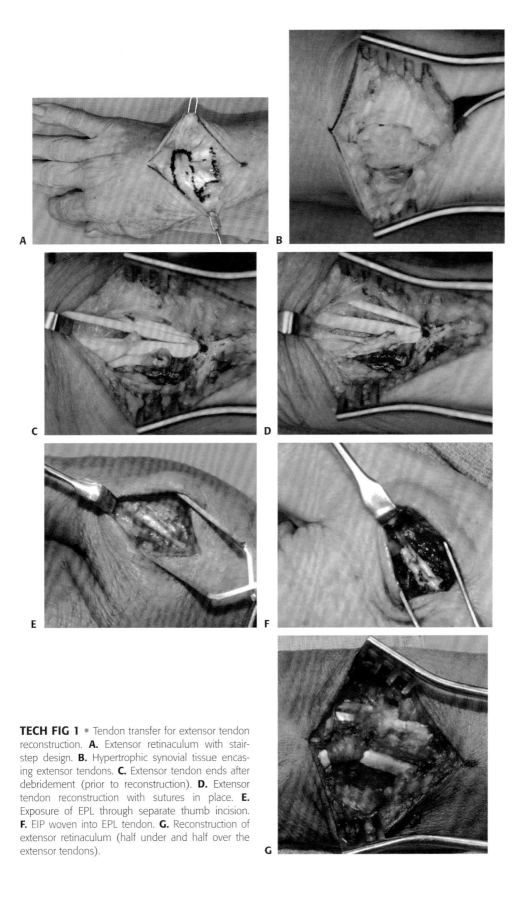

TECH FIG 1 • Tendon transfer for extensor tendon reconstruction. **A.** Extensor retinaculum with stairstep design. **B.** Hypertrophic synovial tissue encasing extensor tendons. **C.** Extensor tendon ends after debridement (prior to reconstruction). **D.** Extensor tendon reconstruction with sutures in place. **E.** Exposure of EPL through separate thumb incision. **F.** EIP woven into EPL tendon. **G.** Reconstruction of extensor retinaculum (half under and half over the extensor tendons).

TECHNIQUES

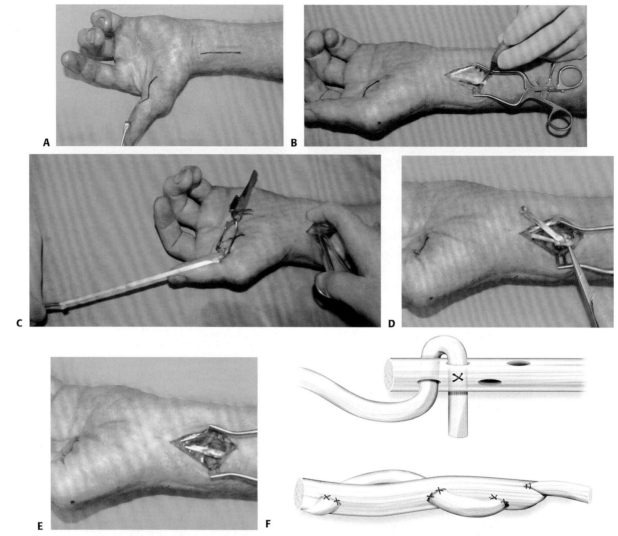

TECH FIG 2 • Ruptured flexor pollicis longus tendon reconstruction with PL. **A.** Planned skin incisions. **B.** Ruptured FPL tendon is identified at the wrist. **C.** FPL with excellent excursion. **D.** FPL is attached to PL. **E.** PL to FPL tendon reconstruction. **F.** Pulvertaft weave.

- The FDS is then delivered into the flexor tendon sheath of the thumb using a pediatric feeding tube.
- Nonabsorbable braided suture is then used to sew the FDS tendon to the distal FPL tendon (**TECH FIG 3D**). Tension should be set so that IP extension occurs with wrist flexion, and full flexion into the palm occurs with wrist extension.

Isolated FDS or FDP Ruptures

- If an isolated FDS rupture occurs within the palm or carpal tunnel, an end-to-side suture using a Pulvertaft weave to an adjacent FDS is performed, along with flexor tenosynovectomy and the smoothing of any sharp bony edges.
  - However, if the FDS rupture occurs within the finger, a tenosynovectomy with resection of the FDS should be performed.
- Similarly, if an isolated FDP rupture occurs within the palm or wrist, an end-to-side suture to an adjacent FDP is performed.

- If FDP rupture occurs within the finger, as long as FDS is still functional, the FDP is resected.
- If the DIPJ hyperextends during pinch or grip, DIP arthrodesis is performed as well.

Combined FDS and FDP Ruptures

- If occurring within the palm or wrist, the combination rupture of both FDS and FDP is treated with end-to-side suturing of the FDP to an adjacent tendon.
  - Alternatively, a bridge graft from the ruptured FDS can be used to repair the FDP tendon.
- If both FDS and FDP have ruptured within the flexor tendon sheath, a staged reconstruction should be considered, though outcomes in patients with RA are often disappointing due to limited recovery of motion.
- In patients with IPJ arthritis, the best option is arthrodesis of the PIP and DIP joints in a functional position, with preservation of some finger motion at the MCPJ via the intrinsic system.

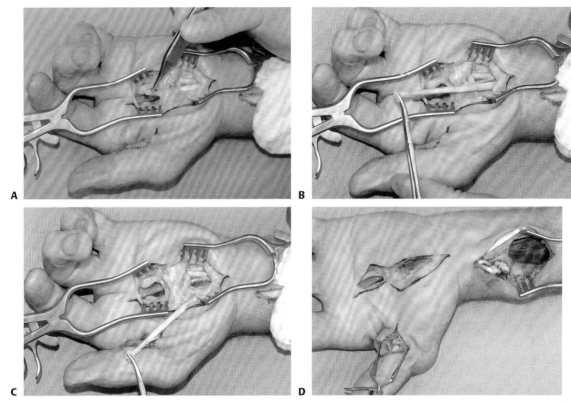

TECH FIG 3 • Long finger FDS tendon transfer for ruptured flexor pollicis longus tendon reconstruction. **A.** Long finger FDS is identified through a palmar incision. **B.** The FDS is divided and retracted into palmar wound. **C.** The FDS is transferred from the long finger to the FPL tendon through a Bruner incision on the thumb. **D.** The reconstructed FPL tendon is shown.

■ Postoperative Care

- If tendon transfers are performed for flexor reconstruction, the hand and fingers are immobilized in a dorsal blocking splint to take tension off the transfers for 3 to 4 weeks.
- After this period, ROM exercises are gradually initiated, as guided by the hand therapist.

■ Correction of Swan-Neck Deformity

- It is imperative to understand the anatomy of the extensor apparatus of the finger (see **FIG 5**).

Correction of PIPJ Hyperextension (Type I to III Deformities)

FDS Tenodesis ("Lasso")

- This is the authors' preferred technique.
- A slip of FDS is divided proximal to the A2 pulley (**TECH FIG 4A**).
- A hole is made in the distal third of the proximal phalanx, from the volar to lateral surface (**TECH FIG 4B**).
- The FDS slip is passed through the hole, from volar to lateral (**TECH FIG 4C**), and is sutured with the PIPJ at 20 to 30 degrees of flexion (**TECH FIG 4D**).
- This procedure can be combined with removal of a small ellipse of skin at the PIPJ to reinforce the tenodesis, particularly in lupus patients.

Retinacular Ligament Reconstruction

- The ulnar lateral band at the midproximal phalanx is divided and dissected distally (**TECH FIG 5A**).
- It is passed volar to the Cleland ligament, such that the ulnar lateral band can maintain the PIPJ in flexion (**TECH FIG 5B**).
- The lateral band is sutured to the A2 pulley or into the bone of the proximal phalanx to maintain PIPJ flexion at 20 to 30 degrees (**TECH FIG 5C**).
- An extension block pin is placed to protect the reconstruction.

Bone Anchor Repair of Volar Plate

- A Bruner (zigzag) incision is made on the volar finger surface.
- The accessory collateral ligament is identified and incised in order to retract the volar plate and flexor sheath laterally, exposing the head of the proximal phalanx.

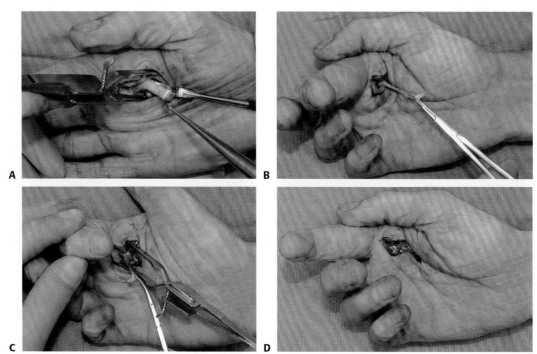

TECH FIG 4 • FDS tenodesis for correction of swan-neck deformity. **A.** An FDS slip is divided proximal to A2 pulley. **B.** A hole is drilled in the proximal phalanx (distal third), from volar to lateral surface. **C.** FDS slip is passed through the hold from volar to lateral. **D.** FDS slip is sutured with PIPJ at 15 to 20 degrees of flexion.

- A drill hole is made in the center of the volar surface of the proximal phalanx, approximately 5 to 7 mm proximal to the joint line.
- A bone anchor, which is connected to two needled sutures, such as the Mitek Mini (Mitek Surgical Products Inc., Norwood), is placed into the hole.
- One needled suture is passed from the dorsolateral volar plate, emerging at the central volar plate, and then

passed through the edge of the previously divided accessory collateral ligament. The suture is tied with the goal of maintaining 10 degrees of PIPJ flexion.
- The other needled suture is then passed in a similar fashion on the other side and then tied with the PIPJ at about 20 to 30 degrees of flexion.
- Note that this procedure is technically difficult to perform and is not the authors' preferred technique.

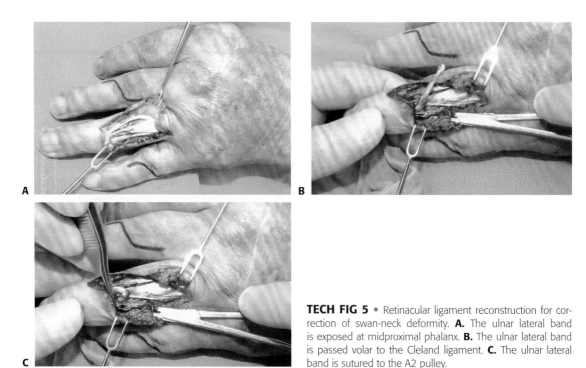

TECH FIG 5 • Retinacular ligament reconstruction for correction of swan-neck deformity. **A.** The ulnar lateral band is exposed at midproximal phalanx. **B.** The ulnar lateral band is passed volar to the Cleland ligament. **C.** The ulnar lateral band is sutured to the A2 pulley.

Correction of DIPJ Flexion Deformity (Type I to IV Deformities)

Dorsal Tenodermodesis of the DIPJ

- A transverse ellipse of skin is excised at the dorsal DIPJ.
- A 3-0 nylon horizontal mattress suture is placed through the skin and underlying extensor tendon in order to close the skin gap. With the DIPJ held in extension, the suture is tied.
- A K-wire is inserted obliquely through the extended DIPJ and is cut off beneath the skin.
- In general, this technique is not preferred because patients have thin skin and tend to experience complications.

DIPJ Arthrodesis

- An H- or Y-incision over the dorsal DIPJ is made to expose the extensor tendon.
- The extensor tendon and collateral ligaments are divided, allowing the joint to be hinged open.
- The joint surfaces are sculpted with a small bur, creating a "trough" distally and a "crest" proximally.
- The bone is fit together, and a compression screw is placed across the joint to support bony fusion. (See chapter on Degenerative Disease of the Hand and Wrist for details).

Correction of a Stiff Swan-Neck Deformity (Type III Deformity)

Lateral Band Mobilization

- A curved incision is made over the extensor apparatus overlying the proximal phalanx to the mid middle phalanx (**TECH FIG 6A**).

- The lateral bands are typically found to be dorsally displaced and adherent to the central slip, causing the extension contracture. The lateral bands are sharply dissected from the central slip (**TECH FIG 6B**), distal to proximal, preserving a wide central slip, particularly when the demarcation between the central slip and lateral bands is unclear.
  - A wider central slip can better resist accidental rupture during joint manipulation and is easier to lengthen.
- Next, the PIPJ is flexed to enable the lateral bands to move laterally and volarly (**TECH FIG 6C**).
  - If it is difficult to flex the PIPJ, the dorsal capsule and dorsal aspects of the collateral ligaments may need to be release.
  - Care must be taken to monitor the tension of the central slip during PIPJ manipulation to avoid rupture.

Step-Cut (Z) Central Slip Lengthening

- This procedure can be considered if the central slip continues to restrict PIPJ flexion after release of the lateral bands and attempted PIPJ manipulation. It is generally not necessary, however, because the central slip tends to stretch over time with therapy.
- A Z-incision of the central slip is made, starting 3 to 4 mm proximal to its insertion at the middle phalanx. It is extended 1 to 1.5 cm proximally.
- If not yet performed, the dorsal capsule and dorsal portions of the collateral ligaments are sharply released.
- With the PIPJ in slight flexion, the central slip is then repaired with at least three or four horizontal mattress sutures to prevent rupture during early mobilization.

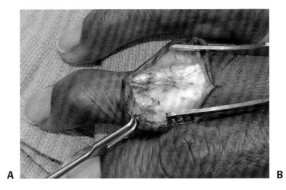
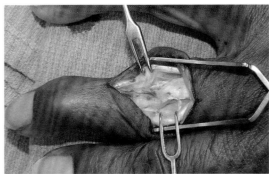
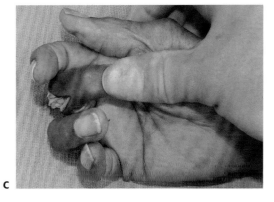

TECH FIG 6 • Lateral band mobilization for correction of stiff swan-neck deformity. **A.** Exposure of extensor apparatus from proximal to mid middle phalanx **B.** The lateral bands are identified and separated from the central slip **C.** The PIPJ is flexed, allowing the lateral bands to fall volarly

■ Postoperative Care

- Active motion is initiated on the 2nd postoperative day.
- A dorsal extension block splint is applied for 2 weeks until the skin has healed. Then, a thermoplastic figure-eight splint is applied for an additional 8 weeks.

- After lateral band mobilization and manipulation of the PIPJ for a type III deformity, the PIPJ should be splinted in flexion in order to stretch the dorsal soft tissue.
- Patients should continue active flexion exercises, except in cases in which central slip lengthening was also performed.

■ Ligament Reconstruction to Correct Boutonniere Deformity

- Once the patient is made comfortable with a wrist or digital block, a dorsally placed curved incision over the PIPJ is made to expose the extensor apparatus.
- The lateral bands and transverse retinacular ligaments are identified.
- The radial and ulnar transverse retinacular ligaments are sharply divided from their insertions on the volar plate of the PIPJ.
- The transverse retinacular ligaments are then turned over dorsally on either side of the PIPJ and sutured together.

  - Tension of the suture is determined by asking the patient to actively extend the PIPJ.
  - Tension should be set at the near-full extended position.
- Next, active flexion of the DIPJ must be checked. If DIPJ flexion is limited, small transverse cuts into the lateral bands to lengthen them between the PIPJ and DIPJ (overlying the distal half of the middle phalanx) should be made, until the DIPJ can be actively flexed to 30 degrees.
- The PIPJ is then immobilized in full extension with a K-wire for 2 weeks.

■ Postoperative Care

- Within 3 days of surgery, active DIPJ flexion exercises are initiated, while the PIPJ remains immobilized.
- At about 2 weeks, active PIPJ flexion exercises are begun, while active extension exercises should be avoided.

- To keep the PIPJ in full extension, a daytime dynamic splint and nighttime static splint should be provided.
- The splint is gradually weaned, and active finger exercises are slowly advanced under the guidance of a hand therapist.

■ Silicone Metacarpophalangeal Joint Arthroplasty

- The patient is positioned supine with the extremity abducted on a hand table.
- Under tourniquet control, a transverse incision is made over the heads of the second through fifth metacarpals, taking care to preserve the dorsal veins and sensory nerves (**TECH FIG 7A**).
- The radial sagittal bands are divided to expose the MCPJs. Synovectomy is performed sharply.
- The collateral ligaments are divided at the metacarpal neck, taking care to preserve the radial collateral ligament insertion on the proximal phalanges for later reconstruction.
- With an oscillating saw, the metacarpal heads are resected at the proximal origin of the collateral ligaments (**TECH FIG 7B**).
  - After metacarpal head resection, the fingers are brought into alignment.
  - Using a twisting motion, an awl is used to perforate the medullary cavities of the metacarpals and proximal phalanges (**TECH FIG 7C**).
- Next, sequentially sized broaches are used to enlarge the medullary cavities of the proximal phalanges first, then the metacarpals, since the size of the phalangeal cavity usually determines the implant size to be used.
  - The exception is the ring metacarpal, which is typically narrower than the ring finger proximal phalanx and

should thus be prepared first to avoid over-reaming the proximal phalanx.
  - It is important that the broach is inserted straight without twisting, making a rectangular trough to accommodate the shape of the silicone implants.
- The largest implants that will fit into the medullary cavity are then selected.
- Prior to implant insertion, two drill holes are made with a 0.035-in. K-wire on the radial edge of the metacarpal (**TECH FIG 7D**)
  - 3-0 braided permanent sutures are placed through these drill holes to reconstruct the radial collateral ligaments (**TECH FIG 7E**).
- Next, the implants are inserted (**TECH FIG 7F**).
- The radially placed sutures are used to reattach the radial collateral ligament, bringing the fingers into slight radial deviation (**TECH FIG 7G**).
- If still tight, the ulnar lateral bands can be released, though this is usually not necessary.
- The position of the extensor tendons should be re-evaluated. If they cannot be centralized easily, the ulnar sagittal bands may also need to be released.
- Next, the extensor tendons are centralized by imbricating the radial sagittal bands with 3-0 braided horizontal mattress sutures.
- The tourniquet is released, and hemostasis is achieved.
- The skin is closed with absorbable dermal sutures followed by 4-0 horizontal mattress nylon sutures (**TECH FIG 7H**).
- A volar resting short-arm splint is applied.

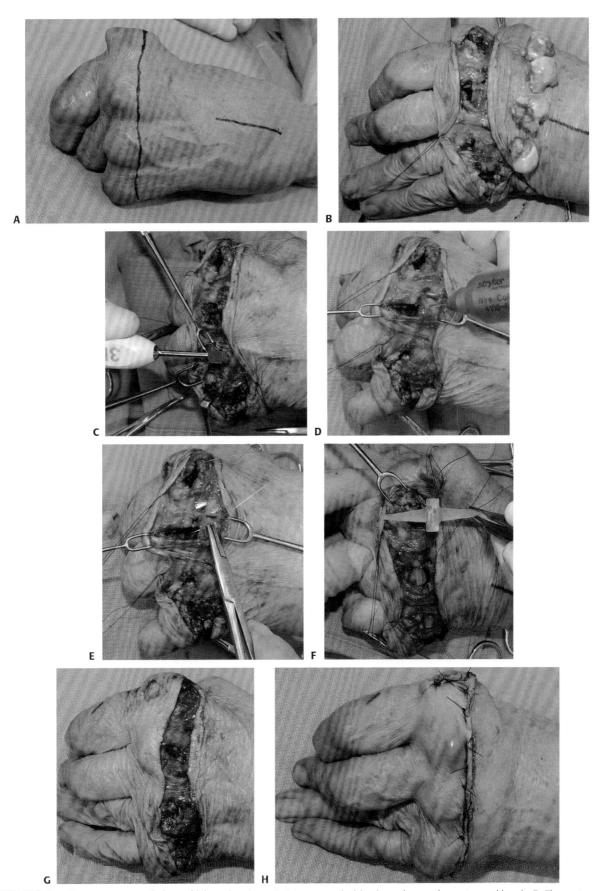

TECH FIG 7 • Silicone metacarpophalangeal joint arthroplasty. **A.** A transverse incision is made over the metacarpal heads. **B.** The metacarpal heads are resected with an oscillating saw. **C.** An awl is used to perforate the medullary cavities of the metacarpals and proximal phalanges. **D.** Two drill holes are made on the radial edge of the metacarpal. **E.** Sutures are placed through the drill holes. **F.** The silicone implants are inserted. **G.** The sutures are tied down, thereby reconstructing the radial collateral ligament. **H.** Skin closure, improved alignment of fingers

■ Postoperative Care

- The patient is placed in a dynamic extension splint 1 week postoperatively.

- While in the splint, the patient is to begin active flexion exercises for 6 weeks under the guidance of a hand therapist. The splint is adjusted as necessary to align the fingers.

■ Crossed Intrinsic Transfer for Correction of Ulnar Deviation Deformity

Pertinent Anatomy

- The radial and ulnar sagittal bands stabilize the extensor tendon over the dorsal midline of the MCP joint (see **FIG 5A**). When the radial sagittal band is attenuated, the extensor tendon subluxes ulnarly, leading to ulnar deviation of the finger (see **FIG 5C**).
- On the ulnar side of the digit, the common intrinsic tendon is formed by the tendons of the palmar and dorsal interosseous muscles. On the radial side, the common intrinsic tendon is formed by the tendons of the interosseous muscles as well as the lumbrical.
- The common intrinsic tendon then passes volar to the MCP joint and divides into a medial band (which inserts into the central slip at the dorsal base of the middle phalanx) and a lateral band (which inserts at the dorsal base of the distal phalanx).
- Thus, intrinsic muscle contraction results in MCP joint flexion and IP joint extension.
- In a cross intrinsic transfer, the common intrinsic tendon is divided distally (slanted lines) and sutured to the extensor tendon of the adjacent finger (**TECH FIG 8**).

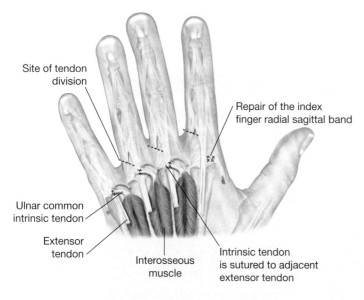

Site of tendon division

Repair of the index finger radial sagittal band

Ulnar common intrinsic tendon

Extensor tendon

Interosseous muscle

Intrinsic tendon is sutured to adjacent extensor tendon

TECH FIG 8 • Cross intrinsic transfer for repair of the index finger radial sagittal band. The common intrinsic tendon is divided distally (*slanted lines*) and sutured to the extensor tendon of the adjacent finger (*arrows*).

■ Transfer Procedure

- Under tourniquet control, the extensor apparatus over the MCP joint is exposed through a lazy-S incision if only one finger is involved or through a dorsal transverse incision over the MCP joints if multiple fingers require correction (**TECH FIG 9A**).
- A longitudinal incision paralleling the extensor tendon is made through the attenuated radial sagittal band (**TECH FIG 9B**).
- The MCP joint is opened. A synovectomy is performed.
- On the ulnar side, the common intrinsic tendon is identified (**TECH FIG 9C**) and divided from its attachment to the extensor mechanism at the midproximal phalanx.

- The tendon is rerouted across the adjacent web space to reach the extensor tendon of the digit ulnar to it (**TECH FIG 9D**). It is then passed through a slit made at the midportion of the extensor tendon overlying the MCP joint and sutured to itself using 3-0 braided nonabsorbable suture.
  - Note that the ulnar common intrinsic tendon of the index finger is used to correct the long finger; the tendon of the long finger is used to correct the ring finger; and the tendon of the ring finger is used to correct the small finger.
- The index finger is then corrected by a double-breasted repair of the radial sagittal band (**TECH FIG 9E**).
- The skin is closed with simple interrupted horizontal mattress sutures (**TECH FIG 9F**).

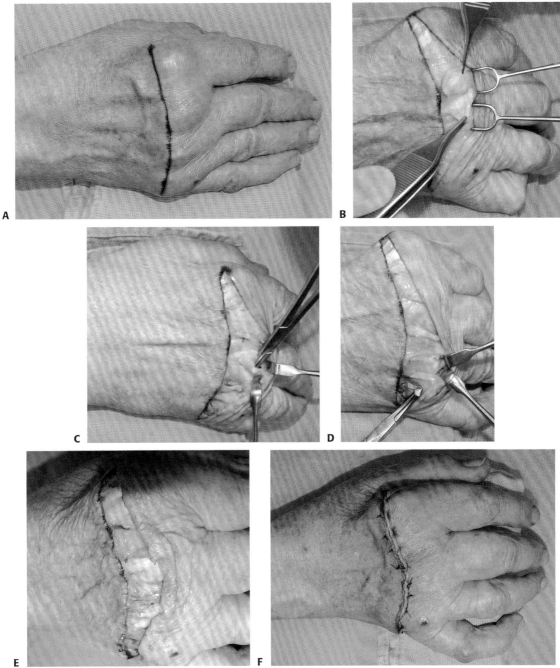

TECH FIG 9 • A. Planned skin incision over the MCP joints. **B.** The attenuated radial sagittal band of the long finger is incised to access the MCP joint to facilitate synovectomy. **C.** The ulnar common intrinsic tendon of the long finger is identified. **D.** The ulnar common intrinsic tendon of the ring finger has been rerouted to the small finger to be sutured to the extensor tendon. The intrinsic tendon is being held by the clamp in this photo. **E.** Final appearance of multiple cross intrinsic tendon transfers to the long, ring, and small fingers. A double-breasted repair of the radial sagittal band of the index finger is also shown. **F.** Skin closure.

■ Postoperative Care

- A volar hand splint is placed to support the reconstruction with the MCP joint in extension.

- At 10 days, a removable splint is placed.
- At 4 weeks, a gradual mobilization protocol is initiated with protective splinting for another 4 weeks.

PEARLS AND PITFALLS

TENDON TRANSFERS FOR TENDON RUPTURES

Extensor tendon exposure	▪ Skin flaps are raised superficial to the extensor retinaculum, taking care to preserve the longitudinal dorsal veins (improves postoperative swelling) and superficial sensory nerve branches. ▪ Skin must be handled as gently as possible, as skin quality and vascularity are already impaired by rheumatoid disease and/or medications.
Stair-step incision of extensor retinaculum	▪ Facilitates closure of the extensor retinaculum at the end of the case, as swelling under retinaculum is common. ▪ Can be useful to shield the extensor tendons from the radiocarpal joint in cases of bony erosion (half the retinaculum is placed under the extensor tendons, and the other half is used to close over them).
Treatment of combined ring and small finger extensor tendon ruptures	▪ Treatment options include EIP transfer or end-to-side repair of the ring and small finger extensor tendons to the long finger extensor tendon. ▪ EIP transfer is preferred due to the line of pull. ▪ End-to-side repair to the long finger extensor tendon results in an oblique pull that can cause unwanted abduction of the small finger.
Transferring FDS tendons	▪ For extensor tendon reconstruction, a subcutaneous transfer is preferred over a transfer through the interosseous membrane (high risk of adhesions). ▪ A subcutaneous transfer on the radial side is preferred over the ulnar side, because the direction of pull helps to correct the ulnar deviation deformity.
Thumb interphalangeal joint (IPJ) fusion	▪ Can be considered as long as the MCPJ is stable and functional and the strength of intrinsic muscles is adequate. If not, the patient will not achieve satisfactory pinch strength.
Darrach procedure	▪ Defined as the resection of the head of the ulna. ▪ May be required if the distal ulna is the source of tendon attrition and rupture. ▪ If performed concomitantly with tendon reconstruction, a supination splint should be placed for 4 weeks postoperatively.

CORRECTION OF SWAN-NECK DEFORMITY

Exposure	▪ Avoid injury to the digital nerve at the tip of the flap where it is just beneath the skin by identifying the nerve at the base of the flap.
Dorsal DIPJ tenodermodesis	▪ Generally, soft tissue reconstruction for DIPJ extension is discouraged, and arthrodesis is preferable. ▪ However, tenodermodesis combined with DIPJ pinning for greater than 2 months can create a generally stiff DIPJ allowing for slight motion.

LIGAMENT RECONSTRUCTION TO CORRECT BOUTONNIERE DEFORMITY

Preoperative management	▪ Passive PIPJ mobility is critical to optimize surgical outcomes after correcting a boutonniere deformity. ▪ If a severe PIPJ flexion contracture is present, rehabilitation and extension splinting should be performed prior to surgery.
Imaging	▪ Radiographs are required to evaluate MCJP, PIPJ, and DIPJ status prior to surgery. PIPJ destruction indicates the need for arthrodesis or arthroplasty, as opposed to ligament reconstruction. ▪ MRI may be helpful in identifying synovitis of the PIPJ but is expensive and not usually necessary to make the diagnosis.
Anesthesia: wrist or digital block	▪ The surgery is done under a wrist or digital block such that the patient can perform active finger motion during the operation to allow for proper tension setting.
Tension setting	▪ The transverse retinacular ligaments are sutured together at the dorsal aspect of the PIPJ when it is in near-full extension. ▪ If set too tight, the tension may lead to extension contracture of the PIPJ and DIPJ.
PIPJ contracture	▪ If a contracture exists at the PIPJ, the accessory collateral ligament and proximal volar plate should be released to obtain full passive PIPJ extension. ▪ Care must be taken to preserve the true collateral ligaments to prevent PIPJ instability.
Achieving DIPJ flexion	▪ In some cases, dividing the oblique retinacular ligament is necessary to obtain DIPJ flexion. ▪ Avoid releasing the lateral bands too far, as this can result in DIPJ extension lag.
PIPJ synovectomy	▪ For patients with active RA, PIPJ synovectomy is required.

PEARLS AND PITFALLS (Continued)

SILICONE METACARPOPHALANGEAL JOINT ARTHROPLASTY

Surgical considerations	■ If the patient's fingers are ulnarly drifted without evidence of MCPJ dislocation, soft tissue reconstruction can be performed instead of SMPA.
	   ■ A crossed intrinsic transfer may be performed to correct finger misalignment of the small, ring, and long fingers (see crossed intrinsic transfer for ulnar deviation technique below).
	   ■ For the index finger, the radial sagittal band must be tightened to centralize the extensor tendon, given that there is no ulnar intrinsic tendon available for transfer.
	 ■ Thumb MCPJ laxity is best treated with MCPJ fusion.
	 ■ Patients with wrist collapse and radial deviation of the metacarpals should first have their wrists addressed by fusion or arthroplasty. Not only will this enhance the outcome of SMPA, but also it will prevent early postoperative ulnar subluxation of the fingers after SMPA.

Imaging	■ PA, lateral, and oblique radiographs of the hand and wrist are important in order to evaluate joint alignment, joint congruity, and bony erosions.
Metacarpal head resection	■ Resection of the metacarpal heads decreases the tightness of the ulnar intrinsic tendons that contribute to ulnar deviation of the fingers. As such, ulnar lateral band release is usually not necessary.
Preparing the medullary canals for implant insertion	■ The medullary canals of the proximal phalanges, which are typically narrower than those of the metacarpals, should be prepared first since they usually determine the implant size to be used. ■ The exception to this rule is the ring finger. The ring metacarpal typically has a narrower canal than does the proximal phalanx and should therefore be prepared first to avoid over-reaming the proximal phalanx.

CROSSED INTRINSIC TRANSFER FOR CORRECTION OF ULNAR DEVIATION DEFORMITY

Indications	■ The crossed intrinsic transfer may also be considered for lupus patients with ulnar deviation deformities, as they do not have underlying joint destruction.
Surgical tips	■ Try to preserve longitudinal dorsal veins during surgical exposure to minimize postoperative swelling. ■ Avoid dividing the common intrinsic tendon too proximally, as it may not reach the extensor tendon of the adjacent finger if too short. ■ Take care to preserve the neurovascular bundle volar to the common intrinsic tendon. ■ Division of the abductor digiti minimi for correction of a small finger ulnar deviation deformity may be necessary. ■ A double-breasted repair of the radial sagittal band is facilitated by leaving a 2- to 3-mm cuff of the sagittal band when longitudinally incising it at the beginning of the case.

OUTCOMES

■ Tendon transfers in patients with preserved MCPJs reliably achieve restoration of MCPJ extension. However, in patients with volarly subluxed and arthritic MCPJs, arthroplasty and soft tissue reconstruction to restore joint alignment prior to performing tendon transfers are critical for optimizing outcomes.
- In general, tendon transfers for extensor tendon reconstruction achieve good results, though more extension lag is observed when more tendons are involved. For flexor tendons, patients with isolated ruptures in the palm or wrist have the potential to maintain good finger function, provided that their prerupture finger function was good. However, if preruptured function was limited, outcomes will be poor regardless of the treatment provided.
- Outcomes after the combined rupture of FDS and FDP are also poor, regardless of prerupture finger function or method of treatment.

- To optimize outcomes, correcting the underlying causes of tendon rupture, such as extensor tenosynovitis, rough bony surfaces, and the caput ulna deformity, is critical in preventing the rerupture of reconstructed tendons.
■ For advanced swan-neck deformities, the results of surgery can be unpredictable. Still, even if motion is lost, the flexed PIPJ position is functionally preferable to the hyperextended position. As such, as long as PIPJ hyperextension is prevented, there should be no hesitation in performing surgery for advanced swan-neck deformities.
■ Patients who undergo SMPA typically gain 30 to 40 degrees of active motion at the MCPJ. Grip strength and pinch strength are unaffected by surgery, while ulnar drift, extension lag, and arc of motion significantly improve (**FIG 11**).
■ The crossed intrinsic transfer can provide long-term correction of ulnar deviation deformities but may be associated with decreased active ROM at the MCP joint.

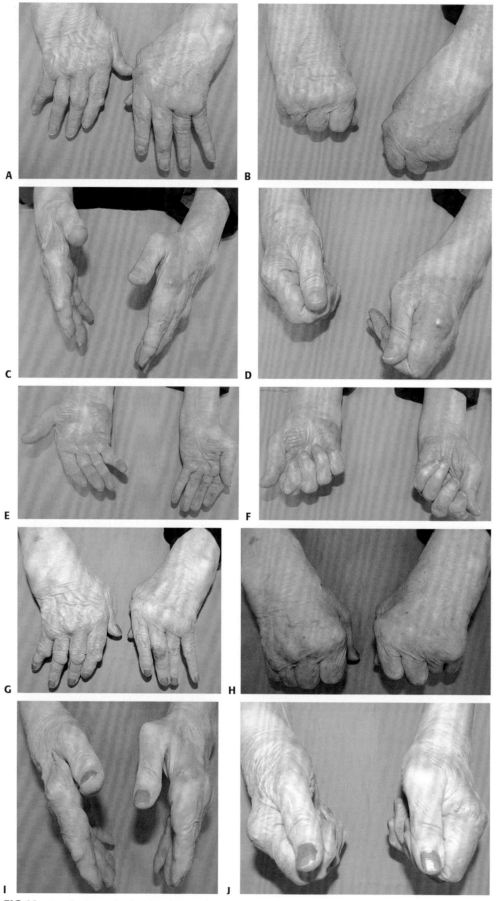

FIG 11 • Results 2 months **(A–F)** and 5 months **(G–L)** after silicone metacarpophalangeal joint arthroplasty.

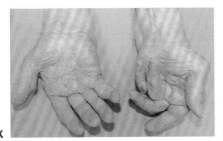
K

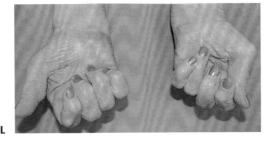
L

FIG 11 (Continued)

REFERENCES

1. Stastny P. Association of the B-cell alloantigen DRw4 with rheumatoid arthritis. *N Engl J Med*. 1978;298(16):869-871.
2. Feldmann M, Brennan FM, Maini RN. Role of cytokines in rheumatoid arthritis. *Annu Rev Immunol*. 1996;14:397-440.
3. Kirkham BW, Lassere MN, Edmonds JP, et al. Synovial membrane cytokine expression is predictive of joint damage progression in rheumatoid arthritis: a two-year prospective study (the DAMAGE study cohort). *Arthritis Rheum*. 2006;54(4):1122-1131.
4. Arnett FC, Edworthy SM, Bloch DA, et al. The American Rheumatism Association 1987 revised criteria for the classification of rheumatoid arthritis. *Arthritis Rheum*. 1988;31(3):315-324.
5. Nishimura K, Sugiyama D, Kogata Y, et al. Meta-analysis: diagnostic accuracy of anti–cyclic citrullinated peptide antibody and rheumatoid factor for rheumatoid arthritis. *Ann Intern Med*. 2007;146(11):797-808.
6. Aletaha D, Neogi T, Silman AJ, et al. 2010 Rheumatoid arthritis classification criteria: an American College of Rheumatology/European League Against Rheumatism collaborative initiative. *Arthritis Rheum*. 2010;62(9):2569-2581.
7. Nam JL, Winthrop KL, van Vollenhoven RF, et al. Current evidence for the management of rheumatoid arthritis with biological disease-modifying antirheumatic drugs: a systematic literature review informing the EULAR recommendations for the management of RA. *Ann Rheum Dis*. 2010; 69(6):976-986.
8. Rehim SA, Chung KC. Applying evidence in the care of patients with rheumatoid hand and wrist deformities. *Plast Reconstr Surg*. 2013;132(4):885-897.
9. Nalebuff EA, Millender LH. Surgical treatment of the boutonniere deformity in rheumatoid arthritis. *Orthop Clin North Am*. 1975;6(3):753-763.

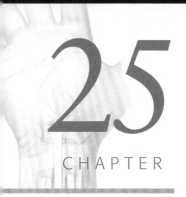

25 CHAPTER

Section VII: Degenerative Disease

Degenerative Disease of the Hand and Wrist

Shoshana W. Ambani and Kevin C. Chung

DEFINITION

- Osteoarthritis (OA) is a noninflammatory degenerative joint condition of the hand and wrist that clinically affects 3% to 7% of adults.[1]
- The hallmark of OA is the loss of articular cartilage, leading to joint destruction and osteophyte formation (**FIG 1**).

PATIENT HISTORY AND GENERAL FINDINGS

- OA is more common in women and usually presents in patients over 40 years of age.
- Patients generally complain of pain, swelling, and stiffness of the affected joint. Pain is usually activity related.
- Examination confirms swelling, tenderness, limited range of motion (ROM), and decreased function. Crepitus with passive ROM may also be noted.
- Thumb carpometacarpal joint (CMCJ) arthritis often leads to thumb weakness due to pain.
- Examination may reveal a positive grind test, in which pain is produced upon axial compression of the joint.
- Regarding the fingers, patients may display classic Heberden nodes on the dorsal distal interphalangeal joints (DIPJs) or Bouchard nodes on the dorsal proximal interphalangeal joints (PIPJs) (**FIG 2A**).
  - Mucous cysts can also present at the DIPJ and cause nail deformities (**FIG 2B,C**).
- Pain with loss of wrist ROM compared to the contralateral side is indicative of wrist arthritis.

- Provocative testing of the distal radioulnar joint (DRUJ) with dorsal and palmar stress (a shuck test) may indicate DRUJ involvement.

IMAGING

- Standard three-view radiographs of the hand and wrist are typically sufficient for evaluation of OA.
  - Further imaging such as CT scan or MRI is usually not routine but may be useful in select situations, such as evaluating the wrist for midcarpal arthritis.
- OA is characterized by narrowed joint spaces due to loss of radiolucent articular cartilage.
  - In addition, osteophytes and loose bodies may be present.
  - Subchondral cysts and sclerosis are signs of more advanced disease (see **FIG 1**).
- Patient symptoms do not always correlate with the radiographic severity of disease. As such, interventions should be based on patient complaints and general goals.

PATHOGENESIS AND ETIOLOGY

- In *primary*, or *idiopathic*, *OA*, there is no identifiable cause.
  - In *secondary OA*, articular loss is a result of traumatic injury, such as intra-articular fractures, ligamentous injuries that lead to unfavorable articular load-bearing characteristics, or joint infections.
- Generally, OA develops as a result of an imbalance between the destruction and repair of articular cartilage.

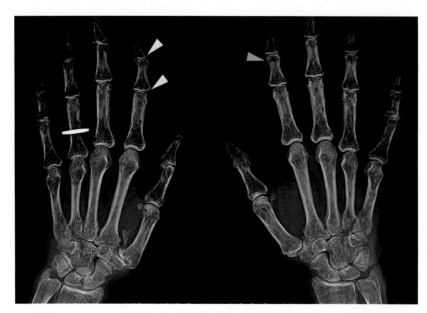

FIG 1 • Radiograph of bilateral hands displays typical characteristics of osteoarthritis, including joint space narrowing (*yellow arrowheads*), osteophyte formation (*blue arrowhead*), and subchondral cyst and associated sclerosis (*red arrowhead*).

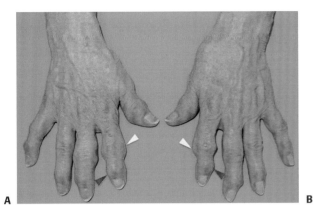
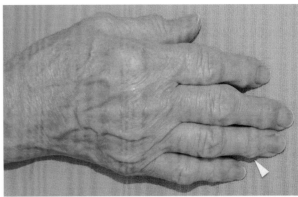
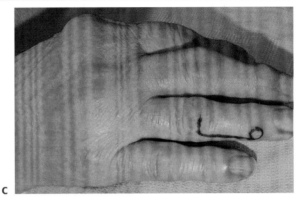

FIG 2 • **A.** Example of Heberden nodes (*red arrowheads*) and Bouchard nodes (*yellow arrowheads*). **B.** Mucous cyst on dorsal DIPJ of ring finger (*arrowhead*). **C.** A circular incision was used to excise the cyst down to the joint. An osteophyte was removed at the base of the cyst. A skin flap (*marked*) was advanced to close the remaining defect.

- Clefts in the articular surface and a decrease in cartilage thickness eventually progress to exposure of the subchondral bone.
- Bone density increases, as demonstrated by sclerotic changes seen on radiographs, and overly exuberant bone formation may produce osteophytes at the joint periphery. In addition, the synovial membranes become inflamed as cartilage fragments are embedded within them.
- Because of these mechanical factors and pain, joint motion is progressively lost, leading to joint stiffness as the capsule and associated ligaments contract.
- Hand
  - In the hand, OA most commonly affects the DIPJs of the fingers and the CMCJ of the thumb.
  - OA then affects the PIPJs and metacarpophalangeal joints (MCPJs), respectively.
- Wrist
  - Scaphotrapeziotrapezoid (STT) joint arthritis is one of the most common presentations of idiopathic OA of the wrist.
  - Other causes of primary wrist OA include avascular necrosis of the lunate (Kienbock disease) or the scaphoid (Preiser disease), which can lead to degenerative changes later on.
  - Congenital conditions, including Madelung deformity, can also alter the articular load, leading to wrist OA.
  - Secondary OA is usually trauma related and most frequently develops after distal radius fractures (DRFs), scaphoid fractures, and scapholunate ligamentous injuries.
  - Intra-articular DRFs can lead to a 91% incidence of arthritis if any degree of articular step-off remains after fracture reduction, but only an 11% incidence if a congruent articular reduction is achieved.
    - Extra-articular DRFs can also lead to wrist OA due to the development of abnormal load-bearing patterns across the wrist.

- Up to 11% of DRFs are associated with instability of the DRUJ, leading to DRUJ arthritis.[2]
  - Of note, rheumatoid arthritis is the most common inflammatory arthritis to involve the DRUJ.
- Scaphoid fractures may fail to heal in 5% to 10% of cases, leading to a pattern of carpal instability termed *scaphoid nonunion advanced collapse* (SNAC) arthritis.
  - SNAC wrist typically starts with arthritis at the radial styloid-scaphoid articulation (stage 1) and progresses to the radioscaphoid and scaphocapitate articulations (stage 2) and finally the lunocapitate articulation (stage 3).
- Similarly, a scapholunate ligament injury can initiate progressive carpal instability and arthritis starting at the radial styloid (stage 1) and progressing to the proximal scaphoid and scaphoid fossa of the radius (stage 2) and finally the midcarpal joint at the lunocapitate articulation (stage 3).
  - This is cumulatively known as *scapholunate advanced collapse* (SLAC) arthritis.
  - The radiolunate joint is typically spared in the SLAC wrist because of the unique congruency of this joint.

NONOPERATIVE MANAGEMENT

- Because there is no cure for OA and no effective method to alter disease progression, the mainstay of treatment is nonoperative and focuses on symptom management.
- Patients may engage in lifestyle modifications, hot and cold therapy, splinting, oral or topical anti-inflammatory medications such as nonsteroidal anti-inflammatory drugs (NSAIDs), or alternative methods such as acupuncture or electrostimulation.
- Steroid injections into the affected joints may provide short-term relief.

SURGICAL MANAGEMENT

Preoperative Planning

- As OA patients are typically older with multiple comorbid conditions, a full medical workup is recommended prior to surgery.

Positioning

- The patient is positioned supine on the operative table and padded comfortably.
- The upper extremity is abducted onto the attached hand table.
- A tourniquet is placed on the upper arm.

Approach

- The indications for surgery in OA patients include refractory pain, loss of motion, and/or joint instability leading to decreased function.
- Surgical methods for the treatment of OA generally involve joint debridement, arthrodesis, arthroplasty, and load-altering procedures.

Fingers

- Because the DIPJs are the most commonly affected joints in OA, surgery typically involves the removal of an enlarged osteophyte and/or excision of a mucous cyst.
  - If the joint is destroyed, arthrodesis at about 5 to 10 degrees of flexion is preferred.
- The PIPJs are treated with arthrodesis or arthroplasty.
- For the radial digits, arthrodesis of the PIPJs with K-wires, screws, or tension banding is preferred in order to provide a strong post for pinch.
- The PIPJ of the index finger should be fused at 25 degrees of flexion, advancing by 5 degrees with each finger ulnarly, if required, for the most functional posture.
- The PIPJs of the ulnar digits require more motion for grip, however, and should be considered for arthroplasty.
  - Silicone arthroplasty provides limited motion to the PIPJs (30–60 degrees) and has a high fracture rate but can easily be revised.
  - Pyrocarbon implants provide greater motion, but implant dislocation may occur, and high complication rates have led to this approach falling out of favor for PIPJs.
  - We have abandoned the pyrocarbon implant in favor of the silicone implant using the volar approach for the PIPJ.

Thumb

- As the second most commonly affected joint in OA, the thumb CMCJ (ie, the trapeziometacarpal [TM] joint) is surgically treated with volar ligament reconstruction, arthroplasty, or arthrodesis.
  - Although the initial treatment may consist of splinting or steroid injections, most patients presenting to surgeons already have sufficient joint destruction to warrant surgery.
- The Eaton classification[3,4] (Table 1) of TM osteoarthritis describes and categorizes the radiographic progression of the disease. However, surgical planning is based on patient symptoms and complaints, not Eaton classification.
- For early OA (Eaton stage I), which may be characterized symptomatic instability or laxity of the thumb TM joint, volar ligament reconstruction is indicated (Eaton-Littler procedure).
- For Eaton stage II to IV disease, loss of articular cartilage precludes the possibility of joint salvage. Surgical options fall into four major categories:

Table 1 Eaton Classification of Trapeziometacarpal (TM) Osteoarthritis[3,4]

Stage	Radiographic Characteristics
I	• Normal or slightly widened TM joint • TM subluxation up to 1/3 of articular surface • Normal articular contours
II	• Decreased TM joint space • TM subluxation up to 1/3 of articular surface • Osteophytes or loose bodies less than 2 mm
III	• Decreased TM joint space • TM subluxation greater than 1/3 of articular surface • Osteophytes or loose bodies greater than or equal to 2 mm • Subchondral cysts or sclerosis
IV	• Pantrapezial arthritis with stage III features • Involvement of the scaphotrapezial, trapeziotrapezoid, and/or the trapezio-index metacarpal joints

- Trapeziectomy alone
- Trapeziectomy with soft tissue arthroplasty via ligament reconstruction and tendon interposition (LRTI) or an abductor pollicis longus (APL) suspensionplasty
- Arthrodesis
- Prosthetic arthroplasty
- Because of high complication rates with prostheses and lack of outcomes data to show their effectiveness over autologous options, we do not advocate the use of a prosthesis for the thumb TM joint.
  - For heavy laborers, thumb TM arthrodesis is preferred for joint stability and strength.[5] In these cases, the thumb TM joint should be fused at 30 to 40 degrees of abduction, 15 to 20 degrees of extension, and 15 degrees of pronation to allow tip-to-tip pinch.
  - In any case, the presence of thumb MCPJ instability or hyperextension greater than 30 to 45 degrees may also warrant concomitant volar plate advancement or MCPJ fusion to avoid failure of the reconstructed TM joint.

Wrist

- Surgical treatment of wrist OA is focused on pain reduction. The specific treatment is formulated based on the patient's symptoms, arthritic pattern, and functional demands.
  - The selected approach should always account for future additional procedures should the most current option fail.
  - In general, surgical options include joint debridement, denervation, arthroplasty, partial vs total wrist arthrodesis, or a combination thereof.
- A radial styloidectomy can be performed for arthritis at the radial styloid.
- Wrist denervation is an option that has been shown to provide partial pain relief in patients and can be considered if selective blocks of the anterior interosseous nerve (AIN) and posterior interosseous nerve (PIN) prove favorable.
- A proximal row carpectomy (PRC), in which the scaphoid, lunate, and triquetrum are removed, is an option when there is no arthritis at the midcarpal joint or radiolunate joint.
- Midcarpal and radiocarpal arthritis can be treated with a scaphoidectomy and four-corner fusion, in which the scaphoid is removed and fusion of the lunate, capitate, triquetrum, and hamate is performed.

- For the arthritic DRUJ, surgical options include resection arthroplasties, including the Darrach procedure, hemiresection ulnar arthroplasty, the Sauve-Kapandji procedure, and prosthetic replacement of the ulnar head or DRUJ.[2]
  - The Darrach procedure involves resection of the entire distal ulna and has been advocated for low-demand elderly patients.
  - The Sauve-Kapandji procedure preserves the head of the ulna while fusing the DRUJ to prevent ulnar translocation of the carpus.
  - Hemiresection ulnar arthroplasty, in which the radio-carpal joint surface of the ulna is resected while maintaining the triangular fibrocartilage complex (TFCC), is often preferred over the Darrach procedure because of improved postoperative wrist stability. Prosthetic replacement of the ulnar head or DRUJ is a less common option for the arthritic DRUJ.
- In cases of significantly advanced arthritis, wrist arthroplasty or fusion may be the only remaining surgical options.
  - Wrist arthroplasty provides motion at the expense of strength and is considered only in select patients with low-demand wrists or who have fusion of the contralateral wrist. Patients with OA tend to fit this profile, as opposed to those with OA.
  - Total wrist fusion is the ultimate salvage option for all types of wrist arthritis, achieving both pain relief and strength.

■ Distal Interphalangeal Joint Arthrodesis

- The distal interphalangeal joint (DIPJ) is exposed dorsally with a T-shaped incision (**TECH FIG 1A**).
- The extensor tendon is transversely divided, leaving a 5-mm distal stump for later repair.
- The radial and ulnar collateral ligaments are divided, allowing the joint to hinge open.
- Joint debridement is performed using a small rongeur, removing inflamed capsule, ganglions, osteophytes, and residual cartilage.
- A rongeur is used to fashion a concave "trough" at the base of the distal phalanx and a convex "crest" at the head of the middle phalanx until the surfaces align (**TECH FIG 1B**).
- With the joint reduced and compressed at 5 to 10 degrees of flexion, a K-wire is driven through the joint from distal to proximal in a retrograde fashion.
  - A second K-wire is inserted to prevent rotation.
  - The angle is checked with fluoroscopy.
  - A third K-wire may be inserted for further stabilization.
- The extensor tendon is then repaired with a 5-0 absorbable suture, and the skin is closed with interrupted nonabsorbable suture (**TECH FIG 1C**).
  - Soft bulky dressings are applied.
  - The fused joint is supported in a splint for about 6 to 8 weeks until radiographs show bony union (**TECH FIG 1D,E**).
    - At that point, strengthening exercises may be initiated.

T E C H N I Q U E S

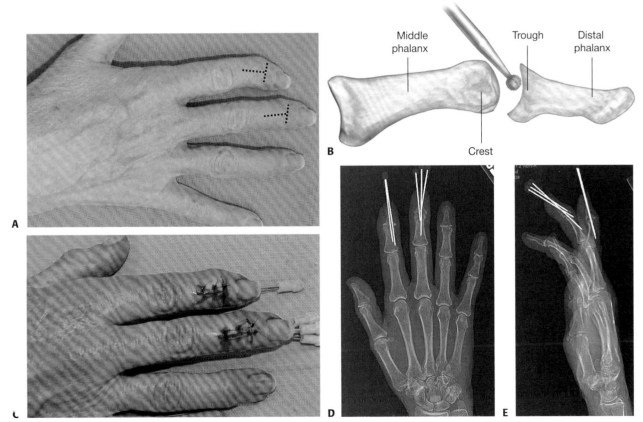

TECH FIG 1 • A. Skin incision. **B.** Bur is used to create a crest and trough. **C.** Skin closure with K-wires in place. **D,E.** Postoperative radiographs show K-wires in place, fusing the DIPJs of the index and long fingers.

■ Volar Approach to Proximal Interphalangeal Joint Arthroplasty

Silicone Implant

- Patients who do not want proximal interphalangeal joint (PIPJ) fusion for their osteoarthritic pain may consider silicone PIPJ arthroplasty with the understanding that a limited range of motion of 30 to 60 degrees is expected postoperatively.
  - Important prerequisites to PIPJ arthroplasty include good bone quality for implant insertion, supple soft tissue coverage, adequate finger sensibility and blood flow, and normal tendon gliding. The best candidate for surgery is a patient with painful PIPJ motion but good stability and normal tendon function.
  - We prefer using silicone over pyrocarbon implants given the lower complication rate and the ability to revise the joint more easily if complications arise.
- A V incision over the volar PIPJ is made (**TECH FIG 2A**).
  - Skin flaps are elevated, identifying and preserving the ulnar and radial neurovascular bundles (**TECH FIG 2B**).
  - The A3 pulley is incised and elevated. The flexor tendons are retracted volarly.

- The volar plate is then incised proximally to expose the arthritic head of the proximal phalanx (**TECH FIG 2C**).
- The head of the proximal phalanx and the base of middle phalanx are excised with an oscillating saw (**TECH FIG 2D–F**).
- The medullary cavity is broached and reamed (**TECH FIG 2G**).
- An appropriately sized implant is then placed (**TECH FIG 2H**).
- Motion at the joint is checked.
- The volar plate is reattached using 4-0 absorbable braided suture.
- The A3 pulley is repaired.
- After skin closure (**TECH FIG 2I**), the hand is placed in a volar splint.
- The patient is seen in the clinic 3 or 4 days after surgery to initiate gentle active range of motion exercises at the PIPJ.
- Splint protection is maintained for approximately 3 weeks to preserve joint alignment and encourage joint encapsulation for additional stability.

Pyrocarbon Implant

- Steps for PIPJ pyrocarbon arthroplasty through a dorsal incision are shown in **TECH FIG 3**.

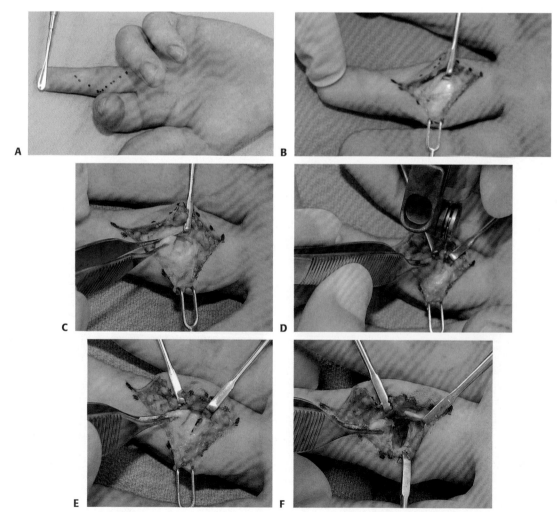

TECH FIG 2 • PIPJ silicone arthroplasty–volar approach. **A.** A V incision. **B.** Skin flap elevation. **C.** Exposure of the arthritic head of the proximal phalanx. **D–F.** Excision of head of proximal phalanx and base of middle phalanx with oscillating saw.

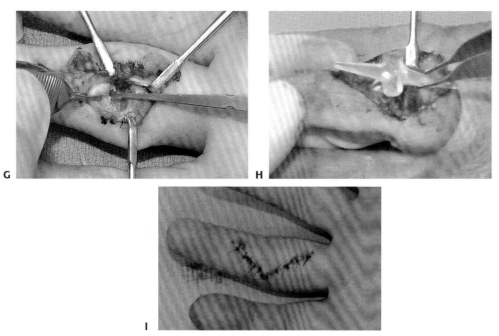

TECH FIG 2 (Continued) • **G.** The medullary cavity is broached and reamed. **H.** Placement of implant. **I.** Skin closure.

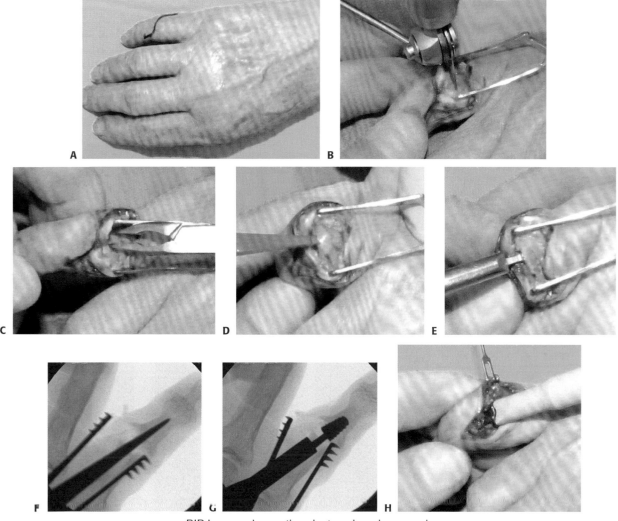

PIPJ pyrocarbon arthroplasty—dorsal approach

TECH FIG 3 • **A.** Incision. **B,C.** Excision of head of proximal phalanx and base of middle phalanx. **D,E.** Medullary cavity of proximal phalanx is broached. **F,G.** Fluoroscopy. **H,I.** Implant is seated into the medullary cavity.

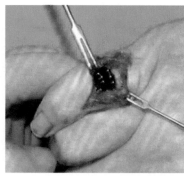
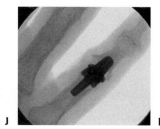
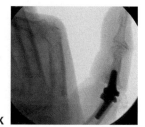

TECH FIG 3 (Continued) • **J,K.** Fluoroscopy.

◼ Thumb Metacarpophalangeal Joint Fusion for Osteoarthritis

- Patients with instability and pain at the thumb metacarpophalangeal joint (MCPJ) due to osteoarthritis are candidates for arthrodesis.
- A plate is used to achieve long-lasting joint stability for patient comfort.
- A 4-cm incision over the dorsum of the thumb MCPJ is made (**TECH FIG 4A**).
  - The interval between the extensor pollicis longus (EPL) and the extensor pollicis brevis (EPB) tendons is entered (**TECH FIG 4B**).
  - The joint capsule is incised to expose the joint.
- The articular surfaces are removed with a rongeur.
- A low-profile T-plate is selected and bent to fit the MCPJ with about 30 degrees of flexion.
- As the bony surfaces are compressed, the T-plate is fixed to the plate with screws (**TECH FIG 4C**).
  - Fluoroscopy is used to check hardware placement.
- The capsule is closed with 4-0 absorbable suture, and the skin is closed with 4-0 nonabsorbable suture.
- A thumb spica splint is placed.
- The patient is immobilized for 6 to 8 weeks or until radiographic union occurs (**TECH FIG 4D,E**).
  - At 2 weeks, the patient can start engaging in light activities of daily living while wearing the splint.

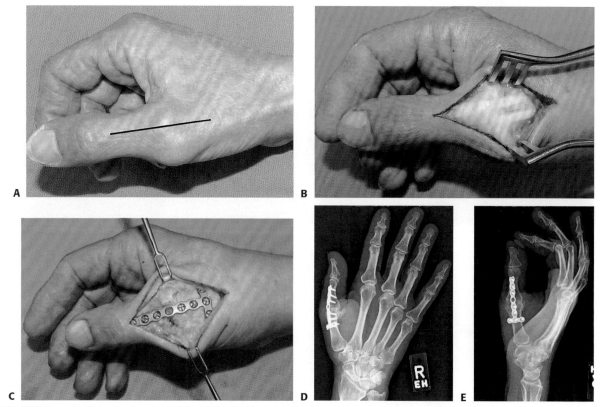

TECH FIG 4 • Joint fusion for thumb MCPJ instability. **A.** Skin incision. **B.** Interval between EPL and EPB. **C.** Plate placement. **D.** Radiograph of fused MCPJ (AP view). **E.** Radiograph of fused MCPJ (lateral view).

T
E
C
H
N
I
Q
U
E
S

Reconstruction for Thumb Trapeziometacarpal Instability Using Flexor Carpi Radialis: Eaton-Littler Procedure

- The Eaton-Littler procedure is reserved for thumb trapeziometacarpal (TM) instability in the setting of intact articular surfaces.
- A modified Wagner incision is made at the junction of glabrous and nonglabrous skin along the border of the thenar eminence (**TECH FIG 5A**).
  - The radial edge of the thenar musculature at its insertion on the metacarpal is identified and elevated to expose the metacarpal base and trapezium (**TECH FIG 5B**).
  - The dorsal cortex of the metacarpal base is further exposed through the interval between the EPL and EPB.

- Using a small bur, a hole is made at the base of the metacarpal, from dorsal to volar, starting at about 1 cm from the joint in a plane perpendicular to the axis of the thumbnail (**TECH FIG 5C**).
  - The exit site should be at the apex of the volar beak of the metacarpal.
- For harvest of the flexor carpi radialis (FCR), short transverse incisions centered over the tendon are made at 2- to 3-cm intervals proximal to the volar wrist crease.
  - The FCR sheath is entered through these incisions to isolate the radial half of FCR, which is transected at about 6 cm proximal to the wrist crease and separated longitudinally from the other half of the tendon (**TECH FIG 5D**).
- At the wrist crease, the FCR slip is traced to its insertion at the base of the index metacarpal.
  - The free end of the FCR is brought out through the thenar incision (**TECH FIG 5E**).

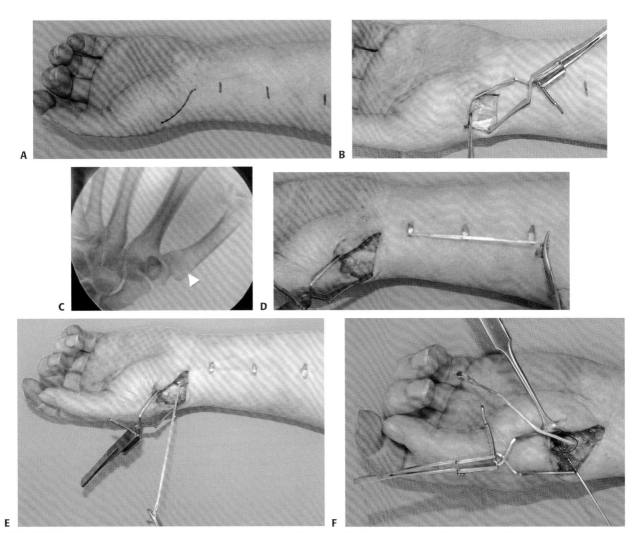

TECH FIG 5 • Reconstruction for thumb trapeziometacarpal instability using FCR (Eaton-Littler). **A.** Skin incision. **B.** The trapeziometacarpal joint is exposed. **C.** A hole is drilled through first metacarpal base (*arrow*). **D.** Harvest of radial half of FCR. **E.** The FCR slip is traced to its insertion at the base of the index metacarpal and brought out the thenar incisions. **F,G.** The tendon is directed through the hole at the base of the first metacarpal, from volar to dorsal, using a wire-loop tendon passer.

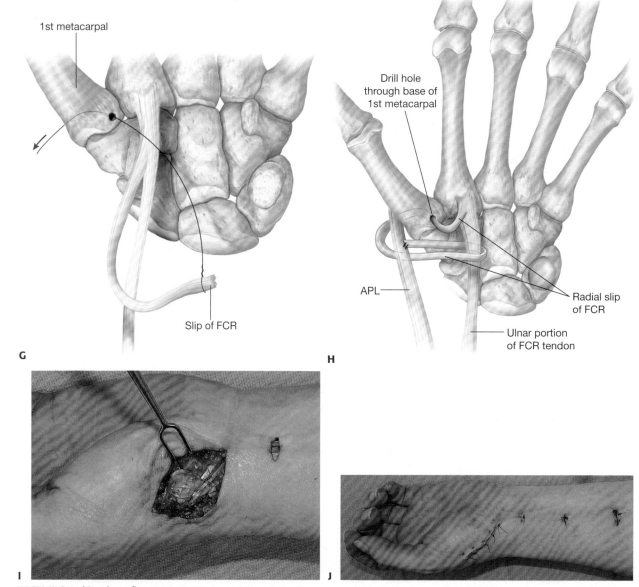

1st metacarpal

Slip of FCR

G

Drill hole through base of 1st metacarpal

APL

Radial slip of FCR

Ulnar portion of FCR tendon

H

I

J

TECH FIG 5 (Continued) • **H.** The FCR is passed through the first metacarpal. **I.** Final reconstruction. **J.** Skin closure.

- Using a wire-loop tendon passer, the tendon is directed through the hole at the base of the thumb metacarpal, from volar to dorsal (**TECH FIG 5F,G**).
- Under direct vision, the joint is reduced and held in extension and abduction, seating the metacarpal well against the trapezium.
- The tendon is pulled taut and sutured to the dorsal periosteum with a 3-0 braided nonabsorbable suture.
- The tendon is then passed around the metacarpal base, deep to EPB and abductor pollicis longus (APL), through a small spit in the intact FCR tendon proximal to its

insertion, and finally back across the joint and sutured to the APL tendon (**TECH FIG 5H,I**).
- Additional sutures are placed at the junction through the FCR tendon.
- The thenar musculature is reattached using 3-0 braided absorbable suture.
  - The skin is closed with 4-0 nylon horizontal mattress sutures (**TECH FIG 5J**).
- A thumb spica splint is placed and worn for 4 weeks, at which point gentle active ROM exercises are initiated.
  - At 8 weeks, strengthening exercises are begun.

Trapeziectomy and Abductor Pollicis Longus Suspensionplasty

- A trapeziectomy with APL suspensionplasty is our preferred technique for thumb TM (carpometacarpal joint [CMCJ]) arthroplasty, as it is faster and technically easier than the Eaton-Littler procedure yet provides comparable outcomes.[6]
- The first incision is made over anatomic snuffbox and TM joint (**TECH FIG 6A**).
    - The radial sensory nerve branches are identified and retracted. The EPL tendon is found at the ulnar aspect of the anatomic snuffbox.
    - The radial artery is identified in close proximity to the TM joint capsule and is mobilized and retracted inferiorly (**TECH FIG 6B**).
    - The TM joint capsule is incised and sharply elevated to expose the scaphotrapezial joint, the trapezium, and the thumb metacarpal base (**TECH FIG 6C**).
- The trapezium is cut longitudinally into three pieces using an oscillating saw followed by an osteotome.
    - The pieces are removed with a rongeur (**TECH FIG 6D,E**).
    - Osteophytes and loose bodies embedded in the surrounding soft tissues must also be removed meticulously.
    - Care is taken to avoid injury to the FCR tendon as it passes volar to the trapezium at its proximal radial corner.
- The surface of the trapezoid that articulates with the scaphoid is inspected, and if arthritis is present, a partial proximal trapezoidal resection is performed.
- The second incision is made over the first extensor compartment to identify the musculotendinous junction of the APL, which has multiple slips (**TECH FIG 6F**).

- The most radial slip of APL is divided at this junction (**TECH FIG 6G**), passed under the skin bridge into the thumb incision with a hemostat, and traced to its insertion at the thumb metacarpal base (**TECH FIG 6H**).
- The extensor carpi radialis longus (ECRL) tendon is identified ulnarly where it inserts into the base of the index metacarpal, deep to the EPL tendon.
    - A small incision is made longitudinally in the ECRL tendon (**TECH FIG 6I**).
- The APL tendon is then passed volar to EPL and through the hole in the ECRL into a tendon weave (**TECH FIG 6J**).
- The tension is set such that the thumb metacarpal base is suspended at the level of the index metacarpal base.
- The tendon weave between APL and ECRL is secured using 3-0 braided nonabsorbable horizontal mattress sutures (**TECH FIG 6K,L**).
- The remaining tendon is cut, fashioned into a ball with 4-0 absorbable suture, and placed in the trapeziectomy space (**TECH FIG 6M**).
- The joint capsule is closed with 4-0 braided absorbable suture.
    - The skin is closed with 4-0 absorbable monofilament dermal sutures and a 4-0 absorbable monofilament running subcuticular suture (**TECH FIG 6N,O**).
- A thumb spica splint is placed and worn for 4 weeks.
    - Hand therapy is then initiated for passive and active ROM exercises, with the splint worn between exercises.
    - At 6 weeks, light strengthening exercises are begun. At 8 weeks, the splint is weaned and heavy strengthening with grip and pinch exercises is initiated.
    - Studies show that patients experience significant improvements in activities of daily living, work, satisfaction, and pain at 1 year postoperatively.

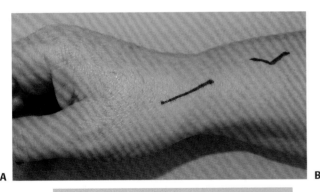
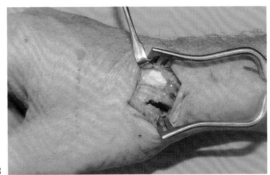
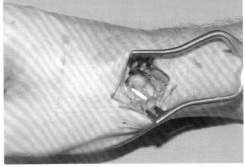
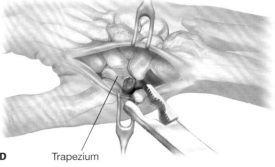

Trapezium

TECH FIG 6 • Trapeziectomy and APL suspensionplasty. **A.** First skin incision. **B.** Radial artery is preserved. **C.** Trapezium is exposed. **D.** A rongeur is used to remove the trapezium.

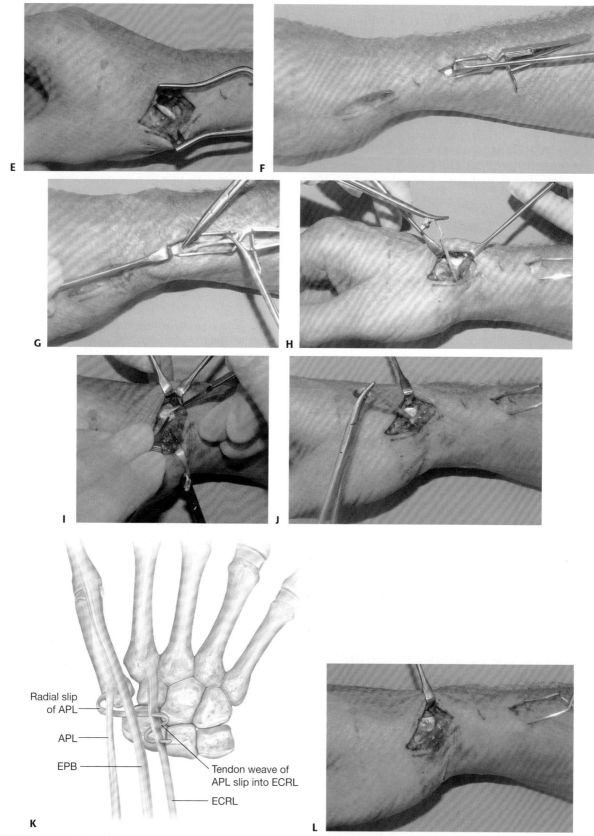

TECH FIG 6 (Continued) • **E.** Trapezium has been removed. **F.** APL is identified via second incision. **G.** The radial slip of APL is divided at the musculotendinous junction. **H.** The slip of APL is brought into the thumb incision and traced to its insertion on the thumb metacarpal base. **I.** A small incision is made in the ECRL tendon. **J,K.** The slip of APL is passed volar to EPB and EPL and through the hole in the ECRL into a tendon weave. **L.** Completed APL tendon weave with ECRL.

TECHNIQUES

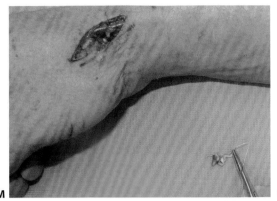

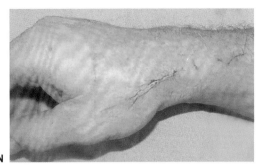

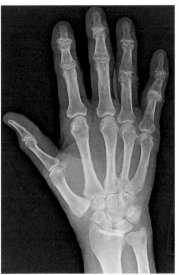

TECH FIG 6 (Continued) • **M.** The excess APL tendon is cut, sutured into a ball, and inserted into the trapeziectomy space. **N.** Skin closure. **O.** Postoperative x-ray.

■ Arthrodesis of the Thumb TM Joint (Thumb CMCJ Arthrodesis)

- Osteoarthritis of the thumb TM joint (ie, CMCJ) can be addressed with joint fusion, particularly in manual laborers who require greater stability than can be achieved with trapeziectomy and ligament reconstruction.
  - Arthrodesis is also indicated in patients with substantial joint laxity and deformity. In the past, nonunion rate is high using the traditional plating system.
  - We have applied the locking plate and screw design for this joint to provide even more rigid fixation that may enhance fusion.
  - Using locking system is the preferred approach to fuse the thumb CMCJ.
- A 4- to 6-cm dorsal longitudinal incision is made over the TM joint at the base of the thumb metacarpal (**TECH FIG 7A**).
  - The interval between the EPL and EBP tendons is entered, exposing the joint capsule. Care is taken to preserve and retract the radial artery.

- The joint capsule and periosteum are incised, and periosteal flaps are elevated off the trapezium and metacarpal (**TECH FIG 7B,C**).
- Using a combination of rongeur and osteotome, the articular cartilage and subchondral bone are resected (**TECH FIG 7D**).
- A 2.3-mm locking T-plate is selected and positioned with the T-portion centered on the trapezium and the longitudinal portion centered along metacarpal.
  - Screws are applied with the joint in compression (**TECH FIG 7E**).
  - Plate position is confirmed with fluoroscopy.
  - If any bony gaps exist, cadaveric bone graft is applied.
- The periosteal flaps and joint capsule are closed over the plate using 4-0 absorbable braided suture (**TECH FIG 7F**).
  - After skin closure, a thumb spica splint is placed.
- The patient is immobilized in a thumb spica splint for 6 weeks to allow for bony fusion, after which gentle active ROM exercises are initiated (**TECH FIG 7G–I**).

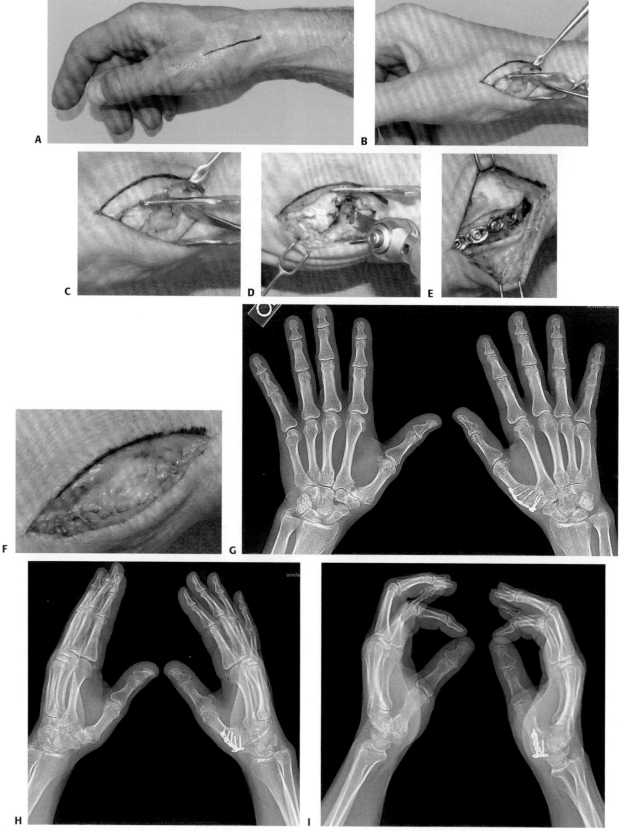

TECH FIG 7 • Thumb CMC arthrodesis. **A.** Incision. **B,C.** Radial artery retracted and thumb CMC joint identified. **D.** Chevron-type osteotomy made through base of metacarpal and trapezium. **E.** Thumb CMC fusion with Synthes locking T-plate. **F.** Interval between EPB and EPL closed over plate. **G–I.** Six weeks postoperative x-rays.

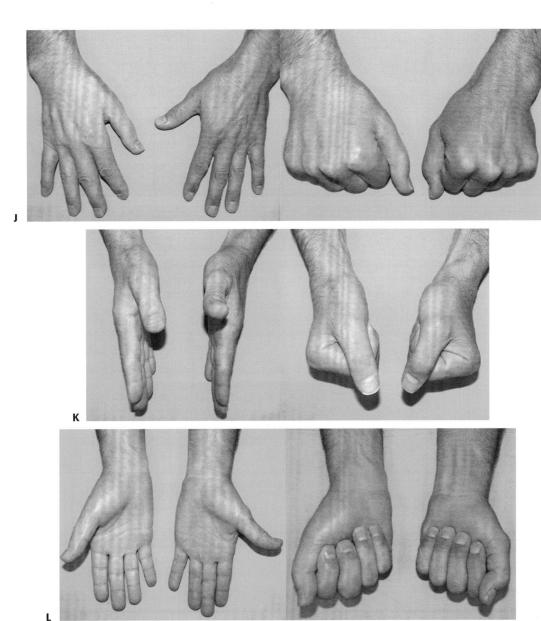

TECH FIG 7 (Continued) • **J–L.** Results 6 weeks postoperatively.

■ Darrach Procedure for Distal Radioulnar Joint Arthritis

- A dorsal incision is made longitudinally over the distal ulna, just proximal to the extensor retinaculum, taking care to preserve the dorsal ulnar sensory nerve (**TECH FIG 8A**).
  - The interval between the extensor carpi ulnaris (ECU) and extensor digiti minimi (EDM) is entered (**TECH FIG 8B**).
  - The periosteum is incised, and radial and ulnar periosteal flaps are raised.
- An oscillating saw is used to resect 2 cm of distal ulna at a 45-degree angle, such that the long end of the oblique cut is in the ulnar border to minimize impingement against the radius.
- The loose ulnar head is sharply excised from its soft tissue attachments (**TECH FIG 8C**).
  - Sharp edges of bone and synovitis within the sigmoid notch are removed with a rongeur.

- Ulnar stump stability is then assessed.
  - If stable, the tourniquet is release, and hemostasis is achieved with cautery.
  - If unstable, an ECU tenodesis is performed.
- Then, with the wrist fully supinated, the dorsal wrist capsule is imbricated with 2-0 braided nonabsorbable horizontal mattress sutures, ensuring that the ulnar is not dorsally prominent in this position.
- The skin is closed with 3-0 absorbable monofilament dermal sutures and a 4-0 nonabsorbable (**TECH FIG 8D**).
- A sugar-tong splint is applied with the forearm fully supinated for 4 weeks, keeping the fingers free for ROM.
  - Gentle active ROM is started at 4 weeks, but if an ulna stabilizing procedure has been performed, pronation and supination are delayed until 6 weeks (**TECH FIG 8E**).
  - Full activities may be resumed as tolerated at 6 to 8 weeks.

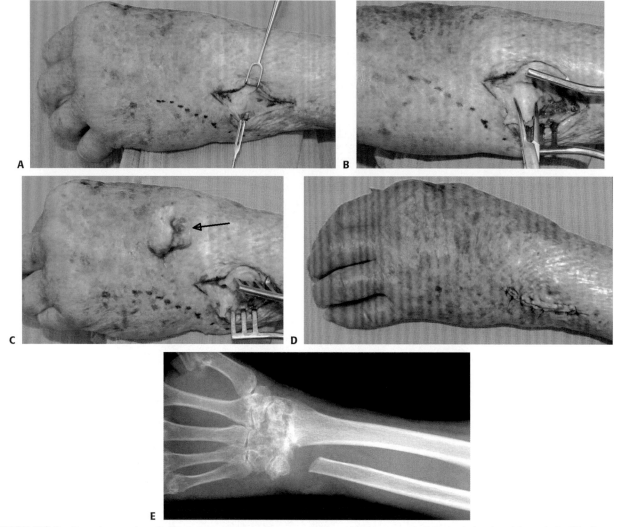

TECH FIG 8 • Darrach procedure. **A.** Skin incision. **B.** Interval between ECU and EDM is entered. **C.** Excised ulnar head (*arrow*). **D.** Skin closure. **E.** Postoperative x-ray.

■ Hemiresection Arthroplasty of the Distal Ulna

- We prefer hemiresection ulnar arthroplasty over the Darrach procedure for patients with wrist pain due to distal radioulnar joint (DRUJ) osteoarthritis, as it is associated with less postoperative wrist instability[7] and better wrist range of motion, grip strength, and pain relief.[8]
  - In this procedure, the ulnar attachments of the TFCC (triangular fibrocartilage complex) are preserved.
  - Resection of the radial and dorsal margins of the distal ulna is performed such that the resected bone corresponds with the articular surface of the sigmoid notch.
  - This "matched resection" is performed to prevent radioulnar impingement during forearm rotation.[9]
- The distal ulna is exposed in a similar manner as for the Darrach procedure (see above for details) while maintaining the ulnar TFCC (**TECH FIG 9A–C**).

- Using a miniature C-arm, a Freer is used to delineate the dorsal radial cut of the distal ulna to match the curvature of the sigmoid notch.
- An oscillating saw is used to remove this portion of the ulna (**TECH FIG 9D–F**).
- Pronation and supination are checked to ensure no impingement of the distal ulna on the radius.
- The dorsal capsular sheath over the ulna is imbricated to further stabilize the distal ulna using buried 2-0 nonabsorbable braided horizontal mattress sutures.
- After skin closure (**TECH FIG 9G,H**), the extremity is splinted with the forearm in supination.
- The postoperative supination splint is maintained for approximately 4 weeks to stabilize the DRUJ.
  - After 4 weeks, gentle pronation and supination exercises are initiated.

Title

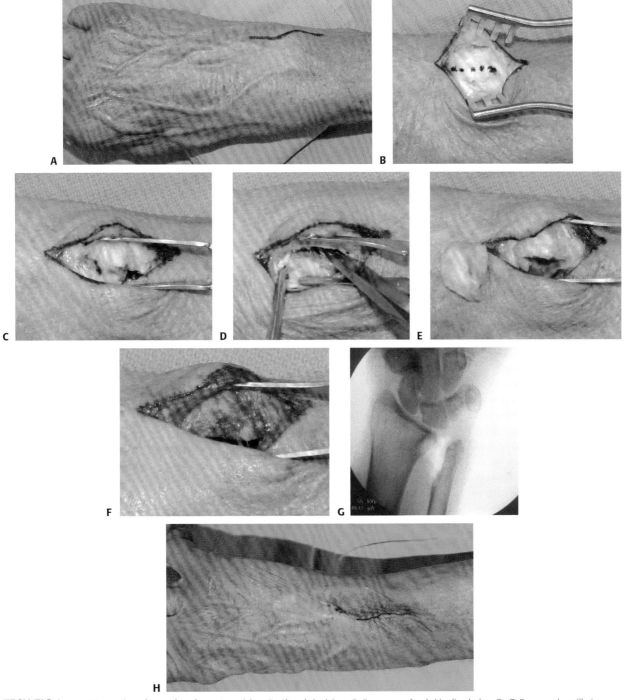

TECH FIG 9 • Hemiresection ulnar arthroplasty. **A.** Incision. **B.** Sheath incision. **C.** Exposure of arthritic distal ulna. **D–F.** Freer and oscillating saw is used to remove distal ulna. **G.** Fluoroscopy. **H.** Skin closure.

■ Total Wrist Fusion

- A dorsal midline incision is made, centered at the radio-carpal joint and extending from the third metacarpal neck to about 5 cm proximal to Lister tubercle (**TECH FIG 10A**).
  - The skin flaps are elevated, taking care to preserve the cutaneous nerves.
  - The third extensor compartment is entered, and the EPL tendon is transposed.

- The extensor retinaculum is incised, exposing the second through fifth extensor compartments.
- The posterior interosseous nerve (PIN) is identified on the floor of the fourth compartment and excised.
- The dorsal wrist capsule is incised along the dorsal intercarpal and dorsal radiocarpal ligaments, creating a radially based capsular flap and elevating it off the dorsal triquetrum.

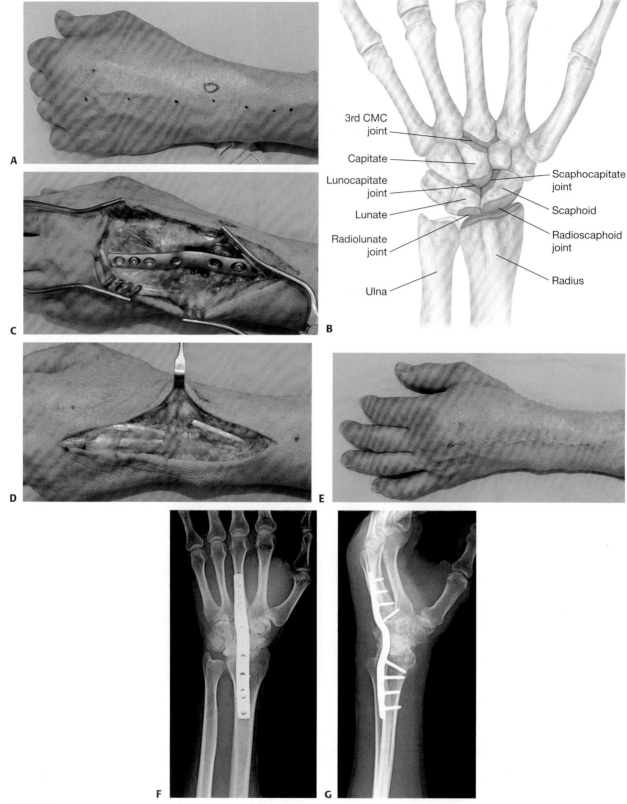

Labels in B: 3rd CMC joint • Capitate • Lunocapitate joint • Lunate • Radiolunate joint • Ulna • Scaphocapitate joint • Scaphoid • Radioscaphoid joint • Radius

TECH FIG 10 • Total wrist fusion. **A.** Skin incision. **B.** Dorsal wrist anatomy showing areas decorticated and removed of cartilage in preparation for fusion: third CMC, radioscaphoid joint, radiolunate joint, scaphocapitate joint, lunocapitate joint. **C.** Fusion plate placed. **D.** Wrist capsule and extensor retinaculum are repaired. **E.** Skin closure. **F,G.** PA and lateral postoperative x-rays.

- The dorsal radius, carpus, and third metacarpal are then exposed via a subperiosteal dissection and further decorticated with an osteotome.
- Lister tubercle is removed to allow the plate to seat well on the radius.
- The articular cartilage and subchondral bone are removed from the radioscaphoid, radiolunate, scapho-capitate, lunocapitate, and third carpometacarpal joints to prepare them for fusion (**TECH FIG 10B**).
  - Care is taken to maintain carpal height by avoiding over-resection of bone.
- Soft tissues are released as needed to permit joint reduction and alignment at about 10 degrees of extension and slight ulnar deviation.
- The surface of the radius is contoured to fit the curvature of the fusion plate.
- The prepared joint spaces are filled with the bone graft.
  - For healthy patients, we use cadaveric bone graft, whereas for smokers or those at risk for wound healing delay, we prefer using bone autografts from the iliac crest.
- The fusion plate is applied, spanning from the distal radius to the third metacarpal.
  - A screw affixing the plate to the third metacarpal is placed in a neutral, unrotated position.

- With the wrist joint compressed, the plate is further affixed to the radius (**TECH FIG 10C**).
  - The remaining screws are placed.
  - Hardware placement is check with fluoroscopy.
  - Full forearm rotation and passive digital ROM should be intact.
- Once the plate is secured, additional bone graft is packed into the prepared joint spaces.
- The wrist capsule is closed over the plate.
  - The extensor retinaculum is repaired, leaving the EPL transposed over the retinaculum.
  - The skin is closed with absorbable monofilament dermal and subcuticular running sutures (**TECH FIG 10E–G**), and a bulky volar wrist splint is applied.
- Typically, at 2 weeks postoperatively, a removable wrist splint is provided for full-time wear and may be removed transiently for personal hygiene.
  - The splint is worn for 3 months.
  - However, if the fixation is tenuous or patient compliance is questionable, a postoperative cast should be placed.
  - Digital ROM and edema control are encouraged throughout this time frame.
  - Upon surgical recovery, patients should expect pain relief, full digital ROM, full forearm rotation, and the ability to complete most activities of daily living.

PEARLS AND PITFALLS

DIPJ ARTHRODESIS	
Exposure	■ Avoid injury to the germinal matrix of the nail fold. ■ If the joint deformity is fixed, adequate soft tissue release must be performed to reduce the joint in an optimal position. This includes release of the volar plate, if necessary.
Shaping the bone	■ As an alternative to burring a "crest-and-trough" configuration, the bone ends can be cut with the distal bone at 0 degrees and the proximal bone at the desired angle of fusion. ■ Avoid excessive bony removal to preserve length and retain good quality bone for healing.
Other techniques for DIPJ arthrodesis	■ The two other most commonly reported techniques for DIPJ fusion include the use of headless compression screws or interosseous cerclage wires. Although evidence is insufficient to support any particular technique, the technique with the least reported complications is K-wiring.[10] ■ If a headless compression screw is placed across the joint, it should be aimed from proximal to distal and slightly palmar to avoid the nail matrix.
SILICONE PIPJ ARTHROPLASTY	
Preoperative assessment of collateral ligaments	■ The collateral ligaments of the PIPJ must be assessed for stability preoperatively. ■ If deficient, the patient may require collateral ligament reconstruction at the time of surgery or may eliminate patient candidacy for arthroplasty.
Finger selection	■ Avoid the use of silicone implants at the index and long finger PIPJs, particularly in young, active patients, because repetitive stresses on the radial collateral ligaments during key or chuck pinch can result early implant failure.
Alternative implants: pyrocarbon	■ Pyrocarbon, or pyrolytic carbon, implants have enhanced lateral stability that makes implantation into the index finger PIPJ more attractive compared to silicone. ■ However, pyrocarbon implants have fallen out of favor due to complication rates as high as 30%. ■ If performed, pyrocarbon PIPJ arthroplasty can be done through a lateral or dorsal approach (see TECH FIG 3A–K).

(Continued)

PEARLS AND PITFALLS (Continued)

THUMB MCPJ FUSION

Techniques for thumb MCPJ fusion	▪ Thumb MCPJ fusion can be accomplished with a variety of techniques, depending on surgeon preference: 　▪ Tension band wiring 　▪ Crossed K-wire fixation 　▪ Plate fixation 　▪ Intramedullary implant placement ▪ For patients with RA, K-wire placement is the author's preferred technique given that thumb MCPJ fusion is often combined with a number of other procedures dealing with the rheumatoid hand.
Angle of fusion	▪ The fused position of the thumb MCPJ should be at about 5–15 degrees of flexion for optimal functionality. ▪ Slightly more flexion at 20–40 degrees may be considered in patients at risk for developing/worsening OA at the thumb CMCJ.

THUMB TM LIGAMENT RECONSTRUCTION WITH FCR

Anatomy of the thumb CMCJ	▪ The thumb CMCJ is the articulation between the trapezium and the thumb metacarpal. It is also known as the trapeziometacarpal (TM) joint. ▪ It is a biconcave saddle-shaped joint that permits thumb flexion, extension, abduction, adduction, and opposition. ▪ The volar beak ligament is the primary stabilizer of the thumb CMCJ. It extends from the ulnar base of the thumb metacarpal onto the trapezium.
Harvest of FCR	▪ The radial half of the FCR tendon is harvested. ▪ The radial artery and sensory nerve branches must be identified and protected. ▪ Injury to the palmar cutaneous branch of the median nerve, which lies 1 mm ulnar to the FCR tendon, must be avoided. ▪ Care should be taken to separate the radial half of FCR from the ulnar half as to avoid accidental transection. Scissors should not be used to slide down the tendon and instead to make deliberate cuts from proximal to distal.
Postoperative course	▪ Thumb CMCJ stiffness is expected for 4–6 wk after surgery but can last up to 4 mo. ▪ Patients can expect near-complete pain relief and minimal progression of degenerative arthritis at the CMCJ provided that the surgery is performed prior to onset of articular cartilage destruction.

TRAPEZIECTOMY WITH APL SUSPENSIONPLASTY

MCPJ laxity	▪ Remember to assess the patient's thumb MCPJ for hyperextensibility during pinch. ▪ If laxity greater than 30–40 degrees is present and unaddressed, ligament reconstruction will be stressed by obligatory metacarpal adduction. ▪ Hyperextensibility at the MCPJ can be addressed with joint capsulodesis, volar plate advancement, or fusion. We advocate MCPJ fusion in these cases because soft tissue imbrication tends to attenuate over time, whereas fusion has a more predictable outcome.
Carpal tunnel syndrome	▪ Up to 43% of patients with TM joint arthritis have concomitant carpal tunnel syndrome. If present, a carpal tunnel release should be performed as well.
Eaton classification	▪ The Eaton classification of TM osteoarthritis (see Table 1), which is based on radiographic findings, often does not correlate with patient symptoms.
Radiographs	▪ A stress view of the TM joint is useful to assess joint space loss and subluxation in patients with symptomatic joint laxity (Eaton stage I). This is obtained by pressing the thumb tips together with a 30-degree posteroanterior view.
Arthritic involvement of the trapezoid	▪ If degenerative changes are present between the trapezoid and the scaphoid, concomitant partial resection of the trapezoid is recommended. This is done to ensure that no contact between the scaphoid and trapezoid occurs with axial loading. ▪ Traction on the index and long fingers after trapeziectomy will allow visualization and assessment of the scaphotrapezoid joint.
Exposure of the trapezium	▪ A dorsal approach provides easy access to the trapezium. ▪ Identify and protect these four structures: 　▪ Radial sensory nerve branches 　▪ Extensor pollicis longus (EPL) tendon 　▪ APL tendon 　▪ Radial artery (located deep to the fatty tissue between EPL ulnarly and APL radially) ▪ Thumb traction can help facilitate exposure of the trapezium.

PEARLS AND PITFALLS (Continued)

THUMB TM JOINT ARTHRODESIS

Anatomy	■ One must protect the radial sensory nerve during exposure of the thumb TM joint. ■ The radial artery must be protected in the interval between the EPL and EPB tendons where it lies deep to the subcutaneous fat.
Plate selection	■ A 2.3-mm locking T-plate is preferred, with the T-portion centered on the trapezium. ■ Utilization of a locking plate is important in the setting of poor bone stock. The trapezium is often devoid of strong cortical bone necessary to secure traditional screws and plates.
Functional thumb position	■ The thumb should be fixed at 30–40 degrees of palmar abduction, 15–20 degrees of extension, and 15 degrees of pronation. ■ This functional position facilitates tip-to-tip pinch.

DARRACH PROCEDURE

Indications	■ Post-traumatic DRUJ arthritis, rheumatoid arthritis, or osteoarthritis without pre-existing radiocarpal instability in patients who are older and sedentary ■ Caput ulna syndrome with TFCC destruction and painful pronation-supination of the DRUJ ■ Preferred in patients with no ulnar translation of carpus who are at low risk of translation in the future ■ Can be performed concomitantly with partial or total wrist fusion in setting of radiocarpal instability ■ Notably, we tend to avoid the Darrach procedure in osteoarthritis, as it weakens the wrist. We prefer hemiresection arthroplasty of the distal ulna (see Technique no. 8).
Caput ulna syndrome	■ Combination of ulnar head dorsal dislocation, ECU volar subluxation, and carpal supination seen in patients with rheumatoid arthritis ■ The fifth extensor compartment (containing EDM) crosses the ulnar head.
Extent of ulnar head resection	■ The pronator quadratus (PQ) is a dynamic stabilizer of the distal ulna, originating at the distal radius and inserting on the distal ulna. ■ Ulnar head excision should be performed at the level of the sigmoid notch in order to preserve the ulnar attachments of the PQ.

Ulna-stabilizing procedure	■ Prior to closing the wrist capsule, the distal ulna stump is tested for stability with pronation-supination.
	■ If unstable, an ulnar stabilizing procedure is indicated (ECU tenodesis):
	  ▪ A hole in the dorsal cortex of the distal ulnar stump is drilled with a 3-mm bur.
	  ▪ The distally based ulnar half of the ECU is harvested and brought from inside the ulnar canal and out the hole dorsally.
	  ▪ The ECU is then sutured to itself with the ulnar stump reduced palmarly and wrist in 15-degrees of extension and 15-degrees of ulnar deviation.
	  ▪ The wrist capsule is then closed as described in the text.

HEMIRESECTION ARTHROPLASTY OF THE DISTAL ULNA

Relative contraindications	■ Hemiresection ulnar arthroplasty should be considered with caution in younger patients because it may lead to loss of support for the ulnar carpus over time. ■ Ulnar-positive variance is a relative contraindication for hemiresection ulnar arthroplasty because it increases the risk of impingement between the ulnar styloid and triquetrum. ■ Other contraindications to hemiresection ulnar arthroplasty include pre-existing ulnar carpal translation (may exacerbate the ulnar translation) and irreparable damage to the TFCC (no benefit over a Darrach procedure).
Technical points	■ Avoid excessive resection of the ulnar head. ■ Preserve the foveal attachments of the TFCC. ■ If necessary, debride the TFCC. ■ Consider ulnar shortening if positive variance is present.

(Continued)

PEARLS AND PITFALLS (Continued)

TOTAL WRIST FUSION

Indications	■ Painful wrist with limited ROM due to osteoarthritis, inflammatory arthritis, and post-traumatic arthritis ■ Multiple joint involvement ■ Failed partial wrist fusions or soft tissue reconstructions ■ Carpal instability patterns (eg, SLAC/SNAC arthritis) ■ Contraindications for joint arthroplasty or failed arthroplasty ■ Desire for a one-stage definitive treatment.
Dorsal wrist capsule	■ The wrist capsule can be elevated as a radially based flap (as described in the text) or via a straight midline longitudinal incision. ■ A thick capsular flap should be maintained for good coverage of the fusion plate. ■ The ECRL and ECRB tendons can be released from their metacarpal insertions and used to augment soft tissue coverage of the hardware.
The fusion mass	■ Bony fusion involves the radius, scaphoid, capitate, lunate, and third metacarpal bones. ■ Not included in the fusion mass are the ulnar joints (lunotriquetral and triquetrohamate joints).
Proximal row carpectomy (PRC)	■ Performing a PRC may help to facilitate joint alignment before fusion, particularly in cases of chronic and severe carpal deformity.
Fusion plate	■ A dynamic compression plate is used for wrist fusion and must be contoured appropriately to allow for 10 degrees of wrist extension and slight ulnar deviation. ■ In patients with poor bone stock, locking screw fixation can be used.
Postoperative splinting	■ A supportive wrist splint is applied at the end of the case. ■ Avoid MCPJ extension in the splint, which may result in intrinsic tightness and loss of digital ROM.

COMPLICATIONS

- Inadequate pain relief
- Wound healing delay
- Nonunion
- Hardware failure
- Failure of reconstruction
- Infection
- Need for further surgery

REFERENCES

1. Kozlow JH, Chung KC. Current concepts in the surgical management of rheumatoid and osteoarthritic hands and wrists. *Hand Clin.* 2011;27(1):31-41.
2. Nacke E, Paksima N. The evaluation and treatment of the arthritic distal radioulnar joint. *Bull Hosp Joint Dis (2013).* 2015;73(2):141-147.
3. Eaton RG, Glickel SZ. Trapeziometacarpal osteoarthritis: staging as a rationale for treatment. *Hand Clin.* 1987;3:455-471.
4. Eaton RG, Littler JW. Ligament reconstruction for the painful thumb carpometacarpal joint. *J Bone Joint Surg Am.* 1973;55:1655-1666.
5. Rizzo M. Thumb arthrodesis. *Tech Hand Up Extrem Surg.* 2006;10(1):43-46.
6. Chang EY, Chung KC. Outcomes of trapeziectomy with a modified abductor pollicis longus suspension arthroplasty for the treatment of thumb carpometacarpal joint osteoarthritis. *Plast Reconstr Surg.* 2008;122(2):505-515.
7. Sauerbier M, Fujita M, Hahn ME, et al. The dynamic radioulnar convergence of the Darrach procedure and the ulnar head hemiresection interposition arthroplasty: a biomechanical study. *J Hand Surg Br.* 2002;27(4):307-316.
8. Minami A, Iwasaki N, Ishikawa J, et al. Treatments of osteoarthritis of the distal radioulnar joint: long-term results of three procedures. *Hand Surg.* 2005;10(2-3):243-248.
9. Watson HK, Ryu JY, Burgess RC. Matched distal ulnar resection. *J Hand Surg [Am].* 1986;11(6):812-817.
10. Dickson DR, Mehta SS, Nuttall D, Ng CY. A systematic review of distal interphalangeal joint arthrodesis. *J Hand Microsurg.* 2014;6(2):74-84.

Carpal Tunnel Release

26
CHAPTER

Angelo B. Lipira and Jason H. Ko

DEFINITION

- Compression of the median nerve at the level of the wrist is the most common compression neuropathy, with a prevalence of 1% to 3%.[1]
- Patients present with numbness or paresthesias in the distribution of the median nerve (thumb, index finger, middle finger, radial half of ring finger).
- Long-standing carpal tunnel syndrome (CTS) can result in weakness and atrophy of the thenar musculature; sensory fibers are preferentially affected earlier in the process.
- CTS is diagnosed clinically. It is often confirmed with electrodiagnostic studies, which can also indicate the severity of nerve injury.

ANATOMY

- The median nerve provides sensation to the thumb, index finger, middle finger, and radial half of the ring finger, as well as the skin of the thenar eminence via the palmar cutaneous branch. It provides motor function to the thenar musculature via the recurrent motor branch and radial two lumbricals via the proper (first lumbrical) and common (second lumbrical) digital nerves (**FIG 1A**).
- The carpal tunnel is an anatomic space bounded by the transverse carpal ligament (TCL) volarly; the hamate, triquetrum, and pisiform ulnarly; the scaphoid and trapezium radially; and the lunate and capitate dorsally (**FIG 1B**).
- The carpal tunnel contains the median nerve and nine flexor tendons (four flexor digitorum superficialis [FDS], four flexor digitorum profundus, and flexor pollicis longus).
- The recurrent motor branch innervates the abductor pollicis brevis, opponens pollicis, and superficial head of flexor pollicis brevis. Most commonly, it arises from the median nerve distal to the TCL (extraligamentous, 46%) but may be subligamentous (31%) or transligamentous (23%). Variants that arise from the ulnar aspect of the median nerve and cross over the TCL are at highest risk of injury, particularly in endoscopic techniques.[2]
- The palmar cutaneous branch usually branches from the radial aspect of the median nerve 5 to 8 cm proximal to the wrist crease and travels distally between the flexor carpi radialis (FCR) and palmaris longus.
  - Therefore, thenar sensation is typically preserved in CTS.
  - However, the palmar cutaneous branch can also show variation, including a variant where it branches from the ulnar aspect of the median nerve.[2] The branch becomes superficial at the wrist level and is vulnerable during incisions.

PATHOGENESIS

- Increased pressures within the carpal tunnel lead to vascular congestion, edema, and ischemia of the median nerve.
- Demyelination occurs first, followed by axonal degeneration in more severe cases. Sensory nerve fibers are affected earlier than motor fibers.

PATIENT HISTORY AND PHYSICAL FINDINGS

- Patient history
  - Patients will often report numbness of the entire hand, rather than localizing it to the median nerve distribution.[3]
  - Classically, patients will report being awakened by paresthesias and pain, as symptoms often worsen at night because during sleep, the wrist relaxes and is often flexed for prolonged periods of time, leading to elevated pressure in the carpal tunnel. Furthermore, many will sleep with their hands and wrists under the head, which also contributes to nerve compression.
  - They may report weakness or clumsiness in more advanced presentations with motor weakness.
  - Investigate associated conditions including diabetes mellitus, rheumatoid arthritis, obesity, gout, hypothyroidism, and pregnancy.[1,4]
  - Take a good occupational history, identifying predisposing and repetitive tasks that may contribute to increased carpal tunnel pressure.
  - Inquire about past therapies including splinting and steroid injections.
- Physical examination
  - Inspect the hand, looking for atrophy of the thenar musculature and differences in temperature and sweat patterns in the median nerve distribution.
  - Test and document two-point discrimination (static and dynamic) on both the radial and ulnar aspects of all digits (normal values: static less than 6 mm, moving 2–3 mm).
  - Provocative maneuvers are used in an attempt to reproduce the patient's symptoms[4]:
    - Phalen test: The wrists are held in a flexed position for up to 1 minute. Record the time it takes to precipitate their usual symptoms.
    - Tinel sign: The examiner percusses over the median nerve at the wrist. If tingling paresthesias are elicited in the fingers, the test is considered positive.
    - Durkan carpal compression test: Direct pressure is applied over the carpal tunnel with the examiner's thumb. Apply just enough pressure to blanch the overlying skin. Record the time it takes to precipitate their usual symptoms.[5]

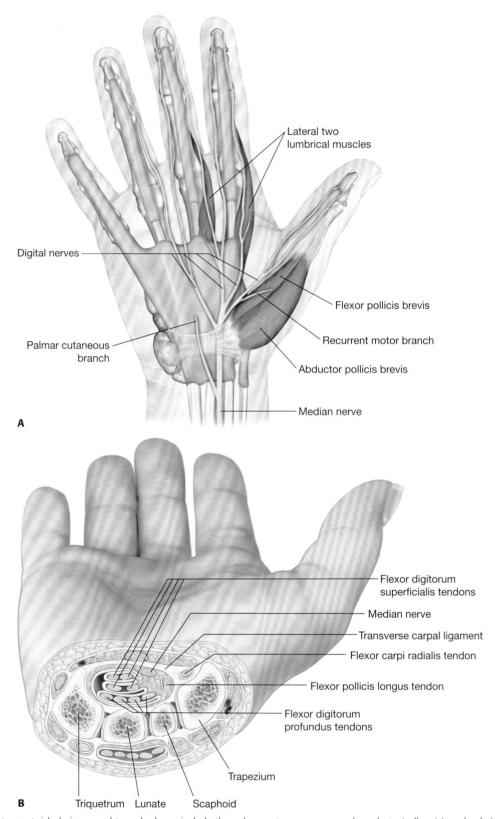

FIG 1 • A. Structures at risk during carpal tunnel release include the palmar cutaneous sensory branch, typically arising ulnarly just proximal to the transverse carpal ligament (TCL), and the recurrent motor branch, typically arising radially just distal to the TCL. **B.** Anatomic boundaries of the carpal tunnel include the TCL volarly; hamate, triquetrum, and pisiform ulnarly; lunate and capitate dorsally; and the scaphoid and trapezium radially. The carpal tunnel contains nine flexor tendons—four flexor digitorum superficialis, four flexor digitorum profundus, and flexor pollicis longus—and the median nerve.

IMAGING AND OTHER DIAGNOSTIC STUDIES

- The diagnosis of CTS is usually made clinically, and electrodiagnostic studies are frequently employed to confirm the diagnosis and rate the severity.
- Imaging is not routinely performed for CTS but may be indicated if there is suspicion of a mass lesion or other rarer presentations.
- Electrodiagnostic studies focus on assessing the conduction velocities and amplitude of the median nerve across the wrist. The ulnar and radial nerve are also often evaluated to compare values in a nerve outside the carpal tunnel and rule out effects of temperature, polyneuropathy, and other factors.
- Nerve conduction studies may demonstrate increased sensory or motor latency (demyelination) and decreased sensory and/or motor amplitude (loss of axons).[4] Sensory latencies are compared to an unaffected nerve (ulnar or radial) and are generally considered abnormal if the difference exceeds 0.3 to 0.5 ms. Motor conduction is assessed by stimulating the median nerve at the wrist and measuring at the abductor pollicis brevis. Latency of over 4.5 ms is generally considered abnormal.[6]
- The combined sensory index (CSI) is a useful composite value that is obtained by measuring the difference in latency between the thumb, palm, and ring fingers and the ulnar or radial nerve and summing these three values together. A CSI of 1 ms or more is considered abnormal.[7] Higher CSIs have been associated with greater frequency of symptom resolution following carpal tunnel release (CTR).[6]
- There is evidence that preoperative electrodiagnostic studies may increase costs and delay time to surgical treatment. Although the American Association of Orthopaedic Surgeons (AAOS), in a prior proactive guideline, recommended electrodiagnostic studies if surgery is being considered, a substantial portion of hand surgeons do not routinely obtain them.[8]

DIFFERENTIAL DIAGNOSIS

- Proximal median nerve lesion (eg, compression from pronator teres, FDS arch, or an accessory muscle such as Gantzer muscle)
- Polyneuropathy
- Central nervous system lesion (tumor, CVA, multiple sclerosis)
- Arthritis

NONOPERATIVE MANAGEMENT

- Nonoperative therapies for CTS include avoidance of provocative maneuvers, wrist immobilization (splinting), nonsteroidal anti-inflammatory drugs (NSAIDs), and corticosteroid injection.
- Wrist braces should hold the wrist in a neutral position. Wrist flexion or extension increases pressure in the carpal tunnel. However, the active position of the wrist is 30 degrees of extension, so neutral splints can make tasks more difficult.
- Although corticosteroid injection leads to transient relief in many patients, the majority will recur within 1 year.[9] Some surgeons believe that relief with steroid injection is predictive of relief with operative CTR and thus holds diagnostic value.
- Dexamethasone is the preferred corticosteroid, as it appears to be less deleterious than hydrocortisone or triamcinolone if inadvertently injected into the nerve substance.[10]

SURGICAL MANAGEMENT

- CTR is commonly performed using both open and endoscopic techniques.
- There is currently no consensus supporting the superiority of one technique over the other.

Preoperative Planning

- Preoperative planning is based on the patient's history and physical exam, as well as review of electrodiagnostic studies, if available.
- Considerations include conducting unilateral vs bilateral releases, anesthesia plan (local, regional block, sedation), and special considerations in the case of recurrent CTS (see below).
- A recent study showed that patients undergoing bilateral simultaneous CTR have increased difficulties with certain activities compared with unilateral CTR, but self-care was unaffected, and the differences did not persist past two postoperative days.[11]
- Open CTR can be performed under local anesthetic block with or without sedation or regional block such as Bier intravenous block (**FIG 2**).
  - General anesthesia is not typically required.
- Endoscopic CTR can be difficult to perform under local anesthetic, as the liquid in the carpal tunnel can obscure visualization, so one of the other anesthetic techniques is recommended.
- In cases of recurrent or persistent CTS following CTR, be sure to rule out other etiologies of symptoms, such as cervical radiculopathy, proximal median nerve or brachial plexus lesions, and polyneuropathy.
  - If the patient has hypersensitivity directly over the carpal tunnel without evidence of palmar cutaneous branch injury, or if the median nerve is found to be adherent to the TCL intraoperatively, we consider the interposition of a hypothenar fat pad flap at the time of reoperation.[12]

Positioning

- The patient is positioned supine on an OR table or stretcher, with the operative extremity on a hand table.
- A well-padded, nonsterile tourniquet is placed on the upper arm prior to prep and drape.
- The surgeon is seated with his or her dominant hand more proximal relative to the operative extremity so that they are working distally down the carpal tunnel.
- A sterile folded towel is placed under the wrist to slightly extend the wrist (15–20 degrees), which moves the median nerve away from the TCL.
- For positioning considerations specific to endoscopic CTR, see section below.

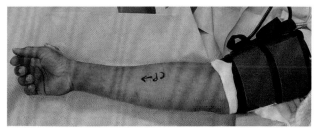

FIG 2 • Typical setup for Bier block anesthesia. Note the intravenous line in the dorsum of the hand and the double tourniquet.

Approach

- Techniques can be broadly divided into open or endoscopic. Open approaches include numerous described incisions, including limited incision and minimally invasive approaches.
- Although numerous variations of incisions for open CTR have been described, most agree that it should be in line with the ring finger, thus slightly ulnar to the axis of the median nerve and less likely to cause injury to the palmar cutaneous branch.
  - We prefer a 2- to 3-cm longitudinal curvilinear incision, staying 2 mm ulnar to the thenar crease to avoid the palmar cutaneous branch. The distal extent is well short of Kaplan cardinal line, which identifies the location of the palmar arterial arch (**FIG 3**).
- Endoscopic approaches include single-portal[13] and two-portal[14] techniques.
  - We prefer the single-portal (Agee) technique, and the proximal incision is typically a 1- to 1.2-cm transverse incision placed in the distal flexion crease of the wrist, just ulnar to the palmaris longus tendon (halfway between FCR and flexor carpi ulnaris [FCU] tendons).

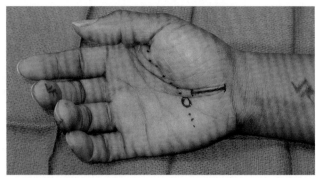

FIG 3 • Incision placement for open carpal tunnel release. It is typically 2 to 3 cm long, in line with the ring finger, and at least 2 mm ulnar to the thenar crease to avoid the palmar cutaneous branch. *Circle* denotes hook of hamate, a palpable landmark. Note incision terminates proximal to Kaplan cardinal line (*dotted line*), which is drawn by extending the ulnar border of the abducted thumb ulnarly and denotes the location of the palmar arterial arch.

■ Open Carpal Tunnel Release

- Mark a 2- to 3-cm longitudinal curvilinear incision 2 mm ulnar to the thenar crease.
- Exsanguinate the arm with an Esmarch bandage, and inflate the tourniquet to 250 mm Hg (or 100 mm Hg over systolic blood pressure).
- Incise full thickness through skin incision with a 15-blade scalpel.
- An assistant retracts the skin with two Senn retractors while dissection is carried down sharply through the subcutaneous tissues until the transverse carpal ligament (TCL) is encountered. During this dissection, be mindful of ulnar variants of the palmar cutaneous branch that may be encountered (**TECH FIG 1A**).
- Using a no. 15 blade, carefully incise the TCL, using a controlled "push," rather than a slicing motion.
- Once the median nerve is visualized, complete as much of the release of the TCL under direct visualization with the use of a scalpel blade.
- Then use tenotomy scissors to spread both superficial and deep to the TCL, being careful to separate the median nerve (which can be quite adherent) from the deep surface of the TCL. Insert one tine of the tenotomy scissors and divide the TCL distally until the palmar fat surrounding the superficial vascular arch of the palm is reached (**TECH FIG 1B,C**).
- Attention should now be turned toward dividing the proximal TCL and contiguous antebrachial fascia.

The surgeon should change positions so that he or she is now seated at the end of the hand table for optimal visualization. Extend the skin incision proximally if necessary (**TECH FIG 1D**).

- Again dissect both superficial and deep to the TCL, separating the median nerve from the deep surface of the TCL. Under direct visualization, release the proximal end of the TCL.
- Continue spreading and dissecting proximally, exposing the deep antebrachial fascia. It is important for the surgical assistant to use two Senn retractors to lift away the skin and subcutaneous tissue to expose the antebrachial fascia proximally. Use tenotomy scissors to release the antebrachial fascia proximally for at least 1 cm proximal to the distal wrist crease.
- Consider lifting the flexor tendons in the carpal tunnel using a Ragnell retractor, and inspect for any mass lesions, such as ganglia, within the tunnel.
- Inject bupivacaine (0.25% with epinephrine) locally into the incision.
- Deflate the tourniquet while holding pressure on the incision.
- Attain meticulous hemostasis.
- Close the incision with 4-0 nylon simple interrupted or horizontal mattress sutures.
- Apply a soft, bulky dressing consisting of nonstick gauze, fluffs, and Kerlix or Ace wrap. Allow for immediate postoperative motion.

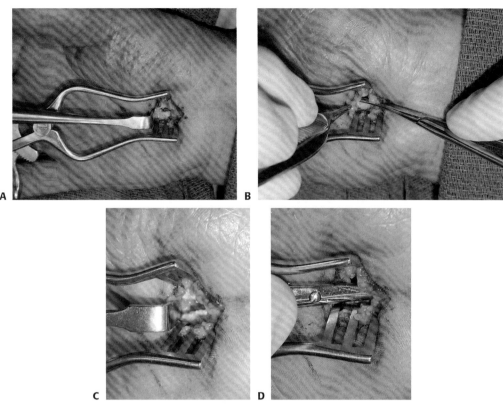

TECH FIG 1 • Open carpal tunnel release. **A.** A small self-retaining retractor and a Ragnell retractor provide exposure of the TCL. **B.** After bluntly spreading above and below the TCL, it is divided with the tenotomy scissors. **C.** Distal division of the TCL has been completed to the level of the distal palmar fat. **D.** The proximal antebrachial fascia is exposed by bluntly spreading above and below and then divided with the tenotomy scissors.

■ Endoscopic Carpal Tunnel Release

Preparation and Incision

- To avoid fogging of the lens, the lens can be placed in warm water or saline for several minutes prior to use. Otherwise, defogging solution can be applied to the lens immediately prior to use.
- Position the monitor at the distal end of the hand table. Assemble the blade/scope unit and then white-balance the camera (can use a white surgical sponge). Test the camera and endoscopic device blade prior to proceeding. Have defogging solution available on a sponge to defog the lens, if needed. Place a folded OR towel under the wrist to extend it.
- Mark a transverse incision approximately 1 to 1.2 cm in length at the distal transverse wrist crease, slightly ulnar to the palmaris longus (if present) (**TECH FIG 2**).
- Exsanguinate the arm with an Esmarch bandage, and inflate the tourniquet to 250 to 300 mm Hg (or 100 mm Hg over systolic blood pressure).

Accessing the Carpal Tunnel

- Incise the skin with a 15 blade, and use bipolar cautery to coagulate small subcutaneous vessels.

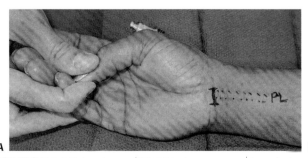
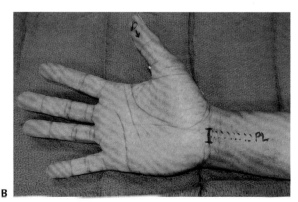

TECH FIG 2 • **A,B.** Incision marking for endoscopic carpal tunnel release. The palmaris longus tendon (when present) is often palpable when the thumb and small finger are opposed and the wrist flexed. The incision is marked transversely in the distal flexion crease of the wrist, slightly ulnarly translated over palmaris longus (PL, Palmaris longus).

- If excessive fatty tissue is present, perform a direct subcutaneous lipectomy.
- Use tenotomy scissors to release the superficial antebrachial fascia.
- Two Ragnell retractors are then used to bluntly spread through the subfascial tissue to expose the TCL.
- Pick up the TCL with Adson forceps distally (**TECH FIG 3A**), and make a small transverse fasciotomy with a no. 15 blade scalpel until the underlying nerve is visualized.
- Once the fascial incision is large enough to insert the tips of tenotomy scissors, use the scissors to extend the fasciotomy transversely with a single, large spreading motion.
  - Then, make a longitudinal fascial incision along the ulnar aspect of the fasciotomy for about 5 mm to create an L-shaped flap.
- Use a small double-skin hook to lift the L-shaped flap of the proximal TCL (**TECH FIG 3B**).
- With a synovial elevator, using gentle pushing motions (not scraping), clear off the deep surface of the TCL, which helps to effectively push the oft-adherent median nerve away from the TCL.

- Advance the elevator until it can be passed into the palm and palpated there with your left hand. This should be done in line with the ring finger (**TECH FIG 3C,D**).
- Sequentially introduce two progressively larger sound dilators into the dissected space between the median nerve and the TCL (**TECH FIG 3E,F**).
- Take the light off standby, and again check the blade engagement mechanism and make sure the blade recedes back into the blade sheath upon trigger release.

Inserting and Advancing the Endoscope

- Insert the assembled scope and blade in line with the ring finger.
  - Rotate the blade sheath slightly ulnarly while introducing it beneath the L-shaped fascial flap.
- If using hot water to eliminate fogging of the camera, after placing the blade/endoscope unit deep to the TCL, remove the scope from the sheath and immerse it in hot water. Rub it dry with a 4 × 4 Raytec gauze. Turn the room lights down, and reintroduce the scope into the blade unit.

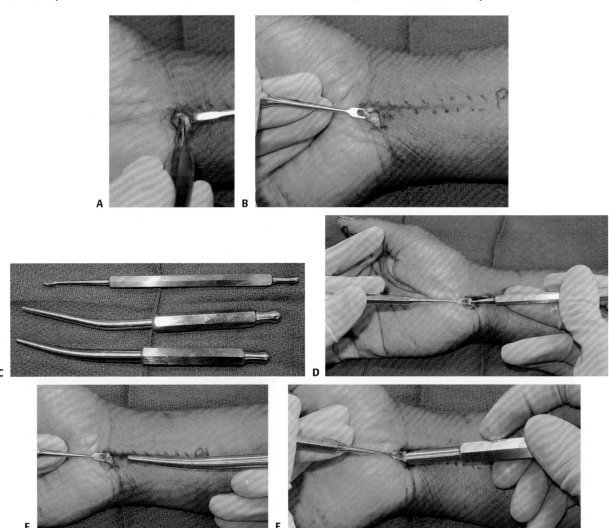

TECH FIG 3 • Accessing the carpal tunnel. **A.** Once exposed, the TCL is grasped with forceps, and a small transverse nick is made with a no. 15 blade. Next, a blunt spread of the tenotomies under the TCL clears the median nerve from its undersurface, and the incision is extended longitudinally along the ulnar aspect to create an L-shaped flap. **B.** A small double hook is used to retract the L-shaped flap. **C.** From top down: synovial elevator, small dilator, large dilator; to be used in that sequence. **D.** Using the synovial elevator, gentle pushing motions (not pulling) clear the synovium from the deep surface of the TCL. **E,F.** The smaller dilator is then passed through the carpal tunnel, followed by the larger dilator. The tunnel is now prepared for insertion of the endoscopic device.

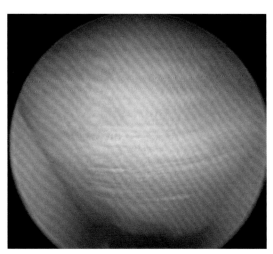

TECH FIG 4 • Endoscopic view showing the TCL forming the roof of the carpal tunnel, predivision. Note that it has been cleared of adherent synovium. Also note the palmar fat visible at the distal extent of the tunnel.

- ▪ If using defogging solution, this step can be skipped.
- ▪ Advance the scope until the distal aspect of the TCL is visualized, usually corresponding to the 3.5-cm measurement on the sheath.
- ▪ While watching the video monitor, the surgeon's hand that is not controlling the scope can be used to push on the palm repeatedly to determine where the distal edge of the TCL is located, since the tight TCL will minimize motion of the tissues even upon deep palpation.
  - ▪ However, the tissue distal to the TCL will "bounce" more easily with palpation (**TECH FIG 4**).

Releasing the Carpel Tunnel and Completion

- ▪ Ensure that the hand is completely flat against the towel (with the thenar eminence firmly pushed down by the assistant) to tighten the TCL while moving the nerve as far away from the blade as possible.
- ▪ Engage the blade and slowly pull the scope proximally to cut the distal end of the TCL, stopping at approximately halfway (**TECH FIG 5A**).

- ▪ Disengage the blade and readvance the scope to visualize the distal aspect of the TCL, ensuring no uncut bands remain distally. Any residual fibers can be cut at this time (**TECH FIG 5B**).
- ▪ The scope is pulled proximally again, and the blade is engaged again just before reaching the proximal, uncut edge of the TCL.
  - ▪ Continue pulling the device proximally to divide the remainder of the ligament while applying pressure to the palm with the hand not controlling the scope, which "pushes" the TCL into closer approximation with the blade.
- ▪ The scope can be reintroduced to visualize any residual fibers of TCL, though after release of the TCL, the superficial fat can obscure the view seen on the monitor.
- ▪ Remove the scope.
- ▪ Introduce closed tenotomy scissors under the cut TCL (superficial to the nerve).
  - ▪ Using a bimanual palpation technique, the tips of the tenotomy scissors can be gently run along the deep surface of the palm to determine if any fibers of TCL remain while the surgeon's other hand follows the tips of the tenotomy scissors on the surface of the palm.
- ▪ Attention should now be turned toward dividing the proximal antebrachial fascia, which is a very important part of the endoscopic carpal tunnel release.
  - ▪ The surgeon should change positions to be seated at the end of the hand table for optimal visualization.
- ▪ Retract the skin and fat above the proximal superficial and deep antebrachial fascia using a Ragnell retractor, and divide the antebrachial fascia proximally with tenotomy scissors for approximately 2 cm.
- ▪ The incision can be approximated with 4-0 nylon suture in a simple or horizontal mattress fashion.
- ▪ Infiltrate a 0.25% bupivacaine with epinephrine into the incision, along with the area of the released TCL and antebrachial fascia.
- ▪ Apply a soft dressing of fluffs and a 4-in. Kling wrap.
- ▪ Apply firm pressure at the incision site through the dressing while deflating the tourniquet.

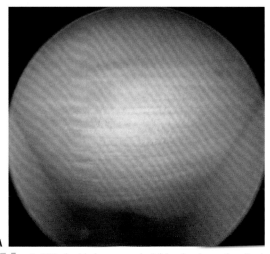

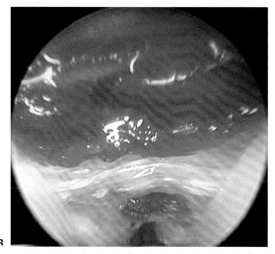

A   **B**

TECH FIG 5 • **A.** With the blade engaged, division begins at the distal extent of the TCL by slowly withdrawing the device. **B.** Following the initial pass of the blade, much of the TCL has been divided, exposing the overlying pink palmar fascia. Note the band of intact TCL that must be divided with a second pass.

■ Hypothenar Fat Flap

- In cases of recurrent or recalcitrant carpal tunnel syndrome (CTS), excessive scar formation may contribute to entrapment of the nerve. The hypothenar fat flap is a technique to interpose healthy, vascularized tissue over the nerve to prevent recurrence from aggressive scar formation.
- Exsanguinate the arm with an Esmarch bandage, and inflate the tourniquet to 250 mm Hg (or 100 mm Hg over systolic blood pressure).
- Make a linear incision just radial to the hypothenar eminence, and carry dissection down to the carpal tunnel to identify the median nerve.
  - Typically, the hypothenar fat flap is used for the treatment of recalcitrant CTS, so the incision can be made through the previous surgical scar (**TECH FIG 6A**).
- Perform external neurolysis of the median nerve.
- Using sharp dissection, develop a subdermal plane over the adipose tissue of the hypothenar region, being cautious not to make the cutaneous flap too thin. Carry this dissection to the dermal insertion of the palmaris brevis[12] (**TECH FIG 6B**).

- Perform deep dissection under the fat pad, directly over the hypothenar musculature, until the ulnar nerve and artery are visualized.
- Check if the flap has been sufficiently mobilized to be advanced to the radial wall of the carpal tunnel (**TECH FIG 6C,D**).
- If not, carefully perform additional dissection, being careful to preserve the vascular pedicles of the flap and the ulnar neurovascular structures.
- Retract the carpal tunnel contents ulnarly, and place the hypothenar fat pad flap volar to the median nerve and deep to the radial leaf of the TCL. Place horizontal mattress sutures through the flap and into the radial wall of the carpal tunnel. Tag these sutures and sequentially tie them once all have been placed.
- Irrigate the wound and deflate the tourniquet. Achieve meticulous hemostasis.
- Approximate the skin using 4-0 nylon suture in a simple interrupted or horizontal mattress fashion. Apply dressings as described above.

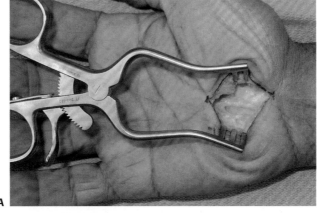

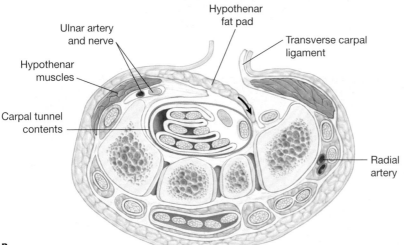

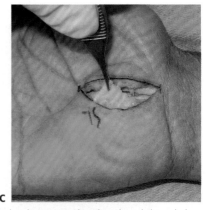

TECH FIG 6 • Hypothenar fat pad flap. **A.** The carpal tunnel has been released, the median nerve has been neurolysed, and a subdermal plane has been developed over the adipose of the hypothenar region. **B.** The hypothenar fat pad flap must be mobilized sufficiently to reach the radial wall of the carpal tunnel. The subdermal plane is developed to the dermal insertion of palmaris brevis, and the deep dissection is carried out just over the musculature until the ulnar neurovascular bundle is visualized. **C.** The elevated hypothenar fat pad flap, prior to inset.

PEARLS AND PITFALLS

Incomplete release	▪ Be sure to adequately release the distal TCL in the palm to the level of the palmar fat pad, and the antebrachial fascia for 1–2 cm in the forearm. In endoscopic CTR, check for bands of undivided TCL by palpating with closed tenotomy scissors.
Palmar cutaneous branch injury	▪ Make incision ulnar to axis of ring finger. Look out for ulnar cutaneous branch variant.
Recurrent motor branch injury	▪ Subligamentous and transligamentous variants are at increased risk specifically with endoscopic CTR. Rare variant that exits median nerve ulnarly and curves distally around TCL is highest risk.[2]
Superficial palmar arch injury	▪ Located 2–26 mm from the distal edge of TCL, contained in palmar fat pad[15]
Radially located ulnar artery	▪ In some patients, the ulnar artery is located radial to the hook of hamate, making it vulnerable during CTR.[15]
Visualization on endoscopy	▪ Watch the monitor closely at all times while the endoscopic device is entering, exiting, or within the carpal tunnel.
Anesthesia	▪ Endoscopic release is very difficult with local anesthesia, as the liquid anesthetic obscures visualization.

POSTOPERATIVE CARE

▪ We do not use postoperative splinting, but rather a soft dressing that the patient removes after 24 to 48 hours. We encourage use of the hand right away to encourage nerve gliding and prevent adhesion formation.

▪ We do not routinely refer our patients to hand therapy postoperatively. Therapy can be useful in specific cases such as desensitization for abnormal postoperative hypersensitivity or if there is stiffness or immobility.

OUTCOMES

▪ A Cochrane systematic review found that both surgical and nonoperative treatments of CTS are effective, but surgery produces a longer-lasting relief of symptoms than nonoperative therapies.

▪ Surgical release yields continued improvement for around 12 months postoperatively, whereas improvements from nonoperative therapies plateau at around 3 months.[1]

COMPLICATIONS

▪ Postoperative recurrence has been reported in 3% to 20% of cases.[16,17]

▪ Etiologies of persistence or recurrence include incompletely released TCL, abundant scar formation from a number of causes, neuropathy of other etiology (eg, polyneuropathy), and psychosocial factors.[16]

▪ Serious complications are rare but include injury to the median nerve, recurrent motor branch, or palmar cutaneous branch.

▪ Other complications include painful or hypertrophic scar, hematoma, infection, and wound healing problems.

REFERENCES

1. Shi Q, MacDermid JC. Is surgical intervention more effective than non-surgical treatment for carpal tunnel syndrome? A systematic review. *J Orthop Surg Res.* 2011;6:17.
2. Lanz U. Anatomical variations of the median nerve in the carpal tunnel. *J Hand Surg [Am].* 1977;2:44-53.
3. Stevens JC, Smith BE, Weaver AL, et al. Symptoms of 100 patients with electromyographically verified carpal tunnel syndrome. *Muscle Nerve.* 1999;22:1448-1456.
4. Robinson LR. Electrodiagnosis of carpal tunnel syndrome. *Phys Med Rehabil Clin N Am.* 2007;18(4):733-746.
5. Durkan JA. A new diagnostic test for carpal tunnel syndrome. *J Bone Joint Surg Am.* 1991;73(4):535-538.
6. Robinson LR. Entrapment neuropathies of the median and ulnar nerves. *AANEM Course.* 2011;27-30.
7. Robinson LR. Role of neurophysiologic evaluation in diagnosis. *J Am Acad Orthop Surg.* 2000;8:190-199.
8. Sears ED, Swiatek PR, Hou H, Chung KC. Utilization of preoperative electrodiagnostic studies for carpal tunnel syndrome: an analysis of national practice patterns. *J Hand Surg Am.* 2016;41(6): 665-672.e1.
9. Blazar PE, Floyd WE, Han CH, et al. Prognostic indicators for recurrent symptoms after a single corticosteroid injection for carpal tunnel syndrome. *J Bone Joint Surg.* 2015;97:1563-1570.
10. Mackinnon SE, Hudson AR, Gentili F, et al. Peripheral nerve injection injury with steroid agents. *Plast Reconstr Surg.* 1982;69:482-490.
11. Osei DA, Calfee RP, Stepan JG, et al. Simultaneous bilateral or unilateral carpal tunnel release? A prospective cohort study of early outcomes and limitations. *J Bone Joint Surg.* 2014;96:889-896.
12. Strickland JW, Idler RS, Lourie GM, Plancher KD. The hypothenar fat pad flap for management of recalcitrant carpal tunnel syndrome. *J Hand Surg [Am].* 1996;21:840-848.
13. Agee JM, McCarroll HR, Tortosa RD, et al. Endoscopic release of the carpal tunnel: a randomized prospective multicenter study. *J Hand Surg [Am].*1992;17:987-995.
14. Chow JC. Endoscopic carpal tunnel release: two-portal technique. *Hand Clin.* 1994;10:637-646.
15. Cobb TK, Knudson GA, Cooney WP. The use of topographical landmarks to improve the outcome of Agee endoscopic carpal tunnel release. *Arthroscopy.* 1995;11:165-172.
16. Louie D, Earp B, Blazar P. Long-term outcomes of carpal tunnel release: a critical review of the literature. *Hand.* 2012;7:242-246.
17. Cobb TK, Amadio PC. Reoperation for carpal tunnel syndrome. *Hand Clin.* 1996;12:313-323.

27
CHAPTER

Ulnar Tunnel Syndrome

Mary Claire Manske and Jason H. Ko

DEFINITION

- Ulnar tunnel syndrome, first described by DuPont et al. in 1965, is a compressive neuropathy of the ulnar nerve at the wrist that presents with a variable constellation of sensory and motor symptoms, depending on the site of nerve compression within the ulnar tunnel.[1]
- The ulnar tunnel is commonly referred to as Guyon canal after Jean Casimir Felix Guyon, a French surgeon who first described this anatomic space in 1861.[2]

ANATOMY

- The ulnar tunnel is a fibro-osseous canal that extends from the proximal edge of the volar carpal ligament to the hook of the hamate and the fibrous arch of the hypothenar muscles distally.
- Medially, it is bordered by the pisiform, flexor carpi ulnaris (FCU), and abductor digit minimi; laterally, it is limited by the hook of the hamate, transverse carpal ligament, and extrinsic flexor tendons.

- The roof of the ulnar tunnel is composed of the volar carpal ligament, palmaris brevis, and hypothenar fascia; the floor is formed by the transverse carpal ligament, pisohamate ligament, pisometacarpal ligament, and opponens digiti minimi[3] (**FIG 1A**).
- The contents of the ulnar tunnel include the ulnar nerve, ulnar artery and venae comitantes, and fat. The ulnar nerve is ulnar and dorsal to the ulnar artery.
- In the distal forearm, the ulnar nerve travels volar to the flexor retinaculum before entering the ulnar tunnel. Although variations exist,[4] the ulnar nerve bifurcates within the tunnel into superficial and deep branches approximately 6 mm distal to the distal pole of the pisiform.
- The superficial branch innervates the palmaris brevis and then continues as a sensory nerve, providing sensation to the hypothenar eminence, small finger, and ulnar side of the ring finger.
- After passing through the ulnar tunnel, the deep motor branch of the ulnar nerve runs through the pisohamate hiatus just distal to the ulnar tunnel, which is bordered by the

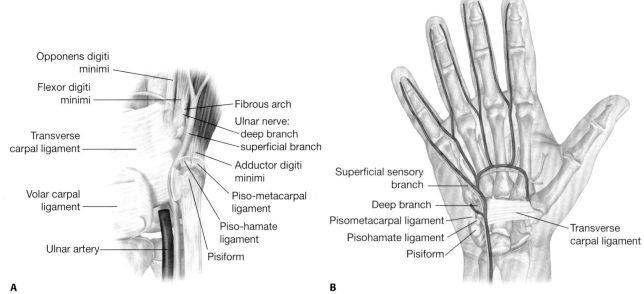

A   **B**

FIG 1 • **A.** Anatomy of the ulnar tunnel. The ulnar tunnel is defined dorsally by the transverse carpal ligament; volarly by the volar carpal ligament; ulnarly by the pisiform, FCU, and ADM; and radially by the hook of the hamate. **B.** Anatomy of the ulnar nerve in the ulnar tunnel. The dorsoulnar fibers of the ulnar nerve become the deep motor branch innervating the intrinsic hand muscles, while the volar-radial fibers provide sensory fascicles to the small finger and ulnar side of the ring finger.

pisohamate ligament dorsally and by the fibrous arch of the hypothenar fascia volarly. The deep motor branch curves around the hook of the hamate to innervate the abductor digiti minimi (ADM), flexor digiti minimi, opponens digiti minimi, interossei, third and fourth lumbricals, adductor pollicis, and flexor pollicis brevis (**FIG 1B**).

- The ulnar nerve at the wrist has been divided into three zones, which can be used to correlate clinical symptoms to the site of compression.[2,5,6]
    - Zone I: From the proximal edge of the volar carpal ligament to the bifurcation of the ulnar nerve into motor and sensory branches. Compression in zone I results in intrinsic muscle weakness and sensory deficits over the hypothenar eminence and small and ring fingers.
    - Zone II: From just distal to the bifurcation to the fibrous arch of the hypothenar muscles and contains the deep motor branch of the ulnar nerve. Compression in this zone presents with ulnar-innervated intrinsic motor weakness and intact sensation in the ulnar nerve sensory distribution.
    - Zone III: Also begins just distal to the bifurcation and includes the sensory branch of the ulnar nerve. Compression at this level results in diminished sensation in the volar aspect of the small finger and volar ulnar ring finger.

PATHOGENESIS

- Many cases of ulnar tunnel syndrome are idiopathic.[7] Space-occupying lesions, aberrant musculature, carpal tunnel syndrome, and acute and chronic trauma have also been implicated in the pathogenesis of ulnar nerve compression at the wrist.
    - Space-occupying masses in the ulnar tunnel are reported to cause compression of the ulnar nerve or its branches, including ganglia, lipomas, ulnar artery thrombosis, ulnar artery pseudoaneurysm, hemangioma, osteoarthritis and rheumatoid arthritis, edema, proliferative synovitis, and bony deformity.
    - Hypertrophic hypothenar muscles or anomalous muscles (hypothenar adductor) may cause ulnar nerve compression.
    - Carpal tunnel syndrome may cause compression of the ulnar nerve distally, as increased pressure in the carpal tunnel is transmitted to the adjacent ulnar tunnel.
        - Seventy-one percent of patients with ulnar tunnel syndrome have a concomitant diagnosis of carpal tunnel syndrome.[7]
    - Fractures and dislocations
        - Hook of hamate fractures: Fracture displacement or associated hematoma and edema may compress the ulnar nerve.
        - Dorsally displaced distal radius fractures and other carpal fractures can cause ulnar nerve palsies secondary to traction on the ulnar nerve or edema.
    - Chronic compression
        - "Handlebar palsy" in long-distance cyclists who place prolonged pressure on the hypothenar area
    - Chronic repetitive microtrauma or vibration
        - "Hypothenar hammer syndrome" in patients who use high impact vibratory equipment with the wrist extended (eg, jackhammer) results in direct trauma to the ulnar artery leading to thrombosis, which may compress the ulnar nerve and/or cause ischemia.

PATIENT HISTORY AND PHYSICAL FINDINGS

- History and physical examination findings may be purely sensory, purely motor, or mixed sensory and motor, depending on the location of pathology.
- History
    - Sensory complaints: numbness and/or paresthesias in small and ring finger
        - Patients with ulnar tunnel syndrome do not present with sensory disturbance over the dorsal aspect of the hand, given that the dorsal sensory branch of the ulnar nerve supplying this area branches from the ulnar nerve proximal to the ulnar tunnel.
        - Cold intolerance or pain in the ring and small fingers
    - Motor deficits: clumsiness, loss of coordinated hand function, weakness of pinch and grasp, clawing
    - History of trauma
        - Acute: direct blow or sports injury (consider fractures, dislocation)
        - Chronic: use of power tools, cycling (consider ulnar artery thrombosis, pseudoaneurysm, or compression)
    - Comorbid medical conditions: rheumatoid arthritis, osteoarthritis, diabetes mellitus, carpal tunnel syndrome
- Physical Examination
    - Inspection: intrinsic muscle atrophy/wasting or clawing; mass or fullness; ecchymosis, swelling, or other evidence of trauma; compare to contralateral upper extremity
    - Palpation: tenderness may indicate fracture; identify presence of a mass (ganglia, lipomas)
    - Sensory exam: decreased sensation to light touch in small and ulnar ring finger; Semmes-Weinstein monofilament or two-point discrimination test
    - Motor exam: intrinsic motor weakness, index finger abduction (assessment of the first dorsal interosseous muscle), or the cross-finger test (asking the patient to cross the middle finger over the index finger to assess the first volar and second dorsal interossei)
    - Special motor tests
        - Froment sign: Positive test when patient is unable to use adductor pollicis for lateral pinch. Instead, patients compensate with the median nerve innervated flexor pollicis longus to flex the thumb interphalangeal joint. Positive test indicates dysfunction of ulnar nerve motor fibers, although it does not localize the site of the lesion.
        - Jeanne test: Test is positive, indicating ulnar motor neuropathy, when the patient hyperextends the metacarpophalangeal joint to compensate for weak adductor pollicis during lateral pinch.
        - Wartenberg sign: Inability to adduct the small finger secondary to paralysis of the third palmar interosseous muscle. Positive test indicates an ulnar motor neuropathy.
    - Vascular exam: palpation of radial and ulnar artery pulses, bruits, or thrills; Doppler examination of radial and ulnar artery; Allen test to assess ulnar artery patency
    - Provocative tests: Tinel and Phalen test over pisiform (Phalen test over pisiform is more sensitive than Tinel for ulnar tunnel syndrome)[8]
    - Must rule out alternative sites of nerve compression: cubital tunnel syndrome, carpal tunnel, cervical radiculopathy, thoracic outlet syndrome

IMAGING

- Electrodiagnostic studies are indicated in nearly all patients with a suspected diagnosis of ulnar tunnel syndrome. The need for additional imaging is determined by the suspected structural etiology of the patient's ulnar tunnel symptoms; bony pathology requires x-ray and/or CT scan; vascular pathology should be evaluated with ultrasound or contrast arteriography; soft tissue masses should be worked up with an MRI. In addition, elbow or cervical spine imagine (x-rays, MRI) may be indicated if there is concern for more proximal pathology.
  - Electrodiagnostic studies are useful to confirm and localize ulnar nerve entrapment.
    - Conduction velocity of the ulnar nerve across the elbow and the wrist can determine the location of ulnar nerve entrapment (elbow, wrist, zone I, II, or III).
      - The most sensitive electrodiagnostic study for ulnar tunnel syndrome is the distal motor latency to the first dorsal interosseous combined with conduction velocity across the wrist (90% sensitivity).[9]
      - Zone I lesions are characterized by decreased sensory responses and prolonged latency to the first dorsal interosseous and ADM. Zone II lesions show prolonged latency to the first dorsal interosseoi (and possibly hypothenar muscles) with normal sensory findings. Zone III lesions show only decreased ulnar sensory responses without motor deficits.[10]
- Radiographic studies
  - Posteroanterior, lateral, and oblique views of the wrist are useful when fracture or dislocation is the suspected etiology of the patient's ulnar nerve symptoms.
  - A 30-degree supinated oblique view with the thumb abducted or carpal tunnel view is useful when there is clinical concern for pisotriquetral joint pathology or hook of the hamate fracture, respectively.
- The indication for obtaining a CT scan in the setting of ulnar tunnel symptoms is similar to that for x-rays. CT scan is particularly useful in detecting hook of hamate fractures.
- Magnetic resonance imaging is useful for identifying and localizing soft tissue masses, aberrant musculature, vascular anomalies, and hook of hamate fractures.
- Ultrasound has similar indications to MRI but is less costly.[11]
- Arteriography serves as the standard for evaluated ulnar artery pathology (eg, thrombosis, pseudoaneurysm).[12]

DIFFERENTIAL DIAGNOSIS

- Cubital tunnel syndrome or proximal compression of the ulnar nerve
- Carpal tunnel syndrome
- Cervical radiculopathy
- Neuromuscular disorders (Charcot-Marie-Tooth, amyotrophic lateral sclerosis)
- Malignant peripheral nerve sheath tumors
- C8-T1 brachial plexopathy
- Central nerve system lesion
- Poliomyelitis

NONOPERATIVE MANAGEMENT

- Nonoperative management consisting of activity modification, rest, and a short course of bracing in a neutral wrist splint may be considered in patients without motor symptoms.
- Activity modification for ulnar tunnel symptoms secondary to hypothenar eminence compression. Cyclists with handlebar palsy may modify the position of their handlebars to prevent the compression of the ulnar base of the palm.
- Patients with hypothenar hammer syndrome without thrombosis and symptoms of digital ischemia may attempt nonoperative intervention, consisting of the following:
  - Smoking cessation, avoidance of trauma, protective gloves, change of occupation, cold avoidance, and calcium channel blockers[13]
- Cortisone injections are not indicated for ulnar tunnel syndrome because inflammation is rarely the cause of ulnar tunnel syndrome and there is a high risk of neurovascular injury when injecting into this confined space.

SURGICAL MANAGEMENT

- Indications:
  - Failure of nonoperative intervention
  - Loss of two-point discrimination
  - Presence of intrinsic muscle weakness or atrophy
  - Severe electrodiagnostic abnormalities
- Operative intervention for ulnar tunnel syndrome consists of ulnar nerve decompression through the distal ulnar tunnel. Additional procedures may be performed as needed to address the causative pathology.
  - Space-occupying mass requires mass excision in addition to ulnar nerve decompression in the ulnar tunnel.
  - Ulnar artery thrombosis or aneurysm should be treated with artery reconstruction and ulnar nerve decompression.
  - Ulnar tunnel syndrome secondary to carpal tunnel syndrome often improves with carpal tunnel release alone, and additional release of the ulnar tunnel is not recommended.
- Optimal outcomes are achieved when all sources of pathology are addressed.

Preoperative Planning

- Indications for operative intervention include failure of nonoperative intervention, motor weakness or loss of two-point sensibility in the ulnar nerve distribution due to ulnar nerve compression distally, or severe electrodiagnostic changes involving the ulnar nerve at the wrist.
- Electrodiagnostic studies should be reviewed to confirm the precise location of ulnar nerve compression and appropriate site of decompression.
- Relevant imaging studies must be reviewed to allow the surgeon to address all etiologies of ulnar nerve symptoms.

Positioning

- Patients are positioned supine on a well-padded operating table with the affected limb on a hand table.
- The operating table is turned so that the hand table faces the center of the room.
- A nonsterile tourniquet is applied to the affected upper extremity.

Approach

- A volar approach to the ulnar nerve at the wrist is the most direct approach and allows accesses to the relevant pathology.

■ Ulnar Tunnel Release and Ulnar Nerve Decompression

Exposure

- Operative limb is elevated and exsanguinated with an elastic bandage immediately prior to tourniquet elevation.
- Alternatively, or in addition to a tourniquet, 0.25% bupivacaine with epinephrine can be injected into the planned incision site for postoperative comfort and intraoperative hemostasis.
- Identify landmark for incisions: The pisiform is easily palpated in the ulnar base of the palm. The hook of the hamate is located 1 cm distal and 1 cm radial to the pisiform and can be palpated.
- A no. 15 blade scalpel is used to make a 4-cm longitudinal or curvilinear incision through the skin paralleling the thenar crease between the pisiform and hook of the hamate, approximately 6 mm ulnar to the thenar crease (**TECH FIG 1**).
  - To extend proximally into the forearm, the incision should cross the wrist crease obliquely and may continue proximally adjacent to the flexor carpi ulnaris tendon.
  - To extend the incision distally into the palm, the incision may be extended in a zigzag or Bruner fashion.

Dissection

- Tenotomy scissors are used to dissect through the subcutaneous tissue, and gentle skin retraction is provided by two double-prong skin hooks.

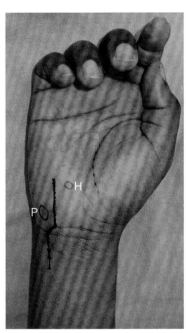

TECH FIG 1 • Incision for ulnar tunnel release. In the palm, a longitudinal incision is centered between the pisiform and hook of the hamate. The incision crosses the wrist flexion crease obliquely before continuing proximally adjacent to the flexor carpi ulnaris (FCU) tendon. P, pisiform; H, Hook of hamate.

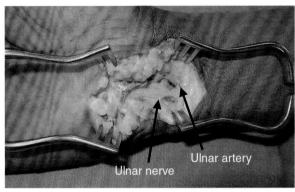

TECH FIG 2 • In the forearm, the ulnar neurovascular bundle is identified deep to the antebrachial fascia between the FCU tendon and tendons of the finger flexors. At this location, the ulnar nerve is deep and ulnar to the artery.

- A cutaneous branch of the ulnar nerve crosses the distal aspect of the incision in 15% of patients. Care must be taken to identify and protect this nerve to avoid a painful neuroma if injured.
- Dissection continues until the volar carpal tunnel and palmaris brevis are identified.
- Proximally in the forearm, the ulnar neurovascular bundle is identified deep to the antebrachial fascia between the flexor carpi ulnaris and the finger flexor tendons. The ulnar nerve is located ulnar and deep to the ulnar artery (**TECH FIG 2**).

Ulnar Nerve Decompression

- The ulnar nerve is carefully dissected from proximal to distal, through the ulnar tunnel.
- The volar carpal ligament and palmaris brevis (roof of the ulnar tunnel) are incised, staying ulnar to the hook of the hamate, so as not to inadvertently enter the carpal tunnel.
- Within the ulnar tunnel, the ulnar nerve is gently retracted medially to identify and decompress the deep motor branch.
- To identify the deep motor branch, locate the oblique fibers of the proximal edge of the hypothenar fascia. Immediately proximal to this leading edge, 1 to 2 mm of the deep motor branch is visible as it dives deep to the hypothenar fascia to enter the pisohamate hiatus and curves around the hook of the hamate.
- A small blunt elevator may be placed deep to the proximal edge of hypothenar fascia to protect the deep motor branch, and this fascia is then released (**TECH FIG 3A**).
- The deep motor branch is then followed around the hook of the hamate, and all tendinous bands of the hypothenar musculature must also be divided (**TECH FIG 3B**).
  - If the deep motor branch is compressed more distally in the palm, it may be followed along the interosseous fascia (deep to the flexor tendons and superficial palmar arch) to its terminus in the adductor pollicis.

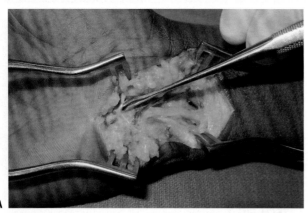
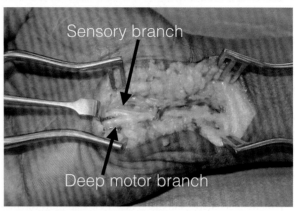

TECH FIG 3 • A. A Freer elevator has been placed beneath the leading edge of the hypothenar fascia. **B.** The sensory branch and deep motor branch of the ulnar nerve have been decompressed.

- Within the canal, care must be taken to protect the small vessels running with the motor branch.
- After releasing the ulnar nerve and the deep motor branch, the floor of the ulnar tunnel is evaluated for masses or anomalous muscles, which are then excised. In the case of a ganglion cyst, the stalk of the cyst is identified and ablated at its origin.
- After the ulnar nerve and its distal branches have been decompressed, the wound is thoroughly irrigated with sterile saline and the tourniquet deflated. Meticulous hemostasis is achieved with bipolar electrocautery.

Wound Closure and Dressing

- The incision is closed with 4-0 nylon suture in a horizontal or simple interrupted fashion.
- If local anesthetic, such as 0.25% bupivacaine, has not previously been injection, it may be injected into the incision site at this time for postoperative comfort.
- A nonadherent dressing is applied directly to the wound, and a sterile, bulky soft dressing is placed.
- Typically, a splint is not needed, unless a ganglion cyst was excised or the dissection was extensive.

PEARLS AND PITFALLS

Diagnosis	Evaluate for extrinsic sources of compression based on suspected pathology. ■ Osseous pathology: radiographs, CT ■ Vascular pathology: Ultrasound, contrast arteriogram ■ Soft tissue mass: MRI
Incision	■ Fifteen percent of patients have a cutaneous branch of the ulnar nerve in the distal aspect of this incision. Avoid injury to the nerve here to prevent a painful neuroma.
Entering the ulnar tunnel	■ Stay ulnar to the hook of the hamate to avoid entering the carpal tunnel.
Identification of the deep motor branch	■ Identify the oblique fibers of the hypothenar fascia at the proximal edge of the hypothenar muscles and carefully release these fibers to expose and decompress the ulnar motor branch.
Release of the deep motor branch	■ Ensure complete nerve decompression, including complete release of the tendinous bands of the hypothenar muscles.
Hemostasis	■ Preserve the small vessels running with the deep motor branch to avoid having to cauterize vessels adjacent to the nerve.

POSTOPERATIVE CARE

- Apply a soft bulky dressing to the wrist postoperatively, and active range of motion can be initiated immediately to minimize scarring around the nerve.
- The bulky surgical dressing is removed on postoperative day 1 or 2 and replaced with a clean gauze dressing or bandage, if necessary.
- Night splinting with the wrist in a neutral position may be used for 2 weeks for patient comfort.

- Strengthening exercises may be initiated at 4 to 6 weeks. Patients may gradually increase activities as tolerated at this time.

OUTCOMES

- There are limited data on the outcome of ulnar tunnel release and decompression.
- Murata et al. retrospectively reported their outcomes in 31 patients with ulnar tunnel syndrome with a variety of causes treated with ulnar tunnel decompression.[7]

- The authors reported improvement in subjective symptoms and two-point discrimination in all patients (from a preoperative mean of 7.0 and 6.9 mm in the ring and small fingers, respectively, to 5.4 and 5.3 mm postoperatively), although no statistical analysis was provided.
- Five patients had persistent symptoms in the ring and/or small fingers.

COMPLICATIONS

- There are few studies reporting the type and incidence of complications of ulnar tunnel release.
- Potential complications include the following:
  - Incomplete relief of symptoms (persistent numbness, weakness)
  - Iatrogenic injury to the ulnar nerve or artery branches, especially to the deep motor branch as it enters the pisohamate hiatus
  - Hematoma resulting from injury to vascular plexus around the ulnar nerve branches and failure to achieve hemostasis prior to wound closure
  - Wound infection
  - Wound dehiscence
- Meticulous hemostasis, careful dissection, and knowledge of the ulnar nerve and artery branching anatomy and its variations are helpful in avoiding complications.

REFERENCES

1. Dupont C, Cloutier GE, Prevost Y, Dion MA. Ulnar tunnel syndrome at the wrist. *J Bone Joint Surg Am.* 1965;47:757-761.
2. Maroukis BL, et al. Guyon canal: the evolution of clinical anatomy. *J Hand Surg [Am].* 2015;40(3):560-565.
3. Chen S, Tsai T. Ulnar tunnel syndrome. *J Hand Surg [Am].* 2014;39(3):571-579.
4. Murata K, Tamai M, Gupta A. Anatomic study of variations of hypothenar muscles and arborization patterns of the ulnar nerve in the hand. *J Hand Surg [Am].* 2004;29(3):500-509.
5. Shea JD, McClain EJ. Ulnar-nerve compression syndromes at and below the wrist. *J Bone Joint Surg Am.* 1969;51(6):1095-1103.
6. Gross MS, Gelberman RH. The anatomy of the distal ulnar tunnel. *Clin Orthop Relat Res.* 1985;(196):238-247.
7. Murata K, Shih J, Tsai T. Cause of ulnar tunnel syndrome: a retrospective study of 31 subjects. *J Hand Surg [Am].* 2003;28(4):647-651.
8. Grundberg AB. Ulnar tunnel syndrome. *J Hand Surg Eur Vol.* 1984;9(1):72-74.
9. Seror P. Electrophysiological pattern of 53 cases of ulnar nerve lesion at the wrist. *Clin Neurophysiol.* 2013;43:95-103.
10. Earp BE, Floyd WE, Louis D, et al. Ulnar nerve entrapment at the wrist. *J Am Acad Orthop Surg.* 2014;22(11):699-706.
11. Kowalska B, Sudoł-Szopińska I. Ultrasound assessment on selected peripheral nerve pathologies. Part I: Entrapment neuropathies of the upper limb—excluding carpal tunnel syndrome. *J Ultrason.* 2012;12(50):307-318.
12. Higgins JP, McClinton MA. Vascular insufficiency of the upper extremity. *J Hand Surg [Am].* 2010;35(9):1545-1553.
13. Yuen JC, Wright E, Johnson LA, Culp WC. Hypothenar hammer syndrome: an update with algorithms for diagnosis and treatment. *Ann Plast Surg.* 2011;67(4):429-438.

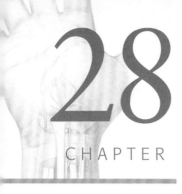

Cubital Tunnel Syndrome

Mary Claire Manske and Jason H. Ko

DEFINITION

- Cubital tunnel syndrome is symptomatic ulnar nerve dysfunction resulting from a combination of compression, traction, friction, and nerve instability at or near the elbow.
- The cubital tunnel is a fibro-osseous canal through which the ulnar nerve passes at the level of the medial elbow and is thought to be the most common site of nerve pathology.

ANATOMY

- The ulnar nerve is composed of fibers from the C8 and T1 nerve roots, although additional contributions from the C5, C6, C7, or T2 roots are common.
  - It arises from the medial cord of the brachial plexus and enters the arm by passing deep to the pectoralis major muscle, medial to the brachial artery.
- At 8 to 10 cm proximal to the medial epicondyle, the nerve pierces the medial intermuscular septum from anterior to posterior and descends through the arm along the posterior aspect of the medial intermuscular septum.
  - At this location, there is often a thick fascial band (the internal brachial ligament) spanning from the medial intermuscular septum to the medial head of the triceps, commonly referred to as the arcade of Struthers (**FIG 1**).
- The ulnar nerve travels posterior to the elbow via the cubital tunnel to enter the anterior forearm. The cubital tunnel is a fibro-osseous space bordered by the medial epicondyle anteriorly, the olecranon posteriorly, the oblique and posterior bands of the ulnar collateral ligament medially (the "floor"

of the tunnel), and Osborne (or arcuate) ligament laterally (the "roof" of the tunnel). Within the cubital tunnel, the ulnar nerve commonly provides articular branches to the elbow and motor branches to the flexor carpi ulnaris (FCU) (between 1 and 4 branches, arising from 4 cm proximal to the elbow to 10 cm distal to the medial epicondyle). The ulnar nerve provides motor branches to the ulnar two flexor digitorum profundi, which arise approximately 3 cm distal to the medial epicondyle.
- After passing though the cubital tunnel, the ulnar nerve travels deep to the fibrous aponeurosis of the FCU to pass between the two heads of the FCU and into the forearm along the undersurface of the FCU into the distal forearm.

PATHOGENESIS

- Four pathogenic mechanisms have been implicated in cubital tunnel syndrome: compression, traction, friction, and instability.
  - Compression: The ulnar nerve may be compressed anywhere along its course, but the most common clinical sites of compression are the arcade of Struthers, the median intermuscular septum, medial epicondyle, anconeus epitrochlearis (if present), the cubital tunnel, and the deep flexor-pronator aponeurosis
    - The cubital tunnel is round and spacious with elbow extension but narrows and becomes elliptical with the elbow flexed, decreasing the volume of the tunnel by 55%.[1,2]
    - Decreased cubital tunnel volume results in a four- to fivefold increase in extra- and intraneural pressure of the ulnar nerve.[3]
    - Both blood flow and axonal transport are impaired with external nerve compression; as pressure increases, the nerve tissue thickens and nerve conduction is impaired.[1,4–6]
    - Less common sources of ulnar nerve compression include soft tissue masses (eg, ganglia, tumors), hypertrophic synovium, cubitus valgus, and osteophytes.
  - Traction[7]: The course of the ulnar nerve around the medial epicondyle places tension on the ulnar nerve where it crosses the elbow and enters the forearm.
    - The ulnar nerve elongates by 4 to 8 mm when the elbow is flexed. This stretch is further increased with the shoulder abducted and the wrist extended.
    - Stretch of the ulnar nerve results in both reduced blood flow and impaired conduction.
  - Friction: Although the nerve naturally experiences some traction and excursion with elbow motion, repetitive elbow motion or subluxation of the nerve can cause traction neuritis, inflammation, and endoneurial edema, decreasing the nerve's ability to glide smoothly.[1]

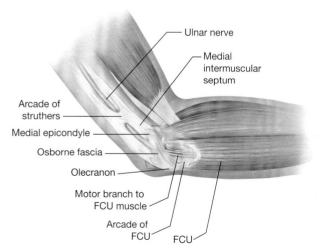

FIG 1 • Anatomy of the cubital tunnel.

Labels: Ulnar nerve; Medial intermuscular septum; Arcade of struthers; Medial epicondyle; Osborne fascia; Olecranon; Motor branch to FCU muscle; Arcade of FCU; FCU

- Instability: Subluxation of the ulnar nerve out of the cubital tunnel or over the medial epicondyle may result in elbow pain, a snapping sensation, numbness, or intrinsic motor weakness.

PATIENT HISTORY AND PHYSICAL FINDINGS

- Sensory
  - Numbness and paresthesia in the ring and small finger
  - Dorsoulnar hand numbness helps differentiate cubital tunnel syndrome/proximal ulnar nerve compression from ulnar tunnel syndrome at the wrist.
  - Presence of numbness or paresthesia in the medial forearm distinguishes C8 radiculopathy from cubital tunnel syndrome.
  - Depending on severity and chronicity, numbness may be intermittent or constant.
- Motor
  - Hand clumsiness, loss of dexterity
  - Weakness of pinch and grip
  - Inability to adduct or abduct the fingers
  - Intrinsic muscle atrophy, clawing of the ulnar two digits, with severe ulnar nerve compression
  - Pain in the medial elbow or forearm
- Physical exam
  - Inspection: Intrinsic muscle atrophy/wasting or clawing; compare to contralateral upper extremity
  - Palpation: Medial elbow tenderness; subluxation or perching of ulnar nerve over medial epicondyle with elbow flexion and extension
  - Sensory exam: Decreased sensation to light touch in small and ulnar ring finger; decreased sensation over dorsoulnar hand. Semmes-Weinstein monofilament or 2-point discrimination test
  - Motor exam: Intrinsic motor weakness indicates compromise of ulnar motor nerve fibers. Assess by testing index finger abduction (first dorsal interosseous muscle) or performing the cross-finger test (asking the patient to cross the middle finger over the index finger to assess the first volar and second dorsal interossei).
  - Additional motor tests:
    - Froment sign: Positive test when patient is unable to use adductor pollicis for lateral pinch. Instead, patients compensate with the flexor pollicis longus, which is innervated by the median nerve, to flex the thumb interphalangeal joint. Positive test indicates dysfunction of ulnar nerve motor fibers, although it does not localize the site of the lesion.
    - Jeanne test: Test is positive, indicating ulnar motor neuropathy, when the patient hyperextends the metacarpophalangeal joint to compensate for weak adductor pollicis during lateral pinch.
    - Wartenberg sign: Inability to adduct the small finger secondary to paralysis of the third palmar interosseous muscle. Positive test indicates an ulnar motor neuropathy.
  - Provocative tests:
    - Tinel sign at elbow: Percussion over ulnar nerve at medial epicondyle reproduces paresthesias in ring and small finger in patients with cubital tunnel syndrome.
    - Elbow flexion test: Elbow flexion, forearm supination, and wrist extension for 3 minutes elicit paresthesia in ulnar nerve distribution in patients with cubital tunnel syndrome.
    - Pressure provocation test: Manual pressure over ulnar nerve in cubital tunnel elicits ulnar nerve paresthesia.
    - Scratch collapse test[8]: Examiner scratches the skin over the compromised ulnar nerve while the patient performs sustained resisted shoulder external rotation with the arms adducted and the elbow flexed. A positive test is indicated by brief loss of ability to maintain resisted external resistance (ie, collapse).
  - Must rule out alternative sites of nerve compression:
    - Guyon canal (tenderness over hook or hamate or pisiform)
    - Cervical radiculopathy (neck pain, Spurling test, more proximal motor and sensory involvement)
    - Carpal tunnel syndrome (thenar atrophy or weakness; sensory disturbance in radial-sided digits; Tinel, Phalen, Durkan test positive over carpal tunnel)
    - Lower brachial plexus lesion
    - Thoracic outlet syndrome (Roos test, Adson maneuver)

IMAGING

- Electrodiagnostic testing is useful to confirm a diagnosis of ulnar nerve dysfunction, localize the site of compression, and quantify the severity.
  - The following criteria are used to diagnose cubital tunnel syndrome electodiagnostically[9]:
    - Absolute conduction velocity less than 50 m/s
    - Decreased conduction velocity of greater than 10 m/s across the elbow
    - Decreased amplitude of at least 20%
    - Absent sensory response
    - Evidence of motor atrophy
- X-rays should be obtained selectively when there is clinical concern for an osseous abnormality causing ulnar nerve compression.
  - Elbow radiographs are useful in suspected cases of elbow osteoarthritis, rheumatoid arthritis, trauma, or cubitus valgus deformity
  - Chest radiographs may identify a cervical rib causing thoracic outlet syndrome or a Pancoast tumor (suspected in patients with ulnar nerve symptoms, shoulder pain, and history of smoking)
- On ultrasound, patients with cubital tunnel syndrome have an increased cross-sectional area of the ulnar nerve compared to patients without cubital tunnel syndrome.
  - Ulnar nerve cross-sectional area of 0.10 cm^2 or higher on ultrasound of the ulnar nerve within 4 cm of the medial epicondyle is 93% sensitive and 98% specific for cubital tunnel syndrome.[10]
- Morphologic and signal changes in the ulnar nerve have been observed on MRI in cubital tunnel syndrome.
  - MRI has been reported to be both sensitive and specific in diagnosing cubital tunnel syndrome but is not routinely used.[11,12]

DIFFERENTIAL DIAGNOSIS

- Cervical radiculopathy
- Ulnar tunnel syndrome
- Lower brachial plexopathy
- Motor neuron disease (eg, amyotrophic lateral sclerosis, Charcot-Marie-Tooth)

- Guillain-Barré syndrome
- Diabetic neuropathy

NONOPERATIVE MANAGEMENT

- Initial treatment of cubital tunnel syndrome in patients without constant numbness or motor atrophy is nonoperative.
- Nonoperative treatment consists of patient education, activity modification (discontinue triceps exercises, pad medial elbow when resting on a hard surface), postural modification (avoidance of prolonged elbow flexion or resting medial elbow on a hard surface), night splinting (to prevent the elbow from flexing beyond 40 to 50 degrees during sleep), and/or nerve gliding exercises.[13]
- The recommended duration of nonoperative treatment is 3 months in patients with mild or moderate symptoms and 6 weeks in patients with severe symptoms.
- A comprehensive course of nonoperative intervention has been shown to resolve symptoms in 42% of patients with mild cubital tunnel syndrome, 34% of patients with moderate symptoms, and 20% of patients with severe symptoms.[14]
- Steroid injection is not recommended, as this has not been shown to provide any benefit in the treatment of cubital tunnel syndrome and presents a risk of nerve injury.[15]

SURGICAL MANAGEMENT

Preoperative Planning

- Indications for operative intervention include failure of nonoperative intervention, muscle atrophy or weakness, loss of two-point sensibility in the ulnar nerve distribution, or severe electrodiagnostic changes involving the ulnar nerve in the proximity of the elbow.[16]
- Assess stability of ulnar nerve preoperatively, as this guides surgical intervention; patients with ulnar nerve instability are not candidates for in situ decompression.

Positioning

- Patients are positioned supine on a well-padded operating table or stretcher.
- The operative extremity is positioned on a hand table. The patient's shoulder should be placed as close to the hand table as possible.
- We recommend against the use of a nonsterile tourniquet, as this may encroach upon the surgical field when anterior transposition is required.

Approach

- A direct approach to the ulnar nerve on the medial side of the elbow is utilized.

TECHNIQUES

■ In Situ Cubital Tunnel Decompression

- After the operative limb is prepped and draped, a surgical marking pen is used to mark the medial epicondyle, olecranon, and medial intermuscular septum. If a tourniquet is used, a sterile tourniquet should be applied to the upper extremity as proximally as possible. An alternative to the tourniquet is to inject the planned incision subcutaneously with local anesthetic containing epinephrine.
- If a tourniquet is used, the extremity is exsanguinated with an elastic bandage and the tourniquet elevated to 250 mm Hg.
- A 3- to 5-cm incision along the course of the ulnar nerve midway between the medial epicondyle and olecranon is made with a scalpel just through the dermis (**TECH FIG 1A**).
- The subcutaneous tissues are dissected with tenotomy scissors in line with the skin incision down to the level of the deep brachial fascia proximally and the antebrachial fascia distally.
- Care must be taken to identify and protect branches of the medial antebrachial cutaneous (MABC) nerve, which lie within the subcutaneous fat just over the muscle fascia from 6 cm proximal to 6 cm distal to the medial epicondyle.[17]
- The ulnar nerve is identified proximally, deep to the deep brachial fascia and posterior to the medial intermuscular septum.
- The fascia overlying the ulnar nerve proximally is released, beginning 8 cm proximal to the medial epicondyle (**TECH FIG 1B**).
- The nerve is followed distally, releasing the overlying fascia bands to decompress the nerve. Specific structures released include the arcade of Struthers, deep brachial fascia, Osborne ligament, and deep flexor-pronator aponeurosis. Care is taken not to dissect around the ulnar nerve circumferentially.

- The deep flexor-pronator aponeurosis should be released for a minimum of 4 cm distal to where the ulnar nerve enters the forearm between the two heads to the flexor carpi ulnaris (FCU).
- With blunt digital dissection, a finger should be passed along the course of the ulnar nerve as it passes deep to the flexor-pronator mass to ensure that all constricting bands of the deep flexor-pronator aponeurosis have been released (**TECH FIG 1C**).
- Following decompression, the ulnar nerve is not displaced from its bed, nor is a neurolysis performed.
- The elbow is taken through its full arc of motion, and the stability of the ulnar nerve is assessed.
  - If the nerve subluxates or perches on the medial epicondyle, an anterior transposition should be performed.
  - In addition, evaluation for any residual points of ulnar nerve compression should be performed. In particular, the medial intermuscular septum should be examined to ensure the nerve does not kink on the septum with elbow range of motion; if it does, that section of the medial intermuscular septum should be excised, with care to cauterize or ligate the branches of the profunda brachii artery that cross the septum.
- If a tourniquet has been used, it is released and meticulous hemostasis obtained with bipolar electrocautery.
- The skin may be injected with local anesthetic if this was not performed previously.
- The dermis is closed with a 3-0 absorbable suture in a buried interrupted fashion. The skin is closed with an absorbable monofilament suture.
- A bulky soft dressing is applied and elbow range of motion is initiated within the first few days postoperatively. Patients are permitted to perform light activities of daily living (eg, dressing, self-care, feeding) but no heavy lifting or sports for 2 weeks.

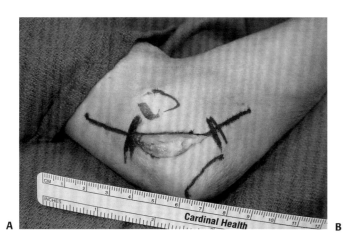

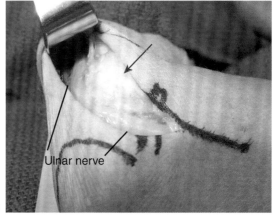

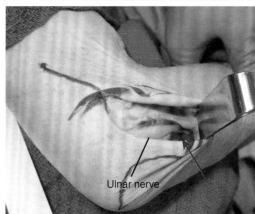

TECH FIG 1 • **A.** A 3- to 5-cm incision is made along the course of the ulnar nerve centered between the medial epicondyle and the olecranon. **B.** The fascia overlying the ulnar nerve proximally is released, beginning 8 cm proximal to the medial epicondyle (*red arrow*) and proceeding distally. **C.** The deep aponeurosis of the flexor-pronator mass is released over the ulnar nerve, as it dives between the two heads of the FCU (*red arrow*). (Proximal is to the left and distal to the right in all parts.)

■ Transposition of the Ulnar Nerve

- Typically, in situ decompression of the ulnar nerve is the first-line treatment for cubital tunnel syndrome.
- However, if there is subluxation of the ulnar nerve, subcutaneous or submuscular transposition of the ulnar nerve may be indicated at the time of decompression.
- For the treatment of recurrent cubital tunnel syndrome, subcutaneous or submuscular transposition of the ulnar nerve is the treatment of choice.
  - Submuscular transpositions are usually reserved for patients who have failed previous subcutaneous transposition.
- The operative extremity is prepped and draped in the usual sterile fashion.
- A sterile tourniquet may be applied to the operative extremity as proximally as possible. An alternative to the tourniquet is to inject the planned incision with local anesthetic containing epinephrine.
- A surgical marking pen is used to mark the anatomic landmarks: medial epicondyle, olecranon, and medial intermuscular septum.
- If a tourniquet is used, the limb is exsanguinated with an elastic bandage and the tourniquet is elevated to 250 mm Hg.
- A 10 cm incision is made over the course of the ulnar nerve centered between the medial epicondyle and olecranon. Proximal to the medial epicondyle, the incision is made along the palpable course of the medial

intermuscular septum. Distally, the incision follows the course of the ulnar nerve as it travels between the two heads of the FCU.
- An ulnar nerve decompression is performed as described above for in situ ulnar nerve decompression.
- A half-inch latex-free Penrose drain is placed around the nerve to allow it to be manipulated atraumatically. The ends of the Penrose drain are sutured together with 4-0 nylon suture.
  - We recommend against using a vessel loop around the nerve or placing a hemostat clamp on the Penrose drain, as both of these may cause unnecessary trauma to the nerve and increase the likelihood of a neurapraxic injury.
- Using tenotomy scissors, the ulnar nerve is circumferentially dissected to free it from surrounding tissues and the bed in which it rests.
- The longitudinally running superior ulnar collateral vessels that accompany the nerve should remain with the nerve as distally as possible, but it is necessary to ligate the vessels as they penetrate the FCU muscle belly.
- To avoid compression of the nerve by the medial intermuscular septum after it is transposed, the distal segment of the medial intermuscular septum should be excised from its insertion on the humerus. Branches of the profunda brachii artery cross the septum, and these need to be ligated or cauterized.

Submuscular Transposition of the Ulnar Nerve

- The subcutaneous tissues are elevated off the flexor-pronator fascia.
- A step-cut is made in the flexor-pronator fascia, such that the anterior musculofascial flap is distally based and the posterior fascial flap is proximally based on the medial epicondyle.
  - The flaps should be approximately 3 cm in length to avoid compression on the ulnar nerve when the flaps are coapted (**TECH FIG 2A**).
- The posterior fascial flap is carefully and sharply elevated from the underlying muscle with a scalpel or tenotomy scissors, with care not to disrupt the base of the fascial flap.
- The anterior musculofascial flap is elevated full-thickness, including the superficial head of pronator teres and the common flexor tendon, using monopolar cautery.
  - This allows the anterior musculofascial unit to slide distally, creating a trough for the ulnar nerve, once transposed.
- Within the muscle of the flexor-pronator mass, there are stout fascial septa that need to be excised to prevent them from compressing the ulnar nerve when it is transposed.
  - Care must be taken to identify FCU motor branches of the ulnar nerve that may cross these septa.
- Monopolar electrocautery is used to dissect through the flexor-pronator muscle in line with the elevated posterior flap to provide a deep muscular bed in which the ulnar nerve may rest.

- Using the Penrose drain, the nerve is gently transposed anteriorly and laid in the previously created muscle trough (**TECH FIG 2B**).
- If the nerve is tethered by motor branches to the FCU, these branches may be separated from the main nerve for up to 6 to 8 cm to allow greater excursion of the ulnar nerve as it is transposed.
- The entire course of the ulnar nerve is examined to ensure there are no points of nerve compression or crimping after it has been transposed.
  - In particular, ensure that all soft tissues proximally have been released, that the nerve is not kinked as it crosses the medial intermuscular septum, and that it is not bending over the superficial or deep flexor-pronator fascia distally.
- Stout, nonabsorbable braided suture is used to coapt the ends of the flaps that were raised from the flexor-pronator fascia, effectively lengthening the musculofascial unit.
  - Figure-of-eight or horizontal mattress suture can be used (**TECH FIG 2C**).
- The elbow is taken through a range of motion from full extension to full flexion.
  - The nerve is inspected to ensure it does not fall out of its bed in the muscle or subluxate posterior to the medial epicondyle.
  - Any dynamic points of compression are also identified and released as necessary.
- If a tourniquet is used, it is now deflated. Meticulous hemostasis is obtained with electrocautery.

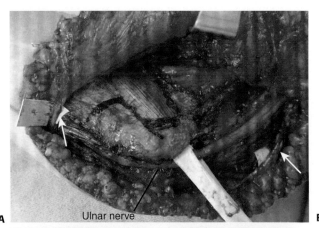

A · Ulnar nerve

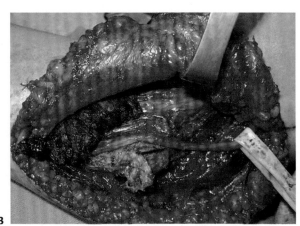

B

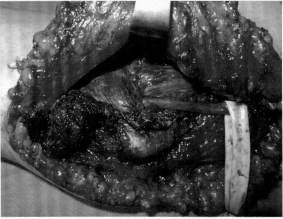

C

TECH FIG 2 • A. A step-cut is made in the flexor-pronator fascia to create an anterior distally based myofascial flap and a posterior proximally based fascial flap. *White arrows* indicate medial antebrachial cutaneous nerve. **B.** Full-thickness myofascial flaps are elevated to create a trough in the muscle bed into which the ulnar nerve is transposed. **C.** The ends of the fascial flaps are sutured together to prevent posterior subluxation of the ulnar nerve and effectively lengthening the musculofascial unit. (Distal is to the left and proximal to the right in all parts.)

- The wound is thoroughly irrigated with normal saline.
- The wound is closed with deep dermal buried interrupted sutures using an absorbable suture material. The skin is closed with a running subcuticular absorbable monofilament suture or a nonabsorbable monofilament in a simple or horizontal mattress fashion.
- A sterile soft dressing is applied to the wound, followed by either a soft compression dressing or a posterior slab long-arm plaster splint, which remains in place for 2 weeks.
  - It is important for the patient to be able to perform gentle active range of motion of the elbow in the immediate postoperative period.

Anterior Subcutaneous Transposition of the Ulnar Nerve

- The subcutaneous tissues are elevated off the flexor-pronator fascia.
- An anteriorly based flap of flexor-pronator fascia is sharply elevated from the medial epicondyle and underlying musculature with a scalpel blade or tenotomy scissors.
  - The fascial flap should be approximately 3 cm in length to avoid compression of the ulnar nerve (**TECH FIG 3A,B**).
- Using the Penrose drain, the nerve is gently transposed anteriorly and positioned superficial to the fascial flap (**TECH FIG 3C**).

- If the nerve is tethered by motor branches to the FCU, these branches may be separated from the main nerve for up to 6 to 8 cm to allow greater excursion of the ulnar nerve as it is transposed.
- The entire course of the ulnar nerve is examined to ensure there are no points of nerve compression or crimping after it has been transposed. In particular, ensure that all soft tissues surrounding the nerve proximally have been released, that the nerve is not kinked as it crosses the medial intermuscular septum, and that the nerve is not compressed by the flap in its transposed position.
- The fascial flap is approximated to the deep dermis on the underside of the anterior skin flap, and that point on the superficial surface of the skin can be marked with a marking pen (**TECH FIG 3D; VIDEO 1**).
- Stout, nonabsorbable braided suture is used to suture the free end of the fascial flap to the deep dermis on the underside of the anterior skin flap. Figure-of-eight or horizontal mattress suture may be used.
  - The flap is approximated quite anteriorly so that when the anterior skin flap is then brought down for closure, the fascial flap acts as a "hammock" for the ulnar nerve, keeping it anterior to the medial epicondyle (**TECH FIG 3E**).

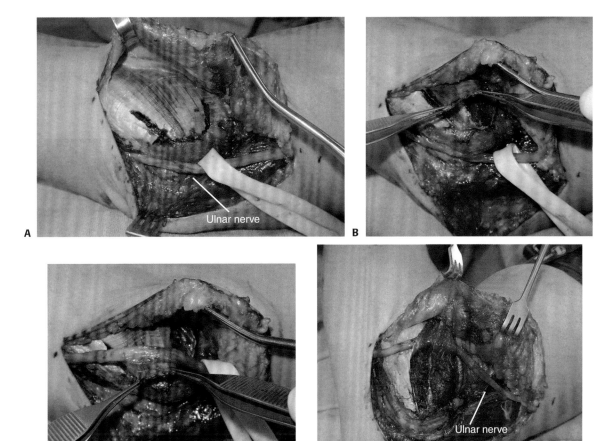

TECH FIG 3 • **A.** An anteriorly based flap of flexor-pronator fascia is designed to form a sling for the transposed ulnar nerve. **B.** The fascial flap then elevated from the medial epicondyle and underlying musculature. **C.** The ulnar nerve is transposed anteriorly over the fascial flap. **D.** The fascial flap is sutured to the dermis of the anterior skin flap to function as a "hammock" for the transposed ulnar nerve to prevent posterior subluxation.

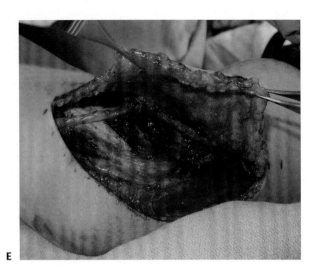

E

TECH FIG 3 (Continued) • **E.** The nerve is evaluated throughout the full range of motion of the elbow to ensure that the nerve does not kink, subluxate, or become compressed in its transposed position. (Distal is to the left and proximal to the right in all parts.)

- The elbow is taken through a range of motion from full extension to full flexion.
  - The nerve is inspected to ensure it does not fall out of its bed in the muscle or subluxate posterior to the medial epicondyle.
  - Any dynamic points of compression are also identified and released as necessary (Video 2).
- If a tourniquet is used, it is now deflated. Meticulous hemostasis is obtained with electrocautery.
- The operative field is thoroughly irrigated with normal saline.
- The incision is closed with deep dermal, buried, interrupted sutures using an absorbable suture material.

- The skin is closed with a running subcuticular absorbable monofilament suture or a nonabsorbable monofilament in a simple or horizontal mattress fashion.
  - If an absorbable subcuticular suture is used, Steri-Strips are applied to the incision.
- A sterile bulky soft dressing is applied to the incision, which remains in place for 2 days.
  - After postoperative day 2, it is important that the patient continue to use a compression dressing to minimize postoperative edema.
- Patients are instructed that they may gently move their elbow and use the extremity for activities of daily living.

PEARLS AND PITFALLS

Superficial dissection	▪ Care should be taken to preserve branches of the medial antebrachial cutaneous nerve to avoid causing a painful neuroma. These branches cross the medial arm from 6 cm proximal to 6 cm distal to the medial epicondyle.
Deep dissection	▪ A Penrose drain is loosely looped around the ulnar nerve to manipulate it atraumatically during dissection and transposition.
Hemostasis	▪ Meticulous hemostasis must be obtained to prevent a hematoma, which could compress the ulnar nerve or lead to wound dehiscence.
Iatrogenic compression	▪ Secondary points of compression may be introduced after ulnar nerve transposition if care is not taken to release them; in particular, the medial intermuscular septum, the deep septa of the flexor-pronator musculature (with submuscular transposition), and the fascial flaps holding the nerve transposed should be inspected to ensure no compression is present.
Nerve stability	▪ Inspect the position of the ulnar nerve throughout the full range of motion of the elbow to ensure the nerve does not rest on or subluxate posterior to the medial epicondyle.

POSTOPERATIVE CARE

- In situ decompression or subcutaneous ulnar nerve transposition
  - Patients are placed in a bulky soft dressing, which may be removed on postoperative day 2. They may begin showering at that point, but it is important to continue the use of a compression wrap to minimize postoperative edema.
  - Patients may move the operative extremity and perform activities of daily living postoperatively. Heavier activities (ie, more than "coffee cup" weight bearing) are prohibited. Patients may move the elbow and forearm as pain permits. Patients are encouraged to move their wrist, hand, and digits to prevent postoperative edema and stiffness.
- Submuscular transposition
  - The use of a bulky soft dressing vs a long-arm splint is at the discretion of the surgeon.
  - It is important for gentle range of motion of the elbow to begin immediately in the postoperative period to minimize scarring along the ulnar nerve.
  - If a long-arm splint is used, it remains in place for 2 week postoperatively. Patients are encouraged to move and use their digits while the splint is in place.
  - If a soft dressing is used, it should remain in place for 2 weeks.
- When the incision is well healed (usually around 2 weeks postoperatively), sutures may be removed if nonabsorbable suture were used. Patients whose incisions are closed with subcuticular absorbable sutures and Steri-Strips are instructed that the Steri-Strips will fall off on their own.
- All patients may allow the incision to get wet in the shower but are restricted from immersing the incision in baths and pools for another week.
- Patients may engage in unrestricted activities as tolerated at 2 weeks postoperatively as long as the incision is well healed.

OUTCOMES

- In situ decompression, subcutaneous transposition and submuscular transposition have all been shown to be effective in the treatment of cubital tunnel syndrome.
  - Most patients experience objective and subjective improvement in sensation, strength, and pain, although persistent subjective sensory abnormalities are common, regardless of surgical technique.
  - Patients express high satisfaction with the outcome of surgical intervention with all procedures.
  - Multiple meta-analyses have demonstrated no difference in outcome in terms of clinical outcomes or conduction velocities.

COMPLICATIONS

- New elbow pain
- Scar tenderness
- Medial elbow and forearm numbness
- Hematoma
- Infection
- Persistent or recurrent symptoms
- The rate of revision surgery following in situ decompression is reported between 3% and 19%.[18,19]

REFERENCES

1. Szabo RM, Kwak C. Natural history and conservative management of cubital tunnel syndrome. *Hand Clin.* 2007;23;311-318.
2. Apfelberg DB, Larson SJ. Dynamic anatomy of the ulnar nerve at the elbow. *Plast Reconstr Surg.* 1973;51(1);79-81.
3. Gelberman RH, Yamaguchi K, Hollstien SB, et al. Changes in interstitial pressure and cross-sectional area of the cubital tunnel and of the ulnar nerve with flexion of the elbow: an experimental study in human cadavers. *J Bone Joint Surg Am.* 1998;80(4):492-501.
4. Aziz W, Firrell JC, Ogden L, et al. Blood flow in a chronic entrapment neuropathy model in the rabbit sciatic nerve. *J Reconstr Microsurg.* 1999;15(1);47-53.
5. Dahlin LB, Rydevik B, McLean WG, et al. Changes in fast axonal transport during experimental nerve compression at low pressures. *Exp Neurol.* 1984;84(1);29-36.
6. Lundborg G, Dahlin LB. The pathophysiology of nerve compression. *Hand Clin.* 1992;8(2);215-227.
7. Wojewnik B, Bindra R. Cubital tunnel syndrome: review of current literature on causes, diagnosis and treatment. *J Hand Microsurg.* 2009;1(2);76-81.
8. Cheng CJ, Mackinnon-Patterson B, Beck JL, Mackinnon SE. Scratch collapse test for evaluation of carpal and cubital tunnel syndrome. *J Hand Surg [Am].* 2008;33(9);1518-1524.
9. American Association of Electrodiagnostic Medicine, American Academy of Neurology, American Academy of Physical Medicine and Rehabilitation. Practice parameter for electrodiagnostic studies in ulnar neuropathy at the elbow: summary statement. *Muscle Nerve.* 1999;22(3);408-411.
10. Wiesler ER, Chloros GD, Cartwright MS, et al. Ultrasound in the diagnosis of ulnar neuropathy at the cubital tunnel. *J Hand Surg [Am].* 2006;31(7):1088-1093.
11. Patel VV, Heidenreich FP Jr, Bindra RR, et al. Morphological changes in the ulnar nerve at the elbow with flexion and extension: a magnetic resonance imaging study with 3-dimensional reconstruction. *J Shoulder Elbow Surg.* 1998;7(4):368-374.
12. Britz GW, Haynor DR, Kuntz C, et al. Ulnar nerve entrapment at the elbow: correlation of magnetic resonance imaging, clinical, electrodiagnostic, and intraoperative findings. *Neurosurgery.* 1996;38(3);458-465.
13. Shah CM, Calfee RP, Gelberman RH, Goldfarb CA. Outcomes of rigid night splinting and activity modification in the treatment of cubital tunnel syndrome. *J Hand Surg [Am].* 2013;38(6);1125-1130.
14. Dellon AL, Hament W, Gittelshon A. Nonoperative management of cubital tunnel syndrome: an 8 year prospective study. *Neurology.* 1993;43(9);1673-1677.
15. Hong CZ, Long HA, Kanakamedala RV, et al. Splinting and local steroid injection for the treatment of ulnar neuropathy at the elbow: clinical and electrophysiological evaluation. *Arch Phys Med Rehabil.* 1996;77(6);573-577.
16. Boone S, Gelberman RH, Calfee RP. The management of cubital tunnel syndrome. *J Hand Surg [Am].* 2015;40(9);1897-1904.
17. Dellon AL, Mackinnon SE. Injury to the medial antebrachial cutaneous nerve during cubital tunnel surgery. *J Hand Surg Br.* 1985;10:33-36.
18. Krogue JD, Aleem AW, Osei DA, et al. Predictors of surgical revision after in situ decompression of the ulnar nerve. *J Shoulder Elbow Surg.* 2015;24;634-639.
19. Gaspar MP, Kane PM, Putthiwara D, et al. Predicting revision following in situ ulnar nerve decompression for patients with idiopathic cubital tunnel syndrome. *J Hand Surg [Am].* 2016;41(3);427-435.

SUGGESTED READINGS

Biggs M, Curtis JA. Randomized, prospective study comparing ulnar neurolysis in situ with submuscular transposition. *Neurosurgery.* 2006;58(2):296-304.
Watts AC, Bain GI. Patient-rated outcome of ulnar nerve decompression: a comparison of endoscopic and open in situ decompression. *J Hand Surg Am.* 2009;34A:1492-1498.

29
CHAPTER

Radial Tunnel Decompression

Joseph Pirolo and Jason H. Ko

DEFINITION

- Radial tunnel syndrome (RTS) is a pain syndrome caused by compression of the radial nerve and its branches in the proximal forearm.
- Generally characterized by lack of muscle weakness and electrodiagnostic findings

ANATOMY

- The radial tunnel is the space through which the radial nerve and its branches pass in the proximal forearm.
- The tunnel extends approximately 5 cm from the radiocapitellar joint to the proximal edge of the supinator muscle.[1-3]
- Tunnel boundaries[1-3]
  - Radial: brachioradialis (BR), extensor carpi radialis longus (ECRL), and extensor carpi radialis brevis (ECRB)
  - Ulnar: brachialis, biceps tendon
  - Floor: radiocapitellar joint capsule, supinator
- Radial nerve branches and sites of compression
  - The radial nerve branches proximal to the superior border of the supinator and forms the radial sensory nerve (RSN) and the posterior interosseous nerve (PIN).
  - The PIN has multiple potential entrapment sites[2,4-6]
    - Arcade of Frohse (proximal tendinous edge of supinator)
    - Proximal edge of ECRB
    - Radial recurrent vessels (leash of Henry)
    - Radiocapitellar joint capsule and osteophytes
    - Supinator distal edge

PATHOGENESIS

- Compression of the radial nerve, PIN, or SBRN by one or more anatomic structures at the radial tunnel, which can be secondary to aberrant anatomy, mass effect, trauma, arthrosis, or idiopathic
- Pathogenesis and pathophysiology of RTS is poorly understood and controversial owing to the fact that it is a compressive neuropathic pain syndrome with no reliably identifiable motor, radiologic, or electrodiagnostic findings.
- Although the PIN is a motor nerve, it does contain group IIA and IV fibers, which have been associated with temperature and nociception.[7] Given that these are not evaluated in standard electrodiagnostic testing, one possibility is that they may contribute to the pain syndrome even though nerve conduction velocities remain normal.
- Occupations that require heavy tool use in full elbow extension have been identified as a risk factor for development of RTS.[8,9]

PATIENT HISTORY AND PHYSICAL FINDINGS

- History
  - Patients complain of pain and fatigue in the proximal dorsal forearm.
  - Pain may radiate and can be aggravated by activities loading a rotated forearm or extended wrist.[1]
  - Muscle weakness is either absent or secondary to pain.[10]
  - Sensory disturbances are usually absent.
- Physical exam
  - The primary finding is localized tenderness over the radial nerve 5 cm distal to the lateral epicondyle.[11]
  - Provocative tests include pain with resisted forearm supination and/or resisted active extension of the middle finger.[10]
  - The "rule of nines" test has been proposed to help localize tenderness to the radial tunnel and help differentiate from other nearby sources of pain. In this test, the proximal volar forearm is divided into nine squares and tenderness with the lateral column marking out the radial tunnel.[12]
  - Examination must take into consideration several other possible sources of proximal forearm pain, especially lateral epicondylar tendinopathy, in which tenderness is located more proximally over the epicondyle.
- Electrodiagnostic studies
  - The results of standard nerve conduction velocity (NCV) and electromyography (EMG) studies are typically normal.
  - Although several modifications to standard NCV testing have been proposed, including testing latencies in different forearm positions and testing motor latencies to different motor groups, these have not been widely adopted in clinical practice.[13,14]
  - Electrodiagnostic studies may be useful to help rule out cervical radiculopathy or other concomitant entrapment neuropathy.

IMAGING

- Plain radiographs are typically nondiagnostic for RTS but can identify radiocapitellar arthrosis, which can lead to a distended, synovitic joint capsule and extrinsic compression at the radial tunnel.
- Magnetic resonance imaging (MRI) is not routinely helpful in the diagnosis of RTS. One study comparing MRI in 25 patients with RTS found that 52% had either edema or denervation atrophy of the supinator, whereas 28% had other aberrant anatomy such as nerve swelling, thickened ECRB, or prominent recurrent vessels.[15]

- The combination of the patient's history, physical exam, and MRI can also help to delineate radial tunnel from lateral epicondylar tendinopathy.

DIFFERENTIAL DIAGNOSIS

- Radial tunnel syndrome
- Lateral epicondylar tendinopathy
- PIN syndrome
- Cervical radiculopathy
- Biceps tendinitis or local muscle strain
- Osteoarthritis of the radiocapitellar joint
- Synovial impingement of the elbow
- Wartenberg syndrome

NONOPERATIVE MANAGEMENT

- Nonoperative treatment using anti-inflammatories, splinting, and activity modification should be exhausted prior to consideration of operative treatment and may lead to resolution of symptoms.[16]
- Although evidence for steroid injections is limited to a single small trial, it may be considered for patients with ongoing symptoms who are poor surgical candidates or those who do not want to consider surgery.[17]
  - When a local anesthetic is mixed with the steroid injection, this can serve as a diagnostic aid and is considered successful if both pain symptoms are temporarily alleviated and a motor block of the PIN is achieved.

SURGICAL MANAGEMENT

- Operative radial nerve decompression is indicated for those patients who have failed to improve after prolonged nonoperative treatment.
- Intravenous regional (Bier block) and axillary block regional are preferred methods of anesthesia.
- Three commonly described dorsal surgical approaches to release potential compression points along the radial tunnel have been described.
  - ECRB-extensor digitorum communis (EDC) interval
  - ECRL-BR interval
  - BR transmuscular splitting approach
- The authors prefer the ECRL-BR interval for the following reasons:
  - It avoids muscle splitting.
  - It allows for easy identification of the radial nerve, PIN, and the sensory branch of the radial nerve to ensure all are free from compression.
    - There is some evidence to support more reliably successful outcomes with decompression of the SBRN, which is best addressed through this interval.[18–20]
    - The most common complication of radial tunnel decompression is neuropraxia of the SBRN, which is best identified and protected in this interval.[20–23]
  - The interval is easily identifiable when marked out in the preoperative area by having the patient flex the elbow against resistance.

■ Radial Tunnel Decompression

Exposure

- In the preoperative area, ask the patient to flex the elbow against resistance to help mark out the interval between BR and ECRL.
  - This causes brachioradialis (BR) to become prominent while the extensor carpi radialis longus (ECRL) is relaxed, making the interval much easier to locate.
- A straight longitudinal or lazy-S incision is made through the skin and dermis (**TECH FIG 1A**).
- Care is taken to identify and protect the posterior cutaneous nerve of the forearm and any posterior branches of the lateral antebrachial cutaneous nerve.

- The fascia overlying BR and ECRL is incised and the interval is developed (**TECH FIG 1B**).
  - BR fascia is thinner, and thus, the BR muscle belly will appear as a brighter red color.
  - The dorsal ulnar edge of BR is also thinner, coming to a tapered edge and lying superficial to the more dorsal central aspect of the ECRL.
  - This interval should open easily and with mostly blunt dissection. If extensive sharp dissection is required, the surgeon has likely strayed out of the appropriate interval.

Release of Entrapment

- Coming down between BR and ECRL will bring the surgeon to a layer of fat containing the SBRN.

TECHNIQUES

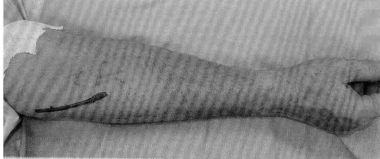
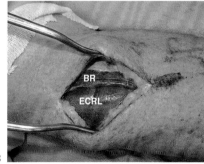

TECH FIG 1 • **A.** Proposed incision over the dorsal proximal forearm marked out at interval between brachioradialis and extensor carpi radialis longus. **B.** Superficial interval between brachioradialis (BR) and extensor carpi radialis longus (ECRL). Note the thinner edge of BR and the more rounded, dorsal central aspect of ECRL.

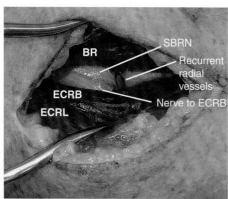

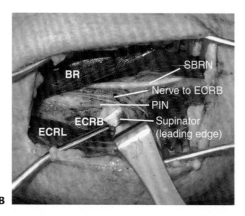

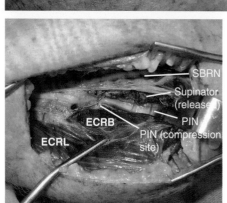

TECH FIG 2 • A. Intermediate interval between extensor carpi radialis longus (ECRL) and extensor carpi radialis brevis (ECRB) ulnarly and brachioradialis (BR) radially. The radial recurrent vessels (leash of Henry) course through and over the radial nerve branches (PIN, SBRN, nerve to ECRB). **B.** Deep interval after limited external neurolysis of radial nerve branches, ligation of crossing vessels, and release of proximal edge ECRB reveals the tight, tendinous leading edge of supinator (arcade of Frohse) directly compressing the PIN. **C.** Release of the supinator reveals a chronic compression deformity of the PIN. (For all parts, proximal is to the left, distal to the right, radial to the top, and ulnar to the bottom.)

- Follow the SBRN proximal, and you will encounter the radial recurrent vessels (leash of Henry) (**TECH FIG 2A**).
  - They must be ligated with suture or clips.
- Dissecting more proximally within this interval, follow the SBRN and you will encounter the posterior interosseous nerve (PIN) and the nerve to extensor carpi radialis brevis (ECRB).
  - Meticulous care to dissect and control crossing vessels is essential.
  - Release any constricting fascial bands over the SBRN as this may increase the likelihood of success.[18–20]
- At this point, you will have identified the SBRN, nerve to ECRB, and the PIN (**TECH FIG 2B**).
  - From radial to ulnar, the orientation will be SBRN, nerve to ECRB, and PIN.
  - The PIN will be larger in caliber and coursing distal and ulnar.
  - The SBRN and nerve to ECRB will be parallel to one another.

- Follow the PIN distally and release the overlying ECRB fascia, which can be a point of compression.
- After ECRB fascia has been released, you will encounter the supinator fascia (arcade of Frohse), which must be released (**TECH FIG 2C**).
  - As ECRB has been implicated in lateral epicondylar tendinopathy, release of the ECRB tendon may be helpful for patients with concomitant "tennis elbow."
- Check proximally and distally to ensure no further entrapment points exist.
  - Proximally, fibrous bands over the radial head can sometimes be found.
- If used, the tourniquet is released to ensure adequate hemostasis.
- Close the skin using a dermal layer with 4-0 absorbable suture followed by a subcuticular layer using 4-0 absorbable suture.
- A long-arm, soft bulky dressing is applied using a thin layer of gauze, sterile cast padding, and a very lightly compressive wrap.

PEARLS AND PITFALLS

Preoperative marking	▪ Marking out the BR-ECRL interval in the preoperative holding area with the patient flexing the elbow against resistance can make surgical orientation much easier.
Hemostasis	▪ Meticulous care to control crossing vessels throughout the case is a part of the decompression, can save time when the tourniquet is let down, and will prevent postoperative hematoma formation.
Adequate exposure	▪ A minimal exposure can lead to inadequate visualization of all compression points and necessitate excessive retraction on the muscular interval, as well as the SBRN, leading to known complications.
Decompression of all radial nerve branches	▪ External neurolysis of the radial nerve, nerve to ECRB, PIN, and SBRN is important to maximize likelihood of success.

POSTOPERATIVE CARE

- Immediate active digital, wrist, and forearm motion is allowed, but with limited weight bearing until the 2-week clinic follow-up.
- The dressing is removed 2 days after surgery.
- The wound is checked and any external sutures are removed at 2 weeks.
- Strengthening allowed at 3 weeks and patients are expected to be back to normal work activities by weeks 4 to 6.

OUTCOMES

- No level 1 evidence exists to guide expected outcomes following radial tunnel release.
- Patients who have had "successful" outcomes following radial tunnel release varies widely in the literature from 32% to 97%[19,21,22] prompting controversy as to the effectiveness of the procedure.
- Known risk factors that lower expected success rates of radial tunnel decompression include
  - Concomitant lateral epicondylitis[22]
  - Multiple entrapment neuropathies[22]
  - Workers compensation/litigation[22]
- A recent study by Lee and colleagues found good results in 86% of patients with isolated RTS, whereas this number dropped to 57% in patients with multiple entrapment neuropathies and 40% in patients with associated lateral epicondylar tendinopathy.[22]
- A thorough examination of available literature makes it clear that appropriate patient selection based on clinical history, exam, and diagnostic workup is crucial to success in the treatment of RTS.

COMPLICATIONS

- Complication rates have been reported in a portion of available retrospective reviews and case series; however, the anticipated rate of these complications is difficult to determine.
- Some reported complications include
  - SBRN neurapraxia or hyperaesthesias[20-22]
  - Paresis of common digital extensors[21,23]
  - Postoperative hematoma[21]
  - Complex regional pain syndrome[20]
  - Infection[20]

REFERENCES

1. Dang AC, Rodner CM. Unusual compression neuropathies of the forearm, part I: radial nerve. *J Hand Surg Am.* 2009;34(10):1906-1914.
2. Eaton CJ, Lister GD. Radial nerve compression. *Hand Clin.* 1992;8(2):345-357.
3. Rosenbaum R. Disputed radial tunnel syndrome. *Muscle Nerve.* 1999;22(7):960-967.
4. Konjengbam M, Elangbam J. Radial nerve in the radial tunnel: anatomic sites of entrapment neuropathy. *Clin Anat.* 2004;17(1):21-25.
5. Portilla Molina AE, Bour C, Oberlin C, et al. The posterior interosseous nerve and the radial tunnel syndrome: an anatomical study. *Int Orthop.* 1998;22(2):102-106.
6. Riffaud L, Morandi X, Godey B et al. Anatomic bases for the compression and neurolysis of the deep branch of the radial nerve in the radial tunnel. *Surg Radiol Anat.* 1999;21(4):229-233.
7. Lin YT, Berger RA, Berger EJ et al. Nerve endings of the wrist joint: a preliminary report of the dorsal radiocarpal ligament. *J Orthop Res.* 2006;24(6):1225-1230.
8. Roquelaure Y, Raimbeau G, Saint-Cast Y, et al. [Occupational risk factors for radial tunnel syndrome in factory workers]. *Chir Main.* 2003;22(6):293-298.
9. van Rijn RM, Huisstede BM, Koes BW, et al. Associations between work-related factors and specific disorders at the elbow: a systematic literature review. *Rheumatology (Oxford).* 2009;48(5):528-536.
10. Lister GD, Belsole RB, Kleinert HE. The radial tunnel syndrome. *J Hand Surg [Am].* 1979;4(1):52-59.
11. Moradi A, Ebrahimzadeh MH, Jupiter JB. Radial tunnel syndrome, diagnostic and treatment dilemma. *Arch Bone Jt Surg.* 2015;3(3):156-162.
12. Loh YC, Lam WL, Stanley JK, et al. A new clinical test for radial tunnel syndrome—the rule-of-nine test: a cadaveric study. *J Orthop Surg (Hong Kong).* 2004;12(1):83-86.
13. Kupfer DM, Bronson J, Lee GW, et al. Differential latency testing: a more sensitive test for radial tunnel syndrome. *J Hand Surg [Am].* 1998;23(5):859-864.
14. Seror P. Posterior interosseous nerve conduction: a new method of evaluation. *Am J Phys Med Rehabil.* 1996;75(1):35-39.
15. Ferdinand BD, Rosenberg ZS, Schweitzer ME, et al. MR imaging features of radial tunnel syndrome: initial experience. *Radiology.* 2006;240(1):161-168.
16. Cleary CK. Management of radial tunnel syndrome: a therapist's clinical perspective. *J Hand Ther.* 2006;19(2):186-191.
17. Sarhadi NS, Korday SN, Bainbridge LC. Radial tunnel syndrome: diagnosis and management. *J Hand Surg Br.* 1998;23(5):617-619.
18. Bolster MA, Bakker XR. Radial tunnel syndrome: emphasis on the superficial branch of the radial nerve. *J Hand Surg Eur Vol.* 2009;34(3):343-347.
19. Jebson PJ, Engber WD. Radial tunnel syndrome: long-term results of surgical decompression. *J Hand Surg [Am].* 1997;22(5):889-896.
20. Lawrence T, Mobbs P, Fortems Y et al. Radial tunnel syndrome: a retrospective review of 30 decompressions of the radial nerve. *J Hand Surg Br.* 1995;20(4):454-459.
21. Atroshi I, Johnsson R, Ornstein E. Radial tunnel release: unpredictable outcome in 37 consecutive cases with a 1-5 year follow-up. *Acta Orthop Scand.* 1995;66(3):255-257.
22. Lee JT, Azari K, Jones NF. Long term results of radial tunnel release—the effect of co-existing tennis elbow, multiple compression syndromes and workers' compensation. *J Plast Reconstr Aesthet Surg.* 2008;61(9):1095-1099.
23. Simon Perez C, Garcia Medrano B, Rodriguez Mateos JI, et al. Radial tunnel syndrome: results of surgical decompression by a posterolateral approach. *Int Orthop.* 2014;38(10):2129-2135.

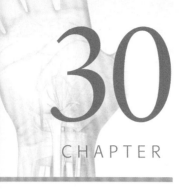

30 Primary Nerve Repair and Nerve Graft for Traumatic Nerve Injuries

CHAPTER

Sonya Paisley Agnew and Jason H. Ko

DEFINITION

- In the setting of acute nerve injuries, the surgeon should abide by the following principles when performing a nerve repair or reconstruction:
  - Debridement of the injured nerve ends to healthy fascicles
  - Correct alignment of fascicles when possible
  - Delicate handling of neural tissue
  - Tension-free repair or reconstruction
  - Prevention of fascicular outgrowth at the coaptation site
- The level of injury, zone of injury, primary nerve function (motor vs sensory), and functional significance of the injured nerve (eg, "critical" nerves such as the ulnar digital nerve to the thumb vs "noncritical" nerves such as the ulnar digital nerve to the long finger) will guide choice of treatment.
- Options for repair include primary repair with or without a conduit vs reconstruction with nerve grafts (autograft vs allograft).[1] Consideration should be given to techniques for bolstering the nerve coaptations (eg, fibrin glue, nerve wraps, nerve tubes).
- The most commonly used techniques for nerve coaptation are an "epineurial repair," which is suturing of the epineurium with no direct manipulation of the fascicles, and a "grouped fascicular repair," which requires reorienting the fascicles and directly placing sutures into the perineurium of the fascicles (**FIG 1**).
  - No studies have documented superiority of one coaptation technique over the other.

ANATOMY

- An understanding of fascicular anatomy of mixed major peripheral nerves can improve the outcomes of nerve repair by aligning proximal fascicles with their distal targets—matching proximal motor fascicles to distal motor fascicles and proximal sensory fascicles to distal sensory fascicles, whenever possible.
- This topographical orientation has been described for major mixed nerves, including the median and ulnar nerves, which can help with fascicular alignment when treating lacerations at various levels in the forearm and hand.[2]
- Anatomic fascicular orientations that have been well-established in the literature[1]:
  - Median nerve in the forearm (**FIG 2**)
    - The motor branches lie peripherally (in the radial and ulnar aspects of the median nerve), with sensory

fascicles located centrally. The recurrent motor fascicle is a separate, distinct fascicle 10 cm proximal to the radial styloid and located radially.
  - Median nerve at the wrist level (see **FIG 2**)
    - Recurrent motor fascicles are located within the volar and radial aspect of the nerve.
    - Digital sensory fascicles are located dorsally along both the radial and ulnar aspects of the nerve.
  - The ulnar nerve in the forearm (see **FIG 2**)

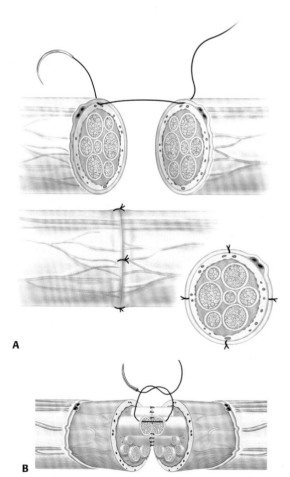

A

B

FIG 1 • Nerve coaptation techniques. **A.** Epineurial repair. **B.** Grouped fascicular repair.

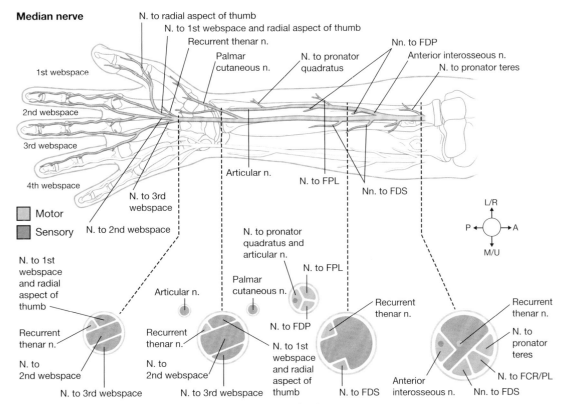

FIG 2 • Intraneural topography of the median nerves at various levels.

- Dorsal sensory branch of the ulnar nerve is located in an ulnar position within the nerve and separates from the main nerve 5 to 8 cm proximal to the radial styloid.
- The intrinsic motor fascicles lie dorsal to the digital sensory fascicles and are distinct 9 cm proximal to the ulnar styloid.
- In the proximal forearm, the motor fascicles (intrinsic and flexor carpi ulnaris [FCU]/flexor digitorum profundus [FDP]) are centrally located, and the sensory fascicles are superficial.
- At the wrist level, the ulnar nerve motor branch is dorsal and ulnar relative to the sensory fascicles—the motor fascicles can be seen as separate and distinct up to 9 cm proximal to the ulnar styloid.[3]
- Grouped fascicular repair should be used in larger mixed nerves, such as the median nerve at the humeral level.[3]
- Care should be taken to avoid bulky perineurial sutures that may become an obstacle to axonal regrowth.
- The less the ends of the nerve are manipulated intraoperatively, the less scarring there will be at the coaptation site.
- Microsutures should be used to repair the epineurium for all nerve repairs. The coaptation sites can be augmented with fibrin glue at the discretion of the surgeon.
- Tension should be avoided at all cost when performing a nerve coaptation. In the authors' opinion, rather than repairing a nerve under tension, the surgeon should reconstruct the nerve with an interpositional nerve graft (autograft or allograft) to achieve a tension-free construct.

PATIENT HISTORY AND PHYSICAL FINDINGS

- Physical exam:
  - A thorough motor examination and evaluation of sensation by two-point discrimination or Semmes-Weinstein monofilament testing will help to localize the nerve injury and adequately counsel the patient regarding postoperative expectations.
  - The location of a Tinel sign will help to pinpoint the site of nerve injury in the acute setting, and an advancing Tinel sign can be used to measure nerve regeneration over time.
  - In the acute setting, the sensory examination may be unreliable due to pain or neurapraxia.
- History: When obtaining the patient's history, certain factors are important for preoperative planning and counseling, including the following:
  - Patient age: Nerve regeneration occurs more rapidly in younger patients. The potential for nerve recovery decreases with age and should be addressed preoperatively with the patient. Older individuals are more likely to have delayed and/or incomplete recovery.
  - Chronicity of injury: In a delayed nerve repair, the surgeon should be prepared for retraction of the proximal nerve stump, in addition to neuroma formation, which may necessitate the use of nerve grafts.

IMAGING

- Ultrasound may be helpful in determining the presence of neuroma-in-continuity or complete laceration of the nerve. It offers the advantage of allowing static and dynamic assessments of the nerve and associated structures.

- MR neurography can also be used to evaluate larger nerves, but it is less effective at visualizing smaller nerves in the palm and fingers.
- Other imaging modalities are not commonly used for traumatic nerve injuries. Operative exploration is the primary method of diagnosis and treatment.

SURGICAL MANAGEMENT

Preoperative Planning

- The patients should be monitored closely to determine the extent of peripheral nerve injury.
  - A penetrating injury with acute nerve deficit warrants operative exploration.
  - A blunt or closed injury with acute nerve deficit may justify a period of monitoring to rule out neurapraxic injury.
- Sharp injury: If addressed acutely, primary nerve repair is possible. Nerve wraps or conduits can be used as adjuncts, if there is minimal tension at the repair site. If primary repair is under tension, then interpositional nerve graft should be used for reconstruction instead.
- Crush injury: The surgeon should be prepared for a broad zone of injury with extensive injury to the nerve. Nerve grafting will most likely be necessary, and the surgeon should consider delayed repair so that the zone of injury in the nerve can be better assessed as the soft tissue heals.
- Poor soft tissue cover: It is important for the surgeon to perform local or distant soft tissue flaps to achieve a stable, well-vascularized soft tissue envelope over the site of a nerve injury. Stable overlying soft tissue is a prerequisite for successful nerve repair or reconstruction.
- Timing: Neuromuscular function disappears 3 to 5 days after nerve transection,[4] whereas nerve action potentials remain for 7 to 9 days after injury.[5] After this time period, the use of intraoperative stimulation to aid in fascicular identification is not possible.

Positioning

- Supine positioning
- For distal nerve injuries in the upper extremity, a well-padded tourniquet is placed on the proximal arm.
  - The authors recommend tourniquet use to maintain a bloodless field, which will more easily identify peripheral nerves, especially in the setting of substantial scarring.
  - However, if intraoperative motor nerve stimulation will be performed, the tourniquet should be released within 30 to 40 minutes to avoid tourniquet neurapraxia.
- The hand table should have a stable base to limit motion during microsurgery.
- If sural nerve grafts are indicated, one or both legs are circumferentially prepared, and a thigh tourniquet should be used. It may be beneficial to harvest the sural nerve from the contralateral leg, which allows a bump to be placed under the contralateral hip.

Approach

- Bruner incisions to cross wrist and digital creases are employed to avoid straight-line incisions across joints.
- For sural nerve harvest, stair-step incisions may be used to decrease the overall length of the harvest site (**FIG 3**). However, longitudinal incisions directly over the entire length of sural nerve can be performed. Endoscopic sural nerve harvest techniques can also be employed.
- Nerve repair and reconstruction requires identification of injured nerve ends. Bruner or mid-lateral incisions should be used to expose the injured nerve(s) on the volar aspect of the palm or fingers. Bruner extensions should be used across all volar joint creases in the upper extremity. Dorsally, longitudinal incisions can be made over joint surfaces.
- Tenotomy scissors should be used to dissect the proximal and distal ends of the injured nerve(s) as atraumatically as possible. Overlying fascia or compression points should be released for better mobilization of the nerve ends.

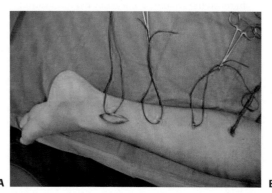
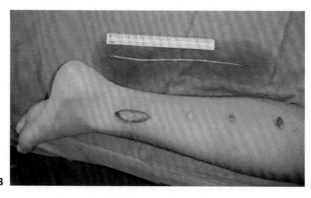
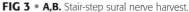

FIG 3 • **A,B.** Stair-step sural nerve harvest.

Primary Nerve Repair

- A direct repair is indicated in a sharp laceration when the nerve ends may be brought together with no tension.
  - Traumatized fascicles should be sharply debrided to healthy-appearing ends and oriented (in cases of larger nerves) appropriately.
  - If the nerve ends cannot be approximated without any tension, direct nerve repair should not be performed—nerve grafting should be used instead.
  - If nearby joints (eg, fingers, wrist, elbow) have to be flexed down to help minimize tension on the nerve repair, the primary nerve repair is too tight and should be abandoned.
- Lining up epineurial vessels proximally and distally can be used to help with orientation at the time of nerve repair. This will make pairing up the proximal and distal fascicles easier.

- Use of an operating microscope is recommended,[6] and 8-0 or 9-0 nonabsorbable monofilament suture should be used for epineurial repair to orient proximal fascicles to their distal targets (**TECH FIG 1A–F**)
- Fascicles that are "outpouching" should be tucked into the epineurial repair and trimmed back if necessary (**TECH FIG 1G,H**).
- A piece of surgical glove, Esmarch bandage, or silicone background can be used like a "burrito" to wrap around the repair into which fibrin glue is applied to bolster the repair. After the fibrin glue has set, the burrito wrap is removed.
- At this point, the surgeon should consider releasing any potential distal compression points (eg, the transverse carpal ligament distal to a median nerve repair in the distal forearm; Guyon canal release after an ulnar nerve repair at the wrist).

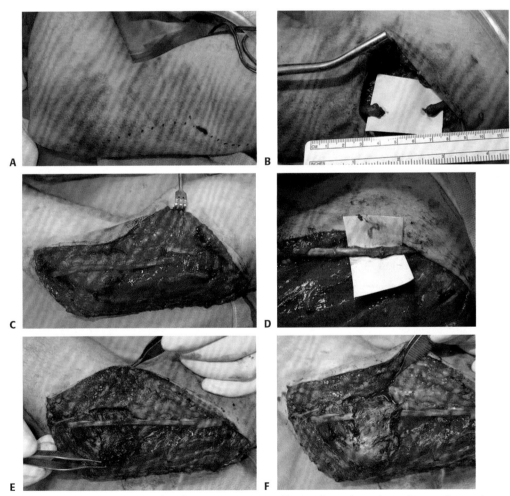

TECH FIG 1 • Ulnar nerve repair proximal to the elbow. Anterior transposition can be performed to reduce tension on the nerve coaptation. **A.** Gunshot wound with suspected ulnar nerve injury. Dotted marks outline possible incision location. **B.** Exploration reveals a complete ulnar nerve transection proximal to the elbow. **C.** Anterior transposition of the ulnar nerve has been performed by extending the skin incision distally and completely releasing the ulnar nerve from the cubital tunnel. **D.** Anterior transposition of the ulnar nerve allows for tension-free primary nerve coaptation. **E.** Fascial sling of the flexor-pronator wad elevated sharply anterior to the medial epicondyle. **F.** The fascial sling is sutured to the deep surface of the anterior skin flap.

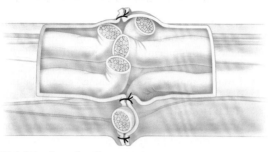
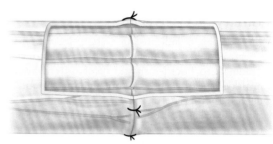

TECH FIG 1 (Continued) • **G.** Outpouching of the fascicles should be avoided to prevent aberrant axonal regeneration. **H.** The fascicles should be trimmed and aligned to maximize regeneration.

■ Repair in the Setting of a Small Nerve Gap in a Small Caliber Nerve

- When the ends of a nerve cannot be brought together without tension despite proximal and distal mobilization, use of a nerve graft is indicated.
- For digital nerve gaps, lateral antebrachial cutaneous (LABC) nerve, medial antebrachial cutaneous (MABC) nerve, and posterior interosseous nerve (PIN) are suitable

sizes for autograft (**TECH FIG 2**). These have the additional benefit of using a donor site in the same surgical area as the nerve reconstruction.
- Alternatively, processed nerve allograft (PNA) of varying lengths and diameters are available as an off-the-shelf option with no donor site concerns (**TECH FIG 3**).
- The proximal and distal ends of both repair sites can be bolstered with absorbable polyglycolic nerve tubes, fibrin glue, or xenogenic wraps (**TECH FIG 4**).

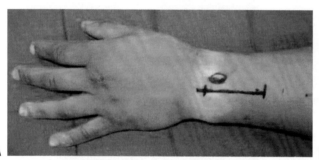
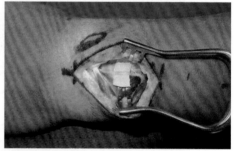

TECH FIG 2 • Posterior interosseous nerve harvest in the dorsal wrist. **A.** Incision site. **B.** Isolation of nerve.

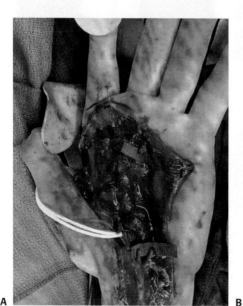
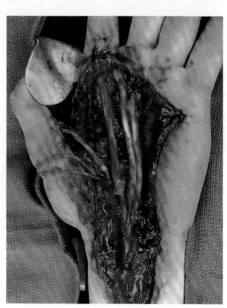

TECH FIG 3 • **A.** A 5-cm nerve gap in the median nerve at the level of the carpal tunnel. **B.** Repair with processed nerve allograft.

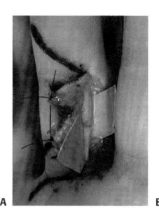
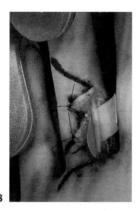

TECH FIG 4 • Direct digital nerve repair **(A)** and after wrapping with xenogenic nerve wrap **(B)**.

A   B

■ Repair of Larger Nerve Gaps or Larger Caliber Nerves

- When a large gap in a nerve exists, either cable grafts or processed nerve allografts are indicated.

Sural Nerve Harvest Technique

- The sural nerve can be harvested in the supine position with a well-padded sterile tourniquet on thigh and the knee flexed.
  - A sterile sandbag and/or an assistant can keep the knee flexed and hip internally rotated.
- If a single sural nerve is to be used, harvesting the contralateral sural nerve will allow a bump or pillows to be placed under the contralateral hip to help gain better access to the posterolateral aspect of the leg, especially more proximally where the sural nerve is deeper.
- If bilateral sural nerves must be harvested, the surgeon should consider performing the sural nerve harvest in the prone position, which would most likely require an intraoperative position change to access the upper extremity.
- Surface landmarks for sural nerve harvest—the lateral malleolus and anterior edge of the Achilles tendon—are marked.
- **FIG 3** depicts the step-cut technique for sural nerve harvesting.
  - The sural nerve is easily located 2 cm superior and posterior to the lateral malleolus. Distal to the malleolus, the nerve begins to branch and becomes significantly smaller.
  - The lesser saphenous vein is intimately associated with the nerve and can be protected or ligated.
  - Gentle traction is placed on the nerve to determine the more proximal incisions.
  - The intervening skin bridges should be short enough that undue traction is not necessary to free the nerve from the surrounding soft tissue.
- The dissection proceeds proximally to the junction of the medial and lateral sural nerves in the mid-leg, where the medial branch pierces the gastrocnemius fascia, and the lateral sural nerve continues superficially.
  - The dissection can continue easily toward the origin of the lateral sural nerve from the common peroneal

nerve or the medial sural nerve in between the two heads of the gastrocnemius muscle.[7]
- Approximately 30 cm of sural nerve can be harvested from one leg.
- A suture or surgical marking pen can be used to signify the proximal end so that the graft is reversed when brought to the recipient site.
  - Graft reversal prevents theoretical loss of axonal regeneration down small side branches and into surrounding soft tissues.

Graft Preparation

- For large defects, multiple sural cables should be prepared, and the number used depends on the number of large groups of fascicles within the injured nerve, in addition to the total length of sural nerve harvested.
- The nearby joints (fingers, wrist, elbow) should be maximally extended when measuring the nerve graft and length of nerve graft needed.
  - This will allow the nerve graft to be placed under no tension, even with early postoperative motion.
- After the length of the nerve defect is measured, the number of cables required is determined by the number of larger groups of fascicles visible that can be matched to accept individual grafts.
- The cables are brought together on a separate operating room table and rolled into a "burrito" as referenced earlier, followed by augmentation with fibrin glue.
  - This technique has been referred to as the "super nerve" technique (**TECH FIG 5A,B**).
- The ends are sharply transected, exposing the grouped fascicles, and one end is coapted to the proximal recipient nerve defect with 8-0 or 9-0 nonabsorbable monofilament suture with the aid of an operating microscope.
- Identical preparation is done for the distal end of the cable graft, and the graft is inset in a similar fashion to the distal recipient nerve (**TECH FIG 5C,D**).
- The central portion of the cable graft is gently draped into the soft tissues with space between the cables to allow for revascularization.
- The upper extremity is taken through a full range of motion to verify that the nerve reconstruction is under no tension.

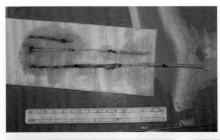
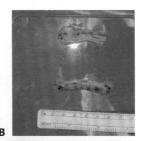
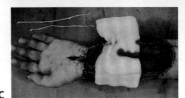
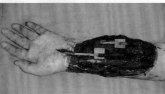

TECH FIG 5 • A,B. Preparation of multiple sural nerve cable grafts on the back table prior to reconstruction—the "super nerve" technique. **C,D.** Ulnar and median nerves grafted with sural nerve cable grafts.

PEARLS AND PITFALLS

Nerve gap	▪ Avoid tension and have low threshold to perform nerve grafting.
Fascicular orientation	▪ When possible, align fascicles at the time of repair.
Positioning	▪ Repair and grafts should be tensioned to allow for "safe" positioning of the fingers/wrist/digits. Flexed postures to accommodate primary repair should be avoided at all costs. When in doubt, use a graft.

POSTOPERATIVE CARE

- For direct nerve repairs, splinting in a position that keeps the nerve repair under no tension should be considered for 2 weeks.
- For nerve reconstructions under no tension, splinting for 2 weeks is optional. A soft dressing is recommended when there is no tension.
- If immobilization is used, range of motion (ROM) begins at 2 weeks.
- Nerve regeneration begins after a period of 30 days and from this point on continues at a rate of 1 mm/d, 1 in./mo, and 1 ft./y.
  - The surgeon should follow the patient for signs of distally migrating sensory recovery and strength testing for motor reinnervation.
- Based on the distance from repair site to distal nerve endings, the surgeon can calculate at what point the patient should begin to experience noticeable recovery, and follow the Tinel sign along the path of the nerve.
  - If the Tinel sign ceases to cross the repair site, consideration should be given to repeat exploration, neurolysis, possible neuroma excision, and grafting.

OUTCOMES

- Positive predictors of sensory recovery include age and time since repair, and data show trends consistent with better outcomes for sharp injuries.

- There is no association between delay in repair and outcome for sensory injuries.[8]
  - For mixed nerve injuries, time to repair is critical as the motor endplates will cease to function after 18 to 24 months, and worse outcomes are seen after a delay in repair of more than 6 to 12 months.[9]
- Similarly, the distance from the injury to the target muscle is an important determinant of outcome.
  - The surgeon may calculate the distance from the injury from the target muscle and determine the time it will take for reinnervation to commence.
  - A commonly reported "satisfactory" result is seen as recovery of M4 (active movement against resistance) or M5 (full power) for motor, and sensation S3+ (static two-point discrimination of 7–11 mm).[10]
- When grafting is required, the results of allograft and autograft nerve appear at this time to be equivalent.

COMPLICATIONS

- Complications of nerve repair are primarily inadequate recovery of sensation or motor function and neuroma formation.
- For inadequate sensory recovery, exploration with neurolysis and possible neuroma excision and grafting may be indicated, although there is no urgency to perform this.
- For suboptimal recovery of motor function, either nerve or tendon transfers may be indicated depending on the nerve injured and the time since injury.

REFERENCES

1. Slutsky DJ. A practical approach to nerve grafting in the upper extremity. *Atlas Hand Clin.* 2005;10:73-92.

2. Planitzer U, Steinke H, Meixensberger J, et al. Median nerve fascicular anatomy as a basis for distal neural prostheses. *Ann Anat.* 2014;196(2-3):144-149.

3. Chow JA, Van Beek AL, Bilos ZJ, et al. Anatomical basis for repair of ulnar and median nerves in the distal part of the forearm by group fascicular suture and nerve-grafting. *J Bone Joint Surg Am.* 1986;68(2):273-280.

4. Landau WM. The duration of neuromuscular function after nerve section in man. *J Neurosurg.* 1953;10:64.

5. Chaudhry V, Cornblath DR. Wallerian degeneration in human nerves: serial electrophysiological studies. *Muscle Nerve.* 1992;15:687.

6. Stančić MF, Mićović V, Potočnjak M, et al. The value of an operating microscope in peripheral nerve repair: an experimental study using a rat model of tibial nerve grafting. *Int Orthop.* 1998;22(2):107-110.

7. Strauch B, Goldberg N, Herman CKJ. Sural nerve harvest: anatomy and technique. *J Reconstr Microsurg.* 2005;21(2):133-136.

8. Mermans JF, Franssen BB, Serroyen J, Van der Hulst RWJ. Digital nerve injuries: a review of predictors of sensory recovery after microsurgical digital nerve repair. *Hand.* 2012;7:233-241.

9. Kabak S, Halici M, Baktir A, et al. Results of treatment of the extensive volar wrist lacerations: 'the spaghetti wrist.' *Eur J Emerg Med.* 2002;9(1):71-76.

10. He B, Zhu Z, Zhu Q, et al. Factors predicting sensory and motor recovery after the repair of upper limb peripheral nerve injuries. *Neural Regen Res.* 2014;9(6):661-672.

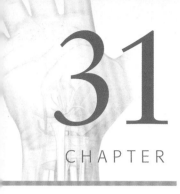

31

CHAPTER

Tendon Transfers for Median Nerve Injury

Rafael J. Diaz-Garcia and Kevin C. Chung

DEFINITION

- Median nerve palsy refers to the loss of motor control and sensation of the hand in the distribution of the median nerve.
- Low median nerve palsy refers to the loss of motor control and sensation of the hand in the distribution of the median nerve. Loss of sensation is the greatest deficit, because it encompasses 70% of the palmar surface. Loss of thenar function, particularly opposition, warrants reconstruction consideration.
- High median nerve palsy has significantly greater disability than does low median palsy due to the variable loss of function in the forearm, which can include pronation and flexion of the thumb, index, and long fingers.

ANATOMY

- The median nerve is a mixed nerve composed of fibers from the C5 through T1 roots, forming as a confluence of the lateral and medial cords of the brachial plexus.
- It travels with the brachial artery in the upper arm, between the biceps brachii and brachialis. It crosses anteriorly to the vessel as it reaches the antecubital fossa. It enters the forearm between the two heads of the pronator teres, innervating it.
- The median nerve travels between the flexor digitorum superficialis (FDS) and flexor digitorum profundus (FDP) in the forearm. It gives off a branch, the anterior interosseous nerve, to innervate the flexor pollicis longus, the radial ½ of FDP, and pronator quadratus.
- The median nerve proper innervates the flexor carpi radialis, FDS, and palmaris longus.
- The palmar cutaneous branch arises 5 cm proximal to the wrist joint, supplying the skin of the thenar eminence.
- The median nerve passes superficially in the carpal tunnel, before giving the recurrent motor branch from the central or radial portion of the nerve. It usually passes distal to the transverse carpal ligament. It passes through the transverse carpal ligament up to 7% of the time.[1] The motor branch goes to the opponens pollicis, abductor pollicis, and the superficial head of the flexor pollicis brevis.
- The sensory branches provide sensation to the radial 3½ digits of the hand.
- Martin-Gruber and Riche-Cannieu connections represent anomalous innervation patterns between the median and ulnar nerves, which may complicate the findings on exam.

PATHOGENESIS

- The pathogenesis of median nerve palsy is most frequently due to compression, attributed usually to long-standing carpal tunnel syndrome.

- Median nerve lacerations happen most commonly at the wrist due to the superficial position of the nerve.
- Lipofibrohamartoma of the median nerve can be seen in pediatric cases.[2]
- Systemic conditions such as Charcot-Marie-Tooth disease can also cause median neuropathy.[3]
- The pathogenesis of high median nerve palsy is most frequently caused by trauma, which can happen from injuries extending from the brachial plexus to the forearm.
- Compression can also cause high median nerve palsy, though it is much more frequently the cause of low median nerve palsy. Sites of proximal compression include the pronator teres, lacertus fibrosis, and supracondylar process.

NATURAL HISTORY

- Compressive causes can have insidious onset symptoms over the period of years or even decades.
- Traumatic cases have a clearer history because of the abrupt onset of sensory disturbance that is noticed by the patient.

PATIENT HISTORY AND PHYSICAL FINDINGS

- Acute injury
  - Patients present with a history of trauma and often a laceration, usually in the volar wrist.
  - Patients present with diminished sensation in the radial 3½ digits of the hand and a positive Tinel sign at the level of injury. There is greater functional loss with high median nerve palsy. There is a loss of opposition, flexion of the thumb through long fingers, and potentially pronation.
  - Palmar abduction may still be present from the intact abductor pollicis longus.
- Chronic compression
  - Patients present with pain, numbness, and paresthesias of the radial 3½ digits.
  - In carpal tunnel syndrome, symptoms may be exacerbated during sleep or activities that require wrist flexion, such as driving or keyboard use.
  - They often complain of "clumsiness" or difficulty with fine motor functions.
  - The most notable finding on physical exam in long-standing low median palsy is thenar atrophy.
  - In pronator syndrome, symptoms may be exacerbated with compression of the proximal forearm over the pronator teres.
- Inability to make an "OK" sign with the thumb and index finger reflects pathology involving the anterior interosseous nerve.
- Lack of pronation reflects pathology proximal to the elbow

IMAGING

- Initial workup for acute median nerve palsy may warrant x-rays to determine if there are any fractures or dislocations in the extremity associated with the acute trauma.
- Nerve conduction studies and electromyography may be helpful in the workup of compressive median neuropathy, helping to determine the level of the lesion.
- Motor and sensory latencies are often increased with chronic compression of the median nerve. Fibrillation potentials indicate denervation of the muscles tested and axonal loss.
- MRI of the brachial plexus may be warranted if there is concern for a lesion at this level.

DIFFERENTIAL DIAGNOSIS

- Carpal tunnel syndrome
- Isolated median nerve injury
- Anterior interosseous syndrome
- Pronator syndrome
- Cervical radiculopathy
- Leprosy
- Charcot-Marie-Tooth disease
- Brachial plexus lesion

NONOPERATIVE MANAGEMENT

- Nonoperative management is indicated in the setting of a brachial neuritis (Parsonage-Turner syndrome), presenting with anterior interosseous nerve dysfunction.
- Work modification may be warranted in a patient with compressive neuropathy secondary to over use in pronator syndrome.
- Thumb adduction contractures must be prevented or treated prior to tendon transfers, as maximum passive motion must be acquired before any tendon transfers.

SURGICAL MANAGEMENT

- There are three key functions that tendon transfers must address in the setting of high median nerve palsy:[9,10]
  - Thumb opposition
  - Flexion of the thumb
  - Flexion of the index and long fingers
- Occasionally, lack of pronation may require biceps rerouting. However, shoulder abduction can often compensate for this deficit enough to not be an issue.

- Unlike nerve transfers, tendon transfers do not have a firm time period in which they must be performed. Tendon transfers can be delayed while awaiting potential nerve recovery.
- The common principles of tendon transfers are as follows:
  - Joint contractures should be treated prior to any transfers.
  - Each muscle transfer should target one specific function.
  - Transferred tendons should glide through a smooth and scar-free surgical site.
- Thumb opposition cannot be reconstructed using FDS or palmaris longus in the setting of high median nerve palsy, as it would be in low median nerve palsy. Examination should be able to determine whether these muscles are functional.[8]
- In isolated low median nerve palsy, all reconstruction options are available. In general, using the extensor indicis proprius is our first choice given the negligible donor morbidity and excellent tendon excursion. The Camitz transfer (palmaris longus) is a good option for elderly patients with long-standing carpal tunnel syndrome. It is simple to execute at the time of carpal tunnel release but creates more palmar abduction than true opposition. The Huber transfer (abductor digiti minimi) is reserved for children and for combined high median and radial nerve palsies.

Preoperative Planning

- Tendon transfers should be delayed until after potential nerve recovery is completed.
- Clinical exam of the patient will allow the surgeon to decide what functions must be recreated and what donor muscles are available for each function.

Positioning

- The patient is placed in the supine position with a tourniquet on the upper arm.
- The OR lights are positioned with one projecting from proximally and one distally from the operative site.

Approach

- Like with all tendon transfers, one should plan for the tendons to glide through a smooth and scar-free wound bed and each transfer should be for one function. If there is scarred tissue along the path of the transfer, it must be replaced by soft supple tissue either through serial scar excision or a flap procedure.

■ Low Median Nerve Injury: Reconstruction of Thumb Opposition

Palmaris Longus to Abductor Pollicis Brevis (Camitz Transfer)

- Confirm the presence of a palmaris longus (PL) tendon and design a longitudinal incision, from the distal wrist crease to the proximal palmar crease, with a Bruner design over the wrist joint (**TECH FIG 1A**).
- Dissect the palmaris longus distally, taking a patch of palmar aponeurosis along with the tendon (**TECH FIG 1B**).
- Make an incision over the dorsoradial aspect of the thumb metacarpophalangeal (MCP) joint.
- Create a subcutaneous tunnel between the PL tendon and the MCP joint with blunt dissection.

- Pass the PL tendon to the thumb incision and suture it to the abductor pollicis brevis (APB) tendon (**TECH FIG 1C,D**) and extensor hood.

Flexor Digitorum Superficialis to Abductor Pollicis Brevis (Bunnell Transfer)

- A transverse incision is made over the ring finger A1 pulley (**TECH FIG 2A**).
- The A1 pulley is exposed and divided longitudinally, preserving the neurovascular bundles.
- The flexor digitorum superficialis (FDS) is divided proximally to the bifurcation with proximal longitudinal traction.
- A Bruner or longitudinal incision is made over the ulnar wrist, just radial to the flexor carpi ulnaris (FCU) tendon and near its insertion.

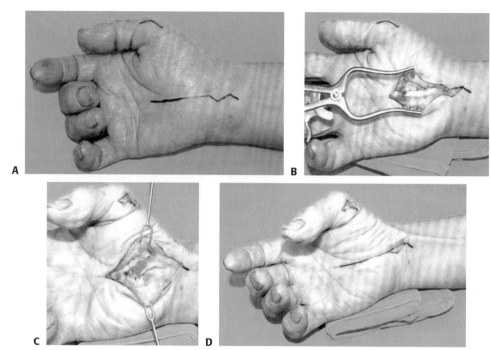

TECH FIG 1 • **A.** Design of incisions for PL transfer to AP. **B.** Exposure of PL at insertion into palmar fascia. **C.** PL tendon is sutured to APB, creating palmar abduction. **D.** PL tendon is sutured to APB, creating palmar abduction.

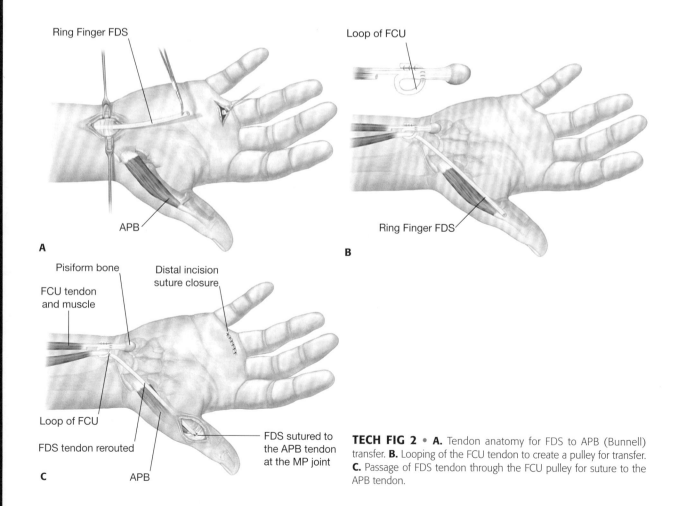

TECH FIG 2 • **A.** Tendon anatomy for FDS to APB (Bunnell) transfer. **B.** Looping of the FCU tendon to create a pulley for transfer. **C.** Passage of FDS tendon through the FCU pulley for suture to the APB tendon.

- The radial half of the FCU tendon is divided and separated from the ulnar half longitudinally.
- The distally based FCU tendon is sutured to itself at the insertion site, creating a pulley (**TECH FIG 2B**).
- A longitudinal incision is made along the radial aspect of the thumb MCP joint.
- A subcutaneous tunnel is created from the thumb incision to the wrist incision.
- The FDS is passed through this pulley and then through the tunnel to the thumb, where it is sutured to the APB tendon and extensor hood with braided suture (**TECH FIG 2C**).

Abductor Digiti Minimi to Abductor Pollicis Brevis (Huber Transfer)

- A Bruner or curvilinear incision is made from the ulnar aspect of the small finger to the radial border of the hypothenar eminence (**TECH FIG 3A**).

- The abductor digiti minimi (ADM) is dissected distally, protecting the ulnar neurovascular bundle to the small finger. It is freed from the underlying flexor digiti minimi, if present (**TECH FIG 3B**).
- The ADM is released from its insertion site on the small finger proximal phalanx with a portion of the lateral band to increase its length.
- From distal to proximal, mobilize the muscle toward and eventually off of the pisiform. Preserve the neurovascular bundle, which comes from the deep and radial surface of the muscle (**TECH FIG 3C**).
- Make an incision along the radial aspect of the thumb MCP joint and use blunt dissection to create a subcutaneous tunnel in the palm, superficial to the transverse carpal ligament.
- Pass the ADM through the tunnel to the thumb and suture it to the APB tendon and extensor hood with permanent braided suture (**TECH FIG 3D**).

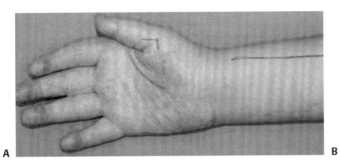
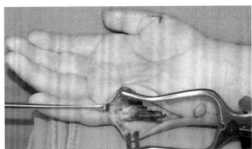
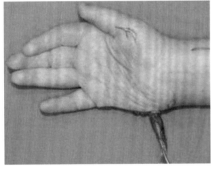
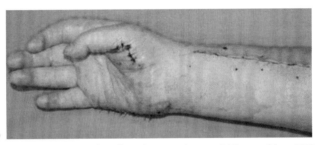

TECH FIG 3 • **A.** Design of incisions for ADM transfer to APB. **B.** Exposure of ADM along hypothenar eminence. **C.** Dissected free ADM muscle, all the way to pisiform. **D.** Final position after transfer, creating both palmar abduction and opposition.

■ High Median Nerve Injury

Reconstruction of Thumb Opposition: Extensor Indicis Proprius to Abductor Pollicis Brevis

- A small longitudinal incision is made along the dorsoulnar aspect of the index MCP joint (**TECH FIG 4A**).
- The extensor indicis proprius (EIP) tendon is identified as the ulnar tendon and released from the index finger extensor hood with a small slip of extensor mechanism. The rent is repaired with permanent suture.
- A longitudinal incision is made over the dorsoulnar wrist, just proximal to the ulnar styloid.

- Dissection is carried radially from this wrist incision to find the EIP tendon, just distal to the extensor retinaculum. The distal aspect of the fourth extensor compartment is divided to fully mobilize the tendon.
- A small incision is made along the radial pisiform and a longitudinal incision along the radial aspect of the thumb MCP (**TECH FIG 4B**).
- A subcutaneous tunnel is created from the dorsal wrist incision to the pisiform incision, attempting to stay deep to the ulnar sensory nerve branch. This tunnel is then dissected from the pisiform to the thumb incision.

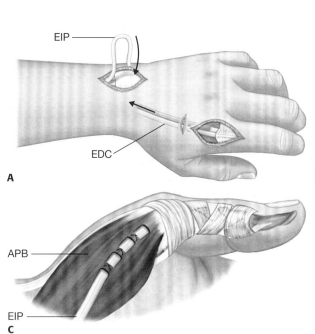

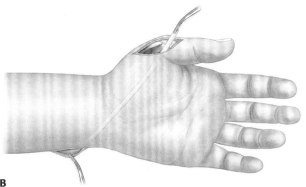

TECH FIG 4 • A. Release of EIP tendon for passage and radial dissection to locate and retrieve EIP tendon for transfer. **B.** Creation of a subcutaneous tunnel from the radial pisiform incision to the longitudinal thumb incision. **C.** EIP suture to APB tendon with braided permanent suture.

- The EIP tendon is passed from dorsal to volar, around the pisiform, and then to the thumb incision. It is sutured to the APB tendon and extensor hood with braided permanent suture (**TECH FIG 4C**).

Reconstruction of Index and Long Finger Flexion: Flexor Digitorum Profundus Side-to-Side Transfer

- A longitudinal incision is made over the distal third of the forearm.
- The flexor digitorum profundus (FDP) tendons are identified, deep to the median nerve (**TECH FIG 5A**).
- The FDP tendons are synchronized to recreate the digital cascade, and one sutures the index through small finger tendons with two rows of braided permanent sutures (**TECH FIG 5B**).

Reconstruction of Thumb Flexion: Brachioradialis to Flexor Pollicis Longus

- A longitudinal incision is made along the distal third of the forearm. The same incision for the FDP transfer can be used (**TECH FIG 6A**).
- The brachioradialis (BR) is released from the radial styloid insertion and mobilized proximally to maximize the excursion (**TECH FIG 6B**).
- The FPL tendon is located under the flexor carpi radialis, in the deep volar compartment.
- The BR is weaved into the flexor pollicis longus (FPL) with multiple passes, after optimizing tension (**TECH FIG 6C,D**). Wrist extension should result in maximal thumb IP joint flexion and lateral pinch.

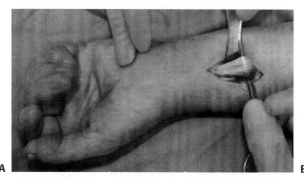

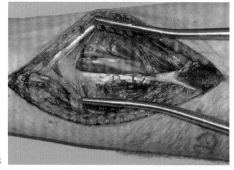

TECH FIG 5 • A. The FDP tendons are localized beneath the median nerve in the distal forearm. **B.** Tension is set between the radial two tendons (median innervated) and ulnar two tendons (ulnar innervated), recreating the digital cascade.

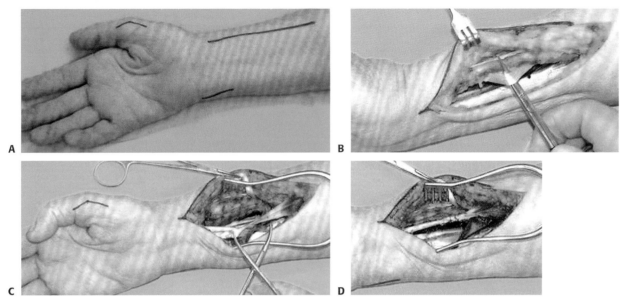

TECH FIG 6 • A. Design of incisions for high median nerve tendon transfers. **B.** Exposure of BR along insertion onto radial styloid. **C.** Tension is set between the BR and FPL. **D.** Final position of thumb after transfer, judging tenodesis with wrist flexion and extension.

PEARLS AND PITFALLS

Preoperative evaluation	▪ Critically assess donor muscle availability and strength.
	▪ Determine patient goals and potential for additional nerve recovery.
	▪ Release any areas of nerve compression for pain control, even if motor recovery is unlikely.
Thumb opposition	▪ Thumb should be in full opposition and IP joint flexed with wrist extension and should relax with wrist flexion.
	▪ Ensure that subcutaneous tunnel is of ample size to allow easy tendon gliding.
Finger flexion	▪ Improvement in finger flexion may not improve grip strength given no additional motor units.

POSTOPERATIVE CARE

▪ Patient is usually splinted with the thumb in full opposition and wrist in flexion immediately after surgery. The fingers are free to move to maintain motion.

▪ At the first postoperative visit, an orthoplast splint is fabricated to maintain thumb opposition and slight wrist flexion. At 3 weeks, gentle active range of motion is commenced several times a day. Passive range of motion is started at 6 weeks. Strengthening is started at 8 weeks.

▪ A knowledgeable hand therapist plays an important role in the surgical outcomes.

▪ Early active range of motion for opposition transfers has been advocated by some surgeons, with quicker recovery and no evidence of pullout of the transferred tendon.[4]

OUTCOMES

▪ Most median nerve palsy patients can perform normal activities of daily living with their hand after complete recovery from surgery. The tendon transfers combine proper direction of action, pulley location, and force for success.[5]

▪ Extensor indicis proprius (EIP) opponensplasty is generally efficacious, with 88% of patients with excellent results—ie, 75% function of the opposite, normal thumb.[6] It works best in the setting of supple hands.[7] EIP is not synergistic with thumb opposition, so retraining can be more difficult than FDS transfers.

COMPLICATIONS

▪ Suboptimal results may be a result of choosing a weak motor for transfer or incorrect vector of pull.

▪ Tendon adhesions can result from prolonged immobilization, particularly if using a pulley to reroute the force of the muscle.

▪ Tendon ruptures can be prevented with patient education and progressive therapy advancement.

REFERENCES

1. Rozin SH. The anatomy of the recurrent branch of the median nerve. *J Hand Surg Am.* 1998;23(5):852-858.
2. Biazzo A, Gonzalez Del Pino J. [Paralysis of the median nerve due to a lipofibrohamartoma in the carpal tunnel]. *Rev Esp Cir Ortop Traumatol.* 2013;57(4):286-295.

3. Michelinakis E, Vourexakis H. Tendon transfer for intrinsic-muscle paralysis of the thumb in Charcot-Marie Tooth neuropathy. *Hand*. 1981;13(3):276-278.

4. Rath S. Immediate active mobilization versus immobilization for opposition tendon transfer in the hand. *J Hand Surg Am*. 2006;31(5):754-759.

5. Cooney WP. Tendon transfer for median nerve palsy. *Hand Clin*. 1988;4(2):155-165.

6. Burkhalter W, Christensen RC, Brown P. Extensor indicis proprius opponensplasty. *J Bone Joint Surg Am*. 1973;55(4):725-732.

7. Anderson GA, Lee V, Sundararaj GD. Opponensplasty by extensor indicis and flexor digitorum superficialis tendon transfer. *J Hand Surg Br*. 1992;17(6):611-614.

8. Jacobs B, Thompson TC. Opposition of the thumb and its restoration. *J Bone Joint Surg Am*. 1960;42A:1015-1026.

9. Sammer D, Chung KC. Tendon transfers, part II: transfers for ulnar nerve palsy and median nerve palsy. *Plast Reconstr Surg*. 2009;124(3):212e-221e.

10. Ratner JA, Peljovich A, Kozin SH. Update on tendon transfers for peripheral nerve injuries. *J Hand Surg [Am]*. 2010;35:1371-1381.

Tendon Transfers for Ulnar Nerve Injury

Rafael J. Diaz-Garcia and Kevin C. Chung

DEFINITION

- Ulnar nerve palsy refers to the loss of motor control and sensation in the distribution of the ulnar nerve.
- Low ulnar nerve palsy refers to isolated loss of intrinsic hand function, whereas high ulnar nerve palsy refers to the additional loss of half the flexor digitorum profundus (FDP) and flexor carpi ulnaris (FCU).

ANATOMY

- The ulnar nerve is a mixed nerve composed of fibers from the C8 and T1 roots via the medial cord of the brachial plexus.
- It lies posteromedial to the brachial artery in the upper arm, prior to piercing the intramuscular septum 8 to 10 cm proximal to the medial epicondyle. It has no branches in the arm.
- It passes through the cubital tunnel into the forearm, running between FCU and FDP, innervating the former and 0.5 of the latter.
- Approximately 6 to 7 cm proximal to the ulnar styloid, the dorsal sensory branch leaves the main nerve to innervate the dorsoulnar hand and dorsal proximal phalanges of the small and ring fingers.
- The ulnar nerve continues into the hand through the Guyon canal at the wrist, splitting into a superficial sensory branch and a deep motor branch. The sensory branch supplies innervation to the small finger and ulnar half of the ring finger. The motor branch supplies the hypothenar muscles, ulnar lumbricals, interossei, adductor pollicis, and the deep head of flexor pollicis brevis.
- Martin-Gruber and Riche-Cannieu connections represent anomalous innervation patterns between the median and ulnar nerves, which may complicate the findings on exam.

PATHOGENESIS

- The pathogenesis of ulnar nerve palsy is most frequently secondary to trauma. Injury may come in the form of a laceration along its course, an axonotmetic injury, or an avulsion of the roots. Proximal injuries that involve the medial cord may also have sensory disturbances in the arm or forearm due to involvement of the medial brachial and antebrachial cutaneous branches.
- Systemic conditions such as Charcot-Marie-Tooth disease, leprosy, and syringomyelia can cause ulnar neuropathy as well.[1] Systemic conditions are unlikely to present with isolated ulnar nerve symptoms.

NATURAL HISTORY

- With prolonged ulnar nerve palsy, secondary deformities of the hand will develop with attenuation of the central slips and flexion contractures of the interphalangeal joints.
- The disability and deformity is directly related to the degree of the nerve injury. If tendon transfers are being considered, nerve recovery is unlikely.

PATIENT HISTORY AND PHYSICAL FINDINGS

- It is important to identify the cause and timing of ulnar nerve palsy to determine if the pathology can be reversed. Acute repair of lacerated nerves, nerve transfers, and decompressions should be done sooner rather than later to prevent irreversible loss of the motor end plates in the innervated muscles.
- Tendon transfers are indicated when no further recovery of the nerve or the ulnarly innervated muscles is expected.
- Working from distal to proximal, testing muscle and sensory function can help localize the level of the lesion. The first dorsal interosseous is the last muscle innervated by the ulnar nerve. Involvement of only motor function implies a lesion in the deep motor branch, distal to the Guyon canal. Loss of sensation along the dorsoulnar aspect of the hand implies a lesion proximal to the takeoff of the dorsal sensory branch. Loss of distal interphalangeal (DIP) flexion of the ring and small fingers implies high ulnar nerve palsy, due to involvement of the FDP. Loss of sensation along the medial arm or forearm implies a lesion in the brachial plexus.
- There are many eponymous physical findings found in ulnar nerve palsy, most of which are functional losses of intrinsic hand muscles:[2,3]
  - Froment sign: hyperflexion of the IP joint of the thumb when attempting forceful adduction, due to substitution of flexor pollicis longus (FPL) for adductor pollicis
  - Jeanne sign: hyperextension of the metacarpophalangeal (MCP) joint of the thumb as a reciprocal result of overuse of FPL
  - Wartenburg sign: abduction of small finger due to paralysis of intrinsics with unimpeded abduction by extensor digiti minimi
  - Duchenne sign: hyperextension of the MCP joints and flexion of the PIP joints, secondary to paralysis of ulnarly innervated interosseous and lumbricals
  - Masse sign: flattening of the metacarpal arch
  - Pollack sign: loss of DIP flexion of the ring and small fingers in high ulnar nerve palsy
- The Bouvier maneuver is a preoperative test to assess IP joint extension if MCP hyperextension is blocked. In theory, a positive Bouvier—that is to say, intact IP extension with MCPs held in flexion—implies that addressing MCP hyperextension with a static procedure should correct claw deformity. In reality, static soft tissue procedures tend to stretch out and most patients would do best with a dynamic tendon transfer.[4]

IMAGING

- Initial workup for an ulnar nerve lesion usually warrants nerve conduction studies and electromyography to determine location and extent of injury.
- MRI of the brachial plexus may be warranted if there is concern for a lesion at this level.

DIFFERENTIAL DIAGNOSIS

- Isolated ulnar nerve compression
- Isolated ulnar nerve injury
- Traumatic lower plexopathy
- Cervical radiculopathy
- Leprosy
- Syringomyelia

NONOPERATIVE MANAGEMENT

- An occupational therapist can be helpful in the nonoperative management of ulnar nerve palsy.
- An anticlaw splint (dorsal blocking at the MCP joint with IP joints free) can be used to preserve extensor integrity while the nerve recovers or as a long-term functional orthosis.
- Flexion contractures must be prevented or treated prior to tendon transfers, as maximum passive motion must be acquired before any tendon transfers.
- Fixed flexion contractures should be addressed with serial casting, if needed.

SURGICAL MANAGEMENT

- There are three key functions that tendon transfers must address in the setting of ulnar nerve palsy:
  - Thumb adduction to recreate key pinch
  - Improved grip by addressing claw deformity and MCP hyperextension
  - Flexion of ring and small finger DIP joints, in those with a high ulnar palsy
- Unlike nerve transfers, tendon transfers do not have a firm time period in which they must be performed. Tendon transfers can be delayed while awaiting potential nerve recovery.

- The common principles of tendon transfers are as follows:
  - Joint contractures should be addressed prior to any transfers.
  - Each muscle transfer should address one specific function.
  - Transferred tendons should glide through a smooth and scar-free surgical site.
- Thumb adduction can be addressed with either extensor carpi radialis brevis (ECRB) or flexor digitorum superficialis (FDS), with the former being our preference. Transfers for adduction require a pulley distal to the pisiform for the transfer to be effective.
- Claw deformity of the fingers can be addressed with either static or dynamic procedures. For static procedures to be indicated, the Bouvier maneuver must be positive. Static procedures prevent hyperextension of the MCP joint but often stretch out over time unless the joint undergoes arthrodesis.[5] Dynamic procedures use FDS, ECRB, extensor carpi radialis longus, or flexor carpi radialis. The FDS transfers are preferable because they do not require tendon grafts, which may be prone to adhesion. High ulnar nerve palsy precludes use of the FDS tendons in the ring and small finger for transfers.

Preoperative Planning

- Tendon transfers should be delayed until after potential nerve recovery is completed.
- Clinical exam of the patient will allow the surgeon to decide what functions must be recreated and what donor muscles are available for each function.

Positioning

- The patient is placed in the supine position with a tourniquet on the upper arm.
- The OR lights are positioned with one projecting from proximally and one distally from the operative site.

Approach

- Like with all tendon transfers, one should plan for the tendons to glide through a smooth and scar-free wound bed and each transfer should be for one function.
- To recreate the intrinsic function of the hand, the transferred tendons should pass volar to the axis of the MCP joint prior to inserting on the dorsal extensor apparatus.

TECHNIQUES

■ Claw Deformity of Digits

Metacarpal Capsulodesis[6,7]

- Indicated only with a positive Bouvier maneuver
- An incision is made in line with the distal palmar crease, over the A1 pulley of the ring and small fingers.
- The A1 pulley is exposed and released longitudinally, protecting the neurovascular bundles and exposing the volar plate of the MCP joint (**TECH FIG 1**).
- A distally based, rectangular-shaped flap of volar plate is created by releasing the proximal attachment off the metacarpal.
- A 30-degree flexion contracture is created with the volar plate advanced proximally, and bone anchors are used to maintain position of the joint.
- As noted before, this procedure can be technically difficult to perform because the exposure is limited and the volar plate cannot be advanced easily. This type

of soft tissue reconstruction does stretch out rather quickly. A truly predictable static procedure is MCP joint fusion.

Flexor Digitorum Superficialis Lasso

- An incision is made in line with the distal palmar crease, over the A1 pulleys of the ring and small fingers.
- The A1 and A2 pulleys are exposed, preserving the neurovascular bundles.
- The FDS insertion is preserved to reduce the likelihood of a swan-neck deformity. The FDS is released at A2 pulley and sutured back to itself proximal to the A1 pulley, creating a tendinous loop (**TECH FIG 2A**).
- Set the tension with the MCP joint at 40 to 50 degrees of flexion with the wrist at neutral, recreating the usual digital cascade of the hand (**TECH FIG 2B**).
- The FDS middle finger can be split into four tails in a more proximal incision and similarly tensioned at each A1 pulley.

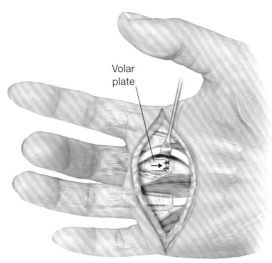

TECH FIG 1 • A1 pulley is released longitudinally and a rectangular-shaped flap of volar plate is created. Flexion contracture is created with the proximally advanced volar plate and bone anchors maintain position of the joint.

Stiles-Bunnell Transfer of FDS to Lateral Bands[8,9]

- One FDS tendon can be used to power two digits or four digits. The ring and small finger FDS is not used in the setting of high ulnar nerve palsy to preserve flexion of the ring and little fingers when the FDP to these two fingers is paralyzed.
- A Bruner incision is made over the proximal phalanx between the A2 and A3 pulleys. A separate longitudinal

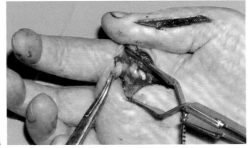

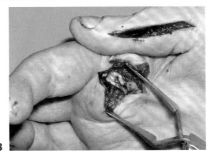

TECH FIG 2 • **A.** FDS tendon is released at distal edge of A2 pulley via Bruner incision. **B.** FDS tendon is sutured back to itself to create a flexion contracture at MCP joint.

incision is made over the proximal phalanx between the glabrous and nonglabrous skin to expose the radial lateral band (**TECH FIG 3A**).
- The FDS is divided just proximal to the insertion and split into four slips as proximally as possible (**TECH FIG 3B**).

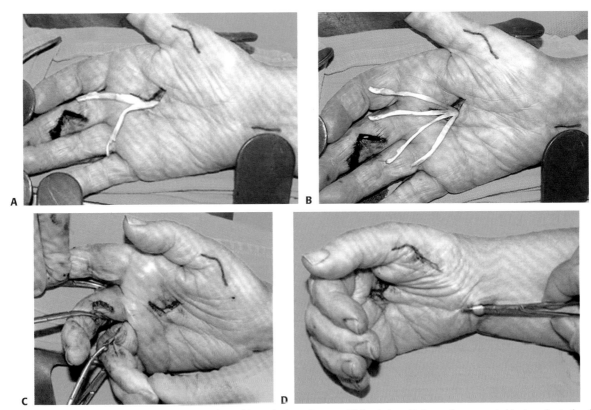

TECH FIG 3 • **A.** The FDS of the middle finger is released from the insertion on middle phalanx. **B.** Four tails are created for transfer to the digits. **C.** FDS is transferred to the lateral bands of each digit, radial of the middle-small and ulnar of the index. **D.** Final position after transfer shows MCP flexion composite with FDS pull.

- FDS slip is passed through lumbrical canal, deep to the neurovascular bundle, with a tendon passer or hemostat to the radial aspect of the middle through small fingers and the ulnar aspect of the index. It is key to stay palmar to the deep metacarpal ligament to maintain the force palmar to the axis of rotation (**TECH FIG 3C**).
- FDS slips are attached to the lateral band with the wrist at neutral, trying to recreate the digital cascade. MCP flexion should be at 50 to 70 degrees and IP joints in full extension (**TECH FIG 3D**).
- Passive wrist flexion should result in full MCP extension.

ECRB to Lateral Bands With Tendon Graft[9,10]

- ERCB is used when the FDS is not available, for example, high median and ulnar nerve palsy when the reinnervated median nerve muscles are too weak to transfer.
- A small transverse incision is made over the third metacarpal base, through which the ECRB is transected at its insertion.
- The ECRB tendon is retrieved proximal to the retinaculum through a separate incision.
- Incisions are made at the metacarpal necks in the second/third metacarpal interval and fourth/fifth metacarpal interval.
  - Excising a small window of paralyzed interosseous muscle creates a path for each tendon graft.
- Longitudinal incisions are made over the proximal phalanges of the index through small fingers, exposing the lateral bands.
- A tendon graft is passed volarly to the intermetacarpal ligament and through the intermetacarpal windows.
- The tendon grafts are sutured to the radial lateral bands of the middle through small fingers and the ulnar lateral band of the index.
- The grafts are sewn to each other and then to the ECRB (**TECH FIG 4**).
  - Tension should be done with the wrist in full extension and the fingers in an intrinsic-plus position.
  - MCP extension should happen with wrist flexion.

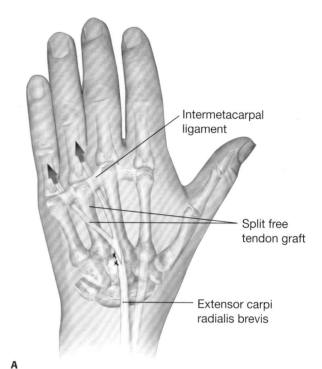

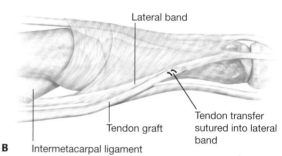

TECH FIG 4 • **A.** Tendon graft is passed volarly to the intermetacarpal ligament and through the intermetacarpal windows. **B.** Tendon grafts are sutured to the radial lateral band of the middle finger and the ulnar lateral band of the index finger. Tendon transfer is sutured into the lateral band.

■ Restoration of Thumb Adduction: ECRB to Adductor Pollicis With Tendon Graft

- A small transverse incision is made over the third metacarpal base, through which the ECRB is transected at its insertion.
- The ECRB tendon is retrieved proximal to the retinaculum through a separate incision.
- A path for the tendon graft is created between the third and second metacarpals, incising skin and excising a small window of paralyzed interosseous muscle.

- A longitudinal incision is made along the ulnar aspect of the thumb MCP joint, exposing the adductor aponeurosis.
- A tendon graft (often palmaris) is passed deep to the adductor pollicis and through the window between the metacarpals (**TECH FIG 5**).
- The graft is tensioned so that the thumb is adducted past the index metacarpal when the wrist is at neutral. In dorsiflexion, the thumb is abducted, and in palmar flexion, it should lie firmly against the palm.

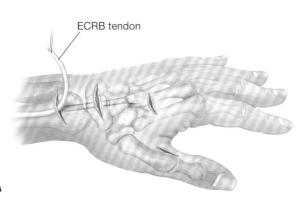

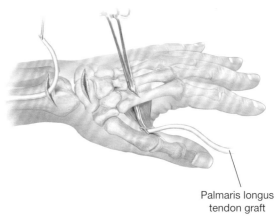

ECRB tendon

Palmaris longus tendon graft

A   B

TECH FIG 5 • A. A transverse incision is made over the third metacarpal base and the ECRB is transected at insertion. The ECRB tendon is retrieved proximal to the retinaculum through another incision. **B.** The palmaris longus tendon graft is passed to the adductor pollicis.

■ Thumb Stabilization: Split Flexor Pollicis Longus (FPL) to Extensor Pollicis Longus (EPL) Tenodesis

- The muscle imbalances of the ulnar paralyzed hand, particularly due to the loss of the adductor pollicis, result in greater flexion of the IP joint and less of the MCP. This creates a Z-deformity in about 60% of patients.[11]

- A radial incision is made over the proximal phalanx of the thumb.
- Preserving the oblique pulley, the FPL and EPL are exposed.
- The radial half of the FPL is released from the distal insertion and weaved into the EPL (**TECH FIG 6**).
- The interphalangeal joint is kept in extension with a 0.045-in. K-wire.

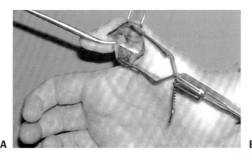

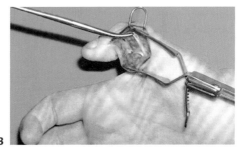

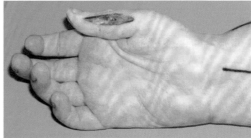

A   B   C

TECH FIG 6 • A. The radial half of the FPL is released from the rest of the tendon at the insertion site. **B.** This radial slip is transferred dorsally. **C.** Final position after transfer shows IP joint stabilization.

■ Restoration of Finger Flexion: Flexor Digitorum Profundus (FDP) Side-to-Side Transfer

- High ulnar nerve palsy results in paralysis of the ulnar 0.1 of FDP, affecting motion of the DIP joints of the ring and small fingers and thus grip strength.

- Side-to-side transfer is an easy way to address this with the median nerve innervated portion of the muscle.
- A longitudinal incision is made over the distal third of the forearm.
- The FDP tendons are identified, deep to the median nerve.
- The FDP tendons are synchronized to recreate the digital cascade, and one sutures the long through small finger tendons with two rows of braided permanent sutures.

PEARLS AND PITFALLS

Preoperative evaluation	■ Critically assess donor muscle availability and strength.
	■ Determine patient goals and potential for additional nerve recovery.
	■ Determine the integrity of the PIP central slip with the Bouvier maneuver.
Thumb adduction	■ The thumb may have joint instability that requires additional procedures such as capsulodesis or arthrodesis.
Addressing claw deformity	■ Static transfers usually stretch over time and should be reserved for combined nerve injuries.
	■ Transfers must pass volar to the MCP joint to address hyperextension.
	■ Dynamic transfers should be sewn into lateral bands if Bouvier maneuver is negative.

POSTOPERATIVE CARE

■ The patient is usually splinted with the MCP joints in 60 to 70 degrees of flexion and the IP joints in full extension (intrinsic plus position) for a total of 4 weeks. Active range of motion exercises are then commenced, with a dorsal blocking splint at the MCP joint.

■ Passive range of motion is started at 6 weeks. Strengthening is started at 8 weeks for the adductor plasty and 10 weeks for the intrinsic transfers.

■ A knowledgeable hand therapist plays an important role in the surgical outcomes.

■ Early active range of motion has been advocated by some surgeons, with quicker recovery and less pain.[12,13]

OUTCOMES

■ Outcome studies are difficult to compare due to the heterogeneity of the patient populations.

■ Static reconstructions often stretch. Less than 50% of the hands treated with capsulodesis see long-term improvement in regard to clawing.[14]

■ Wrist extensor transfers to the lateral bands restore grip strength most effectively, with the highest efficacy in those with short-standing paralysis.[15] However, the need for tendon grafts and scarring through the interosseous muscles makes them less favorable.[16,17]

■ FDS transfers are most efficacious in addressing claw deformity, with minimal improvement in grip strength.[15,18]

COMPLICATIONS

■ Complications are more common with the intrinsic transfers due to the delicate balance in the extensor mechanism.

■ Transfers may be ineffective due to poor tensioning and may need surgical revision to tighten the insertion.

■ Transfers that are too tight can often be addressed with passive range of motion exercises to stretch the transfer.

■ Harvest of FDS results in a swan-neck deformity fairly commonly, with the incidence ranging from 15% to 85%.[15,19,20]

REFERENCES

1. Riordan DC. Tendon transfers for nerve paralysis of the hand and wrist. *Curr Pract Orthop Surg.* 1964;23:17-40.
2. Srinivasan H. Clinical features of paralytic claw fingers. *J Bone Joint Surg Am.* 1979;61(7):1060-1063.
3. Goldfarb CA, Stern PJ. Low ulnar nerve palsy. *J Am Soc Surg Hand.* 2003;3(1):14-26.
4. Wang K, McGlinn EP, Chung KC. A biomechanical and evolutionary perspective on the function of the lumbrical muscle. *J Hand Surg.* 2014;39(1):149-155.
5. Mikhail IK. Bone block operation for clawhand. *Surg Gynecol Obstet.* 1964;118:1077-1079.
6. Zancolli EA. Claw-hand caused by paralysis of the intrinsic muscles: a simple surgical procedure for its correction. *J Bone Joint Surg Am.* 1957;39-A(5):1076-1080.
7. Brown PW. Zancolli capsulorrhaphy for ulnar claw hand: appraisal of forty-four cases. *J Bone Joint Surg Am.* 1970;52(5):868-877.
8. Bunnell S. Surgery of the intrinsic muscles of the hand other than those producing opposition of the thumb. *J Bone Joint Surg Am.* 1942;24(1):1-31.
9. Parkes A. Paralytic claw fingers: a graft tenodesis operation. *Hand.* 1973;5(3):192-199.
10. Brand P. Tendon grafting: illustrated by a new operation for intrinsic paralysis of the fingers. *J Bone Joint Surg Br.* 1961;43:444-453.
11. Palande DD, Gilbie SG. The deformity of thumb in ulnar paralysis. *Lepr India.* 1981;53(2):152-159.
12. Rath S. Immediate postoperative active mobilization versus immobilization following tendon transfer for claw deformity correction in the hand. *J Hand Surg.* 2008;33(2):232-240.
13. Rath S, Selles RW, Schreuders TA, et al. A randomized clinical trial comparing immediate active motion with immobilization after tendon transfer for claw deformity. *J Hand Surg.* 2009;34(3):488-494.
14. Srinivasan H. Dermadesis and flexor pulley advancement: first report on a simple operation for correction of paralytic claw fingers in patients with leprosy. *J Hand Surg.* 1985;10(6 Pt 2):979-982.
15. Ozkan T, Ozer K, Gulgonen A. Three tendon transfer methods in reconstruction of ulnar nerve palsy. *J Hand Surg.* 2003;28(1):35-43.
16. Burkhalter WE. Restoration of power grip in ulnar nerve paralysis. *Orthop Clin North Am.* 1974;5(2):289-303.
17. Burkhalter WE, Strait JL. Metacarpophalangeal flexor replacement for intrinsic muscle paralysis. *J Bone Joint Surg Am.* 1973;55A:1656-1676.
18. Hastings H 2nd, McCollam SM. Flexor digitorum superficialis lasso tendon transfer in isolated ulnar nerve palsy: a functional evaluation. *J Hand Surg.* 1994;19(2):275-280.
19. Brandsma JW, Ottenhoff-De Jonge MW. Flexor digitorum superficialis tendon transfer for intrinsic replacement. Long-term results and the effect on donor fingers. *J Hand Surg.* 1992;17(6):625-628.
20. Reddy NR, Kolumban SL. Effects of fingers of leprosy patients having surgical removal of sublimus tendons. *Lepr India.* 1981;53(4):594-599.

SUGGESTED READINGS

Chase R. Muscle tendon kinetics. *Am J Surg.* 1965;109:277-282.
Omer GE. Tendon transfers for traumatic nerve injuries. *J Hand Surg.* 2004;4(3):214-226.
Riordan DC. Tendon transplantations in median-nerve and ulnar-nerve paralysis. *J Bone Joint Surg Am.* 1953;35-A(2):312-332.

Tendon Transfers for Radial Nerve Injury

Rafael J. Diaz-Garcia and Kevin C. Chung

DEFINITION

- Radial nerve palsy refers to the loss of motor control and sensation of the hand in the distribution of the radial nerve.
- Loss of extensor function of the wrist and digits is the greatest deficit, as the sensation loss is of little consequence in prehension because it is on the dorsum of the hand. Loss of wrist extension affects grip strength.

ANATOMY

- The radial nerve is a mixed nerve composed of fibers from the C5 through T1 roots, forming as a terminal branch of the posterior cord of the brachial plexus.
- It travels initially in the posterior compartment of the arm, where it gives off multiple branches to the three heads of the triceps while coursing along the spiral groove of the humerus. It passes through the intermuscular septum into the anterior compartment, where it lies between the brachialis and brachioradialis (BR), innervating the latter.
  - The BR, extensor carpi radialis longus (ECRL) and, at times, extensor carpi radialis brevis (ECRB) are innervated by the proper radial nerve prior to its entering the supinator, where it then divides into its two terminal branches.
  - The superficial branch of the radial nerve provides sensation to the radial dorsum of the hand and fingers except for the small finger and ½ of the ring finger.
  - The deep branch of the radial nerve innervates the supinator and becomes the posterior interosseous nerve (PIN) as it exits, innervating ECRB, extensor digitorum communis (EDC), extensor carpi ulnaris (ECU), abductor pollicis longus (APL), extensor pollicis brevis (EPB), extensor pollicis longus (EPL), and extensor indicis proprius (EIP).
- Order of innervation is consistent, with EPL and EIP as the last two innervated muscles. This is helpful with clinical examination at time of injury and monitoring recovery.

PATHOGENESIS

- The pathogenesis of radial nerve palsy is most frequently due to traumatic injury, which can happen from injuries extending from the brachial plexus to the forearm.
- Idiopathic and compression causes are rarely seen.
- Radial nerve injury is most commonly seen with humeral shaft fractures, given its location in the spiral groove.[1-3]

NATURAL HISTORY

- The mechanism of injury is an important predictor of potential recovery.

- Open, high-energy, and penetrating injuries should be explored early, as they have demonstrated poor recovery with nonoperative management.[4]

PATIENT HISTORY AND PHYSICAL FINDINGS

- A patient with radial nerve injury will present with potential loss of elbow extension, wrist extension, digital extension, thumb extension, and thumb abduction.
- The BR and ECRL are preserved in PIN palsies, as they are innervated proximal to the elbow.
- Tenodesis on physical exam can differentiate extensor tendon injury vs nerve palsy.

IMAGING

- Initial workup for acute radial nerve palsy may warrant x-rays to determine if there are any fractures or dislocations in the extremity associated with the acute trauma.
- Nerve conduction studies and electromyography may be helpful in the workup of radial nerve palsy, helping to determine the level of the lesion. Axonal loss is evident 3 weeks after injury.
- MRI of the brachial plexus may be warranted if there is concern for a lesion at this level.

DIFFERENTIAL DIAGNOSIS

- Extensor tendon laceration/rupture
- Isolated radial nerve injury
- Cervical radiculopathy
- Volar subluxation of the MCP joint (in inflammatory arthritis)
- Brachial plexus lesion

NONOPERATIVE MANAGEMENT

- Hand therapy is essential to educate the patient in a home exercise program to maintain motion and prevent contracture while waiting for nerve recovery.[5]
- Patients should be given a wrist splint for support to counteract the unopposed wrist flexors. Hand intrinsic muscles can provide some digital extension.

SURGICAL MANAGEMENT

- The goals of reconstruction depend on the level of injury of the radial nerve.
  - Injuries in the arm require reconstruction of independent wrist extension, finger extension, and thumb extension.

- Injuries in the forearm of the PIN will spare the ECRL and sometimes the ECRB, which preserve wrist extension.
- Donor muscles include the pronator teres (PT), flexor carpi ulnaris (FCU), flexor carpi radialis (FCR), flexor digitorum superficialis (FDS), and palmaris longus (PL). The different reconstructions are usually referred to by which transfer is used for reconstruction of digital extension.
- Tendon transfers should be delayed until after potential nerve recovery is completed. However, unlike median or ulnar nerve transfers, sometimes radial nerve transfers are done at the time of nerve repair/reconstruction to minimize need for bracing.

Preoperative Planning

- Clinical exam of the patient helps the surgeon decide what functions must be recreated and what donor muscles are available for each function.
- Hand and wrist joints should be as supple as possible.
  - Wrist motion, particularly flexion, is an important characteristic for radial nerve transfers. That is because additional excursion is obtained with wrist flexion to help the FCR or FCU to fully extend the fingers.
  - If there is significant wrist stiffness, one should consider FDS to EDC transfers for better excursion of the transfer.

Positioning

- The patient is placed in the supine position with a tourniquet on the upper arm.
- The OR lights are positioned with one projecting from proximally and one distally from the operative site.

Approach

- Like with all tendon transfers, one should plan for the tendons to glide through a smooth and scar-free wound bed and each transfer should serve one function.
- If there is scarred tissue along the path of the transfer, it must be replaced by soft supple tissue either through serial scar excision or a flap procedure.

■ Reconstruction of Wrist Extension: Pronator Teres to Extensor Carpi Radialis Brevis

- A radial-sided longitudinal incision is planned over the midpoint of the forearm to expose both the PT and the second extensor compartment (**TECH FIG 1A,B**).
- The pronator teres (PT) is identified inserting on the radial shaft, deep to the brachioradialis (BR) and radial artery.
  - Additional length is acquired by harvesting a strip of distal periosteum along with the distal tendon.
- The proximal PT is freed of its attachments to the other volar muscles to improve the excursion.
- The extensor carpi radialis brevis (ECRB) is localized just distal to the musculotendinous junction. A smooth path is created over the BR and the superficial radial nerve.

- The PT is passed over the BR to the ECRB. The ECRL can also be incorporated into the tendon transfer, but this is typically not done.
- If the ECRL and ECRB has no chance of recovery, the tendon transfer is done in the end-to-end fashion, rather than end-to-side to provide maximum excursion. Tension is set.
- A Pulvertaft tendon weave is done using 2-0 braided nonabsorbable sutures.
- The wrist tendons are reconstructed first to facilitate setting tension for the fingers and thumb.
  - The wrist should be at a neutral posture after the tendon transfer is secured.
  - Each end of the tendon is grasped with a clamp to set the tension, and if the tension is too loose, horizontal mattress sutures are used to "fine-tune" and tighten the transfer (**TECH FIG 1C–E**).

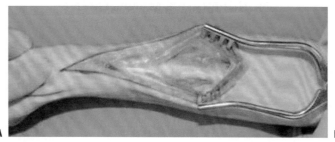
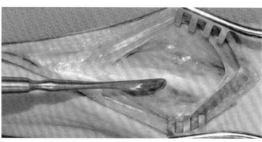

TECH FIG 1 • **A,B.** The PT is identified where it inserts on the radial shaft, deep to the brachioradialis.

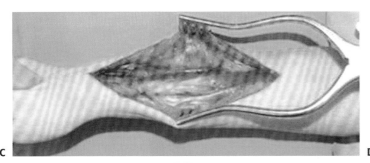
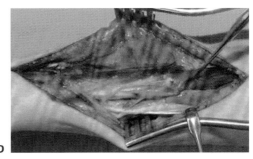

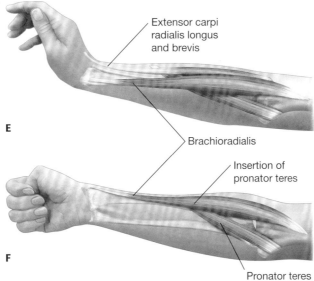

TECH FIG 1 (Continued) • **C,D.** The PT is woven through ECRL and ECRB tendons just distal to the musculotendinous junction. **E,F.** Path of the transfer.

■ Reconstruction of Finger Extension

Flexor Carpi Radialis to Extensor Digitorum Communis[6,7]

- A longitudinal volar incision is used to expose the flexor carpi radialis (FCR) and palmaris longus in the distal forearm.
  - The distal tendon is transected at the distal wrist crease.
- There are two paths of transfer of the FCR.
  - A subcutaneous tunnel in a radial direction to the dorsum of the wrist. This is our preferred transfer, as the path is created for the EPL as well.
  - A tunnel through the interosseous membrane (IOM) to the dorsum of the wrist. This has a more direct line of pull but has a higher incidence of postoperative adhesions.
- Point of insertion on each tendon is chosen to recreate the normal digital cascade by detaching each finger tendon and suture it along the path of the FCR.
- Pulvertaft weaves are held in place with nonabsorbable sutures (**TECH FIG 2A–C**).

- Final tension is set to achieve the tenodesis posture: 30-degree wrist extension is accompanied by 90 degrees of finger flexion; 30 degrees of wrist flexion is accompanied by full finger extension (**TECH FIG 2D,E**).

Flexor Carpi Ulnaris to Extensor Digitorum Communis[8–10]

- A longitudinal incision is made over the distal aspect of the flexor carpi ulnaris (FCU) tendon at the pisiform.
  - The ulnar neurovascular bundle must be identified and protected.
- The FCU is freed from its surrounding attachments to achieve sufficient excursion.
- A broad subcutaneous tunnel is created in an ulnar direction toward the dorsum of the wrist.
- A dorsal incision is made to expose the extensor digitorum communis (EDC) and release the proximal extensor retinaculum.
- Pulvertaft weaves are held in place with nonabsorbable sutures (**TECH FIG 3**).
- Point of insertion and tensioning is done similarly to the FCR transfer.

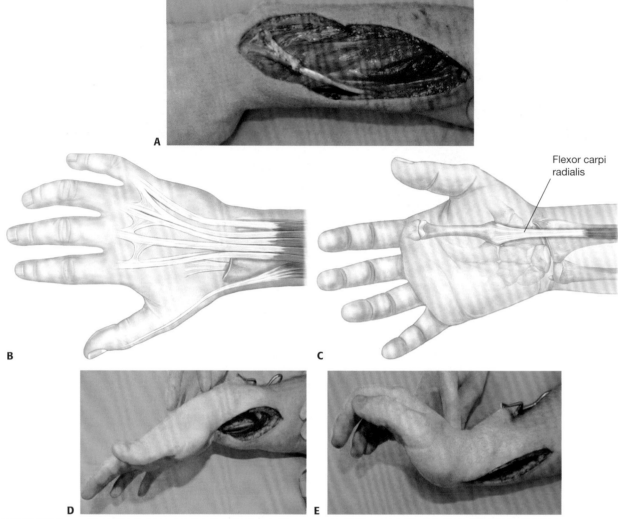

TECH FIG 2 • **A.** The FCR to EDC is completed via a subcutaneous tunnel along the radial side of the wrist. **B,C.** Relationship between the FCR donor and the EDC tendons. The transfer can be either subcutaneous or transinterosseous membrane. **D.** Full digital extension is seen with slight wrist flexion. **E.** Full digital flexion is possible with wrist extension.

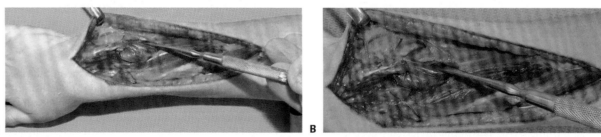

TECH FIG 3 • The FCU to EDC is completed via a subcutaneous tunnel along the ulnar side of the wrist. Care is kept to ensure there is no injury or compression to the dorsal ulnar sensory branch. The distal FCU muscle can be debrided if it makes the weave too bulky.

Flexor Digitorum Superficialis (FDS-IV) to Extensor Digitorum Communis[11]

- FDS to EDC transfer is best suited for patients with poor wrist motion preoperatively.
  - The better excursion of the FDS (70 mm) results in better digital extension.
  - In most patients, wrist motion from tenodesis compensates for the limited excursion of the wrist flexors.

- The FDS tendon is released from the ring finger just proximal to the carpal tunnel via a volar wrist incision.
  - Alternatively, it can be released at the PIP joint through a Bruner-style incision if greater tendon length is needed in the case of tendon rupture or loss.
- For radial nerve palsy, when the extensor tendons are intact, the FDS is transected at the wrist and will be transferred dorsally to attach to the extensor tendons proximal to the extensor retinaculum.

- It is retrieved from the volar forearm incision used to harvest the other tendons.
- The FDS to the long finger is transferred to the index and thumb extensor tendons, coordinating both these digits for precise pinch (**TECH FIG 4A–C**).
- The IOM is exposed proximal to the pronator quadratus.
- Making sure to not disrupt the central band of the IOM, an opening is made to allow for the tendons to pass from volar to dorsal (**TECH FIG 4D**).

- Dorsally, the FDS-IV is transferred to the EDC long through small fingers with a Pulvertaft weave.
- This transfer is grouped in this fashion to coordinate the ulnar digits in power grip.
- Tension is set with the wrist at 30 degrees of extension and the MP joints at full extension (**TECH FIG 4E**).

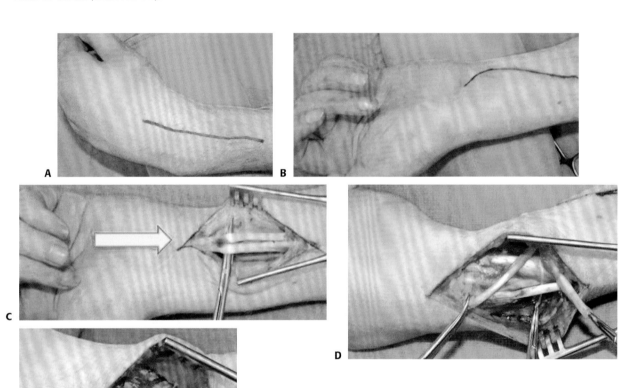

TECH FIG 4 • A,B. Dorsal and volar incisions, respectively, are designed for exposure of tendons. **C.** The FDS to the long and ring fingers are divided just proximal to the carpal tunnel. **D.** The tendons are passed from volar to dorsal via the interosseous membrane. **E.** The FDS-IV is woven into the EDC tendons (*yellow arrow*), and the FDS-III is woven into the EPL and EIP (*black arrow*).

■ Reconstruction of Thumb Extension: Palmaris Longus to Extensor Pollicis Longus

- Palmaris longus (PL) is identified through the volar incision used to expose FCR. It is freed from its surrounding attachments to maximize excursion.
- A subcutaneous tunnel toward the thumb is created below the radial artery and cutaneous nerves along the radial aspect of the wrist (**TECH FIG 5A**).
- If nerve recovery is not expected, the extensor pollicis longus (EPL) tendon is released proximally through the dorsal incision.

- If nerve recovery is expected and transfer is being used as a temporizing measure, the EPL is kept in continuity but released from the third compartment to improve the vector of pull of the transfer.
- A Pulvertaft weave is done between the PL and EPL tendons.
- Tension is set with the thumb fully extended with the wrist in neutral.
- Transfer is secured with nonabsorbable suture (**TECH FIG 5B–D**).

TECHNIQUES

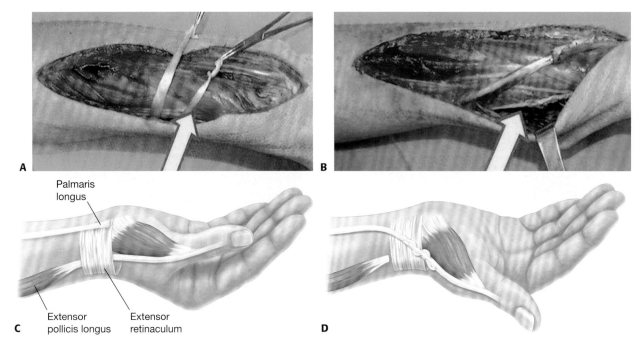

TECH FIG 5 • A. FCR and PL can both be harvested from the same radial incision. **B.** FCR is woven to EDC and PL is woven to EPL. **C,D.** Transfer of PL to EPL.

PEARLS AND PITFALLS

Preoperative evaluation	■ Critically assess donor muscle availability and strength.
	■ Determine patient goals and potential for additional nerve recovery. Tendon transfers for wrist extension and thumb extension may be done even with expected recovery.
	■ Because wrist flexors do not match excursion of finger extensors, preoperative assessment can help determine working range of transfer and how to set tension.[12]
Finger extension transfer	■ Choice between FCR and FCU for digital extension is not straightforward. Neither matches excursion, though FCU has greater force. However, loss of FCU may result in loss of "dart thrower's motion."
	■ Interosseous membrane passage must allow for easy tendon gliding. Prone to greater adhesions.

POSTOPERATIVE CARE

■ The patient is usually splinted with the wrist in 30 to 40 degrees of extension and the MP joints in full extension. The interphalangeal joints can undergo passive range of motion, as the intrinsic hand muscles drive their extension.

■ At the first postoperative visit, an Orthoplast splint is fabricated to wrist and MP extension. At 3 weeks, gentle active range of motion of the wrist is commenced several times a day. Integration of digital extension is added as wrist motion improves. Passive range of motion is started at 6 weeks. Strengthening is started at 8 weeks.

■ A knowledgeable hand therapist plays an important role in the surgical outcomes.

OUTCOMES

■ Most radial nerve palsy patients can perform normal activities of daily living with their hand after complete recovery from surgery.

■ With restoration of wrist extension, grip strength is 40% to 50% of the contralateral side and digital extension is 34% to 75% of normal.[12-14]

COMPLICATIONS

■ Suboptimal results may be a result of choosing a weak motor for transfer or incorrect vector of pull.

■ Radial deviation can result from use of FCR. PIP joint hyperextension or flexion contractures can result from use of FDS tendons.

■ Tendon adhesions can result from prolonged immobilization, but tenolysis should not be considered until at least 9 months out from surgery.

■ Tendon ruptures can be prevented with patient education and progressive therapy advancement. Transfer attenuation may require revision.

REFERENCES

1. Amillo S, Barrios RH, Martinez-Peric R, Losada JI. Surgical treatment of the radial nerve lesions associated with fractures of the humerus. *J Orthop Trauma*. 1993;7(3):211-215.
2. Thomsen NO, Dahlin LB. Injury to the radial nerve caused by fracture of the humeral shaft: timing and neurobiological aspects related to treatment and diagnosis. *Scand J Plast Reconstr Surg Hand Surg*. 2007;41(4):153-157.
3. Burkhalter WE. Early tendon transfer in upper extremity peripheral nerve injury. *Clin Orthop Relat Res*. 1974(104):68-79.
4. Ring D, Chin K, Jupiter JB. Radial nerve palsy associated with high-energy humeral shaft fractures. *J Hand Surg [Am]*. 2004;29(1):144-147.
5. Walczyk S, Pieniazek M, Pelczar-Pieniazek M, Tabasz M. Appropriateness and effectiveness of physiotherapeutic treatment procedure after tendon transfer in patients with irreversible radial nerve injury. *Ortop Traumatol Rehabil*. 2005;7(2):187-197.
6. Brand PW. Biomechanics of tendon transfer. *Orthop Clin North Am*. 1974;5(2):205-230.
7. Ishida O, Ikuta Y. Analysis of Tsuge's procedure for the treatment of radial nerve paralysis. *Hand Surg*. 2003;8(1):17-20.
8. Riordan DC. Radial nerve paralysis. *Orthop Clin North Am*. 1974;5(2):283-287.
9. Riordan DC. Tendon transfers in hand surgery. *J Hand Surg [Am]*. 1983;8(5 Pt 2):748-753.
10. Raskin KB, Wilgis EF. Flexor carpi ulnaris transfer for radial nerve palsy: functional testing of long-term results. *J Hand Surg [Am]*. 1995;20(5):737-742.
11. Chuinard RG, Boyes JH, Stark HH, Ashworth CR. Tendon transfers for radial nerve palsy: use of superficialis tendons for digital extension. *J Hand Surg [Am]*. 1978;3(6):560-570.
12. Lieber RL, Ponten E, Burkholder TJ, Friden J. Sarcomere length changes after flexor carpi ulnaris to extensor digitorum communis tendon transfer. *J Hand Surg [Am]*. 1996;21(4):612-618.
13. Al-Qattan MM. Tendon transfer for radial nerve palsy: a single tendon to restore finger extension as well as thumb extension/radial abduction. *J Hand Surg Eur Vol*. 2012;37(9):855-862.
14. Altintas AA, Altintas MA, Gazyakan E, et al. Long-term results and the Disabilities of the Arm, Shoulder, and Hand score analysis after modified Brooks and D'Aubigne tendon transfer for radial nerve palsy. *J Hand Surg [Am]*. 2009;34(3):474-478.

34 CHAPTER

Tendon Transfers for Combined Median and Ulnar Nerve Injury

Kate Elzinga and Kevin C. Chung

DEFINITION

- Combined median and ulnar nerve injuries cause major impairment of the upper extremity. The ability to perform fine pinch and power grasp is lost. The volar and dorsoulnar hand is insensate. The balance between the flexor and extensor muscle groups of the upper extremity is absent. Prehensile function is greatly reduced.
- Low median and ulnar nerve injuries are the most common combined nerve injury of the upper extremity. Nerve lacerations should be repaired acutely. In the case of a delayed nerve injury presentation or incomplete recovery following nerve repair, tendon transfers can be used to augment function.
- Tendon transfers can be combined with nerve transfers and free muscle transfers to help maximize the function of the injured upper limb. However, in combined nerve injuries, the number of nerves available for transfer is also limited.
- For a successful tendon transfer, a redundant tendon is harvested for transfer, minimizing donor-site morbidity while restoring a lost function. Finding an appropriate donor tendon is more difficult in combined nerve injuries compared to isolated nerve injuries; a greater number of tendons are affected, which results in multiple functional deficits while fewer intact tendons remain for transfer.
- Sensory deficits are also greater in combined nerve injuries (**FIG 1**). Reconstructive outcomes are inferior in combined nerve injuries compared to single nerve injury injuries.
- Donor-site morbidity must be carefully considered prior to tendon harvest for transfer in combined nerve injuries. These patients have a limited number of tendons available for transfer. The patient's individualized goals must be carefully considered. A personalized reconstructive plan is created to best restore the patient's function.
- The patient's physical exam is central in formulating the operative plan. Missing functions, as well as available donor tendons, are documented. Once the functional deficits and available donors have been determined, the donors are matched to the deficits for reconstruction.
- Following the principles of tendon transfers optimizes patient outcomes:
  - Expendable donor
  - Straight line of pull
  - One muscle for one function
  - Similar force of contraction
  - Adequate excursion
  - Synergism

- Skeletal stability
- Stable, supple soft tissue bed
- Full passive range of motion (ROM)
- Synergistic transfers are the most intuitive for patients to learn and offer the quickest return of function. Wrist extension is synergistic with finger flexion, whereas wrist flexion is linked with finger extension.
  - Compared to single nerve injuries, following a combined nerve injury, achieving synergy can be more difficult.
- Ideally, tendon excursion of the donor tendon should match that of the recipient tendon to best restore the biomechanics of the upper extremity. The wrist flexors and extensors have 3.3 cm of excursion, the finger extensors have 5 cm of excursion, and the finger flexors have 7 cm of excursion.[1]
- Staging of procedures is important. Only tendon transfers that can be rehabilitated with hand therapy together should be performed at the same time. Multiple surgeries may be required.

ANATOMY

- Proximally, the median nerve innervates the pronator teres, flexor carpi radialis (FCR), palmaris longus (PL), and flexor digitorum superficialis (FDS).
- The anterior interosseous nerve (AIN) originates from the median nerve 6 to 8 cm distal to the medial epicondyle. It innervates the flexor digitorum profundus (FDP) to the index and middle fingers, flexor pollicis longus (FPL), and pronator quadratus.
- The median nerve continues distally to provide motor innervation to the lumbricals to the index and middle fingers and the thenar muscles (abductor pollicis brevis [APB], flexor pollicis brevis [FPB], and opponens pollicis) and sensory innervation to the thumb, index, middle, and radial half of the ring finger.
  - A low median nerve injury, distal to the origin of the AIN, causes the loss of thumb opposition and sensory deficits in the volar-radial hand.
  - A high median nerve injury affects all of the muscles listed above. In addition to thumb opposition and sensory deficits, forearm pronation is lost, wrist flexion is weakened, flexion of all four proximal interphalangeal (PIP) joints as well as the index and middle finger distal interphalangeal (DIP) joints is lost, and thumb flexion is lost.
- The ulnar nerve innervates, from proximal to distal, the flexor carpi ulnaris (FCU), FDP to the ring and small fingers, hypothenar muscles (abductor digit minimi [ADM], opponens digiti minimi, flexor digiti minimi), lumbricals of the

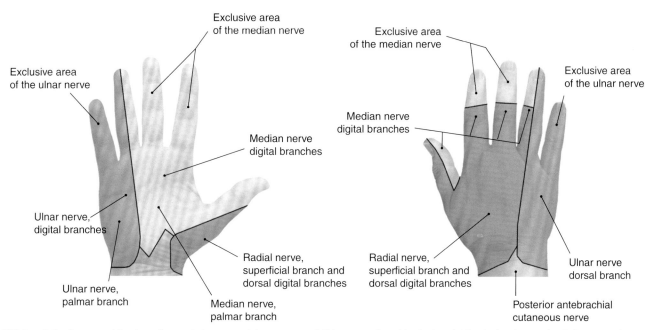

FIG 1 • Following a combined median and ulnar nerve injury, sensory deficits are profound in the hand. All volar hand sensation is lost. Dorsal sensation over the index and middle fingers distal to the PIP joints and over the entire ring and small fingers is also absent. *Yellow*, median nerve; *blue*, ulnar nerve; *pink*, radial nerve.

ring and small fingers, dorsal and palmar interossei, deep head of the FPB, and adductor pollicis (AdP). The ulnar nerve provides sensory innervation to the ulnar ring and bilateral small fingers.

- A low ulnar nerve injury denervates the intrinsic muscles (hypothenar muscles, lumbricals ring and small fingers, interossei, deep head of FPB, AdP) of the hand.
- A high ulnar nerve injury occurs more proximally and denervates the extrinsic muscles (FCU, FDP ring and small fingers) of the hand in addition to the intrinsic muscles.

- Connections are common between the ulnar and median nerves, occurring in 9% to 27% of forearms[1,2] and 83% of hands.[3] However, connections between the radial nerve to either the median or the ulnar nerve have not been reported. In combined median and ulnar nerve injuries, motor and sensory deficits are profound and complete.
  - A combined low median and ulnar nerve injury leads to the loss of thumb opposition and hand intrinsic function (thenar and hypothenar muscles, lumbricals, interossei). Forearm pronation, wrist flexion, and finger flexion are preserved. Hand sensation remains intact in the distribution of the superficial branch of the radial nerve over the dorsoradial hand only.
  - In addition to the deficits of a low combined palsy, a combined high median and ulnar nerve injury results in the loss of forearm pronation, wrist flexion, finger flexion, and thumb flexion.
- The radial nerve innervates, from proximal to distal, the triceps, brachioradialis (BR), extensor carpi radialis longus (ECRL), extensor carpi radialis brevis (ECRB), supinator, extensor carpi ulnaris (ECU), extensor digitorum communis (EDC), extensor digit minimi (EDM), abductor pollicis longus (APL), extensor pollicis longus (EPL), extensor pollicis brevis (EPB), and the extensor indicis proprius (EIP).

- Expendable radial nerve-innervated tendons for wrist and hand reconstruction include:
  - The BR can be transferred if the biceps and/or brachialis are intact to maintain elbow flexion. The biceps and brachialis muscles are innervated by the musculocutaneous nerve and are not affected by median and ulnar nerve injuries.
  - Two of three of the ECRL, ECRB, and ECU can be harvested. One of these tendons must be preserved to maintain wrist extension.
  - The EIP and EDM can be transferred if the EDC is intact to maintain extension of the index and small fingers.
  - The EPB can be harvested if the EPL is intact to provide thumb extension.
  - The APL has multiple slips. As long as one slip of the APL is preserved for thumb abduction, the additional slips can be harvested for transfer.

PATHOGENESIS

- Lacerations to the volar wrist are the most common cause of combined low median and ulnar nerve injuries. The median and ulnar nerves are at increased risk in the distal volar forearm because of their superficial location here compared to their location deep to the muscles in the proximal forearm and arm.
- More proximal injuries, typically resulting from sharp mechanisms, can result in high combined nerve injuries.

PATIENT HISTORY AND PHYSICAL FINDINGS

- Selection of appropriate donor tendons for transfer is critical to restore function while minimizing donor site morbidity.
- A comprehensive history and physical examination is performed to determine the patient's functional deficits and their reconstructive goals.

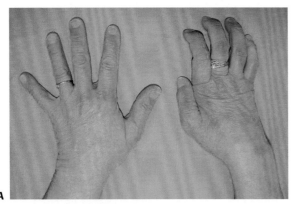
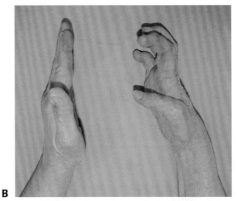

FIG 2 • This patient had a low combined median and ulnar nerve injury of the right hand. A claw hand deformity is viewed from dorsal **(A)** and lateral **(B)**. The finger MCP joints are extended, and the IP joints are flexed.

- The patient's age, handedness, occupation, and avocations are documented.
- Limitations in activities of daily living, recreation, and work are discussed.
  - The patient's goals are explored, including their plans for return to work, their availability and willingness to undergo secondary procedures and hand therapy, and the importance of appearance.
- Discussion with the patient's hand therapist provides further insight into the patient's deficits and can help prioritize reconstructive goals. Reconstruction is focused on providing the most functional benefit to each individual patient.
- The patient's compliance with therapy and their anticipated ability to retrain transferred tendons is assessed by the therapist and considered when determining the reconstructive plan.
- Important considerations from the patient's past medical history include smoking, diabetes mellitus, peripheral vascular disease, connective tissue disorders, arthritis, Dupuytren disease, and previous hand injuries.
- On physical examination, a claw hand deformity is more apparent in a low median and ulnar nerve palsy than in a high injury **(FIG 2)**.
  - In low injuries, FDS and FDP innervation remain intact causing unopposed flexion of the interphalangeal (IP) joints of the fingers due to the denervation of the interossei and lumbricals. The loss of the intrinsic muscles of the hand also leads to a hyperextension deformity of the metacarpophalangeal (MCP) joints due to unopposed extension through the extrinsic finger extensors.
- The Bouvier test is used to assess if the extensor mechanism is functioning normally. The patient's MCP hyperextension is blocked and then he or she is asked to extend their PIP joints **(FIG 3)**.
  - If the MCP flexion facilitates the patient's active PIP joint extension, the test is positive and the claw is defined as "simple," because by procedures to keep the MCP joints flexed, the PIP joints can extend via the extrinsic extensor tendons. However, the word "simple" is a misnomer because other than fusion of the MCP joints in flexion, all the soft tissue procedures applied to flex the MCP joints will stretch out over time.
  - If the patient cannot extend their PIP joints, the test is negative and the claw is "complex." Etiologies of a complex claw include central slip attenuation, central slip adherence to the PIP joint, and volar subluxation of the lateral bands.

IMAGING

- If the patient's clinical history is suspicious for arthritis, plain radiographs are taken of the hand and wrist to assess the joints. Painful arthritic MCP and IP joints are better reconstructed with arthrodesis than with soft tissues procedures such as tendon transfers. Wrist arthrodesis is typically avoided to maintain wrist tenodesis.

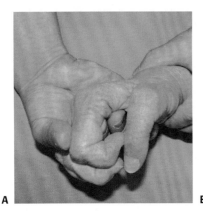
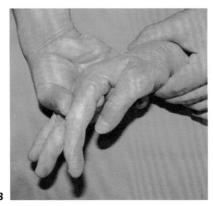

FIG 3 • The Bouvier test is used to assess the extensor tendon mechanism in claw hand deformities. **A.** The examiner holds the MCP joints in flexion to passively correct the MCP hyperextension deformity. **B.** The patient is then asked to extend the PIP joints. If the patient is able to extend, the extensor mechanism is functioning properly and the claw is designated "simple," as shown here. If the patient cannot extend the PIP joints, the claw is designated "complex."

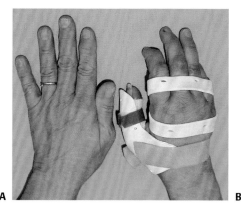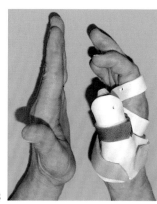

FIG 4 • Thermoplastic splints can be used to correct a claw hand deformity and unopposed thumb extension in combined median and ulnar nerve injuries. Here, the anticlaw splint corrects the patient's simple claw; correcting her MCP hyperextension permits active extension of her IP joints. The dorsal blocking thumb splint prevents the hyperextension deformity of the thumb at the carpometacarpal, MCP, and IP joints. **A** **B**

- Electrodiagnostic studies can be used to assess recovery following incomplete nerve injuries and after nerve repair to aid in planning for tendon transfers.
  - Donor muscles can be tested if there is concern of their integrity. Donor muscles lose one medical research council grade of strength when transferred; grade 5 muscles are normal strength and are preferred as donors.

NONOPERATIVE MANAGEMENT

- Hand therapy is essential to maintain supple joints prior to reconstruction. A tendon transfer will not restore active ROM if the joint is stiff and incomplete passive ROM is present.
  - Passive ROM should be optimized prior to surgery.
  - If necessary, joint contracture release is performed prior to tendon transfer.
- Patients can be taught how to use wrist tenodesis to improve their hand function.
  - Wrist flexion and extension can increase the amplitude of finger extension and flexion by 2.5 cm, respectively.[1]
- Preoperative splinting can be used correct a patient's thumb and finger MCP joint hyperextension following a combined median and ulnar nerve injury (**FIG 4**).
  - If the patient finds the splints helpful, surgical intervention—including thumb MCP arthrodesis and index, middle, ring, and small finger MCP volar capsulodesis or arthrodesis—is indicated.

SURGICAL MANAGEMENT

- Tension of the tendon transfer is critical for restoration of function while preventing the loss of ROM of other joints. In general, when suturing the tendon transfer, the joints as positioned as though the donor muscle is contracting and the transferred tendon is secured under tension.
- To minimize rupture rates, tendon transfers are best secured using three Pulvertaft weaves.[4] The donor tendon is divided distally and the recipient tendon is divided proximally to facilitate adequate tendon weaving.
- The tendon transfer tension is set with one Pulvertaft weave and then wrist tenodesis is checked to ensure adequate passive ROM. Adjustments in tension can be made with the second and third Pulvertaft weaves.
- Tendon transfers can be performed in an end-to-end or end-to-side fashion.

- End-to-end suturing facilitates a direct line of pull and is used if the recipient tendon is not expected to have any spontaneous recovery, for example, after complete denervation from an unrepaired nerve transection.
- If the nerve has been repaired and some muscle recovery is expected, the tendon transfer is performed in an end-to-side fashion to augment existing function.
- A direct line of pull maximizes the power of the tendon transfer. If a direction change is unavoidable, the tendon should be passed around a fixed structure that behaves as a pulley, for example, the EIP tendon around the distal ulna to abduct the thumb.

Preoperative Planning

- When selecting a tendon for transfer, any resulting weakness must be considered. One tendon must remain intact to perform the donor's original function.
- Tendon gliding occurs best in a supple, stable soft tissue bed. If needed, scar contracture releases and flap reconstruction are performed prior to tendon transfers to permit optimal tendon gliding and to minimize tendon adhesions.
- A stable platform with adequate bone and joint stability is required prior to tendon transfer. If required, arthrodesis of select joints is performed prior to tendon transfer.
  - A thumb MCP arthrodesis can be helpful to correct severe thumb hyperextension following the loss of thumb flexion in a median nerve palsy. The MCP is fused in 15 to 20 degrees of flexion and 15 degrees of pronation using headless compression screws, a dorsal plate, or tension band wiring.
- Wrist fusion permits all three wrist extensors (ECRL, ECRB, ECU) to be harvested for transfer; however, this is not typically recommended because it will eliminate wrist tenodesis, which augments the excursion of the remaining tendons.

Positioning

- The patient is positioned supine with the arm extended on a hand table.
- A tourniquet is placed on the upper arm.

Approach

- Loupe magnification is helpful. Incisions are planned prior to inflation of the tourniquet.
- We prefer to use 3-0 polyester suture for our tendon transfers. Two sutures are placed to secure each Pulvertaft weave.

■ Low Combined Median and Ulnar Nerve Palsy

Thumb Opposition

- In a low combined median and ulnar nerve injury, the ADM is denervated, but the FDS, PL, and EIP maintain their innervation and can be used as donor tendons for an opponensplasty. Only the EIP is available in high combined median and ulnar nerve palsies.
- The EIP is our preferred tendon transfer. It has minimal donor-site morbidity and has sufficient length to reach the APB insertion without a tendon graft.
- If the EIP is being used to restore another function of the hand following a low median nerve injury, the ring finger FDS is our second choice for an opponensplasty.
- The ADM is only transferred in cases of congenital hypoplastic thumb or in combined median and radial nerve injuries.

- The PL is primarily used as an adjunct in elderly patients with severe carpal tunnel syndrome and thenar wasting. This tendon transfer provides more thumb abduction than true opposition.

Low Injury: Ring Finger FDS to APB Tendon Transfer

- The FDS is harvested and retrieved via transverse incisions first at the base of the proximal phalanx and then proximal to the carpal tunnel.
- A pulley is created by passing the FDS through a window in the transverse carpal ligament to reroute it obliquely across the palm.
- The FDS is secured to the APB at its insertion on the radial base of the proximal phalanx of the thumb.

Low or High Injury: EIP to APB Tendon Transfer

- The EIP is divided distally over the dorsal index finger MCP joint using a transverse or a V-shaped incision (**TECH FIG 1A**).

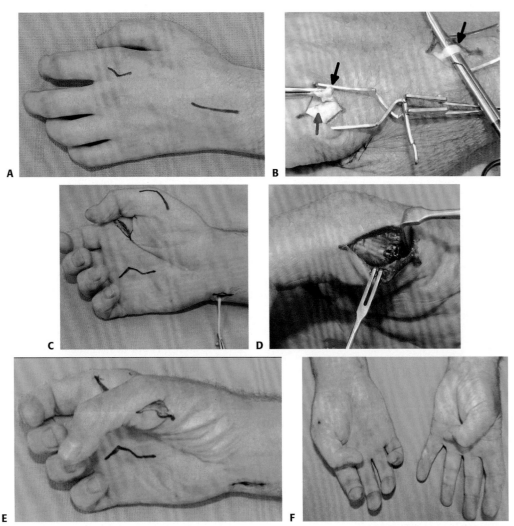

TECH FIG 1 • A. Two incisions are used over the dorsal hand and wrist for EIP harvest. The EIP is first identified over the index finger MCP joint using a transverse or a V-shaped incision. Next, it is identified over the dorsal wrist through a longitudinal incision distal to the extensor retinaculum. **B.** The EIP (*black arrows*) is divided for transfer over the index finger MCP joint. It is located ulnar to the EDC tendon (*red arrow*) in most patients. Next, it is retrieved over the dorsal wrist. **C.** The EIP is rerouted around the ulnar wrist, proximal to the pisiform, and then tunneled subcutaneously to the APB insertion on the radial base of the proximal phalanx of the thumb. **D.** The EIP is secured to the APB tendon at its insertion using three Pulvertaft weaves secured with 3-0 polyester suture. **E,F.** The position of the right thumb is improved following opponensplasty, shown here at the end of the surgery (**E**) and at the 2-month follow-up visit (**F**).

- The EIP is located ulnar to the EDC in most patients (**TECH FIG 1B**); anatomic variations of the EIP and EDC over the MCP joint exist in 19% of patients.[5]
  - The distal stump of the EIP can be sutured end to side to the index finger EDC tendon to prevent an extensor lag of the index finger.
- The EIP is retrieved over the distal wrist, using a longitudinal incision distal to the extensor retinaculum (**TECH FIG 1B**)
- It is then rerouted around the ulnar side of the hand, superficial to the FCU, using an incision proximal to the pisiform (**TECH FIG 1C**).
- After placement through the pulley, the EIP is tunneled through the subcutaneous tissue of the palm, volar to the neurovascular structures, to the APB tendon on the radial base of the proximal phalanx of the thumb.
- The EIP is sutured into the APB with the wrist in neutral and the thumb maximally palmarly abducted (**TECH FIG 1D–F**).
  - Setting tension is unnecessary because the EIP will barely reach the APB; wrist flexion may be required to suture the tendon in place.
  - After the tendon juncture has healed, the wrist is slowly brought to neutral position.

Thumb Adduction: ECRB to AdP With Tendon Graft

- Thumb adduction and pinch can be restored by transferring a tendon to the adductor pollicis (AdP) near its insertion on the ulnar base of the proximal phalanx of the thumb.
- The FDS from the ring finger or the ECRB are commonly transferred; the ECRB must be extended using a tendon graft to reach the AdP.

Low Injury: FDS to AdP Tendon Transfer

- In low median and ulnar nerve injuries, the FDS to the ring finger can be transferred to the AdP. The FDP to the ring finger is intact in these injuries and maintains finger flexion.
- The FDS is divided distal to the A1 pulley using an incision over the volar base of the ring finger proximal phalanx.
- The FDS is then retrieved through a second incision ulnar to the thenar crease at the base of the palm and is passed to the AdP insertion subcutaneously and sutured to the AdP through a third incision over the ulnar base of the thumb proximal phalanx.
- Tension is set with the wrist in neutral, the thumb adducted against the index finger, and the FDS at its resting length (**TECH FIG 2**).[6]

Low or High Injury: ECRB to AdP Tendon Transfer

- The ECRB is divided at its insertion over the dorsal base of the middle finger metacarpal.
- Using a second incision proximal to the extensor retinaculum, the ECRB is retrieved proximally.
- A third incision is used to expose the AdP over the ulnar base of the proximal phalanx of the thumb.
- A tendon graft is secured to the AdP and then passed through the intermetacarpal space between the index and middle finger metacarpals from the volar to the

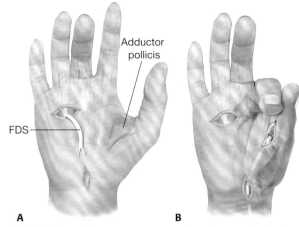

TECH FIG 2 • The ring finger FDS tendon is harvested at the base of the finger **(A)** and then rerouted for transfer to the adductor pollicis tendon on the ulnar proximal phalanx of the thumb **(B)** to restore thumb adduction following an ulnar nerve injury.

dorsal hand using a fourth incision longitudinally over the proximal third of the second intermetacarpal space.
  - This graft is passed deep to the flexor tendons and superficial to the AdP.
- The tendon graft is secured to the distal ECRB over the dorsal wrist with the wrist in neutral and the thumb adducted against the index finger (**TECH FIG 3**).

Index Finger Abduction: APL to First Dorsal Interosseous With Tendon Graft

- In 84% of people, the APL tendon has multiple tendinous slips[7]; up to 14 slips have been recorded.[8] An accessory slip of APL can be harvested as a donor tendon in patients with multiple slips. In the 16% of patients with a single APL tendon, half of the APL tendon can be harvested longitudinally for transfer.
- A slip of the APL can be transferred to the first dorsal interosseous (DIO) tendon near its insertion on the radial index finger metacarpal to restore index finger abduction for pinch.
- A tendon graft is required for the APL to reach the first DIO tendon (**TECH FIG 4**).
  - The palmaris longus, plantaris, extensor digitorum longus (to the second, third, or fourth toes), or flexor digitorum longus (to the second, third, fourth, or fifth toes) can be used as a tendon graft.

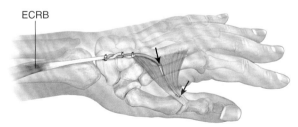

TECH FIG 3 • Thumb adduction can be restored by transferring the ECRB to the adductor pollicis near its insertion on the ulnar base of the proximal phalanx of the thumb (*red arrow*) using a tendon graft. The graft first secured distally, passed through the second intermetacarpal space (*black arrow*), and then secured to the ECRB tendon proximally.

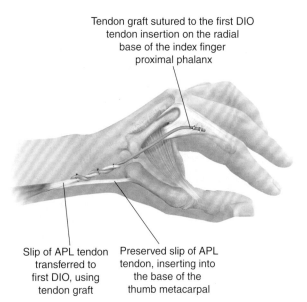

Tendon graft sutured to the first DIO
tendon insertion on the radial
base of the index finger
proximal phalanx

Slip of APL tendon
transferred to
first DIO, using
tendon graft

Preserved slip of APL
tendon, inserting into
the base of the
thumb metacarpal

TECH FIG 4 • To restore index finger abduction and pinch, a slip of the APL is transferred to the first DIO. A tendon graft is necessary for the APL to reach the insertion of the first DIO on the radial base of the index finger proximal phalanx.

- A slip of APL is harvested from its insertion on the radial aspect of the thumb metacarpal base using a longitudinal or V-shaped incision.
- A midlateral incision is made over the radial base of the index finger proximal phalanx to identify the first DIO.
- The tendon graft is secured to the first DIO and then passed proximally over the dorsal hand in the subcutaneous tissues to the proximal incision, where it is secured to the APL tendon.

Finger Clawing: FDS (Low Injury) or ECRL (High Injury) Tendon Transfer to the Lateral Bands of the Index, Middle, Ring, and Small Fingers

- For a simple claw, MCP joint hyperextension can be treated via static procedures such as volar MCP capsulodesis (the volar plate is detached and advanced proximally and secured with a bone anchor to the volar metacarpal to maintain the MCP in 45 degrees of flexion) (**TECH FIG 5**) or the Zancolli lasso (the FDS is divided over the distal proximal phalanx, removed from under the A2 pulley, turned proximally volar to the A1 pulley, and sutured to itself over the MCP joint).

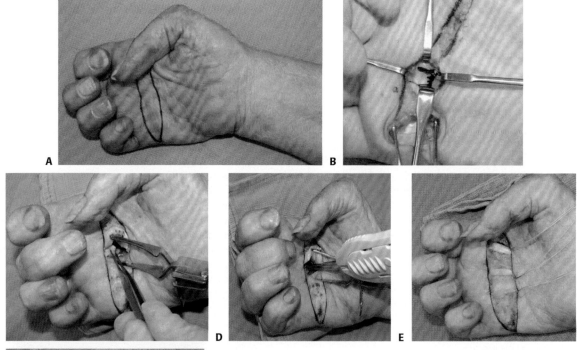

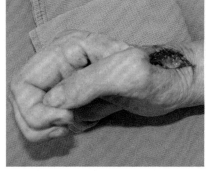

TECH FIG 5 • **A.** This patient had a simple claw identified using the Bouvier test. MCP volar capsulodesis was performed for the index, middle, ring, and small fingers to correct the MCP hyperextension deformity. A volar incision was made over the volar MCP heads. The excess skin was marked for resection here. **B.** The index finger volar plate is shown here, with its proximal extent outlined with a purple marker. **C.** The proximal volar plate was elevated and then advanced proximally and secured to the metacarpal using a bone anchor to maintain the MCP in 45 degrees of flexion to correct the MCP claw hyperextension deformity. **D.** One bone anchor was used to secure each proximal volar plate proximally to the volar metacarpal. The four bone anchors were placed (**E**), and then each volar plate was advanced proximally and secured using the bone anchor suture to hold the MCP joints in 45 degrees of flexion (**F**).

- Restoration of MCP joint flexion in a simple claw permits the patient to extend their IP joints through their extrinsic extensors (EDC, EIP, EDM). The main drawback of these soft tissues procedures is their tendency to stretch out over time.
- Our recommended long-term solution is to fuse the MCPJ in flexion (**TECH FIG 6**) or to perform a dynamic tendon transfer.
- In a complex claw, both MCP joint flexion and IP joint extension reconstruction are required. A dynamic tendon transfer is used. A four-tailed middle finger FDS (low injury) or ECRL (low or high injury) is commonly used as donor tendon for transfer in complex, and simple, claw hands.

- If used, the ECRL must be extended with a tendon graft to enable it to reach the clawed digits.
- Tendon transfers in a simple claw are inserted into the A2 pulley to restore MCP joint flexion only.
- In a complex claw, the insertion is into the lateral bands over the proximal phalanx to restore both MCP joint flexion and IP joint extension.
- The tendon is passed from the distal palm, volar to the deep transverse metacarpal ligament, to the lateral bands of the affected digits.
- The tendon is secured to the ulnar lateral band for the index finger and to the radial lateral band for the middle, ring, and small finger.

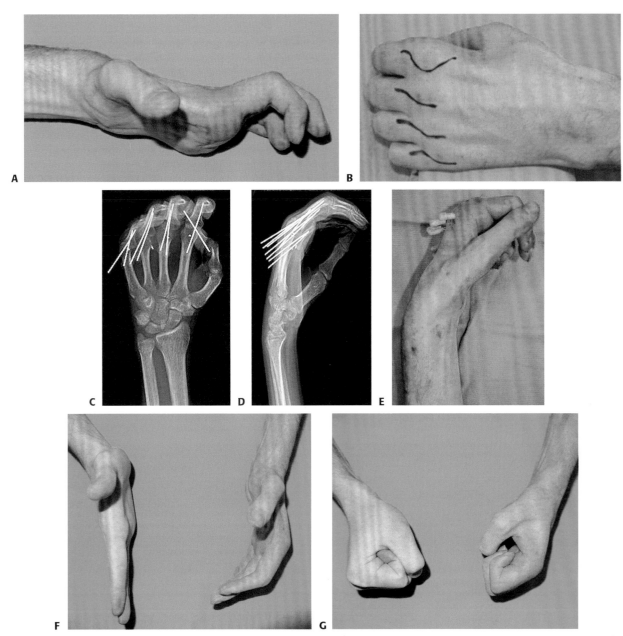

TECH FIG 6 • A. To correct this patient's simple claw deformity of his index, middle, ring, and small fingers following a combined high median and ulnar nerve injury, MCP joint fusions were performed. The MCP joints could be passively flexed, but not actively. **B.** Dorsal incisions were used over the MCP joints. Two K-wires were used to fuse each of the patient's MCP joints in 45 degrees of flexion, as shown here on the PA radiograph **(C)**, lateral radiograph **(D)**, and lateral clinical photograph **(E)**. The K-wires were removed 8 weeks postoperatively. The patient's MCP hyperextension deformity was corrected with MCP joint arthrodesis of the left index, middle, ring, and small fingers, shown here 4 months postoperatively with the fingers in extension **(F)** and flexion **(G)**.

Small Finger Abduction (Wartenburg Sign) Correction: EDM Tendon Transfer

- In a low median and ulnar nerve palsy, the abduction deformity of the small finger occurs due to the ulnar pull of the EDM on the small finger without opposition due to the deinnervation of the third palmar interosseous.
- To correct the ulnar deviation of the small finger, the ulnar half of the EDM is divided from its insertion on the dorsal proximal phalanx of the small finger and then passed volar to the deep transverse intermetacarpal ligament from the dorsal to the volar hand.
- If there is no clawing, the EDM can be sutured to the insertion of the radial collateral ligament of the small finger MCP joint.
- If there is clawing of the small finger, the EDM tendon is passed under the A2 pulley and sutured back to itself to correct the MCP hyperextension deformity.

■ High Combined Median and Ulnar Nerve Palsy

Thumb Flexion: BR to FPL Tendon Transfer

- To restore flexion of the thumb, the BR, ECRL, or ECRB can be transferred to the FPL.
  - We prefer to use the BR, it is the most expendable of these three tendons; its harvest results in minimal donor-site morbidity. This reserves the ECRL for transfer to the FDP for finger flexion and maintains the ECRB as the only remaining wrist extensor.
  - The ECRB is the preferred wrist extensor to preserve because it is the most centrally located over the dorsal wrist.
  - Preserving the ECRL only can lead to radial deviation of the wrist with extension. Similarly, preserving only the ECU can lead to ulnar deviation in extension.
- To transfer the BR, an incision is made over the volar-radial distal radius to identify the insertion of the BR onto the radial styloid as well as the FPL (**TECH FIG 7A**).
- The BR tendon is harvested distally with a 2-cm periosteal extension from the distal radius to increase its length (**TECH FIG 7B**).
- The superficial branch of the radial nerve must be carefully protected; this nerve is the only source of sensation to the hand in patients with combined median and ulnar nerve injures.
- The BR is freed proximally off of the radius to maximize its excursion, moved volarly, and secured to the FPL proximal to the carpal tunnel (**TECH FIG 7C**).

- The tendon transfer tension is set with the elbow flexed at 90 degrees, the wrist in 20 degrees of extension, the forearm fully pronated, and the thumb pulp and PIPJ of the index finger opposed.[9]
- The position of the elbow affects the degree of thumb flexion once the transfer has healed. When the elbow is extended, thumb flexion is stronger than when the elbow is flexed.

Finger Flexion: ECRL to FDP Tendon Transfer

- To restore finger flexion, the ECRL can be transferred to the FDP around the radial side of the wrist.
- An incision is made over the dorsal base of the index finger metacarpal to expose the ECRL insertion (**TECH FIG 8A**).
- The ECRL is divided near its insertion and then rerouted subcutaneously around the radial border of the forearm and sutured into the four FDP tendons proximal to the carpal tunnel using a second incision (**TECH FIG 8B**).
- The tendon transfer is secured to restore the flexion cascade of the digits; the tension is set progressively tighter from the index to the small finger.

Forearm Pronation: Rerouting the Brachioradialis Tendon

- Forearm pronation is lost following a high median nerve injury.
- To re-establish pronation, the biceps tendon insertion can be rerouted around the neck of the radius.[10] Alternatively, the BR can be rerouted and the interosseous membrane can be released if tight.[11]

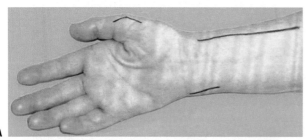

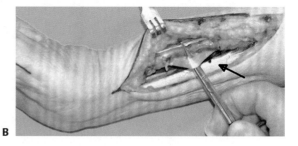

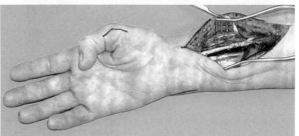

TECH FIG 7 • A. In a patient with a high median nerve injury, an incision is designed over the volar-radial distal radius to identify the BR, FPL, and FDP. The BR is transferred to the FPL to restore thumb flexion. **B.** The ECRL (isolated on scissors) is identified for transfer to the FDP for finger flexion. (Pulling the ECRL causes wrist extension.) The BR (*arrow*) is identified for transfer to the FPL to restore thumb flexion. **C.** The BR is secured to the FPL proximal to the carpal tunnel, restoring thumb flexion.

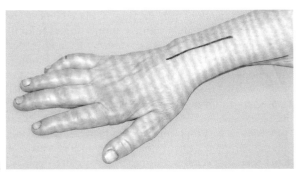
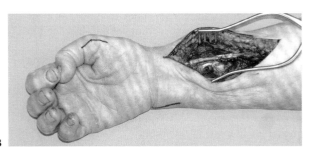

TECH FIG 8 • A. Over the dorsal wrist, an incision is made to identify the ECRL. The ECRL is rerouted around the radial wrist and transferred to the FDP to restore finger flexion. **B.** The ERCL is secured to the FDP, restoring flexion of the index, middle, ring, and small fingers.

- We prefer to reroute the BR, it is less technically challenging than biceps rerouting and it provides greater active pronation than other techniques.
  - Biceps rerouting can cause an elbow flexion contracture.
- To reroute the BR, an incision is made over the volar distal third of the radius. The BR is elevated off the radius at its distal insertion and elevated proximally. It is extended 5 cm distally using Z-lengthening.
- The BR is then passed between the radius and ulna through the interosseous membrane, proximal to the pronator teres, from volar and ulnar to dorsal and radial.
- The elbow is placed in 90 degrees of flexion and the forearm is fully pronated. The BR tendon is secured to the dorsoradial distal third of the radius (**TECH FIG 9**).

Sensory Nerve Transfers

- In combined median and ulnar nerve injuries, all volar hand sensation is lost.
- To restore protective sensation, a branch of the superficial radial nerve can be transferred to the distal median nerve.
- Alternatively, a first dorsal metacarpal artery flap can be used to provide sensation to the volar thumb. A branch of the superficial branch of the radial nerve is contained within this innervated flap.

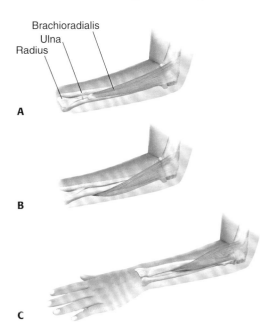

TECH FIG 9 • To restore forearm pronation, the BR can be rerouted around the radius. **A.** The BR tendon is extended 5 cm distally using Z-lengthening. The BR is elevated distally from its insertion on the radius, passed through the interosseous membrane **(B)**, and then secured to the dorsoradial radius with the elbow flexed 90 degrees and the forearm in full pronation **(C)**.

PEARLS AND PITFALLS

Physical findings	■ Creating a chart is helping in determining an individualized surgical plan. The patient's main subjective functional complaints are listed in the first column. In the second column, the patient's objective physical examination deficits are listed. In the third column, the patient's intact, innervated tendons are documented; these are further classified into expendable tendons available for transfer and nonexpendable tendons that must be preserved to prevent donor-site morbidity. ■ The donor tendons are then matched to the functional deficits and the surgical plan is reviewed with the patient. ■ It is beneficial for the patient to meet with a hand therapist prior to tendon transfer surgery for preoperative teaching; rehabilitation protocols and expectations are reviewed.
Technique	■ Proper intraoperative tension setting and postoperative immobilization are necessary to optimize the outcomes of tendon transfers. ■ Wide-awake surgery using local anesthesia can facilitate intraoperative assessment of the tendon transfer tension.
Postoperative	■ The joints crossed by the tendon transfer are immobilized for 4 wk. ■ ROM exercises for the shoulder and unaffected joints of the upper extremity should be resumed immediately postoperatively to minimize stiffness.
Therapy	■ Some authors advocate for early active ROM exercises following tendon transfers secured with 3 Pulvertaft weaves to minimize adhesions. In these cases, tendon gliding exercises are started on postoperative day 2 under the guidance of a hand therapist.[12]

POSTOPERATIVE CARE

- Following a tendon transfer, we prefer to immobilize the affected joints for 4 weeks to permit tension-free tendon healing; casting or splinting is used.
- Above elbow immobilization is used in transfers crossing the elbow. For example, for the BR to FPL transfer, immobilization holds the elbow in 90 degrees of flexion and the wrist slightly flexed or in neutral. Following tendon transfers to correct clawing, the MCP joints are immobilized in flexion and the IP joints in extension.
- ROM exercises are started 4 weeks postoperatively, starting with active ROM and followed by passive ROM. Mobilizing one joint at a time minimizes tension on the tendon transfer.
- 6 weeks postoperatively, muscle retraining and resistance exercises begin.
- 8 weeks following surgery, strengthening exercises begin and splints are weaned.
- At 12 weeks postoperatively, free unrestricted activity can be resumed.

OUTCOMES

- The balance of the flexors and extensors of the hand and wrist is critical for optimal function.
- The transfer of radial nerve-innervated hand and wrist extensors to restore hand and wrist flexion aids in restoring the function of the hand by re-establishing active hand and wrist flexion while weakening hand and wrist extension, improving the overall balance of the hand and wrist.

COMPLICATIONS

- Thorough discussion with the patient, careful physical examination, and thoughtful planning are required to optimize the function of the upper extremity following combined median and ulnar nerve injuries.
- The patient is counseled that his or her volar and dorsoulnar hand will remain insensate following tendon transfers. Worse outcomes are seen in patients with decreased sensation compared to those with intact sensation. Following sensory nerve injury, visual and auditory cues are required to permit the patient to use their injured hand; tactile sensory feedback is absent. Sensory nerve transfers can be performed to restore protective sensation. Ideally, nerve repair at the time of the injury is performed to permit motor and sensory recovery over time.

- Transferred tendons can rupture if placed under excess tension, if inadequately sutured during surgery, and if not sufficiently immobilized after surgery. If rupture occurs, immediate exploration and primary repair are recommended.
- Adhesions frequently form where tendons cross each other and in scarred tissue beds. Frequent, intensive hand therapy is used to optimize passive ROM in these cases. If passive ROM exceeds active ROM, a tenolysis may be beneficial. Tenolysis is performed no sooner than 3 months following the tendon transfer. Patient compliance is critical; daily hand therapy exercises are started 2 days after tenolysis to maintain intraoperative active ROM gains.
- Multiple long incisions are used for tendon transfers; patients must be counseled about postoperative scarring prior to reconstruction. Postoperatively, scar massage and sun avoidance are recommended for scar management.

REFERENCES

1. Erdem HR, Ergun S, Erturk C, Ozel S. Electrophysiological evaluation of the incidence of martin-gruber anastomosis in healthy subjects. *Yonsei Med J.* 2002;43(3):291-295.
2. Kazakos KJ, Smyrnis A, Xarchas KC, et al. Anastomosis between the median and ulnar nerve in the forearm: an anatomic study and literature review. *Acta Orthop Belg.* 2005;71(1):29-35.
3. Kimura I, Ayyar DR, Lippmann SM. Electrophysiological verification of the ulnar to median nerve communications in the hand and forearm. *Tohoku J Exp Med.* 1983;141(3):269-274.
4. Pulvertaft RG. Suture materials and tendon junctures. *Am J Surg.* 1965;109:346-352.
5. Gonzalez MH, Weinzweig N, Kay T, Grindel S. Anatomy of the extensor tendons to the index finger. *J Hand Surg [Am].* 1996;21(6):988-991.
6. Jones NF, Machado GR. Tendon transfers for radial, median, and ulnar nerve injuries: current surgical techniques. *Clin Plast Surg.* 2011;38(4):621-642.
7. Coleman SS, McAfee DK, Anson BJ. The insertion of the abductor pollicis longus muscle; an anatomical study of 175 specimens. *Q Bull Northwest Univ Med Sch.* 1953;27(2):117-122.
8. Thwin SS, Fazlin F, Than M. Multiple variations of the tendons of the anatomical snuffbox. *Singapore Med J.* 2014;55(1):37-40.
9. Fridén J, Reinholdt C, Gohritz A, et al. Simultaneous powering of forearm pronation and key pinch in tetraplegia using a single muscle-tendon unit. *J Hand Surg Eur Vol.* 2012;37(4):323-328.
10. Zancolli EA. Paralytic supination contracture of the forearm. *J Bone Joint Surg Am.* 1967;49(7):1275-1284.
11. Ozkan T, Aydin A, Ozer K, et al. A surgical technique for pediatric forearm pronation: brachioradialis rerouting with interosseous membrane release. *J Hand Surg [Am].* 2004;29:22-27.
12. Sultana SS, MacDermid JC, Grewal R, Rath S. The effectiveness of early mobilization after tendon transfers in the hand: a systematic review. *J Hand Ther.* 2013;26(1):1-20.

Distal Anterior Interosseous Nerve Transfer to Motor Branch of Ulnar Nerve

Shelley S. Noland and Jason H. Ko

DEFINITION

- Ulnar nerve palsy severely limits hand function with loss of dexterity, pinch and grip strength weakness, and claw formation.
- Ulnar-innervated intrinsic muscle recovery after high ulnar nerve injury (above elbow) is poor.
- Distal transfer of the anterior interosseous nerve (AIN) to the motor component of the ulnar nerve can preserve motor endplates and restore motor function.

ANATOMY

- Ulnar nerve
  - After exiting the cubital tunnel, the ulnar nerve enters the forearm between the two heads of the flexor carpi ulnaris (FCU).
  - It travels between the FCU and flexor digitorum profundus (FDP) muscles and gives off the dorsal sensory branch 9 cm proximal to the wrist crease.
  - At the Guyon canal, it enters the hand and divides into the deep motor branch and the sensory branch.
  - Internal topographical anatomy

- Topographical anatomy is critical to the success of this procedure.
- The ulnar nerve has a discrete fascicular pattern.
- At the level of the mid-forearm, the three components are the ulnar-sided sensory component (dorsal sensory branch), the middle motor component (intrinsic motor function), and the radial-sided sensory component (digital ulnar sensation) (**FIG 1**).
- Median nerve
  - After exiting from underneath the lacertus fibrosus, the median nerve travels through the pronator teres.
  - It courses between the flexor digitorum superficialis (FDS) and the FDP and gives off four motor branches in the proximal forearm.
  - It enters the hand at the carpal tunnel and divides into the recurrent motor branch and sensory branches.
  - Anterior interosseous nerve
    - Branches from the median nerve 3 cm distal to the intercondylar line
    - Contains fascicles to the flexor pollicis longus (FPL), FDP (index and middle finger), and pronator quadratus (PQ)
    - Exits the median nerve on the dorsal radial aspect (**FIG 2**)

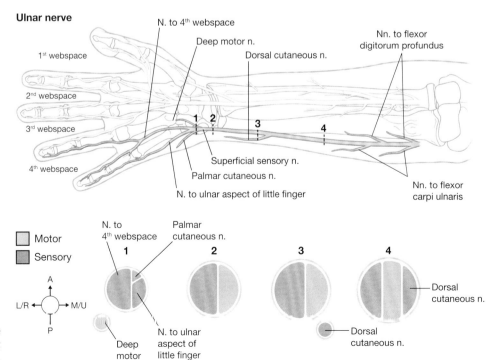

FIG 1 • Internal topography of the ulnar nerve. *A*, anterior; *P*, posterior; *L*, lateral; *R*, radial; *M*, medial; *U*, ulnar.

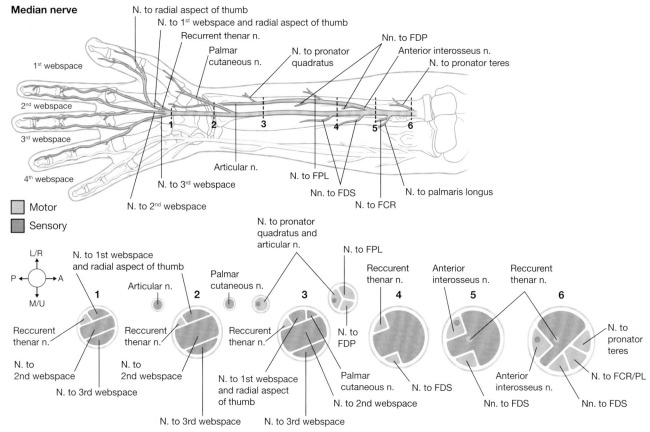

FIG 2 • Internal topography of the median nerve. *A*, anterior; *P*, posterior; *L*, lateral; *R*, radial; *M*, medial; *U*, ulnar.

PATIENT HISTORY AND PHYSICAL FINDINGS

- History
  - Elicit history of trauma, tumor, or other injury to the ulnar nerve or elbow.
  - Elicit location, timing, frequency, and duration of sensory symptoms including numbness and tingling. Elicit correlation with elbow flexion activities (driving, talking on the phone, sleeping).
  - Elicit complaints of weakness or "clumsiness" in the hands, particularly with regard to opening jars, turning door handles, and fine motor tasks.
  - Rule out other causes of symptoms such as cervical spine, shoulder, or brachial plexus issues.
- Physical Examination
  - Sensory disturbances typically involve the dorsal and volar ulnar palm, ulnar half of the ring finger, and small finger.
  - Perform full sensory exam of bilateral upper extremities documenting two-point discrimination and/or Semmes-Weinstein monofilament testing in all nerve distributions.
  - Perform full motor exam of bilateral upper extremities by documenting strength in relevant muscles, clawing of the fingers, intrinsic atrophy/wasting, and presence of Froment (thumb interphalangeal flexion with pinch) or Wartenberg signs (abducted posture of small finger).
  - Perform provocative maneuvers including elbow flexion test and compression at the Guyon canal.

IMAGING

- Obtain nerve conduction studies (NCS) and electromyography (EMG) to help with localization of lesion and to assess severity of ulnar neuropathy.
- NCS may demonstrate a conduction block at the cubital tunnel or Guyon canal.
- EMG can identify the presence and quality of fibrillations, positive sharp waves, and motor unit potentials.
- In setting of trauma, traditional x-rays are recommended to evaluate for fracture, dislocation, or foreign body.
- In setting of tumor, formal imaging studies such as CT or MRI are warranted as appropriate.

DIFFERENTIAL DIAGNOSIS (OPTIONAL)

- Cervical radiculopathy
- Cubital tunnel syndrome
- Guyon canal compression
- Shoulder injury
- Thoracic outlet syndrome
- Polyneuropathy
- Other systemic neuropathy

SURGICAL MANAGEMENT[1-3]

- Distal AIN to motor branch of ulnar nerve transfer should be considered in patients with isolated high ulnar nerve injuries or lesions (above elbow).
- Patient must have intact median nerve and AIN function.

Preoperative Planning

- Patient counseling regarding the timeline of recovery is critical (1 mm/d).
- Need to coordinate care with a hand or physical therapist for postoperative motor re-education.

Positioning

- The patient is positioned supine on operating table with the affected arm extended and supinated on an armboard.

Approach

- The entire procedure is completed through a single incision designed longitudinally or zigzag over the course of the FCU

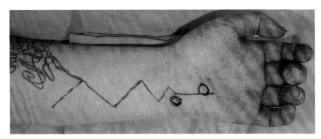

FIG 3 • Surgical approach for AIN to ulnar motor nerve transfer.

and ulnar neurovascular bundle in the distal 1/3 of the volar forearm (**FIG 3**).

TECHNIQUES

■ Distal Exposure Including Identification of the Motor Component of the Ulnar Nerve

- A longitudinal incision is made in the distal 1/3 of the volar forearm over the course of the flexor carpi ulnaris (FCU) and ulnar neurovascular bundle including a short zigzag segment across the wrist crease.
- The pisiform and hook of the hamate are marked, and a longitudinal incision between them is made to approach the Guyon canal. Sharply dissect the overlying fascia at the level of the wrist crease, exposing the ulnar neurovascular bundle.
- The ulnar neurovascular bundle is identified and retracted ulnarly.
- The deep motor branch is released by dividing the leading edge of the hypothenar musculature off of the hook of the hamate.
- The motor branch is then identified and traced proximally. Either manual or visual neurolysis can be

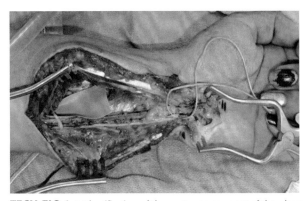

TECH FIG 1 • Identification of the motor component of the ulnar nerve (vessel loop).

performed to identify the motor component of the ulnar nerve 9 cm proximal to the wrist crease.
- The motor component of the ulnar nerve is marked with a vessel loop 9 cm proximal to the wrist crease (**TECH FIG 1**).

■ Proximal Exposure Including Identification of the Anterior Interosseous Nerve

- Through the same incision, identify the finger flexors and retract them radially to identify the pronator quadratus (PQ) muscle. Some muscle fibers of the flexor digitorum profundus (FDP) may have to be released to gain better visualization of the proximal PQ and anterior interosseous nerve (AIN).
- At the proximal edge of the PQ, identify the AIN entering the muscle.
- Carefully divide the PQ with bipolar cautery for 1 to 2 cm (proximal to distal) superficial to the AIN to maximize AIN length for transfer (**TECH FIG 2**).
- Divide the AIN distally just prior to its branching point, which is typically at the halfway point of the PQ.

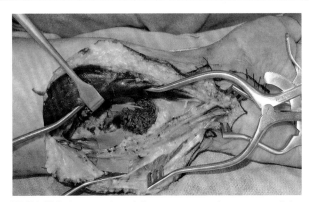

TECH FIG 2 • Division of the pronator quadratus to reveal the distal extent of the AIN (upper *blue* background).

■ End-to-End Transfer of the AIN to the Motor Component of the Ulnar Nerve

- Transfer the AIN ulnarly across the PQ to the ulnar nerve 9 cm proximal to the wrist crease (**TECH FIG 3A**).
- Ensure adequate length to perform transfer with no tension.
- Divide the motor component of the ulnar nerve as proximally as necessary to ensure adequate length to perform transfer with no tension.

- Intrafascicular dissection of the ulnar motor fascicle distally will allow for a tension-free coaptation.
- Perform neurorrhaphy with a microscope using 9-0 nylon suture (**TECH FIG 3B**).
- Evaluate the neurorrhaphy site while performing a full pronation-supination arc to ensure no tension at any forearm position.
- Close skin in standard fashion, and either a soft dressing or volar wrist splint is placed.

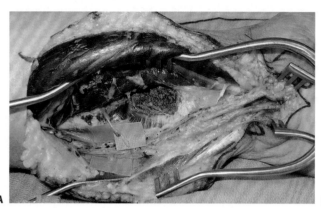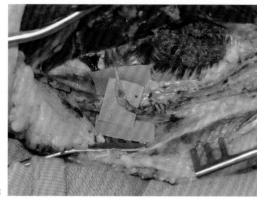

TECH FIG 3 • **A.** Division of the AIN. **B.** End-to-end neurorrhaphy of AIN to motor component of ulnar nerve.

■ Reverse End-to-Side AIN to Ulnar Motor Nerve Transfer[4]

- Consider reverse end-to-side transfer in patients in whom ulnar nerve recovery is ultimately expected. Also, in high ulnar nerve injuries where distal intrinsic recovery is possible, the distal reverse end-to-side AIN nerve transfer can be performed to help "babysit" the motor endplates in the hand until the more proximal regenerating axons can reach the hand.
- When performing a reverse end-to-side nerve transfer, the skin incision should be longer, and the ulnar nerve exposure should be more proximal. To obtain a tension-free reverse end-to-side nerve transfer, the AIN will have

to be transferred more proximally to reach the ulnar nerve than in an end-to-end transfer.
- Instead of dividing the ulnar motor component, create epineurial and perineurial windows in the motor component of the ulnar nerve.
- Transfer the AIN to this epineurial/perineurial window ensuring no tension.
- Perform neurorrhaphy of the AIN to the side of the ulnar motor component with a microscope using 9-0 nylon suture (**TECH FIG 4**).
- Evaluate the neurorrhaphy site while performing a full pronation-supination arc to ensure no tension at any forearm position.
- Close skin in standard fashion, and either a soft dressing or volar wrist splint is placed.

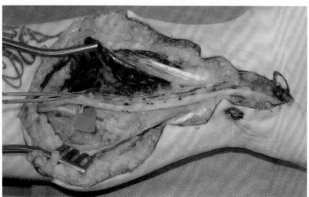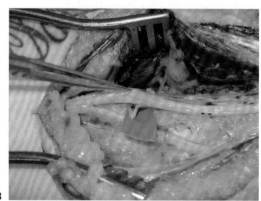

TECH FIG 4 • **A,B.** End-to-side neurorrhaphy of AIN to motor component of ulnar nerve.

PEARLS AND PITFALLS

Nerve transection	■ Remember that the Donor nerve (AIN) is always cut Distal and the recipient nerve (ulnar motor branch) is always cut proximal.
Guyon canal release	■ It is important to perform a full Guyon canal release to prevent a distal conduction block on the recovering nerve.
Reverse end-to-side transfer	■ Consider a reverse end-to-side transfer in patients in whom ulnar nerve recovery is ultimately expected.
Tension	■ Ensure no tension on neurorrhaphy site while observing a full pronation-supination arc.
Postoperative rehabilitation	■ Ensure that you have a hand therapist knowledgeable in motor re-education for optimal outcomes.

POSTOPERATIVE CARE

■ If a splint was used, the postoperative splint can be removed and gentle range of motion can be initiated 1 week after surgery.

■ Once postoperative pain has subsided at 3 to 4 weeks, the patient begins motor re-education under the care of a knowledgeable hand therapist.

OUTCOMES

■ There are limited outcomes data for this procedure, but most case series report return of intrinsic function within 1 year of surgery.

COMPLICATIONS

■ The most common complications are infection, bleeding, and lack of reinnervation of the intrinsic musculature.

REFERENCES

1. Haase SC, Chung KC. Anterior interosseous nerve transfer to the motor branch of the ulnar nerve for high ulnar nerve injuries. *Ann Plast Surg.* 2002;49(3):285-290.
2. Brown JM, Yee A, Mackinnon SE. Distal median to ulnar nerve transfers to restore ulnar motor and sensory function within the hand: technical nuances. *Neurosurgery.* 2009;65(5):966-977.
3. Novak CB, Mackinnon SE. Distal anterior interosseous nerve transfer to the deep motor branch of the ulnar nerve for reconstruction of high ulnar nerve injuries. *J Reconstr Microsurg.* 2002;18(6):459-464.
4. Davidge KM, Yee A, Moore AM, Mackinnon SE. The supercharge end-to-side anterior interosseous-to-ulnar motor nerve transfer for restoring intrinsic function: clinical experience. *Plast Reconstr Surg.* 2015;136(3):344e-352e.

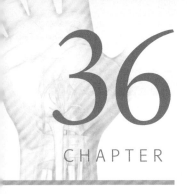

36
CHAPTER

Nerve Transfers for High Radial Nerve Palsy

Shelley S. Noland and Jason H. Ko

DEFINITION

- High radial nerve palsy limits hand and wrist function with loss of wrist, finger, and thumb extension.
- The presence of a wrist drop significantly decreases finger flexion power and grip strength.
- The inability to open the hand to initiate grasp makes tasks of manual dexterity difficult.
- Distal transfer of median-innervated nerve branches to branches of the radial nerve can preserve motor endplates and restore motor function.

ANATOMY

- Radial nerve
  - Originates from the posterior cord of the brachial plexus
  - Courses between the humerus and the triceps and innervates the triceps muscle
  - Travels in the spiral groove posterior to the humerus and exits through the lateral intermuscular septum about 10 cm proximal to the lateral epicondyle
  - Passes between the brachialis and brachioradialis (BR) and gives off the following branches:
    - BR muscle branch

- Extensor carpi radialis longus (ECRL) muscle branch (at the level of the interepicondylar line)
  - Enters the forearm by passing anterior to the lateral epicondyle and gives off the following branches (**FIG 1**):
    - Radial sensory nerve (RSN) branch, which courses underneath the BR
    - Extensor carpi radialis brevis (ECRB) muscle branch (about 3 cm distal to the interepicondylar line)
    - Supinator muscle branches (1–2; just proximal to the leading edge of the supinator)
  - Continues as the posterior interosseous nerve (PIN) and innervates all hand and wrist extensors
- Median nerve
  - Originates from the medial and lateral cords of the brachial plexus
  - Courses anterior and medial to the brachial artery
  - Travels between the brachialis muscle and the medial intermuscular septum
  - Gives off the pronator teres (PT) muscle branch at the level of the interepicondylar line
  - Courses under the lacertus fibrosus, through the superficial and deep heads of the (PT), and underneath the tendinous arch of the flexor digitorum superficialis (FDS) and gives off the following branches (see **FIG 1**):

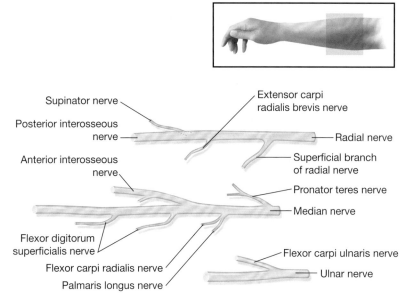

FIG 1 • Anatomy of the median and radial nerves in the forearm.

- FDS muscle branches (2–3) from the ulnar side of the median nerve
- Flexor carpi radialis (FCR) muscle branch
- Palmaris longus (PL) muscle branch (if PL is present)
- Anterior interosseous nerve (AIN) from the dorsal radial side of the nerve
  - Branches 3 cm distal to the intercondylar line
  - Contains fascicles to the flexor pollicis longus (FPL), flexor digitorum profundus (FDP; index and middle finger only), and pronator quadratus (PQ)
  - Palmar cutaneous branch in distal forearm
- Enters the hand at the carpal tunnel and divides into the recurrent motor branch and sensory branches

PATIENT HISTORY AND PHYSICAL FINDINGS

- History
  - Obtain history of trauma, tumor, or other injury to the affected extremity.
  - Ask location, timing, frequency, and duration of sensory symptoms including numbness and tingling.
  - Rule out other causes of symptoms such as cervical spine, shoulder, or brachial plexus issues.
  - Elicit a history of the etiology of the radial nerve palsy.
  - Determine the timeline of injury.
- Physical examination
  - Perform full motor exam of bilateral upper extremities.
  - Assess for a Tinel sign along the course of the radial nerve.
  - Perform a full motor and sensory examination of the entire affected extremity.
    - Determine the level of the injury.
      - If the patient has a wrist drop, it is likely a high radial nerve palsy occurring prior to the innervation of the ECRL and ECRB (**FIG 2**).
      - If the patient can extend the wrist, he or she likely has a PIN palsy with preservation of ECRL and ECRB function.
    - Perform full sensory exam of bilateral upper extremities documenting 2-point discrimination and/or Semmes-Weinstein monofilament testing in all nerve distributions.
      - Sensory disturbances in radial nerve lesions typically involve the dorsal radial aspect of the thumb and hand.
    - Ensure that the injury is isolated to the radial nerve.
      - Test and record function in your potential median-innervated donor nerves including branches to the FCR, FDS, and PL.
      - Test and record function in the median-innervated muscles that may need to be used for tendon transfers in the event there are no nerve transfer options including the PT, FCR, and PL.

IMAGING

- Obtain electrodiagnostic studies to assist with localization of the injury and to assess severity of the radial nerve palsy.

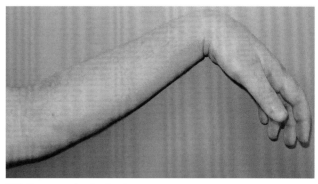

FIG 2 • Example of wrist drop.

- EMG can identify the presence and quality of fibrillations, positive sharp waves, and motor unit potentials. This can be followed over time to determine reinnervation status.
- In setting of trauma, traditional x-rays are recommended to evaluate for fracture, dislocation, or foreign body.
- In setting of tumor, formal imaging studies such as CT or MRI are warranted as appropriate.

SURGICAL MANAGEMENT[1-3]

- Patients should be monitored from the time of injury for reinnervation of wrist, finger, and thumb extensors.
- Patients with no evidence of clinical or electrical reinnervation at 6 to 9 months should be considered for nerve transfers. Alternatively, tendon transfers can be performed in a delayed fashion and will be discussed in Chapter 39 (**FIG 3**).
- The most common nerve transfers for high radial nerve palsy are
  - FCR to PIN
  - FDS to ECRB
  - Lateral antebrachial cutaneous nerve (LABC) to RSN
- Typically, there are redundant motor branches to the FCR and FDS, so using a single-donor nerve branch will still leave some function of the FCR and FDS, which can still be used to power a tendon transfer if the nerve transfer is not sufficient.

Preoperative Planning

- Patient counseling regarding the timeline of recovery after nerve transfers is critical (1 mm/d).
- Need to coordinate care with a hand or physical therapist for postoperative motor re-education

Positioning

- Patient is positioned supine with the arm extended on a hand table.
- Tourniquet can be used if donor exposure and identification can be accomplished within 30 to 40 minutes.
  - After 30 to 40 minutes, tourniquet neurapraxia may preclude the use of nerve stimulation.

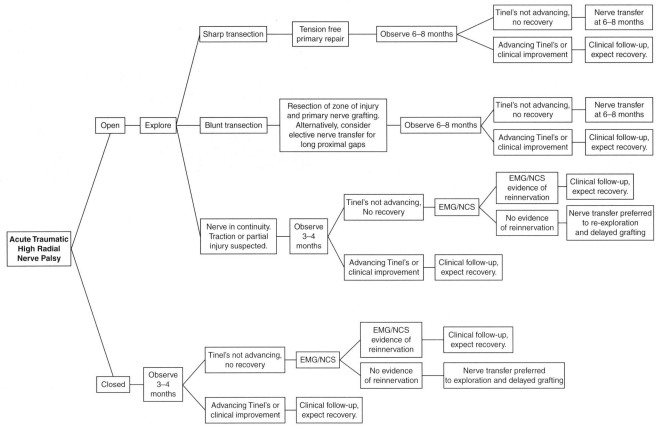

FIG 3 • Algorithm for the management of high radial nerve palsy. Reprinted from Pet MA, Lipira AB, Ko JH. Nerve transfers for the restoration of wrist, finger, and thumb extension after high radial nerve injury. *Hand Clin*. 2016;32(2):191-207 with permission.

■ Identification, Decompression, and Dissection of the Median Nerve

- A straight incision from the lateral antecubital fossa along the medial aspect of the BR to the midpoint of the forearm is utilized, which provides exposure of median and radial nerves (**TECH FIG 1A**).
- Identify and protect the LABC nerve that runs with the cephalic vein.
  - Identify and retract the BR to identify the RSN and radial vessels beneath (**TECH FIG 1B**). This provides visualization of the PT tendon.
- If PT to ECRB tendon transfer will be performed, the skin incision is extended distally to visualize the insertion of the PT on the radius.
  - The insertion of the PT is elevated with a strip of periosteum as distally as possible, and subperiosteal dissection is performed distal to proximal at this stage for later tendon transfer.
- Because it takes 6 to 9 months to begin to see motor recovery after these nerve transfers, the PT to ECRB

tendon transfer acts as an immediate treatment for wrist drop, which can be quite debilitating for patients.
  - This tendon transfer works well and acts as an internal splint until motor recovery occurs.
- If the PT to ECRB tendon transfer is not performed, step-lengthening of the PT tendon should be performed at this point.
  - This allows the superficial head of the PT to be reflected medially, exposing the deep head of the PT.
- Release the deep head of the PT to expose and decompress the median nerve in the proximal forearm.
- Identify and release the tendinous edge of the FDS to further decompress the median nerve and allow direct visualization of the nerve branches.
- Identify the median nerve and dissect it distally to identify the following branches (**TECH FIG 1C**):
  - PT, PL, FCR, FDS, AIN
  - Use of a nerve stimulator will help confirm branch identity.
  - It is helpful to loop each branch with a vessel loop in preparation for later transfer.

TECHNIQUES

TECHNIQUES

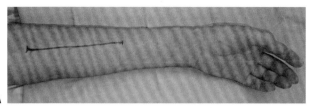

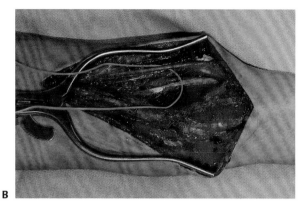

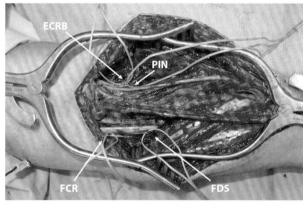

TECH FIG 1 • **A.** Approach for median to radial nerve transfers. **B.** Identification of radial sensory nerve. **C.** Identification of median nerve branches, including flexor carpi radialis (FCR) and flexor digitorum superficialis (FDS), along with radial nerve branches, including extensor carpi radialis brevis (ECRB) and posterior interosseous nerve (PIN).

■ Identification, Decompression, and Dissection of the Radial Nerve

- Retract the BR laterally and follow the RSN proximally until the main radial nerve is identified.
- Divide the transverse radial recurrent vessels that overlie the radial nerve ("leash of Henry").
- Dissect the radial nerve distally and identify the following branches (**TECH FIG 2**).
  - ECRB branch: This branch is small and directly radial to the RSN.

- PIN branch: This branch is larger and radial to the ECRB branch. This branch dives deep to the supinator muscle.
- Use of a nerve stimulator will help confirm branch identity.
- It is helpful to loop each branch with a vessel loop in preparation for later recipient of nerve transfer.
- Release the tendinous leading edge of ECRB and supinator muscles (arcade of Frohse).
  - This is important for maximal mobilization of recipient nerves.

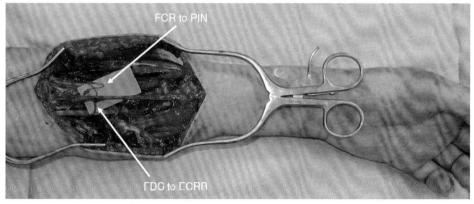

TECH FIG 2 • Coaptation of flexor carpi radialis (FCR) to posterior interosseous nerve (PIN) and flexor digitorum superficialis (FDS) to extensor carpi radialis brevis (ECRB) nerve transfers.

■ Mobilization and Transection of the Donor and Recipient Nerves

- Mobilize FCR, FDS, and LABC branches as distally as possible and transect them distally.

- This will facilitate a tension-free neurorrhaphy.
- Mobilize PIN, ECRB, and RSN branches as proximally as possible and transect them proximally.
  - This will facilitate a tension-free neurorrhaphy.

■ Transfer FCR to PIN

- Oppose the FCR (donor) and the PIN (recipient) to facilitate a tension-free repair (see **TECH FIG 2**).
- Perform end-to-end coaptation using a microscope and 9-0 nylon.

- May use two or three sutures followed by fibrin glue
  - This will minimize trauma and foreign body reaction.
- Perform complete wrist and elbow range of motion to confirm that no tension is present in any arm or wrist position.

■ Transfer of FDS to ECRB

- Oppose the FDS (donor) and the ECRB (recipient) to facilitate a tension-free repair (see **TECH FIG 2**).
- Perform end-to-end coaptation using a microscope and 9-0 nylon.

- May use two or three sutures followed by fibrin glue.
  - This will minimize trauma and foreign body reaction.
- Perform complete wrist and elbow range of motion to confirm that no tension is present in any position.

■ Transfer of LABC to RSN (Optional)

- Oppose the LABC (donor) and the RSN (recipient) to facilitate a tension-free repair (**TECH FIG 3**).
- Perform coaptation using a microscope and 9-0 nylon.
- May use two or three sutures followed by fibrin glue
  - This will minimize trauma and foreign body reaction.
- Perform complete wrist and elbow range of motion to confirm that no tension is present in any position.

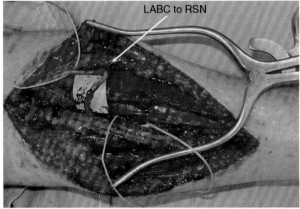

TECH FIG 3 • Example of lateral antebrachial cutaneous nerve (LABC) to radial sensory nerve (RSN) transfer.

■ Tendon Transfer of PT to ECRB (Optional)

- The ECRB tendon is identified in the surgical field.
- The previously elevated distal PT insertion with periosteal strip is identified and dissected proximally.
- An end-to-side tendon transfer of the PT to ECRB is performed using three or four Pulvertaft weaves and secured with 3-0 braided, nonabsorbable suture (**TECH FIG 4**).

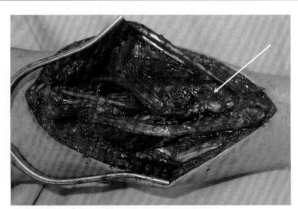

TECH FIG 4 • Example of pronator teres (PT) to extensor carpi radialis brevis (ECRB) tendon transfer (*arrow*).

PEARLS AND PITFALLS

Preservation of critical branches	▪ It is critical to preserve the pronator teres and anterior interosseous nerve branches during this operation.
Pronator teres step-lengthening	▪ This is critical to help with identifying the median nerve and its branches in the proximal forearm.
Decompression of involved nerve branches	▪ Decompression of involved nerves and branches facilitates axonal regeneration.
Nerve transection	▪ Remember that the *donor* nerve is always cut *distal* and the recipient nerve is always cut proximal.

POSTOPERATIVE CARE

- Immediately postoperatively, if no tendon transfer has been performed, a soft dressing is applied, allowing for free motion of the elbow, wrist, and fingers.
- If the PT to ECRB tendon transfer has been performed, a short-arm plaster splint should be applied to stabilize the wrist in an extended position.
- At 2 weeks postoperatively, this should be transitioned to a short-arm cast for an additional 2 weeks.
- If no tendon transfer has been performed, 2 weeks postoperatively, initiate early motor re-education, edema control, scar management, and gentle ROM.
  - It is important to begin motor re-education before reinnervation.

OUTCOMES

- There are limited outcomes data for this procedure, but most case series report return of intrinsic function within 1 year of surgery.

COMPLICATIONS

- The most common complications are infection, bleeding, and lack of reinnervation of the radial-innervated musculature.

REFERENCES

1. Pet MA, Lipira AB, Ko JH. Nerve transfers for the restoration of wrist, finger, and thumb extension after high radial nerve injury. *Hand Clin.* 2016;32(2):191-207.
2. Davidge KM, Yee A, Kahn LC, Mackinnon SE. Median to radial nerve transfers for restoration of wrist, finger, and thumb extension. *J Hand Surg Am.* 2013;38(9):1812-1827.
3. Moore AM, Franco M, Tung TH. Motor and sensory nerve transfers in the forearm and hand. *Plast Reconstr Surg.* 2014;134(4):721-730.

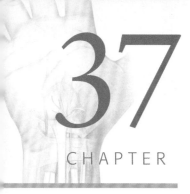

37
CHAPTER

Acute Repair of Flexor Tendon Injuries

Jacques A. Machol IV, Neal C. Chen, and Kyle R. Eberlin

DEFINITION

- Flexor tendon repair has evolved substantially over time. Flexor tendon repair balances strong tendon healing against adhesion formation. There is a complex interplay between tendon repair technique and rehabilitation that dramatically affects the outcome of flexor tendon repair.
- Biomechanical strength of suture technique
  - The strength of most initial tendon repairs ranges between 30 and 150 N.[1]
  - The repair may experience forces up to 50 N during rehabilitation.[2]
  - The strength of flexor tendon repair is related to the number of core strands crossing the repair site.
  - Strength of repair is related to suture caliber.
  - Locking sutures provide greater biomechanical strength than do grasping sutures.
  - Epitendinous sutures provide substantial strength to the tendon repair.
  - Venting of the A2 or A4 pulley can decrease friction in the flexor tendon system and improve clinical results.
  - Similarly, some surgeons elect to excise a slip of the flexor digitorum superficialis (FDS) tendon to reduce bulk and gliding resistance.
- Rehabilitation
  - During the first 1 to 3 weeks, up to 50% of initial repair strength is lost if a tendon is immobilized.
  - Early motion yields superior tensile strengths compared to delayed motion or immobilization.
  - Pyramidal rehabilitation protocols incorporating advancing force and excursion are also being used that are even more physiologically demanding than prior early active motion protocols.
    - Pyramidal protocols begin with the lowest stress force exercises and then progressively advance forces as needed in order to overcome adhesion formation.

ANATOMY

- The FDS muscle belly lies in the superficial anterior compartment of the forearm. It originates from the medial epicondyle of the humerus in the common flexor tendon and also has attachments on the oblique line of the radial head and the proximal ulna. This muscle belly is innervated by the median nerve.
- The FDS tendon to the small finger is congenitally absent in up to 7% of the population.[3]

- The FDS decussates at Camper chiasm. Here, it envelops the flexor digitorum profundus (FDP) and inserts with a 180-degree rotation.
- The FDP originates from the anteromedial surfaces of the ulna, the interosseous membrane, and the deep forearm fascia. It is located dorsal to the FDS.
  - The anterior interosseous nerve of the median nerve in most cases innervates the index and long fingers.
  - The ring and small finger FDPs are innervated by the ulnar nerve.
  - The long, ring, and small FDP tendons share a common muscle belly.
  - The FDP of the index finger is usually separate.
- The common muscle bellies of the long, ring, and small fingers are important clinically because of the quadriga phenomenon. If one of these tendons is shortened, the change in excursion may limit the ability of the other tendons to flex fully.
- The flexor tendons have limited blood supply. They are nourished by segmental, penetrating arteries via the vincular vasculature (**FIG 1A**).
- The digital nerve is volar to the digital artery in the finger.
- A complex pulley system in the distal palm and digits brings the tendons close to the bone, thus increasing the overall mechanical advantage (**FIG 1B**).
- The A5 and C3 pulley systems may require division in zone 1 injuries.
- Flexor tendon injuries are divided into five zones labeled from distal to proximal:
  - Zone 1: Insertion of the FDP to the insertion of the FDS. These are commonly referred to as "jersey fingers." The Leddy-Packer classification is used for zone 1 FDP avulsion injuries:
    - Type 1: The tendon retracts into the palm; surgery is recommended within 7 to 10 days.
    - Type 2: The FDP is at the proximal interphalangeal (PIP) and held by the vinculum; surgery is recommended within 2 to 3 weeks.
    - Type 3: The FDP is located at the A4 pulley and held by the distal phalanx bone fragment; surgery within several weeks may be acceptable, but earlier repair is advocated.
    - It is possible to have a distal phalanx fracture with tendon avulsion off of the bone fragment. These are commonly referred to as Leddy-Packer 4 injuries.

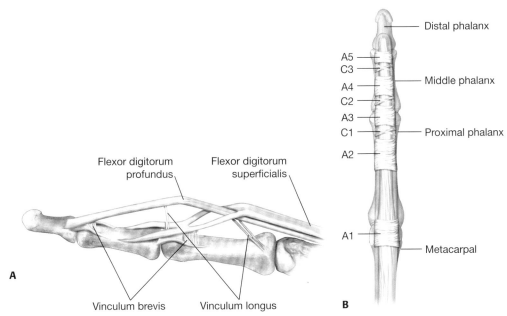

FIG 1 • A. Insertion of flexor digitorum profundus (FDP) and flexor digitorum superficialis (FDS) with vinculum longus (VL) and vinculum brevis (VB). **B.** Flexor tendon pulley systems. *A* indicates annular, and *C* indicates cruciate.

- Zone 2: FDS insertion to the distal palmar crease (A1 Pulley)
  - Much of the study of tendon repair has focused on zone 2 injuries, also termed "no man's land."
  - This area is particularly difficult to repair because of the complexity of the tendons, pulleys, and blood supply in this region.
- Zone 3: Distal palmar crease to the carpal tunnel
- Zone 4: Carpal tunnel
- Zone 5: Wrist to the forearm

PATHOGENESIS

- Zone 1 flexor tendon injuries often are caused by resistive flexion. The ring finger is slightly more prominent than other digits during midflexion. It is theorized this is why jersey fingers affect the ring finger more often than they do other digits.
- Flexor tendon injuries are typically caused by sharp lacerations but may also occur after crush injuries.

PATIENT HISTORY AND PHYSICAL FINDINGS

- The digital cascade should be inspected. The index through small digits should gently point to the scaphoid tubercle.
- A passive tenodesis maneuver can be performed. All digits should flex with wrist extension. If a flexor tendon is injured, it will not reciprocally flex with wrist extension.
- FDP is tested by restricting the metacarpophalangeal (MCP) and PIP joints in extension and asking the patient to flex the digit at the distal interphalangeal (DIP) joint.
- FDS is examined by restricting the adjacent digit(s) in extension and asking the patient to flex the digit. This maneuver utilizes the quadriga effect to limit excursion of the FDP, thereby relying on the FDS to flex the digit at the PIP joint.
- It is important to recognize that incomplete injuries may be missed on clinical exam.

- Sensation of the ulnar and radial digital nerves of each digit should be evaluated. Static two-point discrimination is beneficial in evaluating nerve transection.
- Vascularity of the digit can be evaluated by capillary refill. A digital Allen test can also be beneficial if a single digital vessel injury is suspected.

IMAGING

- Plain radiographs should be obtained to evaluate for underlying fracture or foreign body.
  - These may also be used to locate the distal end of FDP if there is a bony avulsion associated with a jersey finger.
- Ultrasound or MRI can be used if there is question regarding tendon integrity that is not apparent on clinical exam.
  - These studies are not routinely obtained in acute, penetrating trauma.

DIFFERENTIAL DIAGNOSIS

- Usually, the diagnosis is unambiguous based on history and clinical examination, but injuries may be heterogeneous.
- Tendon injuries are often accompanied by digital nerve or arterial injuries.

SURGICAL MANAGEMENT

- There are a large number of tendon repair techniques. We will describe those techniques we most commonly use: Tajima, modified Kessler, locking cruciate (Adelaide), and modified Becker (MGH suture).
  - The Tajima or modified Kessler is biomechanically weaker than the other two suture configurations; however, this suture construct is reasonable in zone 3 to 5 repairs where early motion is not as crucial. We use this suture in cases that may be time dependent, such as multiple digit replantations, to expedite the time expended for tendon repair.

- The locking cruciate offers benefits of a single knot that is buried within the tendon.
- The modified Becker is mechanically stronger than the locking cruciate but requires a larger exposure. One disadvantage is that knots are external to the tendon and may increase the bulk of the repair.
- We perform an epitendinous suture in our zone 2 repairs. With a modified Becker suture, some surgeons place half of the epitendinous suture first before inserting the core sutures.

Preoperative Planning

- Obtain a preoperative digital neurologic and vascular exam to evaluate for injury as these structures are often repaired during the same operative period.
- Wide-awake surgery (WALANT) is helpful to evaluate tendon repair and gliding intraoperatively.
- A pediatric feeding tube is helpful for tendon retrieval and passage through the intact proximal sheath when the tendon is retracted.
  - One trick is to place the feeding tube in a freezer to improve the stiffness of the catheter. There are also various funnels that can be used to help pass the tendon.

Positioning

- The patient is positioned supine with the arm abducted to 90 degrees on a padded hand table.

- A well-padded tourniquet, if used, should be placed on the biceps to avoid compressing the flexor tendon muscle bellies. Excess forearm pressure will affect resting tendon tension.

Approach

- The use of existing lacerations with extensions via Bruner-type incision or midaxial incision will provide adequate exposure for repair.
  - If skin viability/coverage is in question, a midaxial incision is preferable to avoid the acute angle at the tip of the flap that can cause tip flap necrosis and expose the underlying repair.
- It is important to get adequate visualization of the laceration. We commonly expose from the MP joint flexion crease to the DIP flexion crease for a transverse laceration. We find that a large exposure aids in performing an adequate tendon repair and generally does not hamper outcomes.
- Consider extending the incision more proximally, by including a separate carpal tunnel incision if there is concern for retraction into the palm (ie, Leddy-Packer type 1).
- One should preserve most of the pulley system in a way to prevent bowstringing.
  - Some authors will vent the A2 or 4 pulley systems by partially releasing the pulleys to facilitate gliding of repaired tendon and have reported no mechanical problems with this technique.

■ Zone I Repair

Primary Suture

- There should be at least 1 cm of distal tendon stump to use this technique (**TECH FIG 1A**).
- The proximal FDP tendon may or may not be retracted.
- If retracted, it should be passed back through the pulley system. This may be completed using a tendon passer or pediatric feeding tube or via suture to pull through the pulley system.
- Sometimes, the pulley system is very tight, and it is helpful to use a funnel-type device to pull the tendon distally.
  - The funnel helps the tendon end enter the pulley system. We have found this particularly helpful to minimize fraying of the passed tendon, limiting trauma to the tendon and optimizing tendon gliding.
- Wrist and digit flexion will help tendon retrieval.

- A 25-gauge needle is used to maintain the location of the tendon by preventing retraction.
- After pulling the tendon into the repair site, the proximal tendon is skewered with the needle to the tendon sheath to stabilize the tendon (**TECH FIG 1B**).

Pull-Through Button

- The preparation of the proximal tendon is the same as previously described.
- Repair using a pull-through button is indicated if there is no distal stump or bone fragment for fixation.
  - The insertion site is prepared with a small curette to roughen a portion of the volar cortical bone to encourage tendon to bone healing.
  - A 3-0 nonabsorbable suture that can glide such as Prolene is placed at least 1 cm from the distal edge of the proximal tendon in a Bunnell weave fashion.

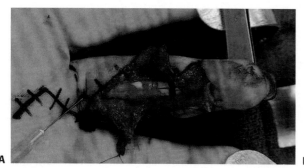 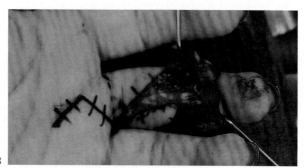

TECH FIG 1 • Zone I repair: primary suture. **A.** Zone 1 flexor digitorum profundus laceration. **B.** Primary repair completed.

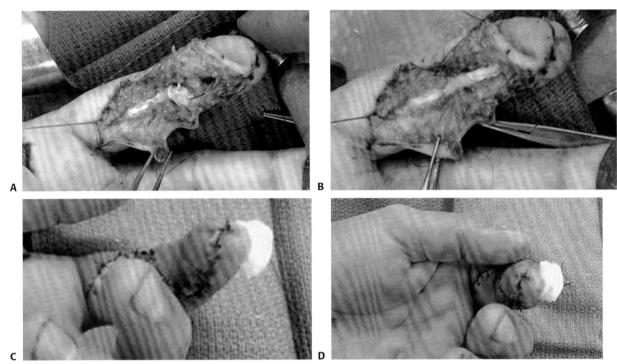

TECH FIG 2 • Zone I repair: pull-through button. **A.** Modified Kessler suture on tendon end (two Keith needles are used to pass the suture through the bone end, not shown). **B.** Suture passed through the distal phalanx. **C,D.** Suture tied over gauze dressing and button.

Prolene is used because this suture will slide and can be pulled out readily during button removal.

- Two Keith needles are then passed through the nail. There are two methods of passing the needles:
  - Some authors pass the needles through bone. They are passed using a drill parallel to each other through the distal phalanx insertion site through the nail plate just distal to the lunula. It is important to pass the K-wires in a relatively acute angle relative to the phalanx (approximately 30 degrees). If they are passed too perpendicular to the nail and too distally, the DIP may assume an excessively flexed position (**TECH FIG 2A,B**).
  - Other surgeons pass needles around the distal phalanx as an alternative to transosseous sutures.

This is performed by pushing Keith needles along the edges of the bone through the nail. The trajectory of the needles should be aimed in a similar manner when passing through the bone as described above.

- The suture is then passed dorsally and tied over a non-adherent dressing and a tendon button after confirmation that the tendon is fully seating within the bone trough (**TECH FIG 2C,D**).
- Another option for repair is the use of bone anchors.
- If there is a large bone fragment on the tendon, this may be amendable to screw fixation into the distal phalanx.
  - This repair can be augmented with a pull-through suture as well.

■ Zone II to V Repair

Tajima

- The Tajima modification of the Kessler uses two suture strands. If the proximal tendon is retracted into the palm, we will use a Tajima suture to draw the proximal tendon stump distally through the pulley system.
- The sutures are passed as they would for half of modified Kessler, but a separate suture is used on each side (**TECH FIG 3**).
- This technique is often applied when multiple tendons are injured. Sutures are passed into all of the injured tendons to allow tagging of proximal structures during exploration of the wound. Usually, once the bony structures are stabilized, the tendons are passed and then tied.

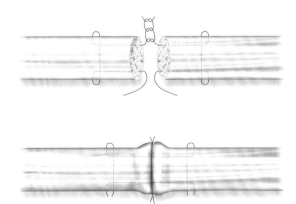

TECH FIG 3 • Tajima suture repair.

Modified Kessler

- The preparation of the zone 2 and 3 repairs may be complicated by the cruciate and pulley system blocking visualization, suturing, or passage. Generous windows should be made to allow the repaired site glide postoperatively.
- Align the proper orientation of the FDP and/or the FDS to prevent twisting and hold the proximal tendon in place with a 25-gauge needle.
- One or two slips of the FDS can be repaired at zone 2.
  - Some authors excise slips to maximize tendon gliding and minimize resistance. Some surgeons always repair the FDS with the rationale that if the FDP ruptures, the patient can preserve FDS function. Some excise the FDS to decrease tendon bulk in within the pulley system.
  - In our practice, we sometimes excise the ulnar slip of the FDS tendon depending on the tendon quality. We make this decision depending on the degree of tendon bulk and resistance after venting the pulleys.
  - The FDS is repaired using a horizontal mattress suture or a figure-of-8 suture using a 4-0 Ethibond or Tevdek suture.
- To start the modified Kessler technique, a suture is passed from the radial cut end of the tendon and exits out the volar surface 1 cm from the end.
- A transverse pass is then made from the radial side of the tendon transversely and out the ulnar side. This pass may be made closer to the cut edge to lock the suture.
- Another loop is made passing the suture back into the volar aspect of the tendon and out the tendon end.
- The mirror image of the suture is passed on the other end and the knot is tied within the tendon ends (**TECH FIG 4**).
- A four-strand repair may be created with the addition of a second suture in the same pattern or with a horizontal mattress suture.

Locked Cruciate

- To begin the locked cruciate tendon suture, a 2-mm longitudinal slit is created 1 cm from the tendon edge and a suture is passed through this out the tendon end.
- The needle is then brought through the opposing tendon end and out 1 cm on the volar aspect.
- The suture is reinserted a few millimeters distal and lateral to the prior exit site and crossed through the tendon without locking.

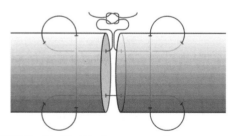

TECH FIG 4 • Modified Kessler suture repair.

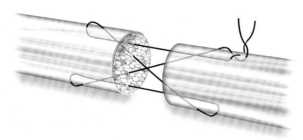

TECH FIG 5 • Locked cruciate suture repair.

- The suture is then reintroduced into the distal end and passed into other lateral edge across from the prior slit site.
- The needle is repassed retrograde a few millimeters distal to the insertion site and brought out the tendon end.
- This is passed into the opposing end again, looped back into the tendon a few millimeters distal, and crossed back into the distal tendon without locking.
- The needle exits the slit and the knot is tied within the tendon (**TECH FIG 5**).
- Slack should be removed from the suture and gapping approximated with each throw.

Modified Becker/Massachusetts General Hospital (MGH) Repair

- This is our preferred core suture technique when possible.
- The suture is introduced from the volar, radial of the tendon 1 cm from the cut end.
- Two epitendinous crisscross sutures are placed on each tendon end, tightened snugly, and the knot is tied on the outside of the tendon.
- A second suture passed in the same fashion is completed on the ulnar side of the tendon creating a four-core suture repair (**TECH FIG 6**).
- This repair can be completed with a single-armed suture, but a double-armed suture will allow safe passes to prevent accidently catching the suture with subsequent passes during placement of the crisscross epitendinous sutures.
- A 5-0 or 6-0 monofilament epitendinous suture is often started dorsally prior to core suture completion. This may be placed after the core suture repair as well.
- The use of an epitendinous suture increases repair strength up to 20% and may improve tendon gliding.

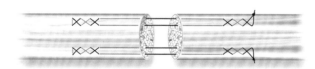

TECH FIG 6 • Modified Becker/Massachusetts General Hospital (MGH) suture repair.

TECHNIQUES

Epitendinous Repair: Running, Running Locking, and Silfverskiold Suture

- Running and running locking sutures are typically done with a monofilament 5-0 or 6-0 suture.
  - The epitendon is grasped with the suture, and a knot is tied approximating the ends. This end may be left free to tie too after completion of the suture technique as well.
  - The suture is then passed from superficial to deep on one end and then out deep to superficial on the other with advancement of each throw.
  - Either the suture is tied to the tail of the first throw or a new knot is created.

- The running locking is completed in the same fashion, but locking loops are used instead.
- The Silfverskiold suture is analogous to a horizontal cross-stitch suture (**TECH FIG 7**).
  - It is performed by placing an anchor stitch and then taking 1- to 2-mm bites perpendicular to the axis of the tendon approximately 1 cm from the repair site. Tendon passes are always taken toward the surgeon.
  - The following suture pass is taken on the other side of the repair site, and the starting point is advanced away from the surgeon.
  - About 10 passes are needed to circumferentially encompass the tendon.
  - The epitendinous suture is then tied to the anchor suture.

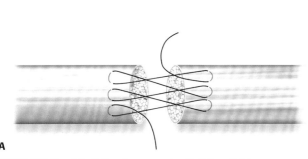
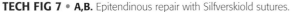
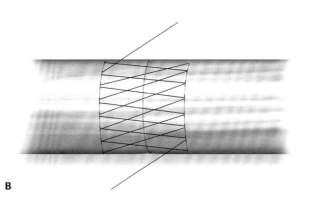

A   **B**

TECH FIG 7 • A,B. Epitendinous repair with Silfverskiold sutures.

PEARLS AND PITFALLS

Technique	■ Use a Tajima suture to retrieve retracted tendons if needed. In the cases of combined injury, the suture is placed during the exploration/ approach, the bone is fixed, and then the suture is passed and tied.
	■ Use a pediatric feeding tube or funnel to help pass sutures through the proximal pulleys.
	■ The primary goal of zone 2 tendon repairs is to repair the tendon with four-core sutures and an epitendinous suture.
	■ Use an epitendinous suture to increase repair strength. Consider placing the dorsal epitendinous suture before the core repair.
	■ Avoid traumatic handling of the tendon to prevent epitendinous injury that may lead to adhesion formation.
	■ The A4 pulley may be vented if the A2 pulley is competent.
Therapy	■ In children, we prefer immobilization in a cast rather than an early motion protocol.
	■ If the tendon repair is strong, begin early motion protocols.
	■ If the tendon repair is tenuous, a less aggressive motion protocol is preferred. Adhesions can be addressed with tenolysis later.

POSTOPERATIVE CARE

- Passive digital flexion-extension results in loads of around 3 N.[4]
- Active digital flexion-extension results in loads of about 30 N.[4]
- Tendon excursion during passive digital flexion-extension ranges from 3 to 8 mm in vivo.[5]

- Hook and straight fist result in greater loads than does composite fist.[6]
- Wrist motion results in greater flexor tendon excursion.
- A postoperative dorsal blocking splint with wrist and digit flexion is applied. This splint is removed at the first postoperative visit and a thermoplastic or like dorsal blocking splint is fashioned to initiate therapy.

- Earlier protocols consisted of immobilization for at least 3 weeks. This resulted in loss of digit motion due to tendon scarring; therefore, newer protocols were established to allow excursion and prevent tendon adhesions
- Kleinert, Duran, and active place-and-hold are commonly employed early motion regimens. There are many modifications of these protocols as well.
- If we have high confidence in the repair, we will begin early motion using the pyramid protocol described by Groth.[7]
- If the repair is tenuous, we will use a modified Duran protocol.
- Overall, the choice of protocol is surgeon and case dependent.

OUTCOMES

- Chesney et al. reviewed multiple rehabilitation regimens for zone II flexor tendon injuries. No significant difference existed between early active and early passive protocols (Duran- and Kleinert-type protocols), and all protocols resulted with high rates of acceptable range of motion. Duran protocols had the lowest rate of ruptures during rehab (2.3%).[8]
- Starr et al. performed a systematic review of early active and early passive protocols for all zones of flexor tendon injury. They found that early passive range of motion protocols had a statistically significantly decreased risk for tendon rupture but an increased risk for postoperative decreased range of motion when compared to early active motion protocols.[9]

COMPLICATIONS

- Adhesions are the most common complication.

- Tendon rupture may occur when loading during rehabilitation exceeds the strength of the repair and the healing tendon. It is sometimes not possible to distinguish between tendon rupture and adhesions if the proximal tendon stump scars to the FDS and the proximal phalanx.
- Quadriga occurs when the FDP is shortened. Because the FDP has a common muscle belly, once the finger with the shortened FDP has fully flexed, the other fingers cannot flex any further.

REFERENCES

1. Jordan MC, Schmitt V, Jansen H, et al. Biomechanical analysis of the modified Kessler, Lahey, Adelaide, and Becker sutures for flexor tendon repair. *J Hand Surg [Am]*. 2015;40(9):1812-1817.
2. Evans RB, Thompson DE. The application of force to the healing tendon. *J Hand Ther*. 1993;6(4):266-284.
3. Allan CH. Flexor tendons: anatomy and surgical approaches. *Hand Clin*. 2005;21:151-157.
4. Schuind F, Garcia-Elias M, Cooney WP III, An KN. Flexor tendon forces: in vivo measurements. *J Hand Surg [Am]*. 1992;17(2):291-298.
5. Horibe S, Woo SL, Spiegelman JJ, et al. Excursion of the flexor digitorum profundus tendon: a kinematic study of the human and canine digits. *J Orthop Res*. 1990;8(2):167-174.
6. Greenwald D, Shumway S, Allen C, Mass D. Dynamic analysis of profundus tendon function. *J Hand Surg [Am]*. 1994;19(4):626-635.
7. Groth GN. Pyramid of progressive force exercises to the injured flexor tendon. *J Hand Ther*. 2004;17(1):31-42.
8. Chesney A, Chauhan A, Kattan A, et al. Systematic review of flexor tendon rehabilitation protocols in zone II of the hand. *Plast Reconstr Surg*. 2011;127:1583-1592.
9. Starr HM, Snoddy M, Hammond KE, Seiler JG III. Flexor tendon repair rehabilitation protocols: a systematic review. *J Hand Surg Am*. 2013;38:1712, 7.e1-14.

Repair of Multiple Flexor Tendon Injury at Wrist Zone V (Spaghetti Wrist)

Jacques A. Machol IV, Neal C. Chen, and Kyle R. Eberlin

DEFINITION

- Volar wrist trauma with tendon, nerve, and arterial injuries is often referred to as a "spaghetti wrist."
- Specific criteria for the definition of a "spaghetti wrist" vary in the literature, with some authors defining it as injury to at least three of the volar wrist structures including at least one nerve,[1,2] with others defining this injury as inclusive of both median and ulnar nerve injuries at the level of the wrist.[3]
  - Other authors have defined this injury as involving a minimum of 10 structures in the wrist.

ANATOMY

- The volar wrist structures include the radial and ulnar arteries, the median and ulnar nerves (along with the palmar cutaneous branch and the dorsal ulnar sensory branch), the flexor pollicis longus (FPL), the four flexor digitorum superficialis (FDS) tendons, the four flexor digitorum profundus (FDP) tendons, the palmaris longus (PL), the flexor carpi ulnaris (FCU), and the flexor carpi radialis (FCR) tendons. Any or all of these structures can be injured with a volar wrist laceration (**FIG 1**).
- The superficial nature of these structures and thin cutaneous coverage render them highly susceptible to penetrating injuries.
- At the wrist, the FDS tendons to the long finger (LF) and ring finger (RF) are volar to the FDS tendons to the index finger (IF) and small finger (SF).
- The FCU is volar to the ulnar artery and ulnar nerve. The ulnar artery is typically superficial (volar) to the ulnar nerve; it is therefore possible to injure the FCU and ulnar artery while sparing the ulnar nerve.
- The palmar cutaneous nerve is often injured.
- Flexor tendon injuries in the spaghetti wrist are in zone V (see Flexor Tendon chapter for details)

PATHOGENESIS

- These injuries are often self-inflicted but also may result from other traumatic causes.[4]
- They often are the result of sharp lacerations but can also be caused by crush injuries.
- The mechanism of injury is most often sharp glass lacerations, followed by knife wounds and saw injuries.
- The median nerve and FDS tendons are the most commonly injured structures, because they are located superficially and centrally in the volar wrist.
- These injuries are more common in males.

PATIENT HISTORY AND PHYSICAL FINDINGS

- A focused history and physical examination is performed with emphasis on the etiology and mechanism of injury, sensory and vascular examination, and examination of each individual tendon in the volar wrist.
- Self-inflicted spaghetti wrist injuries should ideally be identified prior to surgery. Psychiatry consultation is helpful for management.
- A thorough vascular examination should be performed including inspection for color and capillary refill, a Doppler exam with Allen test, and pulse oximetry of the digits.
- A formal nerve examination, including evaluation for light touch and two-point discrimination, intrinsic motor function, and palmar abduction, should be performed.
- The surgeon can glean much information about the status of tendon injuries simply by observing the digital cascade at rest, as the attitude of the digits can reflect the presence or absence of intact tendons.
- In these cases, tenodesis testing is not possible usually because the wrist cannot be flexed or extended because of the injury.

IMAGING

- Plain film radiographs are obtained to assess for fracture and foreign body.

SURGICAL MANAGEMENT

- Early definitive surgical management is recommended, particularly in cases of vascular or nerve injuries.
- Thorough debridement and removal of foreign material with copious irrigation is paramount.
- Identification and labeling of all injured structures is performed; a checklist is helpful to organize one's approach and ensure repair of all injured structures.
- It is important to label the proximal tendons, as the orientation is clear prior to dissection and may be lost with mobilization. The distal tendon ends are easily identified by manual traction intraoperatively.
- The deep structures including the FDP and FPL are repaired first, unless the hand is dysvascular in which case an arterial repair shunting is performed first (usually the radial artery).
- It is important to repair injured structures in a manner that facilitates microsurgical repair of the nerves and/or arteries.

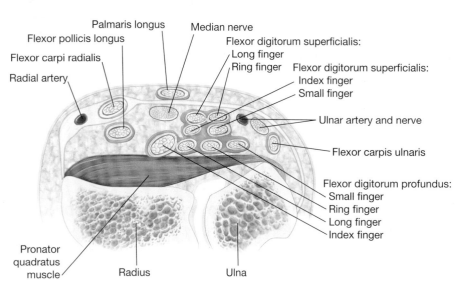

FIG 1 • Distal wrist axial slice anatomy. Flexor carpi radialis (FCR), palmaris longus (PL), flexor digitorum superficialis (FDS), flexor digitorum profundus (FDP), index finger (IF), long finger (LF), ring finger (RF), small finger (SF), and flexor carpi ulnaris (FCU).

- It is important to identify injured structures, repair deep structures, and then progress to more superficial structures.
- If microsurgical repair is anticipated, superficial structures such as the FCR and FCU are repaired last.

Preoperative Planning

- The aforementioned thorough preoperative examination formulates a concrete, definitive operative plan.
- The surgeon and patient should be prepared for vein and/or nerve grafts, depending on the time elapsed and mechanism of injury.

Positioning

- The patient is positioned supine with the arm abducted on a hand table; a tourniquet is used.
- The ipsilateral lower extremity is prepped sterilely for vein or nerve graft(s), if needed.
  - The entire forearm to just above the elbow is prepped. This is particularly germane with distal lacerations near the wrist crease, where the distal tendon ends may retract into the carpal tunnel.
- Skin flaps can be retracted with either elastics/hooks or retraction sutures.

T E C H N I Q U E S

■ Exposure

- The existing wound is extended proximally and distally to provide access to injured structures.
  - Do not try to limit incisions in these cases. Wide exposure is preferred (**TECH FIG 1**).

- Proximally, the incision is extended in linear, longitudinal fashion often in the central aspect of the volar forearm.
- Distally, an extended carpal tunnel incision may aid in mobilization of tendons for repair and is frequently performed to release of the transverse carpal ligament in anticipation of postoperative swelling.

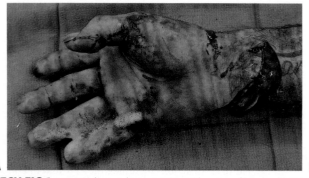

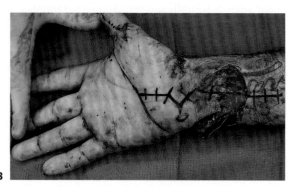

TECH FIG 1 • **A.** Initial wound presentation with exposed injuries. **B.** Extension of the existing wound proximally and distally to provide access to injured structures.

■ Exploration and Tagging of the Structures

- The proximal tendons are exposed and tagged with one-half of the preferred suture technique and labeled (**TECH FIG 2A**). A four-core strand suture technique is commonly used.

- Arteries and nerve are tagged with a small monofilament suture with long tails.
- A checklist is used to ensure repair of all structures (**TECH FIG 2B**).

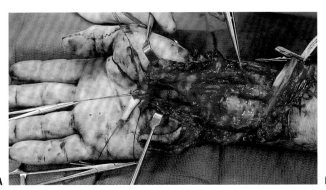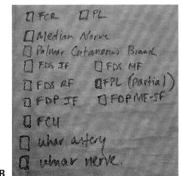

A.   **B.**

TECH FIG 2 • A. Tagging of the proximal structures to ensure proper anatomical repairs. **B.** Checklist ensuring repair of all structures.

■ Repair of Injured Structures

- Tendons are repaired first from deep to superficial, and often from radial to ulnar under tourniquet.
- The choice of tendon repair varies based on surgeon preference and experience but should entail at least four core strands.
  - We prefer a modified Becker, ie, MGH repair for flexor tendons in zone V. Epitendinous repair is not needed because gliding is not impeded in zone V and the surgeon needs to expedite the repairs because of the numerous structures injured.
- Microsurgical repair of the nerves and arteries is then performed.
- The tourniquet can be deflated to visualize arterial inflow and endoneurial bleeding during neurorrhaphy (**TECH FIG 3**).
- Meticulous nerve repair is critical; this should be performed by the most senior surgeon involved in the operation.
  - Care should be taken to avoid fascicular overlap during tension-free neurorrhaphy.

- If there is a single arterial injury, we tend to perform vascular repair even with a perfused hand.
  - We occlude the other major artery for 5 minutes at the time of reperfusion (for instance, the radial artery following ulnar artery repair) to allow for anterograde flow into the hand through the fresh vascular anastomosis.

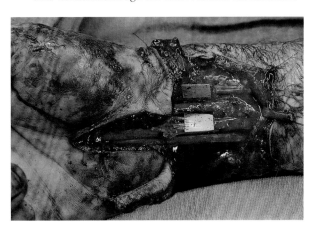

TECH FIG 3 • Status post microsurgical repair.

PEARLS AND PITFALLS

Technique	■ Careful preoperative examination helps surgical planning.
	■ Identification and tagging of proximal tendons will ensure correct repair of structures; a surgical checklist is helpful.
	■ Atraumatic tendon and tissue handling will facilitate gliding of tendons postoperatively.
	■ Meticulous epineurial repair following adequate nerve debridement will optimize chances of neural recovery; care should be taken to avoid fascicular overlap.
	■ Have the contralateral leg prepped if nerve grafts or vein grafts are anticipated.
Physical exam	■ An Allen test and thorough nerve exam should be performed preoperatively.
	■ Inspection of the digits can often reveal the extent of tendon injuries.
Therapy	■ Dedicated occupational/hand therapy is required postoperatively; this will depend on the strength of repair and the patient's motivation and compliance with postoperative instructions.
	■ Patients with self-inflicted lacerations may require a longer period of immobilization, sometimes involving casting.

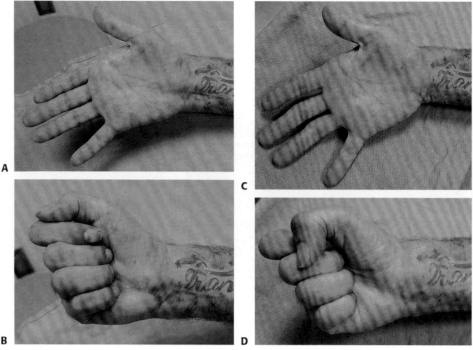

FIG 2 • Eight months **(A,B)** and 2 years **(C,D)** postoperatively.

POSTOPERATIVE CARE

- Patients are placed in a dorsal blocking "clam digger" splint with the wrist in 20 degrees of flexion, MP joints at 90 degrees of flexion, and PIP/DIP joints with mild flexion to off-load the tendon, nerve, and arterial repairs. The splint should extend to the fingertips.
- Strict elevation and non–weight bearing is emphasized, particularly for patients with self-inflicted lacerations.
- Continuous pulse oximetry is utilized for patients presenting with both radial and ulnar artery injuries or dysvascular hands; aspirin is utilized for 1 month postoperatively.
- The specific regimen of postoperative hand therapy is based on the quality of the repairs and the compliance of the patient; we prefer early active motion protocols for sophisticated patients who understand the nature of their injury and 3 to 4 weeks of immobilization for patients with self-inflicted injuries who are unwilling or unable to follow strict postoperative instructions.

OUTCOMES

- Functional outcomes depend on the overall severity of injury and number of injured structures but are often predicated upon the degree of neural recovery (**FIG 2**).
- With sharp injuries, more than 50% of patients will recover protective sensation, but intrinsic dysfunction is common with ulnar nerve injuries.
- Digital range of motion and strength can be satisfactory, particularly with early active motion protocols in compliant patients.[4]

- Patients can be expected to have some degree of dysfunction compared to their premorbid state.

COMPLICATIONS

- Tendon adhesions and/or stiffness, greatest when patients are immobilized for extended periods of time postoperatively
- Tendon rupture, greatest when patients are not compliant with splinting or therapy instructions
- Infection and delayed wound healing, greatest with contaminated wounds
- Pain resulting from neuroma
- Clawing and intrinsic minus hand secondary to poor ulnar nerve recovery
- Arterial insufficiency or cold intolerance

REFERENCES

1. Chin G, Weinzweig N, Mead M, Gonzalez M. "Spaghetti wrist": management and results. *Plast Reconstr Surg.* 1998;102(1):96-102.
2. Puckett CL, Meyer VH. Results of treatment of extensive volar wrist lacerations: the spaghetti wrist. *Plast Reconstr Surg.* 1985;75(5):714-719.
3. Hudson DA, De Jager LT. The spaghetti wrist: simultaneous laceration of the median and ulnar nerves with flexor tendons at the wrist. *J Hand Surg Br Eur.* 1993;18(2):171-173.
4. Wilhelmi BJ, Kang RH, Wages DJ, et al. Optimizing independent finger flexion with zone V flexor repairs using the Massachusetts General Hospital flexor tenorrhaphy and early protected active motion. *J Hand Surg.* 2005;30(2):230-236.

Staged Flexor Tendon Grafting and Pulley Reconstruction

Richard Tosti, Jacques A. Machol IV, and Neal C. Chen

DEFINITION

- Flexor tendon reconstruction refers to the restoration of the flexor mechanism through the use of tendon grafts.
- Pulley reconstruction is the recreation of the flexor tendon sheath in order to prevent bowstringing and optimize strength.

ANATOMY

- Nine flexor tendons originate in the forearm. Flexor pollicis longus inserts at the base of the distal phalanx of the thumb. Four flexor digitorum superficialis (FDS) and four flexor digitorum profundus (FDP) tendons insert on the volar base of the middle and distal phalanges, respectively.
- The FDS tendons are superficial to the FDP in the hand, but as they enter the fibrous sheath, the FDS bifurcates into two slips, which are directed dorsally to their insertion.
- The flexor tendon sheath is a fibrous tunnel through which the flexor tendons glide. Composed of annular and cruciate pulleys, the sheath prevents bowstringing, reduces the flexor moment arm (imparting strength and efficient excursion), and provides nutrition (**FIG 1**). The thumb flexor sheath is composed of annular and oblique pulleys.
- The flexor sheath extends from the metacarpal head to the distal phalanx.

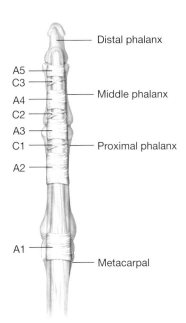

A5
C3
A4
C2
A3
C1
A2

A1

Distal phalanx

Middle phalanx

Proximal phalanx

Metacarpal

FIG 1 • Flexor tendon sheath of a finger consisting of annular and cruciate pulleys.

PATHOGENESIS

- Acute flexor tendon rupture occurs as a result of trauma, including laceration, avulsion, crush, or burn.
- Attritional ruptures may also occur from synovitis, Mannerfelt syndrome, prominent implants, bony prominences, infections, and neoplasms.

NATURAL HISTORY

- Following a rupture, the proximal end of the tendon retracts, leaving an empty space within the sheath.
- In as early as 3 to 6 weeks, irreversible contracture of the muscle tendon unit, degeneration, and scarring within the flexor sheath may occur. The tendon sheath volume will shrink without an intact tendon, which limits passage of tendons through the sheath after tendon repair.

PATIENT HISTORY AND PHYSICAL FINDINGS

- Patients lose the ability to flex the finger at the proximal interphalangeal (PIP) joint or distal interphalangeal joint (DIP) when the FDS or FDP tendons are disrupted.
- Often the cascade of the hand is altered. The affected digit assumes a more extended posture.
- A skin injury overlies the approximate level of tendon injury
- "Tenodesis" effect of the hand is lost. When the wrist is passively extended, the affected finger does not flex.
- Active motion is lost. FDS rupture is detected by observing loss of PIP flexion in the affected digit while holding the adjacent digits in extension. Extending the adjacent digits isolates the FDS because the FDP tendon of the affected digit is placed at a mechanical disadvantage due to the common origin. FDP rupture is detected by stabilizing the PIP in extension and observing a lack of active flexion at the DIP joint.
- "Tenodesis" testing can also help detect flexor tendon injuries. When the wrist is extended, the digits should flex reciprocally if the flexor tendons are intact. If the flexor tendon is lacerated, there will be lack of reciprocal flexion in the injured digits.

IMAGING

- Flexor tendon rupture is usually diagnosed by history and physical exam.
- Radiographs may be helpful to evaluate for avulsion injuries or bony prominences causing attritional rupture.
- Computed tomography may also be useful in evaluating for carpal bone spurs in suspected attritional ruptures.
- Ultrasound or magnetic resonance imaging may be useful in determining the level of proximal tendon retraction.

DIFFERENTIAL DIAGNOSIS

- Adhesions. It is difficult to distinguish between adhesion and rupture clinically.
- Intra-articular injury
- Nerve injury
- Neuromuscular disorders

NONOPERATIVE MANAGEMENT

- Elderly, low-demand patients with comorbidities may not have an outcome worth the overall risk for multiple reconstructive procedures. Additionally, these patients may not be able to complete a rigorous postoperative protocol.
- Physical rehabilitation to maximize passive joint motion is critical prior to tendon reconstruction procedures.
- Although not considered "nonoperative," alternative procedures to reconstruction include joint fusion or digit amputation, which could be considered for patients with injuries to multiple structures within the digit.
- Patients with an intact FDS may have reasonable function even if the FDP has been lacerated. In these situations, no reconstruction is reasonable. If the DIP is unstable, fusion is an option, but in many cases, this is not necessary.

SURGICAL MANAGEMENT

- Direct tendon repair should be performed when possible.
- Single stage tendon grafting can be performed for acute segmental tendon defects or delayed injuries without excessive retraction and good passive motion. An intact flexor tendon sheath is required.
- Two-stage flexor tendon reconstruction is indicated for failed direct repairs in zone II, severe injuries with concomitant injury to the adjacent bone or joint, chronic injuries with excessive scarring, or loss of flexor sheath.
  - Two-stage reconstruction was developed because joint contracture, flexor sheath volume/pulley insufficiency, and tendon length were problems. Two-stage reconstruction allows the surgeon to address these factors prior to addressing the tendon.

- Prior to the first stage, wound healing, and joint contracture are addressed. The first stage allows for reconstitution of the flexor sheath and pulley reconstruction.
  - Once a gliding space is established, the second stage of the reconstruction can be performed with minimal scarring and inflammation.
- If the tendon is too short, patients will have problems with quadriga, ie, the tendon excursion for the injured finger would be shorter than the other digits. When the injured finger was fully flexed, the other fingers would not flex completely because of the common FDP muscle belly.
- If the tendon was too long, some patients developed a lumbrical plus finger. As the FDP contracts, the lumbricals tighten, resulting in paradoxical extension of the PIP joint through the lateral bands.
- Flexor tendon reconstruction, although not a perfect solution, is a method that has more consistent results than these other techniques.

Preoperative Planning

- If autograft is planned for the procedure, one should ensure the presence and integrity of the tendon. Many options are possible, but the most common are palmaris longus, plantaris, and digital long toe extensors of the second, third, or fourth toes. Allograft tendon is also an option.
- Plan for a small-caliber graft (4–5 mm diameter).
- Plan for only one graft.
- Do not sacrifice FDS if it is found intact.
- Perform the repairs outside of the tendon sheath.
- Repair the proximal juncture to the FDP tendon to power the graft.

Positioning

- Position the patient supine on a hand table with a nonsterile upper arm tourniquet.

Approach

- A volar Bruner-style incision is planned along the length of the finger.
- A separate zigzag incision in the palm or distal forearm may be needed as well.

TECHNIQUES

■ Single-Stage Tendon Grafting

- The tendon sheath is approach through a volar Bruner incision (**TECH FIG 1A**) and must be examined for competency particularly for the A2 and A4 pulleys.
  - If an inadequate sheath is found, a staged reconstruction should be performed.
  - If single-stage reconstruction with tendon graft is planned, all the finger joints must have full supple motion and the skin over the tendon sheath must be soft so that the finger can move smoothly during therapy.
- The sheath should be preserved as much as possible.
- Leave FDS intact if it is not disrupted. The graft can be passed anatomically through the decussation.
- Often, both FDS and FDP are disrupted.

- The insertion of FDS can be left with a 1- to 2-cm tail to provide a gliding surface.
- The proximal FDS is transected under traction and allowed to retract (**TECH FIG 1B,C**).
- The FDP insertion is similarly left with a 1- to 2-cm stump. If no FDP stump is available, the graft can be inserted directly into the bone.
- The proximal FDP is often prepared in the palm if no scarring is present but can also be prepared in the distal forearm.
- When in the palm, the FDP is "freshened" with a blade just distal to the lumbrical origin. The proximal tendon graft is woven to the FDP at the level of the lumbrical muscle takeoff to assure that the proper tension can be set to avoid a lumbrical plus finger in which premature contraction of the lumbrical causes PIP joint extension when attempting finger flexion.

TECHNIQUES

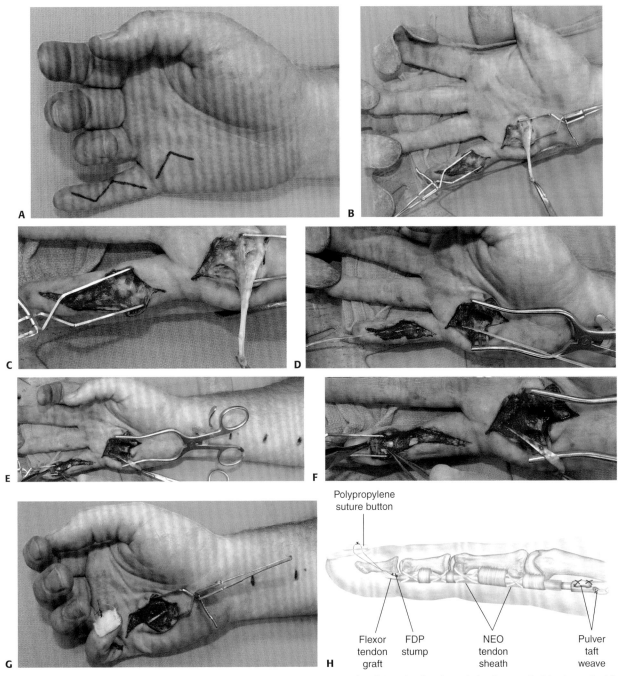

TECH FIG 1 • Single-stage flexor tendon reconstruction. **A.** Bruner incisions in the digit and palm. If needed, a forearm incision is marked for more proximal rod placement. **B,C.** The proximal tendon is excised. **D.** The tendon sheath is intact. **E,F.** The tendon graft is passed through the distal phalanx and tied over a button. **G.** The tendon suture is weaved to the profundus tendon proximally with fingers in slight flexion. **H.** Completed single-stage tendon reconstruction.

- The lumbrical may be released if it is scarred.
- At this point, a moist gauze is placed over the wound, and the graft is harvested.
- The harvested graft may be first secured to the distal or proximal junction first, but we prefer to secure it first distally to facilitate setting tension.
- The graft is sutured. We prefer a smooth 2.0 Prolene or ▓▓▓▓▓▓▓▓▓▓▓▓▓▓▓▓▓▓▓▓▓▓▓▓▓▓▓▓▓▓▓▓▓▓▓▓▓▓ to facilitate easy pullout.

- The sutures are shuttled through the tendon sheath by using a tendon passer (**TECH FIG 1D**). The ends of the suture are brought distally and can be used to slide the tendon graft through the sheath.
- The distal end of the graft is woven once through the FDP stump with the tendon weaver (**TECH FIG 1E,F**).
- A Keith needle is placed into a wire driver and drill across the base of the distal phalanx.

- One suture end is threaded through the eyelet and passed dorsally through the nail plate either through or around the bone, taking care not to pierce the germinal matrix. The other suture is passed the same way.
- The sutures may be tied over a polypropylene button or over the nail plate.
- Alternatively, the graft can be secured with a small suture anchor in the distal phalanx; the anchor is placed in the FDP insertion and angled slightly proximally with care to avoid intra-articular penetration of the DIP joint.

- The graft is then sutured to the distal FDP stump at the distal weave.
- The wrist is positioned in neutral, and the graft is tensioned to place the finger in slight flexion and aligned with the natural cascade (**TECH FIG 1G**). Err on the side of overtensioning rather than undertensioning.
- The proximal end of the graft is then weaved through the proximal FDP tendon at the correct tension (**TECH FIG 1H**).
- We prefer three weaves, each 90 degrees to each other, which are secured with figure-of-8 sutures.

■ Two-Stage Flexor Tendon Reconstruction

Stage 1

- Approach the finger with a volar Bruner incision (**TECH FIG 2A**).
- Assess the flexor sheath and preserve as much as possible.
- If the sheath is deficient, pulley reconstruction is indicated.
- A lacerated sheath may be repaired in this stage as long as it does not hinder the gliding of the rod.
- A stenotic sheath may require dilatation or partial release in order to pass the rod.
- Cut the FDS and FDP leaving a 1- to 2-cm stump at the insertion sites. The excised tendon can be used for pulley reconstruction and should be maintained on the field during the case.
- There are two approaches to rod placement, depending on the anticipated location of the tenorrhaphy. Some surgeons perform the tenorrhaphy in the palm, whereas others perform the tenorrhaphy at the level of the forearm.
  - If there is a large amount of scarring in the palm, forearm placement is preferred.
  - If a forearm tenorrhaphy is used, a palmaris longus tendon is usually too short and a plantaris tendon or other longer tendon may be needed at the secondary reconstruction.
- An incision can be made in the palm or in the distal forearm.
- Identify the FDS and FDP tendons by using a turn-key motion with an Allis clamp. This is performed by

clamping around the tendon and then twisting the clamp so the tendon wraps around the tines. This allows the surgeon to apply a force in line with the tendon and helps avoid pulley rupture.
- The FDS is released and allowed to retract proximally in most cases, but may be retained as the motor for the second stage if the FDP is of poor quality.
- Shorten the FDP but tag it with a suture and sew it side to side to an adjacent FDP tendon to prevent retraction and allow easy identification in stage 2.
- Suture the silicone rod into the distal FDP stump. The size of the rod should fit snugly into the sheath. It is usually 4 to 6 mm.
- Guide the rod through the flexor sheath (**TECH FIG 2B–D**) and allow it to float freely through the carpal tunnel and into the forearm.
- You should observe the rod in the proximal forearm incision, and it should glide smoothly without buckling as the finger is taken through a range of motion.
- Alternatively, the silicone rod can be loosely tacked to the FDP at the level of the palm if it has not retracted proximally.
- Over the course of 2 or 3 months, the gliding silicone rod creates a lubricated pseudosheath.[1]

Stage 2

- Use the previous incisions to identify the silicone rod proximally and distally.
- Obtain the tendon graft. Be sure the length of the graft will be sufficient to span the length of the defect (**TECH FIG 3A,B**).

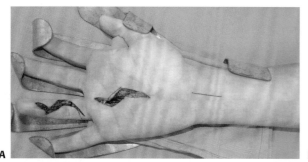
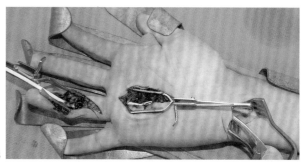

A   **B**

TECH FIG 2 • Stage 1 of two-stage flexor tendon reconstruction. **A.** Volar Bruner incision in the finger and palm. **B.** The Hunter rod placement in flexor sheath.

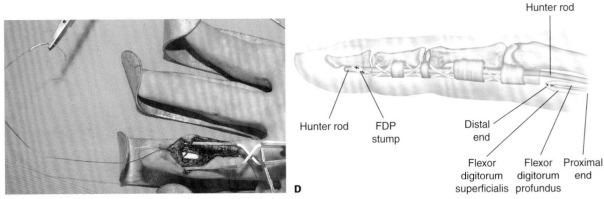

TECH FIG 2 (Continued) • **C.** Hunter rod sutured to the FDP stump. **D.** Completed stage 1 of two-stage tendon reconstruction.

- Identify the rod distally in the finger.
- Cut the sutures between the rod and the FDP stump and suture the distal end of the rod to the proximal end of the graft (**TECH FIG 3C**).
- Pull the rod through the proximal incision, which will shuttle the graft through the sheath.
- Perform a tendon weave on the distal FDP stump as described above for single-stage grafting. If no stump is present, the graft can be inserted into the distal phalanx with transosseous sutures tied over

a button or the nail plate or with a suture anchor (**TECH FIG 3D**).
- Estimate the tension of the graft to produce slight flexion aligned with the natural cascade (**TECH FIG 3E**).
- Err on the side of overtensioning rather than undertensioning.
- Perform a Pulvertaft weave on the proximal FDP using three orthogonal weaves (**TECH FIG 3F**).
- If the proximal FDP stump cannot be identified, a tenodesis to the adjacent FDP tendon can be performed.

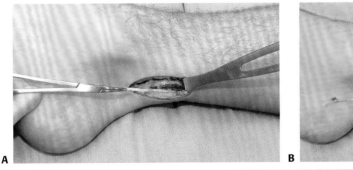

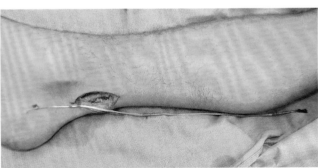

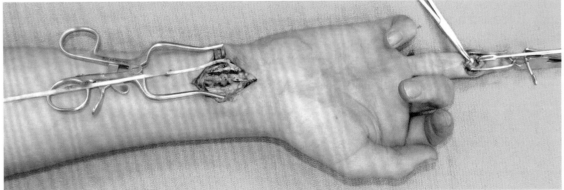

TECH FIG 3 • Stage 2. **A,B.** The tendon graft is harvested. **C.** The sutures are cut between the rod and the FDP stump, and the distal end of the rod is sutured to the proximal end of the graft.

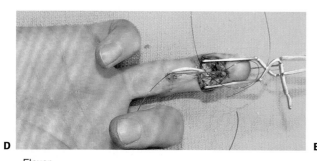

D

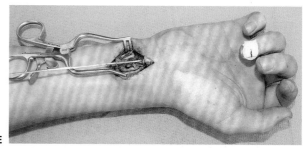

E

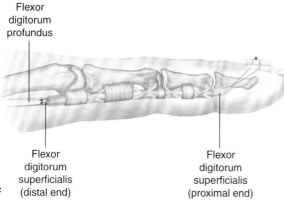

Flexor
digitorum
profundus

Flexor
digitorum
superficialis
F (distal end)

Flexor
digitorum
superficialis
(proximal end)

TECH FIG 3 (Continued) • **D.** A tendon weave is performed on the distal FDP stump. **E.** The tension of the graft is estimated to produce slight flexion aligned with the natural cascade. **F.** Completed stage 2 of two-stage tendon reconstruction.

■ Paneva-Holevich Modification

- Described in 1969, this modification obviates the need for tendon graft harvest in stage 2.[2]
- In stage 1, the volar finger is approached and the silicone rod is secured to the distal FDP or the distal phalanx as described above.
  - The FDS and FDP tendons are both identified in the palm and transected at the level of the lumbrical origin proximal to the A1 pulley. Both distal ends are sutured to each other using a locking core suture technique.

We prefer a Kessler stitch with a running epitendinous stitch.
  - The FDP-FDS "loop" will heal over 3 months.
- In stage 2, the finger is exposed again.
  - The FDS tendon is transected as far proximal as possible. Pull the FDS-FDP loop out of the palm. The proximally cut FDS tendon now becomes the distal end of the graft.
  - Suture the distal end of the tendon graft to the silicone rod and shuttle the graft through the pseudosheath.
  - Tension the graft and secure it as described above.

■ Pulley Reconstruction

- Pulley reconstruction is performed at the first stage of the tendon reconstruction if the A2 and A4 pulleys are deficient (**TECH FIG 4A**).
- We prefer the tendon-wrapping method described by Bunnell.[3]
- Approximately 12 cm of graft may be required to encircle the phalanx twice. Oftentimes this can be obtained from excised flexor tendon.
- The A2 and A4 pulleys should be reconstructed.
- At the level of the proximal phalanx, the graft lies deep to the extensor mechanism and deep to the neurovascular bundle, so that the intrinsic tendons and the finger vascularity are not disrupted.

- Whipstitch one end of the graft with a 4.0 braided suture.
- Use a curved hemostat to dissect around the proximal phalanx deep to the extensor mechanism, and pass the suture into the clamp.
- Pass the graft around the mid shaft of the proximal phalanx twice and suture to itself using 3.0 nonabsorbable suture.
- At the level of the middle phalanx, the graft is passed superficial to the extensor mechanism but still deep to the neurovascular bundle. Encircle the middle phalanx twice and suture the graft to itself (**TECH FIG 4B–D**).
- An alternative method is to shoestring the graft through existing pulley edges. The residual pulley is often stiff enough to support the weave.

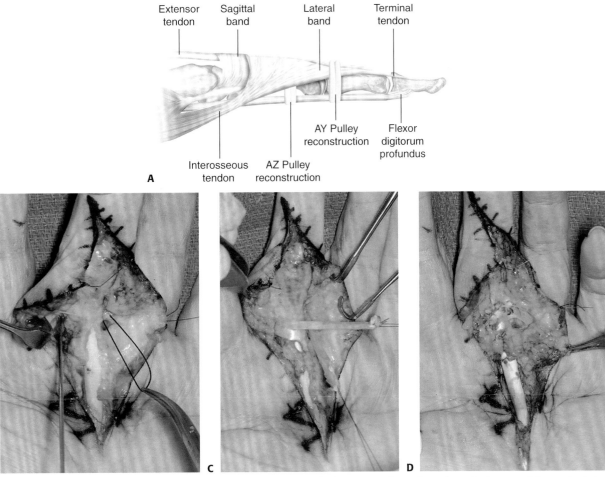

TECH FIG 4 • Pulley reconstruction using tendon autograft. **A.** A2 and A4 pulley location. **B.** The grafts are looped twice around the proximal pha-lanx. **C,D.** The graft is passed under the extensor mechanism for the A2 reconstruction and over the extensor mechanism for the A4 reconstruction.

PEARLS AND PITFALLS

Indications	▪ Single-stage grafting is indicated for a segmental gap in the tendon with an intact sheath. ▪ Two-stage grafting is indicated for a segmental tendon gap with excessive scarring, multistructure injury, failed tendon zone II repair, and/or a deficient sheath. ▪ Digits considered for reconstruction should have adequate vascularity and protective sensation. ▪ Alternatives to tendon reconstruction include adjacent FDS to FDP tendon transfer, arthrodesis, and amputation.
Graft planning	▪ Be sure the desired graft is anatomically present. ▪ Plan for a graft with sufficient length. ▪ If the graft needs to reach the palm, a palmaris graft may be sufficient. ▪ If the graft needs to reach the forearm, a plantaris graft may be necessary. ▪ If a graft is not present, an allograft gracilis or semitendinosus is an acceptable alternative. ▪ The graft should be about 4–5 mm in width to pass through the sheath easily.
Preservation of intact structures	▪ Do not sacrifice an intact FDS to pass a tendon graft. ▪ Preserve as much of the native sheath as possible—not just A2 and A4.

POSTOPERATIVE CARE

Stage 1

- The major goal of stage 1 is to maintain passive range of motion
- 0 to 2 weeks: edema control, dorsal thermoplast splint (wrist neutral, MP joint 60 degrees of flexion, IP joints 0 degrees). Passive flexion and active/passive extension for all joints 6 times per day. If a pulley reconstruction was performed, a thermoplast circumferential pulley ring is worn for 6 weeks.
- 2 to 6 weeks: Remove splint. Buddy strap affected finger to adjacent finger. Continue active and passive exercises until stage 2 is performed (approximately 12 weeks).

Stage 2 (Modified Duran)

- 0 to 3 weeks: Edema control, dorsal thermoplast splint (wrist 20 degrees of flexion, MP joint 60 degrees of flexion, IP joints 0 degrees). Passive flexion and active/passive extension for all joints 6 times per day.
- 3 to 4 weeks: Add active range of motion (AROM), tendon gliding, and place hold exercises in the splint.
- 4 to 6 weeks: Exercises can be performed out of splint. Add blocking exercises to PIP and DIP. Add wrist tenodesis exercises. Add grasp, dexterity, and ADL exercises.
- 6 to 8 weeks: Splint is only worn at night and in crowds. Volar pancake or IP joint extension splints may be added if necessary. Add light resistance exercises.
- 8 to 12 weeks: Discontinue splint. Add progressive resistance exercises and work simulation activities.

OUTCOMES

- Outcomes results are graded by a variety of measures including total active arc of motion (TAM), grip and pinch strength, and scoring systems by Schneider, Stark, and Strickland.[4–6]
- In general, results of primary repair are superior to reconstruction, and fingers with an intact FDS obtain better motion than do those without one.[7] Other factors that portend a better prognosis are younger patient, less soft tissue scar, good preoperative mobility, and at least one intact sensory nerve.[8]
- Grafting through an intact FDS, Stark et al. reported "satisfactory" finger flexion in 20 of 25 patients, defined as a distance of the pulp to distal flexion crease within 3.2 cm and 20-degree active DIP flexion.[5] Using similar criteria, McClinton et al. reported success in 87 of 100 patients with an average of 48 degrees of DIP flexion.[9]

- Two-stage grafting reported by Hunter and Salisbury resulted in pulp to crease flexion within 3.2 cm in 85% of the 69 cases.[10]
- TAM for two-stage grafting ranges from 186 to 206 degrees.[7,11,12]

COMPLICATIONS

- Adhesion of the graft is the most common complication. A tenolysis may be required 3 to 6 months after stage 2 reconstruction.
- Bowstringing, tendon rupture, and infection are also not uncommon complications.
- A tight FDP graft may cause the "quadriga effect," whereby the adjacent digits experience a flexor lag as described earlier.
- A loose FDP graft may cause imbalance in the finger. A swan-neck deformity or a lumbrical plus finger may be the result. Lumbrical plus finger is diagnosed when "paradoxical extension" of the IP joints occurs when the patient attempts to make a fist; the lumbrical originates on the FDP and pulls the IP joints into extension when a retracted FDP contracts. Retensioning the graft or resection of the lumbrical origin may be required.

REFERENCES

1. Hunter JM, Subin D, Minkow F, Konikoff J. Sheath formation in response to limited active gliding implants (animals). *J Biomed Mater Res.* 1974;5:155.
2. Paneva-Holevich E. Two-stage tenoplasty in injury of the flexor tendons of the hand. *J Bone Joint Surg.* 1969;51(1):21-32.
3. Bunnell S. Repair of tendons in the fingers and description of two new instruments. *Surg Gynecol Obstet.* 1918;26:103-110.
4. Schneider LH. Staged flexor tendon reconstruction using the method of Hunter. *Clin Orthop Relat Res.* 1982;171:164-171.
5. Stark HH, Zemel NP, Boyes JH, Ashworth CR. Flexor tendon graft through intact superficialis tendon. *J Hand Surg [Am].* 1977;2(6):456-461.
6. Leversedge FJ, Zelouf D, Williams C, et al. Flexor tendon grafting to the hand: an assessment of the intrasynovial donor tendon: a preliminary single-cohort study. *J Hand Surg [Am].* 2000;25(4):721-730.
7. Tonkin M, Hagberg L, Lister G, Kutz J. Post-operative management of flexor tendon grafting. *J Hand Surg [Br].* 1988;13(3):277-281.
8. Boyes JH, Stark HH. Flexor-tendon grafts in the fingers and thumb: a study of factors influencing results in 1000 cases. *J Bone Joint Surg Am.* 1971;53(7):1332-1342.
9. McClinton MA, Curtis RM, Wilgis EF. One hundred tendon grafts for isolated flexor digitorum profundus injuries. *J Hand Surg [Am].* 1982;7(3):224-229.
10. Hunter JM, Salisbury RE. Flexor-tendon reconstruction in severely damaged hands: a two-stage procedure using a silicone-Dacron reinforced gliding prosthesis prior to tendon grafting. *J Bone Joint Surg Am.* 1971;53(5):829-858.
11. Beris AE, Darlis NA, Korompilias AV, et al. Two-stage flexor tendon reconstruction in zone II using a silicone rod and a pedicled intrasynovial graft. *J Hand Surg [Am].* 2003;28(4):652-660.
12. Coyle MP Jr, Leddy TP, Leddy JP. Staged flexor tendon reconstruction fingertip to palm. *J Hand Surg [Am].* 2002;27(4):581-585.

Tenolysis of Flexor Tendons

Richard Tosti, Jacques A. Machol IV, and Neal C. Chen

DEFINITION

- Total active arc of motion in the fingers is approximately 260 degrees, which is the sum of each individual joint: metacarpophalangeal (MP) joint 85 degrees, proximal interphalangeal (PIP) 110 degrees, and distal interphalangeal (DIP) 65 degrees.
- Flexion contracture is a loss of passive extension. Extension contracture is a loss of passive flexion.
- Flexion lag is a loss of active flexion, but preserved passive flexion. Extension lag is a loss of active extension, but preserved passive extension.
- This chapter will primarily focus on loss of digital motion caused by adhesions of the flexor tendon.

ANATOMY

- The strength and versatility of the hand is dependent upon the balance and gliding of the long flexors and extensors and the intrinsic muscles.
- The extensor apparatus is composed of four lumbrical muscles, four dorsal interossei, three volar interossei, four extensor digitorum communis (EDC) tendons, the extensor indicis proprius (EIP), and the extensor digiti quinti (EDQ).
- The long extensors (EDC, EIP, EDQ) originate in the forearm and insert on the base of their respective proximal phalanx via the sagittal band attachments to the volar plate. The long extensors continue distally to insert on the base of the middle phalanx as the central slip but also give two "lateral slips" that join the intrinsic tendons to form the lateral bands, which insert on the base of the distal phalanx as the terminal tendon.
- The intrinsic muscles originate in the hand and insert on the extensor apparatus. The transverse fibers of the extensor hood link the intrinsic tendon and the proximal phalanx. The oblique fibers of the extensor hood link the intrinsic tendon and the middle phalanx. The tendons of the intrinsic muscles join the lateral slips of the long extensor to form the lateral bands, which insert as the terminal tendon.
- Important to note is the course of the intrinsic tendon relative to centers of rotation at the finger joints. At the MP joint, they course volar to the axis of rotation producing a flexion moment. At the PIP and DIP joints, they course dorsal to the axis of rotation producing an extension moment.[1]

- Nine flexor tendons originate in the forearm. Flexor pollicis longus inserts at the base of the distal phalanx of the thumb. Four flexor digitorum superficialis (FDS) and four flexor digitorum profundus (FDP) tendons insert on the volar base of the middle and distal phalanges, respectively.
- The FDS tendons are superficial to the FDP in the hand, but as they enter the fibrous sheath, the FDS bifurcates into two slips, which are directed dorsally to their insertion.

PATHOGENESIS

- Traumatic or postsurgical stiffness usually begins with edema or hematoma.[2]
- The fluid distends the joints and surrounding structures, becoming a physical barrier to motion.
- The cellular response to injury initiates the inflammatory cascade.
- The inflammatory cascade leads to fibroblast accumulation and fibroblast proliferation into myofibroblasts.
- Reaction to foreign material such as metal plates stimulates adhesion formation as well.
- Persistent motion loss leads to soft tissue contracture.

NATURAL HISTORY

- Contracture or adhesions of dorsal structures generally limit passive flexion. These structures include the dorsal skin, extensor tendons, intrinsic tendons, dorsal capsule, and collateral ligaments.
- Contracture or adhesions of the flexor tendons generally limit active flexion.
- Contracture or adhesions of the volar structures limit passive extension. These structures include the volar skin, flexor tendons, and volar capsule.
- Contracture or adhesions of the extensor tendons limit active extension.

PATIENT HISTORY AND PHYSICAL FINDINGS

- The most common stiff posturing is MP joint extension and IP joint flexion. The MP joint is a cam shape, which holds the greatest fluid volume when in extension. Extension at the MP creates a relative tension on the flexor tendons that brings the IP joints into flexion.
- However, a variety of postures and motion limitations are seen (Table 1).

Table 1 Assessment of a Stiff Finger

Cause	Active Extension	Passive Extension	Active Flexion	Passive Flexion
Extensor tendon adhesion	−	+	−	+/−
Dorsal skin or capsular contracture	+	+	−	−
Flexor tendon adhesion	−	+/−	−	+
Volar skin or capsular contracture	−	−	+	+
Dorsal and volar combined[a]	−	−	−	−
Intrinsic contracture[b]	+	+	−	−

[a]Combined pathology of dorsal and volar structures by adhesion and/or contracture.
[b]Testing of PIP joint with the MP joint extended.

- Begin with assessment of passive and active range of motion (AROM).
- Passive motion greater than active motion suggests a barrier outside the joint (adhesion, rupture, denervation).
- Passive motion of the PIP joint that varies with the position of the MP joint suggests a barrier outside the joint (intrinsic or extrinsic tightness).
- Passive motion barriers may occur from pathology either within the joint or outside the joint.
- Passive motion barriers mask active motion (ability or disability); thus active joint motion can only be assessed after correction of passive motion barrier.

IMAGING

- Stiffness is usually diagnosed by history and physical exam.
- Radiographs may be helpful to rule out bone or joint malalignment as a cause.

DIFFERENTIAL DIAGNOSIS

- Tendon rupture
- Joint contracture

NONOPERATIVE MANAGEMENT

- Prior to any attempt at tenolysis, tissue homeostasis must be achieved. This includes a stable, supple soft tissue envelope, durable bony stability, and edema control.
- It is preferable to gain passive range of motion before a tenolysis procedure if possible.
- Daytime dynamic splints and nighttime static splints can help regain motion. Dynamic splints are typically not worn at night, as they may lose their position.
- Progressive static splints or serial casting can also be successful.

SURGICAL MANAGEMENT

- Surgery may be considered for disability resulting from stiffness if 6 months of nonsurgical management has failed to resolve symptoms.

Preoperative Planning

- Wide-awake surgery under local anesthesia has the advantage of assessing gains in active motion so that intraoperative modifications can be made.
- Hardware removal may be required but should only be performed after bony union has occurred.
- A flexion contracture may be caused by any combination of volar skin contracture, flexor tendon adhesion, or volar capsular contracture; these structures can be addressed by Z-plasty lengthening, flexor tenolysis, or joint release, respectively. Only after the flexion contracture is released can the integrity of the extensor mechanism be assessed.[3]
- An extension contracture may be caused by dorsal skin contracture, extensor tendon adhesion, or dorsal capsule; these structures can be addressed by Z-plasty lengthening, extensor tenolysis, or dorsal capsulotomy/collateral ligament release, respectively. Only after the extension contracture is released can the integrity of the flexor tendons be assessed.[3]
- A flexion lag is often caused by adhesions between the flexor tendon and surrounding bone, soft tissue, and skin. It may only be discovered after release of an extension contracture.
- An extension lag is often caused by adhesions between the extensor tendon and surrounding bone, soft tissue, and skin. It may only be discovered after release of a flexion contracture.

Positioning

- Position the patient supine with the arm on a hand table.
- A nonsterile tourniquet may be used proximally.

Approach

- Dorsal approach to the finger for extensor tenolysis is made through either a longitudinal incision centered over the PIP joint or a radially based curvilinear incision.
- For flexor tenolysis, a volar Bruner incision is the most common approach, although a longitudinal midaxial incision can be considered.
- In patients with a skin contracture, Z-plasty is often helpful.

■ Extensor Tenolysis With or Without Dorsal Capsular Release

- The extensor mechanism is exposed, and any adhesions to the skin are released.
- A Freer elevator can be used to free the extensor hood from the proximal phalanx. This is usually performed from proximally to distally or from laterally to centrally under the lateral bands.
- Caution is taken to avoid detaching the central slip.
- Adhesions to the middle phalanx can also be released from under the lateral bands/extensor hood.
- If there is a PIP joint contracture present, the collateral ligaments can be excised from underneath the lateral bands.
- Adhesions at the level of the metacarpal are approached in a similar manner (**TECH FIG 1**).
- Hardware, if present, should be removed at the time of tenolysis.

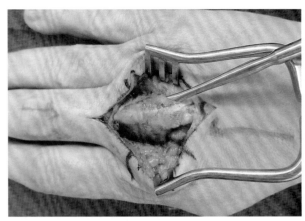

TECH FIG 1 • Extensor tendon adhesions after fixation of metacarpal fracture, dorsal approach showing adhesions of the extensor tendon to the skin and underlying plate.

■ Flexor Tenolysis With or Without Volar Capsular Release

- Open the wound using the prior incisions and identify the neurovascular structures first to protect them (**TECH FIG 2A**).
- The A1 pulley is released and a window is opened over the cruciate and A3 pulleys.
- The A2 and A4 pulleys are preserved as much as possible. If necessary, pulleys may be partially "vented" by making a longitudinal incision along the radial or ulnar border of the sheath.
- The superficialis tendon and the profundus tendon are examined at the level of the A1 pulley using an Allis clamp "turnkey" maneuver (**TECH FIG 2B**).

- Tenolysis knives or a Freer elevator can be used to free adhesions around the tendon. There are often deep adhesions to the bone and between the FDS and FDP (**TECH FIG 2C–G**).
- If a PIP joint contracture exists, the volar plate can be transversely incised and the checkrein ligaments released.[4]
- Rarely, FDS may be sacrificed if dense adhesions and a tight sheath are encountered.
- If contracture of the skin is causing the motion limitation, then preoperative planning should include the design of a longitudinal incision with Z-lengthening at the flexion creases.

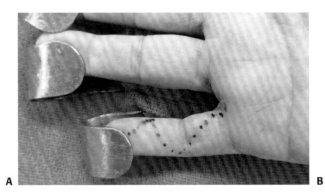

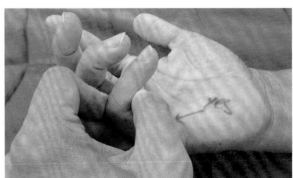

TECH FIG 2 • **A.** Limited flexor tenolysis for adhesions after a pinning of a proximal phalanx fracture. **B.** Turnkey motion demonstrating return of extension. **C.** Both the FDS and FDP tendons were isolated. The A4 pulley was previously excised during the initial repair and was not competent.

TECHNIQUES

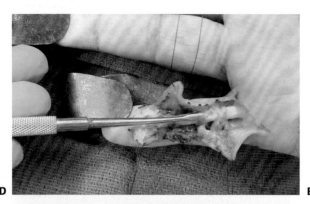
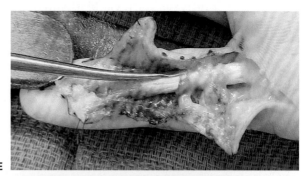
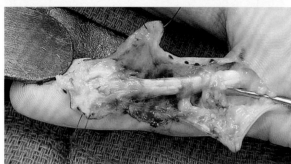
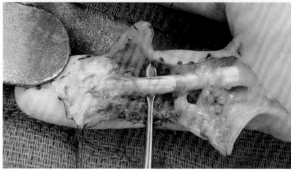

TECH FIG 2 (Continued) • **D–G.** Tenolysis through traction with an Allis clamp was sufficient to disrupt the adhesions and restore motion.

■ Intrinsic Release

- There are two types of intrinsic release:
  - The intrinsics can be released at the extensor hood.
  - The intrinsics can be released proximally off of the metacarpal in the intrinsic slide procedure, typically for intrinsic contracture resulting from compartment syndrome.
- Distal release is indicated for a positive Bunnell intrinsic tightness test. The PIP joint will have less flexion when the MP joint is extended and more flexion when the MP joint is flexed.
- The extensor hood is approached through a single midline dorsal incision or a double midaxial incision.

- The oblique fibers are identified in the distal third of the proximal phalanx.
- A triangular wedge of the oblique fibers is excised.
- Avoid cutting into the transverse fibers, which attach the proximal phalanx to flex the MP joint.
- Proximal release is indicated in patients with severe intrinsic tightness, where the MP joint is also affected.[1]
- Proximal release consists of cutting the intrinsics proximal to the MP joint. Another alternative is an intrinsic slide where the intrinsics are released from the metacarpal. These procedures are typically performed in more severe intrinsic contractures such as those secondary to compartment syndrome.

PEARLS AND PITFALLS

Indications	■ Tenolysis will not improve a stiff finger that has joint incongruity or malalignment. ■ Wounds, swelling, and inflammation should be resolved before surgery. ■ Nonoperative measures should be continued as long as progress is being made. ■ The patient must agree to a strict post-op rehab program before surgery is considered.
Incision	■ For multiple MP joint extension contractures, avoid a single transverse incision, as this will gap during early rehab. ■ Anticipate soft tissue contractures and be prepared to perform Z-plasty or advancement flaps for coverage.
Sequential release	■ Begin with releasing the tendon adhesions from the bone and skin. ■ Release the capsule and then ligaments if necessary. ■ Be mindful that intrinsic tightness may coexist and warrant release.
Rehabilitation	■ Begin rehab immediately after surgery.

POSTOPERATIVE CARE

- All protocols should begin 24 to 48 hours after surgery.
- The quality of the tendon should be noted intraoperatively.
  - Thin, frayed, and poorly vascular tendons are at risk for rupture with an aggressive protocol.[5]

Flexor Tendon Rehabilitation

- Good-quality tendon
  - 0 to 2 weeks: Edema control, volar thermoplast splint (wrist neutral, MP and IP joints 0 degrees) to be worn at night and in between exercises. AROM, tendon gliding, and place-hold exercises to be performed hourly with 10 reps each
  - 2 to 4 weeks: Continue above. Add blocking exercises to PIP and DIP. Add grasp, dexterity, and ADL exercises. Add scar management.
  - 4 to 8 weeks: Continue above. Add sustained gripping and progressive resistance. May add dynamic extension splint if needed.
  - 8 to 12 weeks: Add heavy resistance exercises and work simulation activities.
- Poor-quality tendon
  - 0 to 2 weeks: Edema control, volar thermoplast splint to be worn at night and in between exercises. The splint is fabricated to place the joints in full extension for extensor lag and in resting position for extension contracture. Passive flexion performed hourly.
  - 2 to 4 weeks: Add AROM, tendon gliding, and place-hold exercises to be performed hourly with 10 reps each. The splint is gradually brought to allow MP joint at 0 degrees by 4 weeks. Add scar management.
  - 4 to 8 weeks: Add blocking exercises to PIP and DIP. Add grasp, dexterity, and ADL exercises.
  - 8 to 12 weeks: Add sustained gripping and progressive resistance. May add dynamic extension splint if needed.
  - 12 weeks: Add heavy resistance exercises and work simulation activities.

Extensor Tendon Rehabilitation

- Good-quality tendon
  - 0 to 2 weeks: Edema control, volar thermoplast splint to be worn at night and in between exercises. Fabricate the splint to place the finger joints in extension for extensor lag and in resting position for extension contracture. AROM, gliding, place-hold, and blocking exercises performed hourly.
  - 2 to 4 weeks: Add grasp, dexterity, and ADL exercises. Add scar management.
  - 4 to 8 weeks: Add sustained gripping exercises. At 6 weeks, add progressive resistance. May add dynamic flexion splint if needed.
  - 8 to 12 weeks: Add heavy resistance exercises and work simulation activities.
- Poor-quality tendon
  - 0 to 2 weeks: Edema control, volar thermoplast splint to be worn at night and in between exercises. Fabricate the splint to place the finger joints in extension for extensor lag and in resting position for extension contracture. Tenodesis exercise, gentle AROM, gliding, and place-hold performed hourly.
  - 2 to 4 weeks: Add AROM and blocking exercises. Add scar management.

- 4 to 8 weeks: Add grasp, dexterity, and ADL exercises.
- 8 to 12 weeks: Add sustained gripping exercises and progressive resistance. May add dynamic flexion splint if needed.
- 12 weeks: Add heavy resistance exercises and work simulation activities.

OUTCOMES

- Weeks et al. evaluated 789 stiff MP and PIP joints in 212 patients at a mean 3.4 months after injury. Exercises and dynamic splinting alone were effective in 87% of patients. MP joint range of motion (ROM) improved 32 degrees on average, while PIP joint ROM improved 36 degrees on average. Surgery was required for the remaining 13%.[6]
- Hunter et al. reported on 61 digits with PIP joint contractures treated nonoperatively with exercises and static or dynamic splints. Preoperative motion at the PIP joint range of motion was 24 to 67 degrees, which improved to 8 to 98 degrees.[5]
- Breton et al. reported on 75 digits that underwent postinjury zone II flexor tendon tenolysis. They noted a preoperative total arc of motion of 128 degrees and a postoperative arc of 192 degrees at 3 months. Flexor tendon rupture occurred in seven cases.[7]
- Yamazaki et al. noted that the preoperative range of motion was the strongest predictor of postoperative range of motion in patients undergoing flexor tenolysis after phalangeal fracture.[8]
- Adjunctive treatments such as indwelling local anesthesia catheters and continuous passive motion (CPM) devices have been described; however, limited evidence justifies their routine use. Schwartz and Chafetz noted no difference in gains in total arc of motion with CPM.[9]

COMPLICATIONS

- Tendon rupture can occur if tenolysis performed before repair site is healed.
- Tendon disruption can occur if the tenolysis erroneously strips the insertion site.
- Recurrence can occur if the patient is not compliant with rehab or if the zone of injury is too great.

REFERENCES

1. Smith RJ. Balance and kinetics of the fingers under normal and pathological conditions. *Clin Orthop Relat Res.* 1974;104:92-111.
2. Schneider LH. Tenolysis and capsulectomy after hand fractures. *Clin Orthop Relat Res.* 1996;(327):72-78.
3. Jupiter JB, Goldfarb CA, Nagy L, Boyer MI. Posttraumatic reconstruction in the hand. *Instr Course Lect.* 2007;56:91-99.
4. Watson HK, Light TR, Johnson TR. Checkrein resection for flexion contracture of the middle joint. *J Hand Surg [Am].* 1979;4:67-71.
5. Hunter E, Laverty J, Pollack R. Nonoperative treatment of fixed flexion deformity of the proximal interphalangeal joint. *J Hand Surg Br.* 1999;24:281-283.
6. Weeks PM, Wray RC Jr, Kuxhaus M. The results of non-operative management of stiff joints in the hand. *Plast Reconstr Surg.* 1978;61:58-63.
7. Breton A, Jager T, Dap F, Dautel G. Effectiveness of flexor tenolysis in zone II: a retrospective series of 40 patients at 3 months postoperatively. *Chir Main.* 2015;34(3):126-133.
8. Yamazaki H, Kato H, Uchiyama S, et al. Results of tenolysis for flexor tendon adhesion after phalangeal fracture. *J Hand Surg Eur Vol.* 2008;33(5):557-560.
9. Schwartz DA, Chafetz R. Continuous passive motion after tenolysis in hand therapy patients: a retrospective study. *J Hand Ther.* 2008;21(3):261-266.

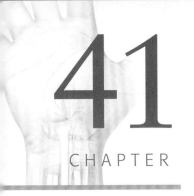

41

CHAPTER

Acute Repair of Extensor Tendon Injuries in Zones I to VI

Michael Smith, Jacques A. Machol IV, and Neal C. Chen

DEFINITION

- The extensor apparatus of the hand is a delicate and complex system that works in synergy with the flexor system to facilitate gross and fine motor activity of the hand and digits.
- Extrinsic extensor function is provided to the digits by the extensor digitorum communis (EDC), extensor indicis proprius (EIP), and extensor digiti minimi (EDM). These muscles work in concert with the intrinsic muscles of the hand to provide extension of the proximal and distal interphalangeal (DIP) joints through the intrinsics' contributions to the extensor mechanism via the lateral bands.
- The extensor apparatus can be injured by blunt or sharp trauma, as well as by attrition from inflammatory conditions.

ANATOMY

- The extensor tendons can be divided into superficial and deep muscle groups.[1]
- The superficial group includes the extensor carpi radialis longus (ECRL), the extensor carpi radialis brevis (ECRB), the EDC, the EDM, and the extensor carpi ulnaris (ECU).
- The deep group includes the extensor pollicis brevis (EPB), the extensor pollicis longus (EPL), and the EIP.
- The extensors are innervated by the posterior interosseous nerve (PIN) with the exception of the ECRB and ECRL, which are innervated by the radial nerve prior to the split into the PIN and the superficial radial nerve.[2]
- The ECRB may sometimes be innervated by the PIN after the radial nerve has split.
- The extensor tendons travel through six separate dorsal compartments at the level of the wrist prior to entering the hand.
- The first dorsal compartment contains the abductor pollicis longus (APL) and the EPB tendons.

- There is septation of this compartment in 20% to 60% of individuals, and it is common for the APL to have multiple tendon slips.[3]
- The second dorsal compartment contains the wrist extensors, the ECRB and ECRL.
  - The ECRB is located ulnarly in relation to the ECRL.
- The third dorsal compartment contains the EPL tendon and is just ulnar to Lister tubercle on the radius.
- The fourth dorsal compartment contains the EIP and EDC tendons. The PIN is also found within the base of this compartment.
  - The EIP can be identified at the level of the hand and wrist in that it:
    - Is ulnar to the index finger slip of the EDC
    - Has the distal most muscle belly
    - Is the deepest tendon proximal to the extensor retinaculum
    - Is not connected by juncturae tendinum
  - The EIP is absent in up to 1% of the population and can have multiple slips in up to 16% of the population.
- The fifth dorsal compartment contains the EDM and overlies the distal radioulnar joint (DRUJ).
  - The EDM is found ulnar to the EDC tendon to the small finger.
  - The EDC tendon to the small finger is often absent, and a double EDM tendon may occur in 80% to 90% of individuals.[4]
- The sixth dorsal compartment contains the ECU tendon.
- At the level of the hand, the tendons become flat and juncturae tendinum provides interconnections between the EDC tendons.
- At the level of the metacarpophalangeal (MCP) joint, the radial and ulnar sagittal bands form a sling around the extensor tendon and attach to the volar plate (**FIG 1A**).
- Distal to the MCP, the intrinsic muscles of the hand join the extensor tendons to form the extensor hood.

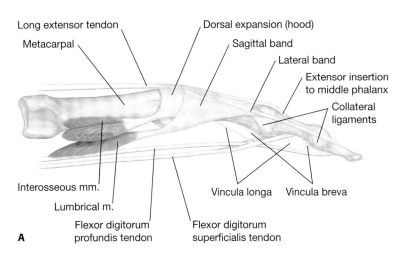

Long extensor tendon
Metacarpal
Dorsal expansion (hood)
Sagittal band
Lateral band
Extensor insertion to middle phalanx
Collateral ligaments
Interosseous mm.
Lumbrical m.
Flexor digitorum profundis tendon
Flexor digitorum superficialis tendon
Vincula longa   Vincula breva

A

FIG 1 • A–C. Extensor apparatus at the digit.

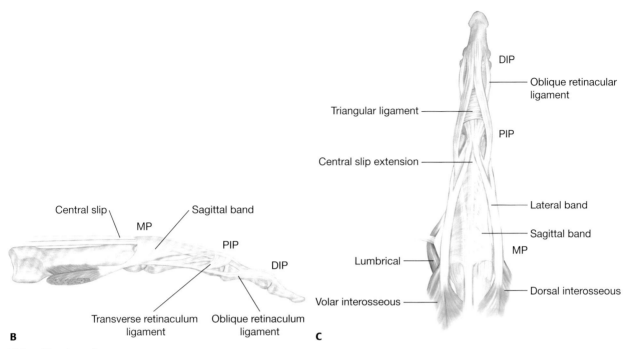

B   **C**

FIG 1 (Continued)

- The central tendon trifurcates at the level of the proximal phalanx, with the radial and ulnar slips becoming the lateral bands and the central slip inserting into the base of the middle phalanx by providing proximal interphalangeal (PIP) joint extension.
- The interossei split into medial and lateral slips. The medial slip will insert into the base of the proximal phalanx and functions to flex the MCP joint. The lateral slip will join with the lateral band of the common extensor tendon to form the conjoined lateral band. The radial and ulnar conjoined lateral bands will form the terminal tendon and insert onto the distal phalanx, extending the DIP joint (**FIG 1B,C**).
- The triangular ligament prevents the conjoined lateral bands from volar subluxation, and the transverse retinacular ligament prevents dorsal subluxation.[1]
- By convention, the extensor tendons are divided into nine zones to assist in classification of extensor tendon injuries. Odd-numbered zones are located over joints, and even-numbered zones are located over the long bones (**FIG 2**):
  - Zone I includes the DIP.
  - Zone II is the middle phalanx.
  - Zone III is the PIP.
  - Zone IV is the proximal phalanx.
  - Zone V is overlying the MCP joint.
  - Zone VI is over the metacarpals.
  - Zone VII includes the carpus and extensor retinaculum.
  - Zone VIII involves the distal forearm, up to the musculotendinous junction of the tendons.
  - Zone IX involves the remaining part of the upper forearm.

PATHOGENESIS

- Extensor tendons can be disrupted in a number of ways.
- Disruption of the terminal tendon in zone I, resulting in a mallet finger, can occur either through an avulsion of the

tendon from its insertion or a fracture of the base of the distal phalanx at the tendon insertion.
- The tendons can also be cut from a sharp laceration, and it is not uncommon to encounter tendon ruptures from attritional wear, from either inflammatory arthritis or other conditions such as prominent hardware.

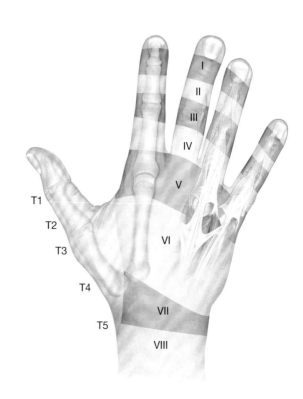

FIG 2 • Extensor tendon zones.

NATURAL HISTORY

- Often, there is an extensor deficit when the tendon is not repaired. In some cases, such as mallet fingers, the patient can still have a functional hand, even with the extensor tendon left unrepaired.
- In other cases, such as a sharp laceration of the EDC at zone VII, there will be residual impairment.

PATIENT HISTORY AND PHYSICAL FINDINGS

- Patients will often present with a history of a recent trauma in the instance of extensor tendon laceration or mallet finger (**FIG 3**).
  - Pain and a history of a pop are common with a mallet finger injury.
  - Patients with attritional rupture, especially patients with inflammatory arthropathy who already have some functional deficits in their hand, may not realize that one of their extensor tendons has ruptured.
- Initial evaluation should include a thorough physical examination, testing all flexor and extensor tendons, in addition to the digital neurovascular bundles.
- Upon initial inspection, attention should be paid to the resting cascade of the digits. If this is disrupted, there is a high likelihood of tendon injury.
- Wounds should be closely inspected and a determination made of the cleanliness, sharpness, size, location, and potential for injury with the wound.
- The function of each extensor tendon should be tested both with and without resistance. Test each finger individually as the juncturae tendinum may mask an injury.
  - To test the EIP and EDM, ask the patient to keep the middle and ring fingers flexed into the palm and extend the index and small fingers.
  - If there is pain and swelling of the PIP joint, coupled with a mild PIP extension lag or weak PIP joint extension against resistance, one must consider a central slip injury.
  - The Elson test, in which the DIP joint will become rigid with attempted extension of the PIP joint from a flexed position, will confirm an early central slip injury. The DIP becomes rigid because the finger extends through the intact lateral slips.
- Active and passive range of motion of all the joints in the hand and wrist should be tested and recorded.

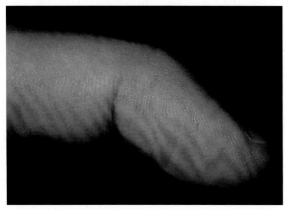

FIG 3 • Clinical appearance of a mallet finger (zone 1 extensor tendon injury). (Courtesy of Philip Blazar, MD.)

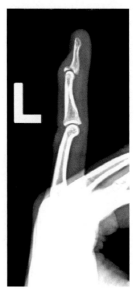

FIG 4 • Radiographic appearance of a bony mallet injury. (Courtesy of Philip Blazar, MD.)

IMAGING

- Radiographs of the hand or digit should be taken in orthogonal planes after an acute extensor tendon injury. This will identify any associated fractures, such as in a bony mallet injury (**FIG 4**), and can also identify any foreign bodies remaining in the extremity after a sharp injury.
- Ultrasound can be a useful adjunct in the setting of a chronic tendon injury to determine the position of the proximal and distal tendon ends if direct repair is being considered.
  - If 4 to 6 weeks have passed since injury, or if the nature of the rupture was secondary to attritional rupture, direct repair often is not possible because of shortening of the proximal tendon, and reconstruction or transfer should be considered.
- MRI can also aid in determining the position of the tendon ends; however, this is an expensive modality and can be time-consuming to obtain in some institutions.
  - In doubtful cases, ultrasound can make a precise determination of the tendon status.

DIFFERENTIAL DIAGNOSIS

- Extensor tendon laceration or disruption
- Adhesions of the extensor tendon system
- Fracture
- PIN palsy
- Radial nerve palsy

NONOPERATIVE MANAGEMENT

- Nonoperative management of extensor tendon disruption is usually considered for soft tissue mallet finger injuries and closed central slip avulsions.
- In closed soft tissue mallet finger injuries, good results can often be obtained with full-time DIP extension splinting.[5] The duration of immobilization varies, but we usually use an extension splint for 8 weeks followed by 4 weeks of night splinting.

- Patient compliance is the most important factor for achieving good outcome with extension splinting of soft tissue mallet injuries. However, patients should be counseled that they will likely have a small extensor lag and dorsal prominence either with or without operative treatment.
- Surgical indications for soft tissue mallet injuries are debated but traditionally include open injuries or mallet fractures with volar subluxation or a fracture fragment larger than 30% to 50% of the articular surface.
- If there is a closed injury to the central slip, the injury can be treated with extension splinting of the PIP joint. One must ensure that the full passive PIP joint extension and DIP flexion can be achieved in the splint.
  - Full-time extension splinting is continued for 6 weeks, followed by 6 weeks of nighttime splinting.
  - Active flexion exercises of the DIP during this period of immobilization can help pull the lateral bands dorsally and prevent volar subluxation of the bands, which can result in a boutonniere deformity.
- If the tendon injury is incomplete, greater than 50% of the tendon is intact, and there is no extensor lag or weakness on physical exam, tendon injuries can be treated nonoperatively with 1 or 2 weeks of splinting.

SURGICAL MANAGEMENT

Preoperative Planning

- Prior to undertaking surgical repair of the extensor tendons, one must ensure that they have performed a complete physical examination of the hand and upper extremity. Other tendon injuries, nerve injuries, fractures, or concomitant conditions that will need to be addressed surgically should be identified preoperatively.
- Radiographs should be obtained to rule out fracture, foreign body, or other etiology of tendon injury such as inflammatory arthritis or prominent hardware.
- If the tendon disruption is chronic, a detailed preoperative plan should be developed to include the possibility of tendon reconstruction or transfer if the tendon cannot be repaired primarily.
- If necessary, pinning of the PIP joint is considered.
- Any additional equipment that may be required to complete and protect a strong repair should be communicated to the operating room staff in advance, including hardware and intraoperative fluoroscopy.

Positioning

- The positioning for the techniques listed below is the same.
- The patient is placed supine on the operating room table.
- A hand and upper extremity table extension is attached to the table.
- A nonsterile tourniquet is applied to the upper arm over padding.
- The arm is pronated to expose the dorsum of the hand.
- One or two OR towels are fluffed and placed in the palm of the hand to keep the fingers extended.

Approach

- There are a number of described surgical approaches to the dorsum of the DIP, PIP, and MCP joints as well as the hand, wrist, and forearm.[6]
- In general, a longitudinal incision is preferred to allow the surgeon to extend the incision distally or proximally should the need arise.
  - We prefer to make a gentle S incision over the DIP joint, a radially based curvilinear longitudinal incision across the PIP and MCP joints and a straight longitudinal incision over the metacarpals, wrist, and forearm.
- The incision should take into consideration possible future procedures.
- If there is a laceration, this is usually extended proximally and distally in a longitudinal manner to fully explore the wound and injured structures.
- Distal to the carpus, there is not much subcutaneous tissue between the skin and the tendon layer. The dissection is brought down sharply to the level of the tendons or extensor retinaculum with care taken to preserve dorsal veins if possible.
- Once the level of the tendon is encountered, full-thickness skin flaps are raised for full exposure of the tendon ends or extensor retinaculum.
  - If the extensor retinaculum is to be opened, we prefer to identify the EPL exiting distally and open the retinaculum in line with the third dorsal compartment to ensure the EPL tendon does not get inadvertently transected.

■ Repair of Open Mallet Injury (Zone I Injury)

- If the terminal tendon has been sharply transected, it is possible to perform a primary repair that is then supplemented with Kirschner wire fixation of the DIP joint in extension.
- Often, the pre-existing laceration can be incorporated into the incision and should be extended distally and proximally.
- Careful sharp dissection of the skin off the terminal tendon is performed, preferably with a flexible scalpel (Beaver Mini-Blade No. 67, Beaver-Visitec Int.).
- Once the terminal tendon has been exposed, insert the K-wire in retrograde fashion under C-arm fluoroscopy to hold the joint in extension while the tendon repair is being performed.
- A determination is made if there is enough remaining terminal tendon in the insertion of the distal phalanx to facilitate direct repair.
  - If there is enough tendon remaining, a four-strand repair is then performed using a 4-0 nonabsorbable braided suture, usually in doubled horizontal mattress configuration if possible or a figure-eight configuration.
  - If there is not enough tendon remaining for a primary repair, the proximal tendon end can be brought back to the insertion site of the distal phalanx and secured over a pullout suture button.
- Repair using one or two microsuture anchors has been described; however, the insertion of the terminal

T E C H N I Q U E S

tendon is immediately adjacent to the origin of the germinal matrix and the risk of iatrogenic injury to the nail bed makes this our less preferred technique.

- A simpler method of repair involves dermatotenodesis (**TECH FIG 1**). With this method, one or two 2-0 nylon sutures are placed through the skin and tendon ends and sutured in a horizontal mattress fashion. The sutures are left for 3 weeks and then removed. Full-time splinting is continued for a total of 6 weeks and nighttime splinting for an additional 6 weeks.

- Once the repair is completed, the wound is copiously irrigated and the skin is closed with interrupted suture.
- The joint is protected with an extension splint for the length of time the pin is in place.
- We pull the pin at 4 to 6 weeks and continue with nighttime splinting for an additional 6 weeks.
- Active and passive range of motion at the PIP and MCP joints is encouraged to prevent stiffness.

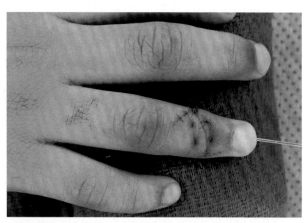

TECH FIG 1 • Example of dermatotenodesis performed in the ring finger after a zone I extensor tendon injury. (Courtesy of Philip Blazar, MD.)

■ Closed Mallet Fracture Pinning

- Ideally, before a closed mallet fracture is brought to the operating room for surgical repair, one should attempt to obtain radiographs with the digit held in extension at the DIP joint to see if fracture reduces easily.
  - If seen acutely, oftentimes the fracture will reduce well with extension of the digit.
- At the beginning of the procedure, the C-arm is brought in and joint is visualized radiographically.
- The DIP joint is then flexed in an attempt to bring the dorsal fragment as far distal as possible.
- One 0.028- or 0.035-in. Kirschner wire (K-wire) is then placed just proximal and dorsal to the dorsal fragment and driven across the DIP joint into the middle phalanx.

- The distal phalanx is then extended, and the K-wire should hold the dorsal fragment in a stable position as the phalanx reduces back to the fragment.
- Once adequate reduction has been achieved, a second K-wire is inserted in a retrograde fashion from the tip of the distal phalanx across the DIP joint and into the middle phalanx.
- The DIP joint is protected with an extension splint throughout the time the pins are in place.
- The pins are pulled in the office at 4 to 6 weeks and nighttime splinting continues for an additional 6 weeks.
- Active and passive range of motion at the PIP and MCP joints is encouraged to prevent stiffness.

■ Zone III Central Slip Repair

- Zone III injuries overlie the PIP joint and involve the insertion of the central slip.
- If left untreated, the lateral bands will migrate volarly and a boutonniere deformity can develop (PIP joint flexion and DIP joint hyperextension).
- Central slip repair can be achieved by either primary repair in open lacerations or injuries or with suture anchors for avulsion injuries.
  - In 1999, Cluett et al.[7] found similar biomechanical strengths for both suture anchor repair and primary repair.
- For lacerations, the laceration is extended proximally and distally to provide full exposure of the central slip and assess for any additional injury to the bone and PIP articular surface.
  - In closed, avulsion-type injuries, a dorsal curvilinear approach is utilized. This avoids making a longitudinal incision directly over the PIP joint.

- Skin flaps are raised sharply, taking advantage of the layer between the skin and the extensor apparatus.
- The injured central slip is identified and the tendon edges sharply debrided.
- The PIP joint is pinned in extension with a single 0.035-in. K-wire.
- If primary repair is to be performed, we prefer to perform the repair using a running, interlocking, horizontal mattress stitch popularized by Lee et al.[8] using a 3-0 or 4-0 braided nonabsorbable suture.
- If suture anchor repair is to be performed, we prefer to place a single mini anchor into the central footprint of the middle phalanx. Care is taken to direct the suture anchor away from the base of the middle phalanx, so as not to penetrate the joint surface with the suture anchor.
- Postoperatively, active DIP motion is allowed. The pin is removed from the PIP joint at 3 weeks. At this point, begin gentle range of motion with hand therapy and nighttime splinting as needed.

■ Zone V Extensor Tendon Repair

- Extensor tendon injury at the level of the MCP joint is the most common location for extensor tendon disruption (**TECH FIG 2A**).[1]
- This zone is also where "fight bite" injuries often occur and special diligence must be made to ensure the MCP joint is thoroughly irrigated to prevent or treat an underlying septic arthritis of the MCP joint.
- There is a high incidence of partial tendon lacerations at this level. Extensor tendon lacerations involving more than 50% of the tendon should be repaired.
- Zone V injuries also must take into account the sagittal bands on the radial and ulnar sides of the MCP joint.
  - If the patient has an acute closed sagittal band rupture, it can often be treated with extension splinting of the MCP joint for 3 to 4 weeks with the PIP joint free.

- Extend the laceration both proximally and distally to ensure there is adequate exposure of the extensor tendon injury at this level and the MCP joint.
- Raise skin flaps with sharp dissection in the plane between the skin and the extensor apparatus.
- With open injuries, the MCP joint should always be explored and irrigated to prevent septic arthritis.
- Evaluate the sagittal band, and if it has been lacerated, perform a primary repair with a braided absorbable suture after the tendon has been repaired.
- At this level, the tendon is beginning to become thicker and may accommodate a core suture. If possible, we prefer to repair the tendon at this level with either a four-strand repair using 3-0 braided, nonabsorbable suture or the running, interlocking, horizontal mattress suture configuration described above (**TECH FIG 2B,C**).
- Postoperatively, there has recently been more emphasis on early, controlled mobilization of the repair.

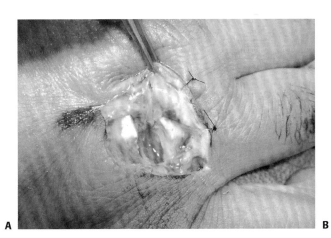
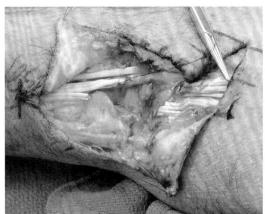
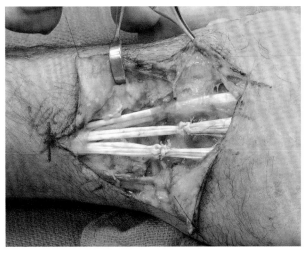

TECH FIG 2 ● A. Initial exploration of a zone V laceration with disruption of the extensor tendon to the ring finger. **B.** Zone VII extensor tendon laceration. **C.** Zone VII extensor tendon repair using core sutures. (Courtesy of Philip Blazar, MD.)

TECHNIQUES

PEARLS AND PITFALLS

Counseling	▪ It is important to set realistic expectations with your patients for the treatment of mallet fingers. Long-term studies have shown that patients undergoing either surgical or nonoperative treatment will likely have some degree of mild extensor lag at the end of treatment.
Technique	▪ The dorsal skin can be thin and friable. Take extra care to handle the tissues delicately and develop full-thickness skin flaps.
Indications	▪ In soft tissue mallet injuries, splinting is preferable to surgical repair as the skin is thin and sometimes can die after surgery. In addition, suture material can be prominent.
Suture anchors	▪ If placing suture anchors into the distal phalanx for a zone I repair, be careful not to place the anchor into the germinal matrix.
Zone V injuries	▪ Always explore the MCP joint in open injuries. Wound cultures should be obtained in "fight bite injuries."

POSTOPERATIVE CARE

▪ Traditionally, extensor tendon repairs have been treated with initial immobilization for longer periods of time when compared with flexor tendon repairs.
▪ There is some evidence that for zone V and VI repairs, there are better short-term functional results with early mobilization protocols. There is some evidence of short-term superiority of early, controlled mobilization of extensor tendon repairs but no evidence of long-term superiority of early motion compared with immobilization[9]; plus, there is a higher risk of tendon repair rupture.[10,11]
▪ For zone I, II, and III repairs, immobilization of the DIP and PIP joints respectively in extension for 6 weeks after repair is reasonable.
  ▪ At that time, range of motion exercises can begin and nighttime splinting initiated for an additional 6 weeks.
  ▪ Be sure to move the remaining joints of the finger to help prevent stiffness of the entire digit.
▪ For zone IV, V, and VI repairs, the MCP joints respectively are immobilized for about 4 weeks in extension, followed by gentle range of motion in conjunction with hand therapy. There is variation regarding immobilizing the PIP joints.

OUTCOMES

▪ Kalainov et al.[12] treated 21 patients with mallet fractures in which greater than one-third of the articular surface was involved with splinting in a 2005 retrospective study. They had good results in terms of pain and function, but their follow-up averaged only 2 years.
▪ Outcomes of surgical treatment for mallet injuries have been comparable across the various techniques. Most patients will have an extensor lag from 2 to 7 degrees and flexion ranged from 67 to 78 degrees.[13–16]
▪ Pratt et al. reported on 27 patients who underwent zone III repairs and were treated with a postoperative protocol that consisted of static immobilization for 3 weeks and early controlled motion for an additional 3 weeks. Twenty-two of 27 patients had good results with mean PIP flexion of 94 degrees. Five fingers had extension lags of an average of 6 degrees.[17]
▪ Newport et al. reported on 101 digits that underwent extensor tendon repair and were treated postoperatively with static splinting.[18] They found that patients with associated injuries (fracture, dislocation, flexor tendon injury) and distal repairs (zones I–IV) did worse than those without injuries and proximal repairs, with flexion loss being the most significant complication.

COMPLICATIONS

▪ Infection
▪ Tendon rupture
▪ Extensor lag
▪ Wound dehiscence
▪ Adhesions and stiffness
▪ Nail deformities

REFERENCES

1. Matzon JL, Bozentka DJ. Extensor tendon injuries. *J Hand Surg [Am]*. 2010;35(5):854-861.
2. Branovacki G, Hanson M, Cash R, Gonzalez M. The innervation pattern of the radial nerve at the elbow and in the forearm. *J Hand Surg Br*. 1998;23(2):167-169.
3. Gonzalez MH, Sohlberg R, Brown A, Weinzweig N. The first dorsal extensor compartment: an anatomic study. *J Hand Surg [Am]*. 1995;20(4):657-660.
4. Celik S, Bilge O, Pinar Y, Govsa F. The anatomical variations of the extensor tendons to the dorsum of the hand. *Clin Anat*. 2008;21(7):652-659.
5. Handoll HH, Vaghela MV. Interventions for treating mallet finger injuries. *Cochrane Database Syst Rev*. 2004;(3):CD004574.
6. Cheah AE, Yao J. Surgical approaches to the proximal interphalangeal joint. *J Hand Surg [Am]*. 2016;41(2):294-305.
7. Cluett J, Milne AD, Yang D, Morris SF. Repair of central slip avulsions using Mitek Micro Arc bone anchors: an in vitro biomechanical assessment. *J Hand Surg Br*. 1999;24(6):679-682.
8. Lee SK, Dubey A, Kim BH, et al. A biomechanical study of extensor tendon repair methods: introduction to the running-interlocking horizontal mattress extensor tendon repair technique. *J Hand Surg [Am]*. 2010;35(1):19-23.
9. Talsma E, de Haart M, Beelen A, Nollet F. The effect of mobilization on repaired extensor tendon injuries of the hand: a systematic review. *Arch Phys Med Rehabil*. 2008;89(12):2366-2372.
10. Mowlavi A, Burns M, Brown RE. Dynamic versus static splinting of simple zone V and zone VI extensor tendon repairs: a prospective, randomized, controlled study. *Plast Reconstr Surg*. 2005;115(2):482-487.
11. Bulstrode NW, Burr N, Pratt AL, Grobbelaar AO. Extensor tendon rehabilitation: a prospective trial comparing three rehabilitation regimes. *J Hand Surg Br*. 2005;30(2):175-179.
12. Kalainov DM, Hoepfner PE, Hartigan BJ, et al. Nonsurgical treatment of closed mallet finger fractures. *J Hand Surg [Am]*. 2005;30(3):580-586.
13. Moradi A, Kachooei AR, Mudgal CS. Mallet fracture. *J Hand Surg [Am]*. 2014;39(10):2067-2069.
14. Hofmeister EP, Mazurek MT, Shin AY, Bishop AT. Extension block pinning for large mallet fractures. *J Hand Surg [Am]*. 2003;28(3):453-459.
15. Fritz D, Lutz M, Arora R, et al. Delayed single Kirschner wire compression technique for mallet fracture. *J Hand Surg Br*. 2005;30(2):180-184.
16. Lu J, Jiang J, Xu L, et al. Modification of the pull-in suture technique for mallet finger. *Ann Plast Surg*. 2013;70(1):30-33.
17. Pratt AL, Burr N, Grobbelaar AO. A prospective review of open central slip laceration repair and rehabilitation. *J Hand Surg Br*. 2002;27(6):530-534.
18. Newport ML, Blair WF, Steyers CM Jr. Long-term results of extensor tendon repair. *J Hand Surg [Am]*. 1990;15(6):961-966.

Stabilization of Extensor Carpi Ulnaris Tendon Subluxation With Extensor Retinaculum

Michael Smith, Jacques A. Machol IV, and Neal C. Chen

DEFINITION

- Symptomatic recurrent extensor carpi ulnaris (ECU) subluxation over the ulnar head with forearm rotation can be a cause of ulnar-sided wrist pain. Not all patients with subluxation of the ECU are symptomatic, and painless subluxation is not an absolute indication for surgery.
- Symptomatic ECU instability manifests in patients who play sports such as tennis, hockey, squash, golf, or baseball.
- It is suspected that snapping of the ECU over the ulnar head with resisted supination, flexion, and ulnar deviation is the mechanism that leads to symptoms.

ANATOMY

- The ECU tendon runs through the sixth dorsal compartment following an angular path across the ulnar head as it travels from its muscle origin on the lateral epicondyle to its insertion on the base of the fifth metacarpal.
- The ECU ulnarly deviates and extends the wrist. The ulnar deviation is counterbalanced by the radially deviating forces of the abductor pollicis longus, extensor carpi radialis longus, and the extensor carpi radialis.
  - The ECU tendon lies just dorsal to the flexion/extension axis of the wrist; therefore, the tendon is at risk for subluxation volar to the flexion/extension axis with hypersupination of the forearm and flexion with ulnar deviation of the wrist.[1]
  - The ECU tendon is stabilized by the extensor retinaculum.
  - The ECU tendon runs through a fibro-osseous tunnel at the level of the distal ulna called the ulnar groove.
    - The average ECU groove depth measures approximately 1.4 mm, and the radius of curvature is approximately 7.0 mm.[2]
- In addition, the ECU has its own subsheath, which consists of an overlying band of connective tissue measuring 1.5 to 2.5 cm in length that functions to keep the ECU tendon within the ulnar groove.
  - There are transverse fibers of the medial wall of the ECU compartment that extend proximally and become confluent with the ECU epimysium. These fibers help prevent volar subluxation of the tendon during supination.[2,3]
  - The ECU subsheath stabilizes the ECU during forearm rotation, while the extensor retinaculum helps prevent bowstringing of the extensor tendons.
  - The ECU subsheath also contributes to the dorsal portion of the triangular fibrocartilage complex.
- The distal subsheath contributes more to ECU stability than does the proximal half of the subsheath.[4]
  - Wrist flexion and supination are positions of relative instability for the ECU subsheath.[4]

PATHOGENESIS

- Incompetence of the ECU subsheath, whether through attritional wear or acute traumatic injury, is thought to lead to ECU instability.
  - Laxity in the ECU subsheath and painless snapping over the ulnar head may be a normal variant, especially in individuals that are ligamentously lax.
- It is proposed that traumatic wrist flexion, ulnar deviation, and supination can result in rupture of the ECU subsheath from its ulnar attachments and lead to the subluxation of the tendon out of the distal ulnar groove.[1]
- Symptomatic patients may demonstrate a snap when the wrist is placed in the at-risk position of flexion, ulnar deviation, and supination.
- ECU instability injuries were classified by Inoue and Tamura and separated into three distinct types.
  - The ECU subsheath can have detachment along the ulnar border (type A), the radial border (type B), or a periosteal detachment with expansion of the sheath, creating a false pouch that allows subluxation of the tendon from the ulnar groove (type C).[5,6]

NATURAL HISTORY

- If left untreated, chronic instability of the ECU tendon can exacerbate ECU tendinopathy as the tendon snaps over the ulnar prominence of the ulnar groove.
- Some authors have theorized that chronic dislocation of the ECU tendon may lead to distal radioulnar joint (DRUJ) instability and eventual degenerative changes at the DRUJ. This phenomenon is uncommon.
- There are some patients who have naturally lax ligaments and have a degree of subluxation of the ECU tendon without previous injury. Their ECU instability is often bilateral and asymptomatic and found incidentally on exam.
  - In general, we recommend observing these patients.

PATIENT HISTORY AND PHYSICAL FINDINGS

- Patients are often younger and participate in stick or racket sports such as tennis, golf, baseball, or hockey.
- Patients will complain of recurrent, painful snapping over the dorsoulnar wrist with wrist supination and pronation that limits their participation in sports, hobbies, or activities of daily living.
- There may be a history of a specific, acute injury.
- On physical exam, the ECU tendon can be palpated subluxating over the ulnar head with circumduction of the wrist.
  - Sometimes, supination and ulnar deviation against resistance are required to produce the snapping.

- If the ECU is irritated, it will often be most painful with full passive radial wrist flexion.
- Occasionally, the clinical exam is inconclusive if the patient is not able to voluntarily subluxate the ECU tendon.
- Painful subluxation of the ECU tendon is an important component of the physical examination, and the surgeon should be cautious if contemplating surgical treatment in the patient who does not have painful demonstrable ECU instability.
- Careful examination of the contralateral wrist should be done to ensure that the patient does not have asymptomatic subluxation of the ECU tendon as a natural variant and the patient's complaints do not have another etiology.
- Other etiologies for the patient's pain are ruled out, such as ulna impaction, ECU tendinosis, DRUJ instability, LT instability, or TFCC tears.

IMAGING

- Routine anteroposterior, lateral, and oblique radiographs of the wrist are obtained to rule out other pathologies that may be causing ulnar-sided discomfort such as fracture or DRUJ arthritis.
  - It is important to note positive ulnar variance, as this can indicate ulnocarpal impaction.
- MRI is an option to evaluate for tendon subluxation; however, this is often a dynamic phenomenon that may not be visualized using a static MRI.
  - Some authors suggest performing an MRI with both wrists positioned in pronation, neutral, and supination. This provides a comparison with the contralateral wrist to show the ECU tendon within the ulnar groove in all three positions. However, the usefulness of this imaging technique is debated.
  - Other pathologies, such as TFCC tears, ECU tendonitis, or longitudinal tears, may be visualized with MRI, but the clinical significance of these findings needs to be considered thoughtfully.
- Dynamic ultrasound may demonstrate ECU subluxation out of the ulnar groove for patients in whom there was not definitive snapping or subluxation elicited during physical exam.[7-9] The role of dynamic ultrasound is still in evolution.

DIFFERENTIAL DIAGNOSIS

- ECU tendonitis
- Triangular fibrocartilage complex tear
- Ulnocarpal impaction
- Carpal instability
- DRUJ instability
- DRUJ arthritis
- Ulnar nerve entrapment

NONOPERATIVE MANAGEMENT

- In acute injuries, 4 to 6 weeks of either a long-arm or Muenster cast immobilization is usually sufficient.
  - Some authors recommend immobilizing in pronation and slight radial deviation, which allows the ECU subsheath to heal to the ulnar edge of the ulnar groove.[1]
- After cast removal, a custom splint is applied and progressive return to activity is begun in conjunction with occupational therapy.

- Full, unrestricted activity is usually achieved by 3 months if the patient is no longer painful.
- After treatment, some patients will have asymptomatic subluxation.

SURGICAL MANAGEMENT

- For patients in whom symptomatic instability of the ECU tendon persists after a period of immobilization and therapy, operative treatment is considered (**FIG 1**).
- If the ECU sheath is incompetent, a retinacular sling reconstruction should be elected. An ulnar groove deepening is performed only if the sheath is competent.
  - Some authors prefer sling reconstruction for all cases.

Preoperative Planning

- If a patient has an MRI present, it is useful to evaluate the anatomic details to understand if there is a type A, B, or C subluxation.

Positioning

- The patient should be positioned supine on the operating room table with the operative extremity on a hand or upper extremity table.
- Prior to draping the arm, perform an exam under anesthesia to recreate the ECU instability. It is important to note the position of instability preoperatively so one can confirm that the stabilization is effective once completed.
- A nonsterile tourniquet is placed on the upper arm to facilitate hemostasis.
- The arm is held in pronation to facilitate a dorsal approach to the ECU tendon.

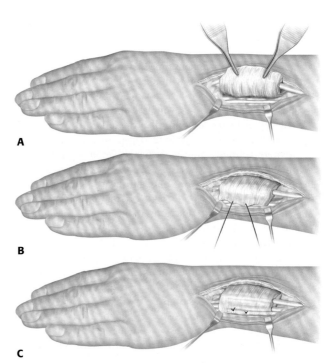

FIG 1 • Anatomic ECU tendon sheath reconstruction. **A.** Exposure of the 6th dorsal compartment and elevation of the extensor retinaculum. **B.** Imbrication of the extensor retinaculum and subsheath. **C.** Final fixation of the extensor retinaculum and subsheath after imbrications.

■ Exposure

- The arm is exsanguinated and the tourniquet is inflated.
- A 5-cm longitudinal incision is made overlying the sixth dorsal compartment and ECU tendon (**TECH FIG 1**).
- After the skin is incised, blunt dissection is carried out through the subcutaneous fat to identify and protect the dorsal cutaneous branch of the ulnar nerve.
- The extensor retinaculum over the sixth compartment should be sharply incised in a longitudinal fashion on its ulnar-most border and the retinaculum carefully dissected off of the underlying ECU subsheath.

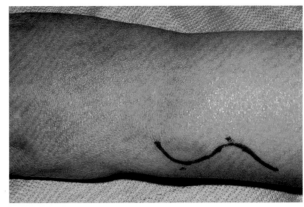

TECH FIG 1 • Marked incision for ECU retinacular sling reconstruction. (Courtesy of Philip Blazar, MD.)

■ Retinacular Sling Reconstruction of the ECU Subsheath

- The extensor retinaculum is carefully dissected from its ulnar border to expose the ECU subsheath (**TECH FIG 2A**).
- Once the ECU subsheath is fully exposed, the type of pathology (type A, B, or C) of the subsheath is noted and the wrist is taken through a full arc of motion from pronation to supination to gauge the behavior of the tendon through wrist range of motion.
- At the level of the ECU subsheath, overlying the ulnar groove, a 3-cm rectangular flap of retinaculum is developed starting at the second compartment; the base of which is the septum between the fifth and sixth dorsal compartments (**TECH FIG 2B**).
- This sling of retinaculum is then passed from radial to ulnar, volar to the ECU tendon, and folded back to the base of the flap (**TECH FIG 2C**).

- A trial stitch should be placed in order to assess the tightness of the sling in pronation, neutral, and supination in both wrist flexion and extension (**TECH FIG 2D**).
- The sling should not constrict the tendon, but it must still prevent subluxation of the ECU tendon about the ulnar head.
- The flap is sutured to itself using 3-0 nonabsorbable, braided suture.
- The remainder of the extensor retinaculum is anatomically repaired to ulnar border of the retinaculum using an absorbable suture.
- The tourniquet is let down, and hemostasis is confirmed.
- The wound is copiously irrigated, the dorsal incision is sutured, and the patient is placed into a sugar-tong splint with the wrist in mild pronation, extension, and radial deviation.

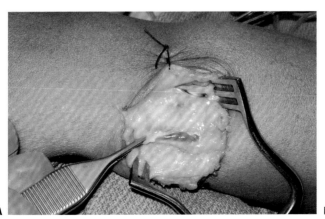

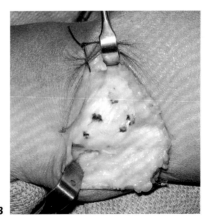

A   **B**

TECH FIG 2 • **A.** The extensor retinaculum flap is carefully dissected off the underlying ECU subsheath; this photograph also demonstrates a tear in the ECU subsheath. **B.** The extensor retinaculum rectangular flap is marked.

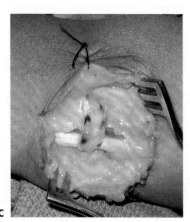 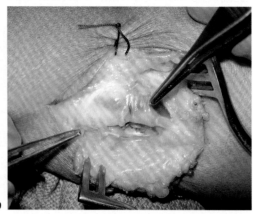

TECH FIG 2 (Continued) • **C.** The extensor retinaculum flap is laid over the ECU tendon in order to ensure adequate length. **D.** The extensor retinaculum flap is provisionally stitched, and stability is confirmed. (Courtesy of Philip Blazar, MD.)

◼ Distal Ulnar Groove Deepening

- A dorsoulnar incision is made along the distal ulna starting 5 cm proximal to the wrist and ending 1 cm proximal to the joint (see **TECH FIG 1**).
- The dorsal sensory branch of the ulnar nerve is identified and protected.
- The extensor retinaculum is divided over the ulnar aspect of the sixth dorsal compartment, and care is taken to preserve flaps of retinaculum for later repair.
- The dissection is taken down sharply to the bone along the volar border of the ECU tendon subsheath.
- The ECU tendon within its subsheath is elevated dorsally by sharp subperiosteal dissection to the radial attachment of the subsheath.
  - The tendon subsheath is not routinely opened. However, if one suspects a longitudinal tear of the ECU tendon or other intratendinous pathology, the subsheath can be opened at this point and the tendon pathology addressed.
- A power bur is then used to deepen the distal ulnar groove by 2 to 3 mm within the central groove. The

groove is deepened until the ECU subsheath no longer subluxates with forearm rotation.
  - An alternative method is to perforate the cortex with a small drill or K-wire and then impact the cortex with a bone tamp so it sits deeper than the adjacent cortex.
- The ECU subsheath is reduced into the reconstructed groove, and two suture anchors are placed along the ulnar margin of the groove to maintain reduction.
  - The suture anchors are passed through the ulnar border of the ECU subsheath in a horizontal mattress pattern, and any redundant sheath is imbricated with the sutures.
- The sutures are tied, and the ECU tendon with its subsheath is secured to the distal ulna.
- The wound is copiously irrigated with normal saline.
- The tourniquet is let down, and hemostasis is obtained.
- The extensor retinaculum is repaired with an absorbable braided suture, and the subdermal and epidermal layers are then closed.
- A long-arm splint is applied with the elbow in 90 degrees of flexion and the wrist in neutral.

PEARLS AND PITFALLS

Approach	◾ Identify and protect the dorsal cutaneous branch of the ulnar nerve throughout the procedure.
	◾ Inspect the ECU subsheath for injury or attenuation and determine if the subsheath can be repaired or will require reconstruction.
Ulnar groove deepening	◾ If the ulnar groove appears shallow, plan to perform an ulnar groove deepening.
Stability	◾ Be sure to check stability in extremes of ulnar deviation and supination with wrist flexion to ensure the ECU is stable before leaving the operating room.
Pitfalls	◾ Avoid injury to the dorsal cutaneous branch of the ulnar nerve with gentle retraction and protection throughout the procedure.
	◾ Avoid overtightening the extensor retinaculum sling. The tendon should glide freely through the sling at the conclusion of the operation.
	◾ Suture anchors placed into the deepened groove may inadvertently capture the ECU tendon.
Postoperative care	◾ Counsel patients that recovery can take 3–6 mo from the date of operation and they will need a period of immobilization and therapy after the operation.

POSTOPERATIVE CARE

- The wrist is initially immobilized in a sugar-tong or long-arm splint in the immediate postoperative period.
- At 2 weeks, the patient is converted to a Muenster-style orthoplast splint to prevent pronation and supination of the forearm but to allow elbow flexion and extension.
- At 6 weeks, occupational therapy is initiated beginning active and active assisted range of motion.
  - Passive range of motion and stretching are added progressively if needed.
  - The patient is advised to avoid forceful supination and flexion and heavy lifting during the rehabilitation period.
- Strengthening activities are initiated around 3 months postoperatively.

OUTCOMES

- A number of case reports and small case series have described the various techniques and outcomes for ECU tendon stabilization, but there is no level I evidence for surgical treatment of ECU instability.
  - Allende and Le Viet reported that 23 of 28 patients had good or excellent results at an average follow-up of 23 months after extensor retinaculum sling stabilization of the ECU tendon.[6]
  - MacLennan et al.[9] reported improvements in DASH scores at 31 months after groove deepening.

COMPLICATIONS

- Injury to the dorsal cutaneous branch of the ulnar nerve
- Recurrent subluxation of the ECU tendon
- Infection
- Complex regional pain syndrome
- Decreased range of motion
- Decreased grip strength

REFERENCES

1. Burkhart SS, Wood MB, Linscheid RL. Posttraumatic recurrent subluxation of the extensor carpi ulnaris tendon. *J Hand Surg [Am]*. 1982;7(1):1-3.
2. Iorio ML, Bayomy AF, Huang JI. Morphology of the extensor carpi ulnaris groove and tendon. *J Hand Surg [Am]*. 2014;39(12): 2412-2416.
3. Taleisnik J, Gelberman RH, Miller BW, Szabo RM. The extensor retinaculum of the wrist. *J Hand Surg [Am]*. 1984;9(4):495-501.
4. Ghatan AC, Puri SG, Morse KW, et al. Relative contribution of the subsheath to extensor carpi ulnaris tendon stability: implications for surgical reconstruction and rehabilitation. *J Hand Surg [Am]*. 2016;41(2):225-232.
5. Inoue G, Tamura Y. Surgical treatment for recurrent dislocation of the extensor carpi ulnaris tendon. *J Hand Surg Br*. 2001;26(6): 556-559.
6. Allende C, Le Viet D. Extensor carpi ulnaris problems at the wrist—classification, surgical treatment and results. *J Hand Surg Br*. 2005;30(3):265-272.
7. Jeantroux J, Becce F, Guerini H, et al. Athletic injuries of the extensor carpi ulnaris subsheath: MRI findings and utility of gadolinium-enhanced fat-saturated T1-weighted sequences with wrist pronation and supination. *Eur Radiol*. 2011;21(1):160-166.
8. Pratt RK, Hoy GA, Bass Franzcr C. Extensor carpi ulnaris subluxation or dislocation? Ultrasound measurement of tendon excursion and normal values. *Hand Surg*. 2004;9(2):137-143.
9. MacLennan AJ, Nemechek NM, Waitayawinyu T, Trumble TE. Diagnosis and anatomic reconstruction of extensor carpi ulnaris subluxation. *J Hand Surg [Am]*. 2008;33(1):59-64.

43

CHAPTER

Trigger Finger Release

Donato Perretta, Jacques A. Machol IV, and Neal C. Chen

DEFINITION

- Trigger digit, also known as stenosis tenosynovitis or tenovaginitis (tendon sheath inflammation), is a pathology characterized by painful locking or clicking of the fingers or thumb as a result of impaired gliding of the flexor tendon at the level of the A1 pulley.

ANATOMY

- The proximal edge of the A1 pulley begins approximately at the level of the metacarpal heads of the fingers. This corresponds to the distal palmar crease.
  - For the index finger, this line can be extrapolated radially.
  - In the thumb, it is at the level of the proximal digital crease.

PATHOGENESIS

- Trigger digit is caused by a thickening of the flexor tendon sheath, specifically the A1 pulley.
- The pathological change in the A1 pulley has been described as fibrocartilaginous metaplasia.[1]
- Over time, the flexor tendon can also undergo degenerative changes consistent with tendinosis.[2] The resulting imbalance in the size of the A1 pulley and the enclosed flexor tendons causes catching and locking.

NATURAL HISTORY

- The thumb is the most commonly involved digit.[3]
- Women are more commonly affected than are men.
- There are no long-term studies documenting the natural history of untreated trigger finger.
- The condition may progress from tenderness at the A1 pulley to painless clicking to painful triggering of the finger that requires passive manual extension.
- Over time, flexion deformities may develop at the PIP joint due to persistent triggering.
- The condition is more common and progresses more often in patients with endocrinopathies and inflammatory arthritides.[2]

PATIENT HISTORY AND PHYSICAL FINDINGS

- Tenderness over the A1 pulley
- Palpable nodule over the A1 pulley
- Painful popping or catching of the digit with flexion
- Inability to actively extend the PIP joint from a flexed position
- Flexion contracture of the PIP joint with long-standing trigger finger

IMAGING

- Imaging is not necessary.

DIFFERENTIAL DIAGNOSIS

- Locked MP joint. The collateral ligament can become entrapped over a metacarpal head osteophyte. This usually presents as inability to extend the digit fully after the collateral is locked.
- Early swan-neck deformity with snapping of lateral bands as they dislocate dorsally
- Subluxation of the extensor tendon after sagittal band rupture. In this situation, the finger can be passively extended and then can be actively maintained in extension. However, if the finger is flexed, the extensor tendon will subluxate and the finger cannot actively extend fully.

NONOPERATIVE MANAGEMENT

- Corticosteroid injection into or superficial to the A1 pulley is the first-line treatment. This is usually performed using a 25-gauge needle with 0.5 cc of 1% plain lidocaine and 5 mg of Kenalog. Injections can eliminate symptoms, but the duration of their effect is unpredictable.
  - One study showed that after injection, 56% of the digits had a recurrence of symptoms within a year. Recurrence was associated with younger age, insulin-dependent diabetes mellitus, involvement of multiple digits, and a history of other tendinopathies.
  - Symptoms often recurred several months after the injection.[4]
  - Taras et al. reported that extra-sheath injections may be more effective than those administered within the sheath.[5]
- Splinting the MCP joint of the affected digit in extension is another commonly used nonoperative measure. Colbourn et al.[6] demonstrated short-term improvement in symptoms with a removable orthoplast splint in 28 patients.

SURGICAL MANAGEMENT

- Percutaneous A1 pulley release is a well-described treatment option that has been reported to be safe and effective.[7] The A1 pulley is released under local anesthesia using a large-bore needle while the patient intentionally triggers the affected finger.
- Open A1 pulley release is our preferred treatment method in a patient with recurrent symptoms after two injections.
- Patients with rheumatoid hand deformity often develop tenosynovitis of the flexor tendons. In this group of patients, A1 pulley release is not recommended, as it can result in increased ulnar drift of the fingers. Instead, annular

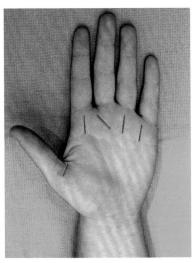 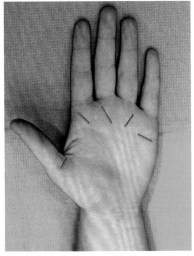 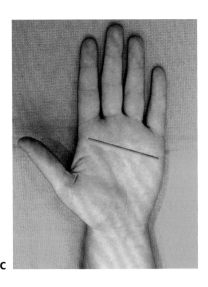

FIG 1 • Trigger finger incisions for single-digit surgery **(A,B)** and for multiple-digit surgery **(C)**.

pulley-sparing tenosynovectomy and carpal tunnel release should be performed. The ulnar slip of the superficialis can be resected from the middle phalanx to reduce the bulk of tendon within the flexor sheath.[8]

Positioning

- Supine with hand table
- The procedure may be performed with a brachial tourniquet with infiltration of local anesthetic into the surgical site.
- Intravenous sedation can be used as an adjunct.

Approach

- If one digit is to be addressed, then a longitudinal or oblique incision is made over the A1 pulley (**FIG 1A,B**). The pulley lies over the metacarpal head.
- If adjacent digits are to be addressed, a transverse incision is used. Often, this is aligned within the distal palmar crease (**FIG 1C**).

■ Open A1 Pulley Release

- After skin incision, blunt dissection is made down to the A1 pulley (**TECH FIG 1A**).
  - Retractors are placed on either side of the pulley to prevent damage to the neurovascular bundles.
- A no. 15 blade is used to incise the A1 pulley in line with the longitudinal axis of the finger in the center of the flexor tendon/pulley (**TECH FIG 1B**).
- Some surgeons describe an A0 pulley proximally or a proximal fascial band that may result in persistent triggering.

- One should be cautious not to release the A2 pulley distally.
- The patient is asked to actively flex the fingers down to the palm, and the presence of triggering is assessed. This can be done passively if the patient is unable to comply.
- If triggering continues once the entire A1 pulley has been released, excision of the ulnar slip of the FDS tendon is an option. This can be performed through a Bruner-type volar incision over the PIP joint.
- The skin is closed with 5-0 nylon interrupted sutures.

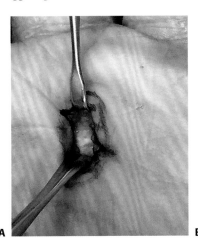 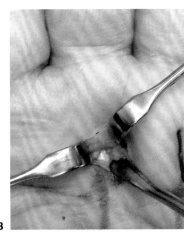

TECH FIG 1 • **A.** Identification of the A1 pulley. **B.** Flexor tendon is visible after A1 pulley release.

T E C H N I Q U E S

PEARLS AND PITFALLS

Incomplete release	▪ The entire A1 pulley should be divided under direct visualization.
Persistent triggering after complete A1 pulley release	▪ There is a band, which some call the A0 pulley, which lies proximal to the A1 pulley. This should be released if the finger still triggers after A1 pulley release. ▪ If triggering is still present after A1 pulley, one slip of the FDS tendon should be excised. Usually, the radial slip is preserved and the ulnar slip excised to help avoid ulnar drift of the digits.
Injury to neurovascular bundle	▪ Care must be made during exposure to protect the neurovascular bundle during A1 pulley release.
Bowstringing	▪ Release of the A2 tendon sheath distal to the A1 pulley may lead to tendon bowstringing.

POSTOPERATIVE CARE

▪ A sterile dressing is placed. It is removed on postoperative day 3, and digital motion is encouraged.
▪ Sutures are removed 10 days after surgery.
▪ No formal therapy is indicated.

OUTCOMES

▪ Outcomes are generally excellent.
▪ Recurrence rates after surgery have been reported at 3%.
▪ Rates of reoperation have been reported at 1% to 2.4%.[3–5]

COMPLICATIONS[9]

▪ Infection (superficial or deep)
▪ Digital nerve or artery injury
▪ Incomplete release
▪ Persistent swelling and pain
▪ Flexion contracture
▪ Tendon bowstringing

REFERENCES

1. Sampson SP, Badalamente MA, Hurst LC, Seidman J. Pathobiology of the human A1 pulley in trigger finger. *J Hand Surg [Am]*. 1991;16:714-721.
2. Lundin AC, Eliasson P, Aspenberg P. Trigger finger and tendinosis. *J Hand Surg Eur Vol*. 2012;37:233-236.
3. Sungpet A, Suphachatwong C, Kawinwonggowit V. Trigger digit and BMI. *J Med Assoc Thai*. 1999;82:1025-1027.
4. Rozental TD, Zurakowski D, Blazar PE. Trigger finger: prognostic indicators of recurrence following corticosteroid injection. *J Bone Joint Surg Am*. 2008;90:1665-1672.
5. Taras JS, Raphael JS, Pan WT, et al. Corticosteroid injections for trigger digits: is intrasheath injection necessary? *J Hand Surg [Am]*. 1998;23:717-722.
6. Colbourn J, Heath N, Manary S, Pacifico D. Effectiveness of splinting for the treatment of trigger finger. *J Hand Ther*. 2008;21:336-343.
7. Ha KI, Park MJ, Ha CW. Percutaneous release of trigger digits. *J Bone Joint Surg Br*. 2001;83:75-77.
8. Ferlic DC, Clayton ML. Flexor tenosynovectomy in the rheumatoid finger. *J Hand Surg [Am]*. 1978;3:364-367.
9. Everding NG, Bishop GB, Belyea CM, Soong MC. Risk factors for complications of open trigger finger release. *Hand (N Y)*. 2005;10:297-300.

First Dorsal Compartment (de Quervain) Release

Donato Perretta, Jacques A. Machol IV, and Neal C. Chen

DEFINITION

- de Quervain syndrome is defined as tenosynovitis of the first dorsal compartment. The first extensor compartment contains the tendons of the extensor pollicis brevis (EPB) and abductor pollicis longus (APL).

ANATOMY

- The first dorsal compartment is the most radial extensor compartment at the level of the wrist and contains the tendons of the EPB and APL. The extensor retinaculum is the ceiling of the compartment.
- The APL may have multiple slips, and there may be separate subsheaths for both the APL and EPB.[1] The APL is more radial and volar, whereas the EPB is more ulnar and dorsal. The separate subsheath for the EPB may be missed if one does not look for it routinely.

PATHOGENESIS

- Although this is commonly described as tendonitis, histologic markers of inflammation are not present. The tendon sheath of the first compartment is thickened, and there is deposition of mucopolysaccharide, an indicator of myxoid degeneration.[2]
- The disease is also common in pregnancy and the postpartum interval. It often is self-limited and resolves with birth or the termination of breast-feeding.[3]

PATIENT HISTORY AND PHYSICAL FINDINGS

- Tenderness at the radial styloid in the first compartment
- Positive Finkelstein test (radial wrist pain with ulnar deviation of the wrist while the thumb is held into the palm)

IMAGING

- Radiographs of the wrist are useful if the diagnosis is in doubt. They can help exclude other degenerative conditions about the wrist and thumb.

DIFFERENTIAL DIAGNOSIS

- Radiocarpal arthritis
- Intersection syndrome (pain and crepitus in the distal forearm at the intersection of the first and second dorsal compartments)
- Thumb basal joint arthritis
- Scaphoid or carpal fracture
- STT arthritis
- Injury or irritation of the superficial branch of the radial nerve

NONOPERATIVE MANAGEMENT

- A forearm-based thumb spica splint is usually the first-line treatment.
- Steroid injection into first dorsal compartment sheath is an effective treatment. Our preference is to use 0.5 cc of 1% lidocaine and 0.5 mg of dexamethasone.
  - About 80% of patients will experience symptomatic improvement after one injection, and half will remain symptom-free at 1 year.[4]
- Steroid injection may be more effective than splinting for breast-feeding mothers.[3]
  - Some pediatricians or obstetricians object to the use of steroid injections while breast-feeding, however, and this should be discussed with other caregivers. There is concern that trace amounts of steroid can enter the breast milk and that lactation can be affected after injection.[5]

SURGICAL MANAGEMENT

- First dorsal compartment release is indicated after failure of nonoperative management.
- Conservative measures such as splinting and injection should be attempted before surgical intervention.

Positioning

- Supine, with hand table, with brachial tourniquet. Local anesthetic infiltration is used.

Approach

- Release of the compartment can be accomplished with a chevron, transverse, or longitudinal incision.

■ First Dorsal Compartment Release

- A 2-cm incision is made 1 cm proximal to the distal extent of the radial styloid (**TECH FIG 1A**).
- The first dorsal compartment is exposed (**TECH FIG 1B,C**).
- Care is taken to avoid injuring the superficial branch of the radial nerve, which travels superficial to the extensor retinaculum.
- Injury to the radial sensory nerve can be minimized with retractors placed proximally and distally rather than dorsally/volarly.

- The first dorsal compartment is released longitudinally at the dorsal edge (**TECH FIG 1D**). This prevents volar subluxation of the tendons.
- The APL and EPB are wholly inspected to ensure that all subsheaths have been released.
  - Up to half of patients may have separate compartments for these tendons. It is theorized that these accessory compartments predispose to de Quervain's.[6]
- Interrupted buried 3-0 absorbable monofilament sutures are used for wound closure, and Steri-Strips are applied.
- A thumb spica plaster splint is applied for 7 to 10 days.

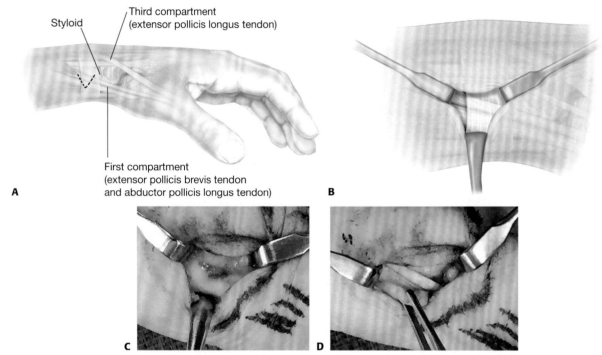

TECH FIG 1 • A. The chevron (*dashed lines*) is the preferred incision for release of the first dorsal compartment. **B.** Sheath of first dorsal compartment exposed. **C.** Once the skin is incised, care is taken to avoid the radial sensory nerve. The blood on the sheath is from the preoperative local anesthetic injection. **D.** First dorsal compartment tendons exposed. The sheath is released from the dorsal side to prevent volar subluxation of the tendons. The forceps are holding the sheath. The APL and EPB are visible, with the APL begin the more volar structure.

PEARLS AND PITFALLS

Nerve injury	■ Identify the superficial branch of the radial nerve. Aggressive retraction results in a problematic injury to the nerve and persistent pain.
Volar tendon subluxation	■ Leave a cuff of tissue volarly when incising the sheath.
Incomplete release	■ Be sure to release both the EPB and APL as they often have separate subsheaths.

POSTOPERATIVE CARE

- The splint is removed in 7 to 10 days, and immediate at-home range-of-motion exercises are initiated. Typically, there is no need for formal therapy.

OUTCOMES

- A consecutive series of 94 patients found symptom resolution in 100% of patients.
  - There were six perioperative complications, including one superficial wound infection, one delayed wound healing, and four transient lesions of the radial sensory nerve.[7]

COMPLICATIONS

- Infection
- Injury to superficial radial nerve
- Scar tenderness

REFERENCES

1. Bahm J, Szabo Z, Foucher G. The anatomy of de Quervain's disease: a study of operative findings. *Int Orthop.* 1995;19:209-211.
2. Clarke MT, Lyall HA, Grant JW, Matthewson MH. The histopathology of de Quervain's disease. *J Hand Surg Br.* 1998;23:732-734.
3. Avci S, Yilmaz C, Sayli U. Comparison of nonsurgical treatment measures for de Quervain's disease of pregnancy and lactation. *J Hand Surg [Am].* 2002;27:322-324.
4. Earp BE, Han CH, Floyd WE, et al. De Quervain tendinopathy: survivorship and prognostic indicators of recurrence following a single corticosteroid injection. *J Hand Surg [Am].* 2015;40:1161-1165.
5. Babwah TJ, Nunes P, Maharaj RG. An unexpected temporary suppression of lactation after a local corticosteroid injection for tenosynovitis. *Eur J Gen Pract.* 2013;15:248-250.
6. McDermott JD, Ilyas AM, Nazarian LN, Leinberry CF. Ultrasound-guided injections for de Quervain's tenosynovitis. *Clin Orthop Relat Res.* 2012;470:1925-1931.
7. Scheller A, Schuh R, Honle W, Schuh A. Long-term results of surgical release of de Quervain's stenosing tenosynovitis. *Int Orthop.* 2009;33:1301-1303.

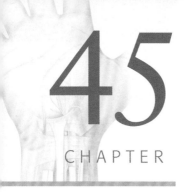

45 CHAPTER

Section X: Flaps and Microsurgery

Flap Coverage of Fingertip Injuries

Kate Elzinga and Kevin C. Chung

DEFINITION

- Fingertip injuries are defined as injuries that occur distal to the insertion of the flexor and extensor tendons of the finger.[1]
- Fingertip injuries are the most common hand injuries; the fingertips are relatively unprotected compared to the rest of the hand.
- The fingertip plays an important role in fine motor skills, precise sensation, and hand aesthetics. Reconstruction of fingertip injuries can restore form and function for injured patients.
- The goals of fingertip reconstruction include the following:
  - Durable coverage
  - Preservation of sensation
  - Preservation of length
  - Maintenance of distal interphalangeal (DIP) joint function
  - Optimized appearance
  - Minimized donor-site morbidity
  - Permitting early return to work and recreational activities
  - Minimizing pain, in the short and long term
- Fingertip flaps are used to cover injuries with exposed bone and tendon. Local (V-Y advancement) and regional (thenar, cross-finger) flaps are useful options.
  - Local flaps, such as the Atasoy-Kleinert V-Y advancement flap,[2] are the simplest flaps used for reconstruction; immobilization is not required and donor-site morbidity is minimal.
  - Regional flaps are employed when local flaps are not available because of the injury geometry (regional flaps are best used for volar oblique injuries) and size (local flaps can only be advanced 1 cm). Regional flaps require two-stage procedures and immobilization of the injured, and often adjacent, finger.

ANATOMY

- The volar fingertip is covered with glabrous skin. The epidermis is thick, and papillary ridges are prominent.
- The fingertip pulp is composed of fibrofatty tissue that is stabilized volarly by fibrous septa that run from the distal phalanx periosteum to the dermis and laterally by Grayson and Cleland ligaments.
- The proper digital nerve trifurcates distal to the DIP joint, sending branches to the nail bed, distal fingertip, and volar pulp. The proper digital artery also trifurcates at this level, sending two branches dorsally and one branch laterally.

PATHOGENESIS

- Trauma is the most common cause of fingertip injuries.[3]
- Common mechanisms of fingertip injuries include sharp injuries from a knife, power tool, or lawn mower and crush injuries from closing a door, a strike with a hammer, dropping a heavy object, becoming trapped in machinery, or sporting activities.

PATIENT HISTORY AND PHYSICAL FINDINGS

- A careful patient history and physical examination help determine which flap options are suitable for a particular patient.
  - Some patients may prefer rapid return to their work and avocations and will refuse fingertip reconstruction, opting for fingertip amputation instead.
- A focused hand history must include age, sex, hand dominance, and occupation and recreational activities. The patients' goals are explored, including their need to return to work, their availability and willingness to undergo secondary procedures and hand therapy, and the importance of appearance.
  - Aesthetic outcome may be more important for females and patients from certain Asian cultures.
- Important considerations from the patient's past medical history include smoking, diabetes mellitus, peripheral vascular disease, connective tissue disorders, arthritis, Dupuytren disease, and previous hand injuries.
  - The presence of comorbidities may affect reconstruction options offered given their effect on flap vascularity and wound healing.
- Key injury factors to consider include the time of injury, mechanism of injury (sharp vs crush), contamination, and associated injuries.
- On physical examination, the defect size is measured. The level of the injury is assessed clinically and using radiographic imaging.
  - Missing tissue (skin, pulp, bone, nail) and exposed structures are documented. The geometry of the injury is assessed and classified as volar oblique, transverse, or dorsal oblique (**FIG 1**).[1]
  - Tissue contamination is assessed, and any early signs of infection are noted.
  - Surrounding tissues and digits are examined as potential donor sites.

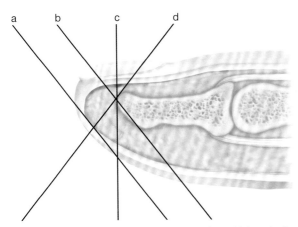

FIG 1 • The angle of amputation is assessed to aid in selection of an appropriate local or regional flap for fingertip coverage. Volar oblique injuries with no exposed bone (*a*) can heal by secondary intention. Volar oblique injuries with exposed bone (*b*) can be reconstructed with regional flaps (thenar flap, cross-finger flap). Transverse (*c*) and dorsal (*d*) oblique injuries with exposed bone can resurfaced with a volar V-Y advancement flap.

- The integrity of the flexor digitorum profundus (FDP) and extensor digitorum communis (EDC) tendons is tested; it is important not to miss an associated jersey finger or mallet finger injury.

IMAGING

- Plain radiographs can identify fractures of the finger and the presence of a foreign body.
- Three radiographic views of the finger and amputated part should be obtained following a fingertip amputation.

NONOPERATIVE MANAGEMENT

- Small defects (less than 1 cm²) with no exposed bone can be treated nonoperatively.[4]
- Dressing changes are performed daily to maintain a clean moist wound bed as the wound heals by secondary intervention over several weeks.
- Outcomes are typically excellent in these cases as glabrous sensate skin heals over the exposed soft tissues.[5]
- Immobilization is not required and range-of-motion exercises are performed throughout.

SURGICAL MANAGEMENT

- Full-thickness skin grafts (FTSGs) can be considered for coverage of large soft tissue avulsion injuries without exposed bone or tendon.
  - The glabrous skin of the hypothenar eminence is the preferred harvest site for volar skin defects. Palmar skin is an excellent donor site for structure and color matching of the fingertip skin; the resultant scar from the palm can be rather imperceptible.
  - Skin grafting promotes faster wound coverage, but sensation, color, and durability are inferior to secondary healing.[5]

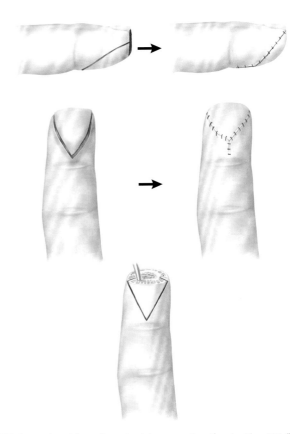

FIG 2 • Volar oblique fingertip defects can be closed with a V-Y flap. Distally, the fibrous septa are released from the undersurface of the flap to allow advancement of the flap distally into the defect, where it is sutured over the wound.

- Replacement of amputated tissue as a composite graft may be considered; outcomes are best for pediatric patients younger than 6 years of age within 5 hours of the amputation.[6]
- Fingertip flaps preserve finger length. Early coverage of exposed bone and tendon decreases the risk of osteomyelitis and tendon desiccation. Protecting the terminal phalanx with a flap preserves bone length that supports the overlying nail.
  - The volar V-Y advancement flap (**FIG 2**) is well suited for transverse and dorsal oblique fingertip injuries.
    - The V-Y flap can cover defects of up to 2 cm² and can be advanced 1 cm.
  - The thenar flap (**FIG 3**) and cross-finger flap (**FIG 4**) provide coverage for volar oblique injuries. The thenar flap provides improved sensory recovery and has a less conspicuous donor site compared with the cross-finger flap but requires greater finger flexion for inset, which can cause joint stiffness, particularly in elderly patients. However, the lack of donor-site morbidity and predictable outcomes makes the thenar flap our first choice, if possible, over the cross-finger flap.
    - The cross-finger flap can be used for defects up to 1.5 × 2.5 cm in size.
    - The thenar flap can be designed to cover the entire pulp with a width of up to 2 cm.

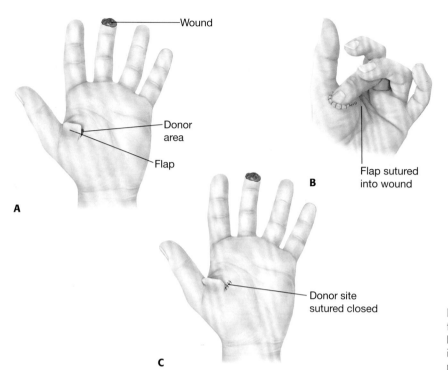

FIG 3 • A. Proximally based thenar flap is elevated from distal to proximal. **B.** Narrow donor sites may be closed primarily. **C.** This is done prior to flap inset to the fingertip defect to facilitate suture placement.

Preoperative Planning

- The risks and benefits of flap coverage for fingertip injuries are discussed with the patient during their initial assessment and reviewed again prior to their surgery.
- Fingertip and/or the removal of exposed bone followed by secondary intention healing are discussed as alternative treatment options.

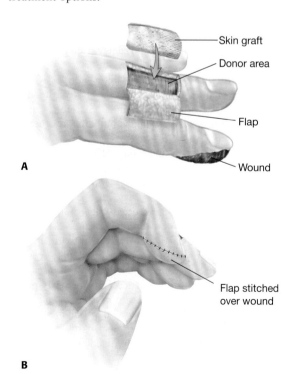

FIG 4 • A. The cross-finger flap is composed of skin and subcutaneous tissue from the dorsal middle phalanx of the adjacent finger. **B.** The flap donor site is closed with an FTSG.

- Benefits of flap coverage include preservation of finger length, provision of durable soft tissue coverage, and good aesthetic results.
  - Drawbacks include the creation of a donor site, the possibility of flap failure, and the need for longer immobilization.
- Cross-finger and thenar flaps require the injured digit to be placed in flexion, which can lead to postoperative stiffness.
  - These flaps are contraindicated in patients at high risk of joint contractures, eg, elderly patients with arthritis or Dupuytren disease.
  - The thenar flap cannot be performed in patients without adequate passive metacarpophalangeal (MCP) and interphalangeal joint flexion.

Positioning

- The patient is positioned supine with the arm on a hand table.

Approach

- Loupe magnification is helpful.
- Incisions are planned prior to inflation of the tourniquet.
- Exposed bone is smoothed out with a rongeur. Minimal shortening is performed.
- Soft tissues are debrided of all nonviable and contaminated tissue. A healthy wound bed is established prior to flap reconstruction.
- The sterile nail matrix should be shortened 2 mm proximal to the tip of the distal phalanx to prevent a hook-nail deformity.[7] A hook-nail deformity can occur when there is a lack of distal support for the sterile matrix.
- The neurovascular bundles and FDP tendon insertion are protected throughout.

V-Y Advancement Flap

- The flap width is marked to match the defect width distally; proximally, it is tapered as a V.
  - The proximal flap edge is traditionally located at volar midline of the distal interphalangeal (DIP) joint crease; proximal extensions have been described (see **FIG 2**).[8]
- The injured finger is exsanguinated, and a finger tourniquet is placed.
- The flap is incised; dissection is performed through the dermis. Once the subcutaneous tissues are exposed, no further deep dissection is required; this prevents injury to the bilateral neurovascular structures (**TECH FIG 1A**).
- Distally, the fibrous septa are divided from the distal phalanx periosteum to permit flap advancement.
- The central undersurface of the flap must not be undermined to maintain flap vascularity.
- The flap is inset into the defect and sutured into place with 4-0 nonabsorbable monofilament suture. The flap is secured to the surrounding intact skin and nail. Tension is avoided at the tip of the finger to lessen the risk of a hook-nail deformity.[9]
- The donor site is closed longitudinally in V-Y fashion (**TECH FIG 1B**). Alternatively, the donor site can be left open to heal secondarily, particularly if flap tension is a concern.[9]
- The tourniquet is released and flap vascularity is assessed (**TECH FIG 1C**). Alternating sutures may be released to lessen tension on the flap; these open areas are left to heal by secondary intention.
- Antibiotic-impregnated gauze is placed over all incisions and covered with sterile gauze. A soft finger dressing is applied.
  - A light dressing can be applied daily until the incisions are healed.
- The sutures are removed 2 weeks postoperatively.
- Range-of-motion (ROM) exercises may be started on postoperative day 2 to prevent finger stiffness.

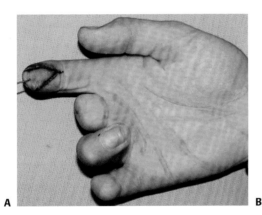
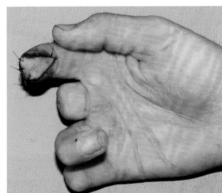
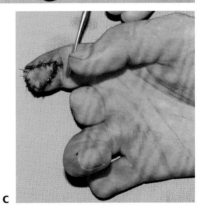

TECH FIG 1 • A. The V-Y advancement is designed with a distal width matching the width of the defect. Proximally, the flap is tapered to a V at the volar midline of the DIP joint crease. The dermis is incised, exposing the subcutaneous tissues below. **B.** The V-Y advancement flap is inset distally to the surrounding intact skin and nail. The donor site is closed proximally in a longitudinal V-Y fashion. **C.** The tourniquet is released, and the vascularity of the flap is assessed. Color, capillary refill, temperature, and turgor of the flap are examined.

Cross-Finger Flap

- A template of the defect is used to mark the flap dimensions on the dorsum of the middle phalanx of the adjacent donor finger (**TECH FIG 2A**).
  - The flap is pedicled on the side of the donor finger adjacent to the defect.
  - The lateral extent of the flap can be marked as far as at the junction of the glabrous and nonglabrous skin for larger defects.
- The arm is exsanguinated and a tourniquet inflated.
- The flap is elevated sharply, just above the paratenon, beginning from the edge of the donor finger farthest from the injured finger (**TECH FIG 2B**). Cleland ligament is divided.
  - The flap remains hinged to the side of the finger closest to the injured finger, along the midaxial line (**TECH FIG 2C**; see **FIG 4**).
- The injured finger is flexed, and the flap is secured to the flap using 4-0 nonabsorbable monofilament sutures (**TECH FIG 2D,E**).

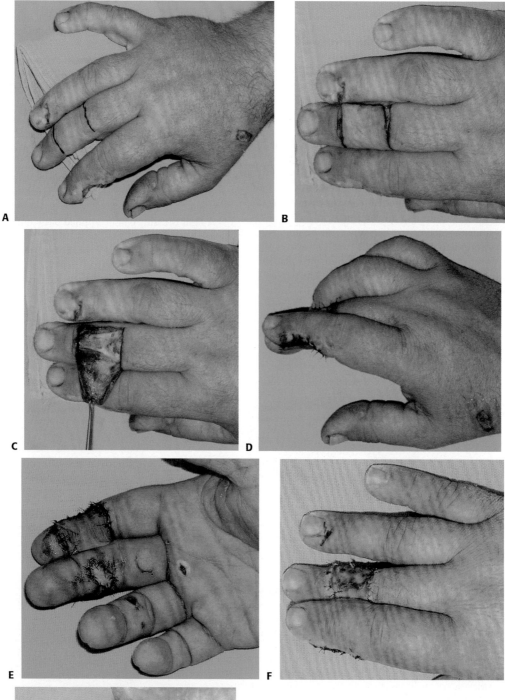

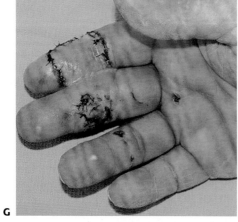

TECH FIG 2 • A. The fingertip defect is marked on the dorsum of the middle phalanx of the adjacent donor finger using a template of the wound. The flap is hinged on the side of the donor finger closest to the defect. **B.** The flap is incised sharply and elevated in the loose areolar place above the paratenon. **C.** The paratenon must be preserved to enable FTSG take at the flap donor site. **D,E.** Volar and oblique views, respectively, of a cross-finger flap from the middle finger after inset into the defect of the index finger. The patient also sustained an injury to the volar middle phalanx of the middle finger that was closed with an FTSG. **F,G.** A dressing change is performed 1 week postoperatively to assess the flap and flap donor site, respectively. The flap provides durable, padded soft tissue coverage for fingertip injuries.

- A full-thickness skin graft (FTSG) is applied to the flap donor site. The FTSG can be inconspicuously harvested from the groin, medial proximal forearm, or nonglabrous hypothenar skin.
- Antibiotic-impregnated gauze is applied to the affected digit and FTSG donor site and covered with sterile gauze. A bolster dressing is applied over the skin graft. A splint is applied to the injured finger and its adjacent donor finger, immobilizing the interphalangeal joints; the metacarpophalangeal (MCP) joints may be left free.
- One week after the first surgery, a dressing change is performed (**TECH FIG 2F,G**). The bolster dressing is removed from the FTSG. A protective splint is reapplied.
- Two weeks after the first surgery, the flap is divided. Immobilization is not typically required after the second surgery, and ROM exercises are started.

■ Thenar Flap

- The injured digit is flexed into the palm (**TECH FIG 3A**). Maximal flexion of the MCP and DIP joints is preferred while minimizing proximal interphalangeal (PIP) joint flexion to decrease postoperative PIP stiffness.
- The flap is marked over the ulnar aspect of the thenar eminence using a template of the defect size (**TECH FIG 3B**).
  - Ulnar flap design is preferred on the thenar eminence to facilitate primary closure of the donor site; skin tension is decreased by adducting the thumb. Furthermore, designing the flap radially over the thenar eminence places the radial neurovascular bundle of the thumb at risk of injury.

- The flap width and length are designed 1.5 times wider and longer, respectively, than the defect length to permit tension-free inset with restoration of the normal rounded contour of the fingertip.
- The flap is proximally or distally based, depending on the geometry of the defect.
- The arm is exsanguinated and a tourniquet inflated.
- The skin and subcutaneous tissues of the flap are sharply incised. The flap is elevated from distal to proximal in the subcutaneous tissue plane, above the level of the palmar fascia, at a depth that matches the defect (**TECH FIG 3C**).
- Once the flap is elevated, the flap donor site is closed longitudinally with 4-0 nonabsorbable monofilament sutures. The thumb is adducted to facilitate primary closure of the donor site.

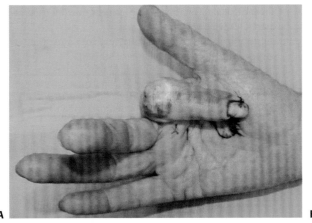
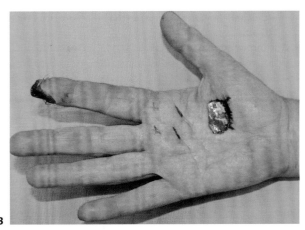
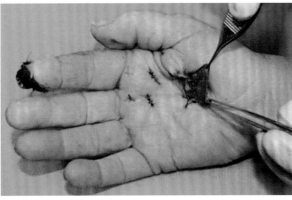
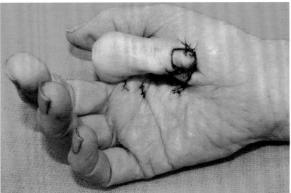

A   B   C   D

TECH FIG 3 • A. The flap is designed over the thenar eminence where the finger meets the palm when flexed. Maximal MCP and DIP joint flexion are preferred rather than PIP flexion to enable the finger to meet the palmar skin. Contractures of the PIP joint are more problematic postoperatively compared to those of the MCP and DIP joints. **B.** A template, cut out of foil, Telfa (shown here), or otherwise can be used to design the flap based on the defect size. **C.** The flap is elevated from distal to proximal in the subcutaneous plane. The palmar fascia is not violated. The finger is flexed to bring the defect to the flap site. **D,E.** Volar and oblique views, respectively, of the flap inset to the intact skin around the defect and the nail.

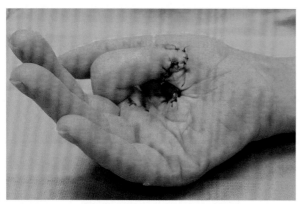
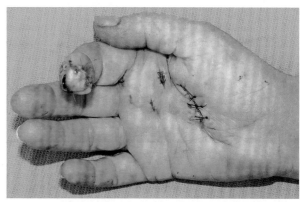

E   **F**

TECH FIG 3 (Continued) • **F.** The thenar flap is divided at its proximal base. The proximal flap edge is inset to the proximal volar edge of the defect with sutures. The thenar donor-site skin is closed.

- An FTSG can be used if the flap donor site is too large for primary closure.
- Next, the injured finger is flexed and the flap is inset over the defect (see **FIG 3**).
  - 4-0 nonabsorbable monofilament sutures are used to secure the flap to the defect; absorbable sutures are at increased risk of breakage and subsequent flap dehiscence.
  - Multiple sutures are used to decrease the chance of accidental fingertip avulsion from the flap site (**TECH FIG 3D,E**).
- Antibiotic-impregnated gauze is placed over all incisions and covered with sterile gauze. A well-padded splint is applied dorsally over the injured finger to prevent accidental avulsion of the fingertip from the thenar eminence.
- Two weeks postoperatively, the flap is divided, and if needed, more skin is removed from the thenar area to cover the entire fingertip that is buried within the thenar pocket.
- The divided flap edge is sutured to the edge of the fingertip defect, and the thenar skin is closed with 4-0 sutures; absorbable or nonabsorbable sutures may be used at this stage (**TECH FIG 3F**).
- Immobilization is not typically required after the second surgery, and ROM exercises are started.

PEARLS AND PITFALLS

Physical findings	■ Carefully assess the flexion and extension of the DIP for patients with a fingertip injury. Associated mallet injury is common.
Technique	■ Handle flaps atraumatically. The blood supply for fingertip flaps is random from small local vessels. ■ Cross-finger flap: The cross-finger flap can be used for resurfacing of fingertip defects of all fingers. A thumb defect is the most difficult to inset using a flap from the index finger because of the pronated position of the thumb relative to the other digits of the hand. Defects of the ring finger are best resurfaced with a flap from the middle finger, rather than the shorter small finger, for adequate inset. A fingertip defect of the small finger requires minimal flexion of the small finger for inset to a flap from the ring finger. ■ Thenar flap: The thenar flap can be used for all fingers; positioning is easiest for the index and middle fingers and most difficult for the small finger. ■ Obtain hemostasis and close the skin while the tourniquet is down to prevent a hematoma to optimize flap and graft survival. ■ Assess flap tension in the operating room with the hand at rest and with passive range of motion. If surgery is performed with local anesthesia only, active range of motion can also be assessed. Splint the hand accordingly; avoid immobilization of uninvolved joints that do not cause undue tension on the reconstruction when moved.
Postoperative	■ Perform second-stage flap division 2 wk after flap inset. Longer periods of immobilization lead to worsening joint stiffness.
Therapy	■ Patients can follow a home therapy program for fingertip desensitization.

POSTOPERATIVE CARE

- Fingertip sensitivity is the most common patient complaint following fingertip injury and reconstruction. Cold sensitivity can be particularly troublesome.
  - Time, reassurance, and hand therapy are beneficial.
  - Massage, desensitization exercises, and cortical retraining of the finger are useful techniques.
- Fingertip protectors can be worn early in the postoperative period when the fingertip is most sensitive. They can be weaned over time as symptoms improve.

OUTCOMES

- V-Y advancement flap
  - Excellent contour of the fingertip can be achieved (**FIG 5**).
  - Near-normal sensation is restored.
- Cross-finger flap
  - Good aesthetic outcomes are achieved following fingertip reconstruction (**FIG 6A,B**).
  - Sensory recovery improves with time; protective sensation is recovered, but tactile gnosis is not.[10]
  - Despite difficulty with cortical relearning and incomplete sensory recovery, particularly in adult patients, patient satisfaction remains high.[11]
  - The donor site is aesthetically unappealing (**FIG 6C**), particularly for female patients, and the flap color match may be poor, especially in dark-skinned patients.
    - A thenar flap is favored for female and dark-skinned patients rather than a cross-finger flap.
- Thenar flap
  - Donor-site tenderness can be problematic; early hand therapy is recommended.
  - Sensory recovery in the injured finger is typically better compared to a cross-finger flap.[12]
  - Aesthetic outcome of the reconstructed fingertip is excellent, and the donor site is hidden in the palm (**FIG 7**).

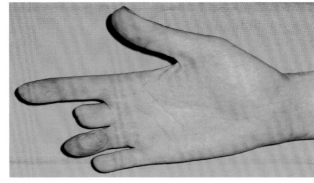

FIG 5 • The V-Y advancement flap of the index finger restores the contour of the fingertip with sensate, durable soft tissue coverage. The donor site is inconspicuous. The incisions over the volar finger pulp can be sensitive; hand therapy may be required postoperatively.

COMPLICATIONS

- A shortened distal phalanx results in the loss of nail bed support. A hook-nail deformity can result. Excision of the sterile nail matrix 2 mm proximal to the shortened bone can help prevent this complication. The patient is taught to trim the nail frequently.
  - If the nail remains troublesome, nail bed obliteration can be performed.
- A V-Y advancement flap creates additional incisions over the volar finger pulp. Hypertrophic and hypersensitive scarring can result.
- With regional flaps, stiffness can be marked postoperatively, particularly for older patients with arthritis and other comorbidities. Patients must be consulted preoperatively on the need for hand therapy following a two-stage flap reconstruction. For severe contractures, static progressive splinting can be used.

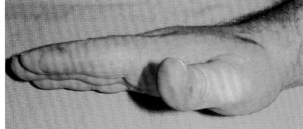

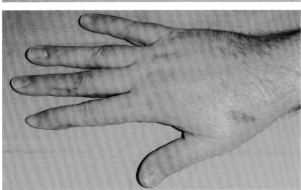

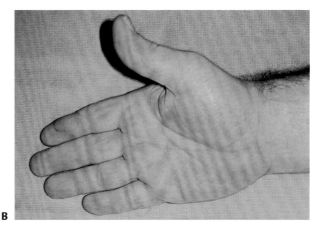

FIG 6 • The cross-finger flap provides excellent resurfacing for a fingertip injury, shown here volarly (**A**) and laterally (**B**) 4 months postoperatively. **C.** The appearance of the FTSG at the donor site, shown 4 months postoperatively, improves with time but remains noticeable over the dorsal middle phalanx of the donor finger. Aesthetic considerations must be discussed with the patient prior to use of this flap.

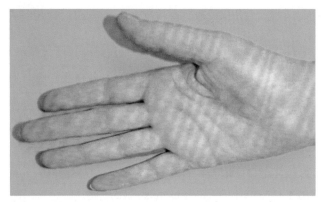

FIG 7 • The appearance of the reconstructed index fingertip and the thenar flap donor site 3 months postoperatively shows satisfactory healing.

■ V-Y advancement and thenar flaps transfer glabrous skin to fingertip injuries; cross-finger flaps do not. Furthermore, cross-finger flaps may transfer hair-bearing skin to the volar skin pulp. Laser hair removal can be used once the flap is healed.

REFERENCES

1. Fassler PR. Fingertip injuries: evaluation and treatment. *J Am Acad Orthop Surg.* 1996;4(1):84-92.
2. Atasoy E, Ioakimidis E, Kasdan ML, et al. Reconstruction of the amputated finger tip with a triangular volar flap: a new surgical procedure. *J Bone Joint Surg Am.* 1970;52(5):921-926.
3. Brown RE. Acute nail bed injuries. *Hand Clin.* 2002;18(4):561-575.
4. Lemmon JA, Janis JE, Rohrich RJ. Soft-tissue injuries of the fingertip: methods of evaluation and treatment: an algorithmic approach. *Plast Reconstr Surg.* 2008;122(3):105e-117e.
5. Holm A, Zachariae L. Fingertip lesions: an evaluation of conservative treatment versus free skin grafting. *Acta Orthop Scand.* 1974;45(3):382-392.
6. Moiemen NS, Elliot D. Composite graft replacement of digital tips. 2. A study in children. *J Hand Surg Br.* 1997;22(3):346-352.
7. Kumar VP, Satku K. Treatment and prevention of "hook nail" deformity with anatomic correlation. *J Hand Surg [Am].* 1993;18(4):617-620.
8. Chao JG HJ, Wiedrich TA. Local hand flaps. *J Am Soc Surg Hand.* 2001;1(1):25-44.
9. Thoma A, Vartija LK. Making the V-Y advancement flap safer in fingertip amputations. *Can J Plast Surg.* 2010;18(4):e47-49.
10. Nishikawa H, Smith PJ. The recovery of sensation and function after cross-finger flaps for fingertip injury. *J Hand Surg Br.* 1992;17(1):102-107.
11. Kleinert HE, McAlister CG, MacDonald CJ, Kutz JE. A critical evaluation of cross finger flaps. *J Trauma.* 1974;14(9):756-763.
12. Melone CP, Beasley RW, Carstens JH. The thenar flap: an analysis of its use in 150 cases. *J Hand Surg [Am].* 1982;7(3):291-297.

Flap Coverage of Thumb Defects

CHAPTER 46

Kate Elzinga and Kevin C. Chung

DEFINITION

- The thumb accounts for over 40% of hand function.[1] Maintenance of length, ideally beyond the neck of the proximal phalanx, is critical for stable pinch and grasp.
- The goals of thumb reconstruction include maximizing length, stability, strength, mobility, sensation, durability of coverage, and appearance while minimizing donor-site morbidity.
- The function of the thumb is optimized following injury by restoring a sensate thumb pulp.[2]

ANATOMY

- The volar thumb is covered by thick, durable, highly innervated, glabrous skin.
- Dorsally, the nail provides protection for the distal phalanx and counterpressure for the pulp during pinch.

PATIENT HISTORY AND PHYSICAL FINDINGS

- Following a thumb injury, important patient factors include age, sex, handedness, comorbidities, medications, allergies, occupation and avocations, and smoking status.
- Injury factors to consider include the time and mechanism of injury, the degree of tissue contamination and necrosis, and any previous hand injuries.
- The patients' goals are explored. Their desire for a rapid return to work and their level of compliance and motivation are considered when formulating a reconstructive plan.
- The thumb wound is examined, noting the level of the injury and tissue loss (skin, soft tissue, neurovascular bundles, tendons, bone, nail). Exposed structures are evaluated and documented.
- The thumb's color, capillary refill, turgor, and temperature are assessed as part of the vascular exam. The digital nerves are assessed using light touch, two-point discrimination, or the ten test.[3]
- The function of the extensor pollicis longus and that of the flexor pollicis longus (FPL) are tested by asking the patient to actively flex and extend the interphalangeal (IP) joint of the thumb.
  - A digital block can be used for patient comfort to facilitate the examination following sensory testing of the thumb.
- Donor sites are examined locally and regionally for thumb reconstruction.

IMAGING

- Plain radiographs are performed for the thumb to assess for bony injury, level of amputation, and presence of a foreign body.

NONOPERATIVE MANAGEMENT

- Small defects, up to 1 cm^2 without exposed bone or tendon, heal well by secondary intention.
  - Ingrowth of glabrous skin results in durable, sensate coverage.
  - Moist, antibacterial dressings are applied daily.
  - Range-of-motion exercises are performed throughout to prevent stiffness.
  - Once healed, early use of the thumb is encouraged to help with desensitization of the fingertip and return of function.
- Elevation of the injured upper extremity and gentle compression decrease edema at the thumb defect site, which expedites wound healing.

SURGICAL MANAGEMENT

- Larger skin and subcutaneous tissue defects, over 1 cm^2 without exposed tendon or bone, can be covered with a full-thickness skin graft (FTSG).
  - Rapid healing occurs, but FTSGs are less durable and have poorer sensory recovery compared with healing by secondary intention.
- When tendon or bone is exposed, coverage with local and regional flaps is necessary.
- To restore sensate, durable coverage over an exposed distal phalanx, flap reconstruction with a local Moberg flap can provide coverage for defects of 1.5 cm in length or up to 2.5 cm in length if a transverse proximal releasing incision is used (**FIG 1**).
- Larger defects can be covered with regional flaps such as the first dorsal metacarpal artery (FDMA) flap (**FIG 2**) or the reverse homodigital flap (**FIG 3**) based on the dorsal radial collateral artery.
  - The FDMA flap can be harvested up to 6 × 3 cm in size.
  - The reverse dorsoradial homodigital flap has been described from 2 × 2 cm up to 5 × 4 cm in size.[4]

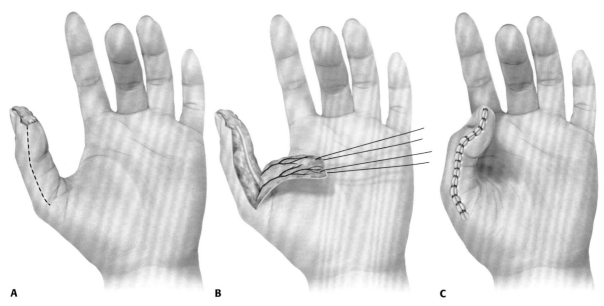

A   **B**   **C**

FIG 1 • The Moberg flap is designed over the volar thumb for coverage of distal thumb defects. **A–C.** Incisions are made at the midaxial line over the radial and ulnar digit up to the volar MCP joint crease. The radial and ulnar digital neurovascular bundles are elevated within the flap. The flap is elevated above the paratenon of the FPL and advanced distally. Flexion of the IP joint facilitates flap inset.

Approach

- The patient is positioned supine with the arm on a hand table.
- Loupe magnification facilitates flap dissection.
- The flap incisions are designed using a template of the defect prior to tourniquet inflation.

- A tourniquet is used for flap elevation to create a bloodless field that facilitates exposure and decreases the risk of injury to the neurovascular structures supplying the flap.
- Following flap elevation, the tourniquet is released. Flap perfusion is assessed. Hemostasis is achieved prior to flap inset to prevent a hematoma that could result in flap compromise.

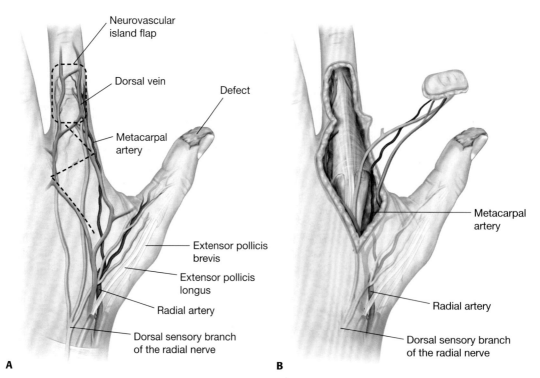

A   **B**

FIG 2 • The FDMA flap is elevated from the dorsal proximal phalanx of the index finger for coverage of thumb defects. **A,B.** The flap can be raised as an island flap, using a straight line, lazy S, or zigzag incision as shown here for elevation of the pedicle back to the flap pivot point, which is found just distal to the EPL tendon.

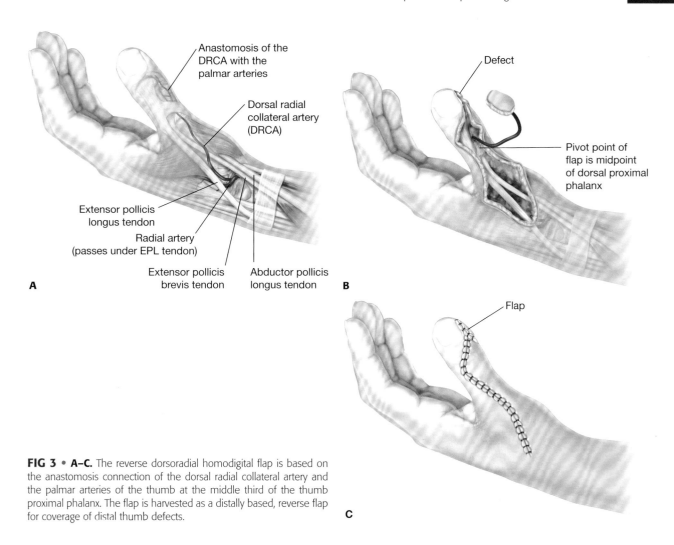

FIG 3 • A–C. The reverse dorsoradial homodigital flap is based on the anastomosis connection of the dorsal radial collateral artery and the palmar arteries of the thumb at the middle third of the thumb proximal phalanx. The flap is harvested as a distally based, reverse flap for coverage of distal thumb defects.

■ Moberg Flap

- Incisions are designed over the midaxial lines of the ulnar and radial thumb, at the junction of the glabrous and nonglabrous skin (**TECH FIG 1A**; see **FIG 1**). Proximally, the flap is marked to the metacarpophalangeal (MCP) joint crease bilaterally. If further advance is necessary, the flap can be extended proximal to the MCP, Burow triangles can be excised at the flap base bilaterally, or the flap can be advanced as a V-Y flap[5] or as an island flap.[6]

- The ulnar and radial digital nerves and arteries are elevated within the flap, which maintains the blood supply to the flap as well as innervation (**TECH FIG 1B**). The dorsal blood supply of the thumb from the princeps pollicis artery permits safe flap elevation without compromising the thumb's perfusion.

- When used as an island flap, a transverse, proximal releasing incision is made over the proximal phalanx (PP), connecting the two midaxial incisions. The radial and ulnar neurovascular bundles are protected. This release is seldom necessary because the thumb interphalangeal

(IP) joint can be flexed sufficiently for the flap to cover the tip of the distal phalanx.

- The flap is raised from distal to proximal, above the paratenon of the flexor pollicis longus (FPL). As dissection proceeds proximally, advancement of the flap can be tested until tension-free inset is achieved. At this point, proximal dissection ceases.

- The flap should not be advanced more than 2.5 cm to avoid traction on the neurovascular bundles. To achieve advancement of 2.5 cm, a transverse proximal releasing incision is required; the flap is then advanced as an island flap (**TECH FIG 1C,D**). Without a proximal releasing incision, the first dorsal metacarpal artery (FDMA) flap can be advanced 1.5 cm.
  - The donor site can be closed with a full-thickness skin graft (FTSG) (**TECH FIG 1E**).

- If needed, the thumb MCP and IP joints are flexed to facilitate flap inset over the distal thumb defect.
  - Rarely, a K-wire is used to maintain the flexed position of the IP joint (**TECH FIG 1F**).
  - For older patients with arthritis, limited flexion is recommended to prevent an IP joint flexion contracture.

T E C H N I Q U E S

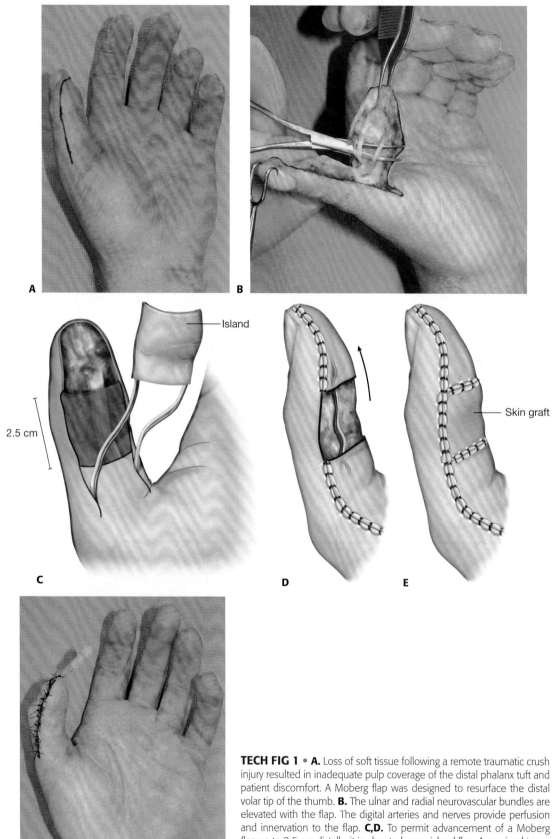

TECH FIG 1 • A. Loss of soft tissue following a remote traumatic crush injury resulted in inadequate pulp coverage of the distal phalanx tuft and patient discomfort. A Moberg flap was designed to resurface the distal volar tip of the thumb. **B.** The ulnar and radial neurovascular bundles are elevated with the flap. The digital arteries and nerves provide perfusion and innervation to the flap. **C,D.** To permit advancement of a Moberg flap up to 2.5 cm distally, it is elevated as an island flap. A proximal transverse incision is used to connect the ulnar and radial midaxial incisions. **E.** The donor site is covered with an FTSG. **F.** A K-wire can be used to maintain IP joint flexion to facilitate flap inset to the distal thumb.

- The flap is inset using 4-0 nonabsorbable monofilament suture. The flap is secured to the intact skin surrounding the defect and to the nail.
- If used, the FTSG is secured with a bolster dressing. Antibacterial gauze is applied to the flap incisions followed by sterile gauze and a well-padded thumb spica splint.

- The splint can typically be discontinued 1 week postoperatively, and range-of-motion (ROM) exercises are started for the MCP joint. Two weeks postoperatively, if present, the K-wire can be removed and IP ROM is initiated.

■ First Dorsal Metacarpal Artery Flap (see FIG 2)

- Over the dorsal hand, distal to the anatomic snuffbox, the radial artery gives off three branches: the dorsal carpal arch (radial branch), the princeps pollicis (middle branch), and the FDMA (ulnar branch). After giving off the FDMA, the radial artery dives deep between the two heads of the first dorsal interosseous (DIO) and joins the deep palmar arch.
- The FDMA travels within or just above the fascia of the first DIO radial to the index finger metacarpal. A branch of the dorsal sensory branch of the radial nerve travels with the FDMA.
- The FDMA flap provides innervated vascularized soft tissue coverage for large thumb or first web space defects (**TECH FIG 2A,B**).
  - It is designed over the dorsal PP of the index finger. Typically, the flap is designed from the proximal interphalangeal joint to the MCP joint; proximal extensions are possible for coverage of larger defects (**TECH FIG 2C**).
  - Ulnarly and radially, the flap extends to the midaxial lines of the index finger at the junction of the glabrous and nonglabrous skin.
- The pedicle is a proximal adipofascial extension of the flap that contains the FDMA, two dorsal veins, a branch of the dorsal sensory branch of the radial nerve, subcutaneous adipose tissue, and the fascia of the first DIO.
  - Alternatively, the pedicle may be designed as a dermofascial flap extension with a 1-cm strip of overlying skin (**TECH FIG 2D**). In these cases, the skin donor-site defect from the pedicle harvest can be closed primarily.
- The pivot point of the flap is marked distal to the extensor pollicis longus at the junction of the metacarpal bases of the thumb and index finger. A handheld Doppler ultrasound (US) can be used to map the course of the FDMA from the dorsoradial index finger PP to the flap pivot point. The course of the FDMA is reliable; US mapping is optional.
- The flap is elevated above the paratenon of the extensor digitorum communis (EDC) and extensor indicis proprius (EIP). It is raised from distoulnar to proximoradial

toward the pedicle that enters the flap base on the radial side of the index finger metacarpal.
- As the dissection approaches the proximoradial aspect of the flap and the first DIO is visualized proximal to the MCP joint, dissection must be continued deep to the fascia of the first DIO to prevent injury to the pedicle.
- When harvested as an island flap, a straight line, a lazy S, or a zigzag incision can be used from the flap base to the flap pivot point for pedicle exposure and elevation. The skin is incised and thin skin flaps are elevated radially and ulnarly in the subdermal plane. The pedicle is raised 1 cm in width. The subcutaneous fat and fascia are included to protect the FDMA and accompanying veins; the FDMA is not skeletonized.
- Our preferred approach is to harvest the flap with a dermofascial pedicle rather than as an island flap. A 1-cm skin bridge is incised. A wider adipofascial strip can be harvested below.
  - Including the dermis helps protect the pedicle below during dissection and lessens the risk of pedicle kinking or compression during flap inset.
- The pedicle is raised with the flap from distal to proximal, just above the first DIO muscle (**TECH FIG 2E**).
- When harvested with skin overlying the pedicle, the flap is inset using a skin incision from the flap pivot point proximally to the thumb defect distally (**TECH FIG 2F**).
- When used as an island flap, the flap can be inset under a tunnel (**TECH FIG 2G**).
  - There is an increased risk of venous congestion of the flap when tunneled compared to inset using a skin bridge.
- Tension-free closure of the flap into the defect is performed using sutures (**TECH FIG 2H–J**).
- An FTSG is used to close the FDMA flap donor site (**TECH FIG 2K,L**). A bolster dressing is placed over the FTSG on the dorsal index finger PP.
- Antibacterial gauze and dry gauze are applied to the flap incisions.
- A well-padded splint is applied, taking care to avoid pressure on the flap or pedicle.
- The splint can typically be discontinued 1 week postoperatively, and ROM exercises are started as long as they do not cause undue tension on the flap.

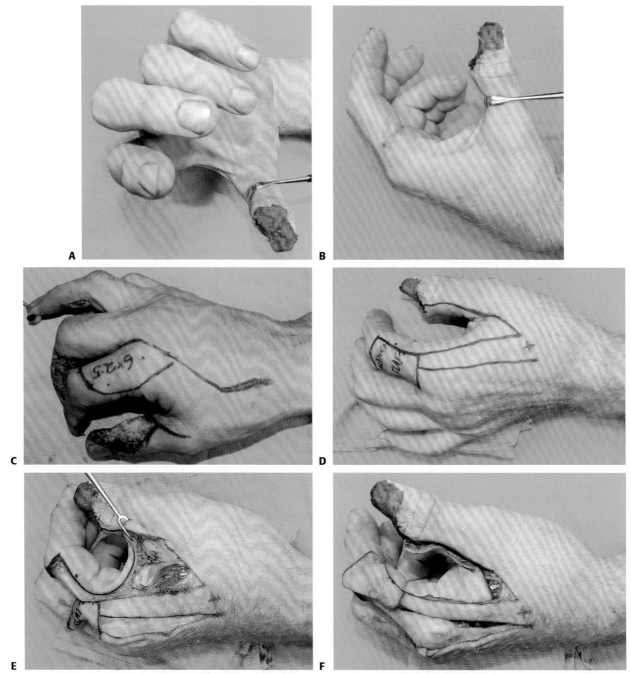

TECH FIG 2 • A,B. A traumatic injury to the ulnar and volar thumb can be resurfaced using a FDMA flap. Prior to reconstruction, the wound should be free of infection and necrotic tissue. **C.** Most commonly, the FDMA flap is designed from the MCP proximally to the proximal interphalangeal joint distally over the dorsal index finger. Proximal extensions can be used as shown here for coverage of larger thumb defects. **D.** The FDMA flap can be raised with a dermofascial pedicle, as shown here, or with an adipofascial pedicle. The flap pivot point is marked here with an "X" at the junction of the first and second metacarpal bases, just distal to the EPL. An incision from the pivot point to the defect is marked for flap inset; alternately, the flap could be tunneled into the defect if an adipofascial pedicle was raised. **E.** The fascia of the first DIO is included with the pedicle to prevent injury to the FDMA and the draining veins of the flap. Here, the first DIO is shown radial to the flap pedicle, exposed but not violated. The paratenon is preserved over the extensor tendons of the index finger, shown ulnar to the flap pedicle. **F.** An incision is made from the flap pivot point to the thumb defect. The flap mobility is tested; tension-free inset is critical for flap survival.

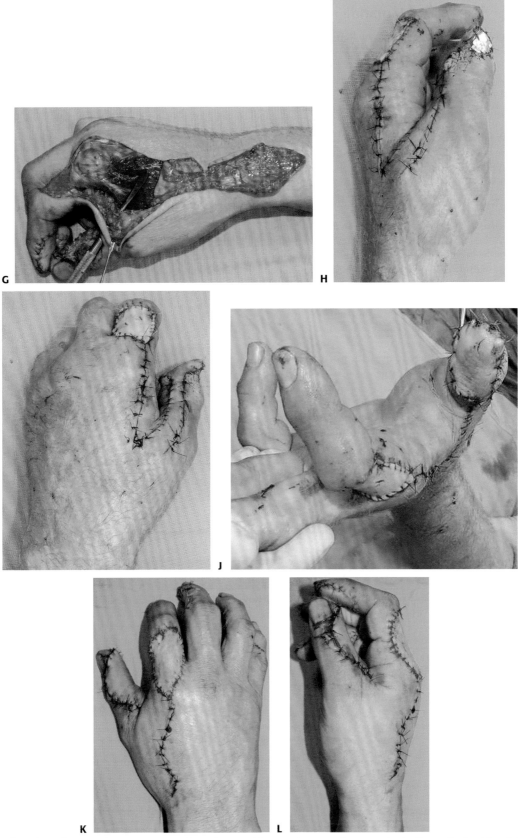

TECH FIG 2 (Continued) • **G.** A different patient is shown here. In this case, the FDMA flap was raised with an adipofascial pedicle and tunneled into the defect. A wide tunnel is created to prevent pedicle compression and venous congestion. **H–J.** The FDMA flap and its dermofascial pedicle are inset using sutures. The nail had been avulsed; a splint was placed into the nail fold. The FDMA flap donor site was closed with an FTSG. **K,L.** For this patient, the flap was tunneled into the defect over the volar-ulnar thumb and sutured into position. The flap donor site and additional superficial wounds over the distal radial index and middle fingers were closed with FTSGs.

■ Reverse Dorsoradial Homodigital Flap

- The reverse dorsoradial homodigital flap is harvested from the dorsoradial side of the thumb metacarpal (see **FIG 3**).
- Its arc of rotation permits coverage of distal volar and dorsal thumb defects and radial defects of the proximal and distal phalanx of the thumb.[7] It is most commonly used for smaller defects over the dorsum of the thumb; the FDMA flap provides more tissue and is better suited for coverage of larger volar defects of the thumb.
- The flap pedicle is the dorsal radial collateral artery, which is a branch of the radial artery over the dorsoradial hand at the anatomic snuffbox. It passes under the extensor pollicis brevis (EPB) tendon as it travels from ulnar to radial. The pedicle is consistent in its course and caliber, traveling distally 1 cm radial to the midline of the dorsal thumb. It communicates with the palmar vessels at the middle third of the PP, permitting this flap to be used reliably as a reverse island flap.
- The course of the dorsal radial artery can be identified using a Doppler US. It runs from the snuffbox to the middle of the dorsoradial PP. The pivot point of the flap is over the middle of the dorsoradial PP.
- Using a template of the defect, the flap is designed over the dorsoradial thumb metacarpal, centered over the dorsal radial collateral artery.
- The skin island is incised, starting at its proximal edge. The dorsal radial collateral artery is identified, and the flap design is adjusted as needed to ensure it is over the pedicle.
  - The flap is raised above the paratenon of the extensor tendons. The incision over the distal flap is made through the dermis, but not deeper, to avoid transection of the pedicle below.

- The flap is elevated from proximal to distal. The dorsal radial collateral artery is divided just distal to where it passes under the EPB.
- A branch of the dorsal sensory branch of the radial nerve runs with the dorsal radial collateral artery. It is divided proximal to the flap to permit flap elevation. This sensory nerve branch can be coapted to the distal radial or ulnar digital nerve of the thumb; however, significant improvement in flap sensitivity has not been demonstrated.[4]
- A skin incision is made from the flap donor site to the defect to permit inset while minimizing the risk of pedicle compression and venous congestion that would occur if the flap were tunneled.
  - A lazy S or a zigzag incision is used.
  - Skin flaps are elevated subdermally radially and ulnarly from the flap donor site to the midpoint of the PP dorsally over the thumb.
- The pedicle is elevated with the surrounding subcutaneous tissue to ensure adequate venous outflow; all nearby venous skin branches are included in the flap elevation. The dorsal radial artery is not skeletonized.
- The flap is inset into the defect and sutured into place. The skin above the pedicle is loosely tackled together to prevent compression and left partially open to heal by secondary intention or covered with an FTSG.
- The flap donor site is closed primarily for flaps up to 4 cm in width. Larger donor sites are closed with an FTSG and covered with a bolster dressing.
- The flap incisions are covered with antibacterial gauze, sterile gauze, and a well-padded, hand-based thumb spica splint.
- The splint can be removed in one week and ROM exercises started.

PEARLS AND PITFALLS

Physical findings	■ The anatomic course of the FDMA and dorsal radial collateral artery is consistent from the radial artery. Doppler US can be used as an adjunct during flap design, but it is not mandatory. Injuries to the dorsal radial hand and wrist preclude the use of these flaps as the flap pedicles may have been damaged. In these cases, an alternate flap should be used.
Technique	■ The FDMA flap donor site leaves a visible donor site over the donor index finger. It can be harvested as an adipofascial flap to minimize the aesthetic morbidity of the donor site; however, the reconstruction of the thumb defect is compromised if the FDMA flap requires an FTSG for coverage. A skin graft on the flap will be less durable and less sensate.
	■ Maintaining the paratenon over the tendons during flap harvest permits FTSG take at the donor site for an island Moberg flap, FDMA flap, and reverse dorsoradial homodigital flap. It also facilitates smooth tendon gliding for the FPL following a Moberg flap harvest, the EDC and EIP after a FDMA flap, and the EPL and EPB after a reverse dorsoradial homodigital flap.
Postoperative	■ The most complete and natural sensation for the thumb pulp is regained using a Moberg flap. Over time, patients will adapt to the sensory input from the FDMA flap; however, cortical retraining is often incomplete and the patient continues to feel as though the dorsal index proximal phalanx is being touched rather than the pulp of the thumb. The homodigital island flap is not innervated. Sensation may be partially regained through the ingrowth of nearby cutaneous nerve fascicles.
Therapy	■ Excessive IP joint flexion, particularly for over 2 weeks, can lead to a flexion contracture following an FDMA flap. Early ROM exercises are recommended, as long as flap viability is not compromised, to minimize IP joint stiffness.
	■ Hand therapy can help a patient regain ROM following a thumb injury. It can also help with desensitization of the reconstructed thumb and donor site.

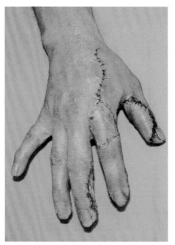 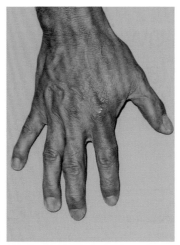 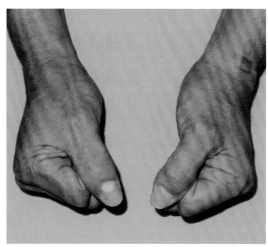

A **B** **C**

FIG 4 • The FDMA flap provides excellent soft tissue coverage for thumb defects. The donor-site aesthetics improve with time. Here, the FDMA flap reconstruction is shown at 2 weeks **(A)** and 16 months **(B,C)** postoperatively.

POSTOPERATIVE CARE

- Nonabsorbable sutures are removed 2 weeks postoperatively.
- The dressings are changed and any FTSG bolster dressings are removed 5 days postoperatively.
- ROM exercises are started 5 to 7 days postoperatively.
- If there is any concern of flap tension, a thermoplastic splint can be used to protect the flap for an additional 1 to 2 weeks between ROM exercises and during sleep.

OUTCOMES

- The Moberg flap best restores sensation to thumb defects. The reverse dorsoradial homodigital flap is not innervated and offers the least complete sensory recovery, averaging 10-mm two-point discrimination.[4]
- The Moberg, FDMA, and homodigital flaps restore the thumb pulp contour well (**FIG 4**).
- The Moberg flap has the least donor site morbidity but can be used only for coverage of smaller thumb defects. The FDMA and homodigital flaps permit coverage of larger defects; the patient must be counseled preoperatively about the visible donor sites on the dorsal hand.

COMPLICATIONS

- Hair growth is rare over the dorsoradial thumb metacarpal. The Moberg and reverse dorsoradial homodigital flaps provide hairless coverage for thumb defects. In contrast, the FDMA flap typically contains hair. Laser hair removal can be used once the flap has healed if hair growth is problematic.

REFERENCES

1. Soucacos PN. Indications and selection for digital amputation and replantation. *J Hand Surg Br.* 2001;26(6):572-581.
2. Margalit M, Shulman S, Stuchiner N. Behavior disorders and mental retardation: the family system perspective. *Res Dev Disabil.* 1989;10(3):315-326.
3. Strauch B, Lang A, Ferder M, Keyes-Ford M, et al. The ten test. *Plast Reconstr Surg.* 1997;99(4):1074-1078.
4. Moschella F, Cordova A. Reverse homodigital dorsal radial flap of the thumb. *Plast Reconstr Surg.* 2006;117(3):920-926.
5. Shah R, Cavale N, Fleming A. A modification of the V-Y Moberg advancement flap for thumb reconstruction. *J Hand Surg Eur Vol.* 2007;32(3):357-358.
6. Mutaf M, Temel M, Günal E, Işık D. Island volar advancement flap for reconstruction of thumb defects. *Ann Plast Surg.* 2012;68(2):153-157.
7. Hrabowski M, Kloeters O, Germann G. Reverse homodigital dorsoradial flap for thumb soft tissue reconstruction: surgical technique. *J Hand Surg [Am].* 2010;35(4):659-662.

47 CHAPTER

Reverse Flow Radial Forearm Flap

Kate Elzinga and Kevin C. Chung

DEFINITION

- The most commonly used regional flap for coverage of volar and dorsal hand and wrist wounds is the reverse radial forearm flap (RRFF). It is a reliable and versatile flap.
- The radial forearm flap can be used as an antegrade flap to cover defects of the elbow.
- The radial forearm flap can also be harvested as a free flap for distant defects.
- The RRFF can be designed up to 35 × 15 cm in size, harvesting up to two-thirds of the circumference of the forearm, from 4 cm distal to the antecubital fossa to the wrist crease.
  - The RRFF's large size makes it suitable for coverage of nearly all wrist and hand wounds. However, the arc of rotation of the flap into the defect typically precludes harvesting the flap extending to the distal forearm.
  - The flap can be pre-expanded to further increase its dimensions proximally in the forearm for adequate use as a reverse flap, although this is rarely necessary.[1]

ANATOMY

- The RRFF is a Mathes and Nahai type B flap; it is supplied by septocutaneous perforators. Its pedicle is the radial artery and its two accompanying vena comitantes. The radial artery is divided proximally. Retrograde flow occurs from the ulnar artery through the deep palmar arch into the radial artery to provide arterial inflow to the flap.
- The radial artery originates from the brachial artery. It travels under the brachioradialis (BR) for most of its course. Distally, it is found in the interval between the BR radially and the flexor carpi radialis (FCR) ulnarly. The radial artery perforators travel within the septum between the BR and FCR to supply the overlying fascia and skin (**FIG 1**).
- There are 6 to 10 septocutaneous perforators arising from the radial artery 2 cm proximal to the radial styloid.[2] A reverse radial artery perforator flap can be elevated on these perforators to preserve the radial artery for patients without an intact palmar arch.[3,4]
- The cephalic vein can be harvested with the RRFF although it does not play a role in the venous drainage of reverse flaps. Venous outflow is through the avalvular oscillating veins.[5] In cases of venous congestion, anastomosis of the cephalic vein within the flap will decompress the venous congestion.
- The RRFF is designed over the proximal and middle volar forearm.
- The RRFF can be harvested as a fasciocutaneous, adipofascial, or fascia-only flap. It may also be raised above the fascia; the subcutaneous tissue and dermis above the fascia are raised suprafascially.

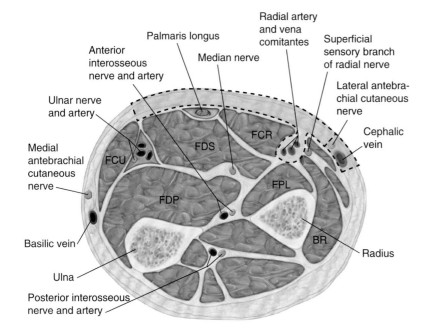

Radial artery and vena comitantes

Palmaris longus

Median nerve

Anterior interosseous nerve and artery

Superficial sensory branch of radial nerve

Lateral antebrachial cutaneous nerve

Ulnar nerve and artery

FCR

Cephalic vein

Medial antebrachial cutaneous nerve

FCU

FDS

FPL

FDP

BR

Basilic vein

Radius

Ulna

Posterior interosseous nerve and artery

FIG 1 • The radial artery and its vena comitantes are found in the distal forearm within the intermuscular septum between the BR radially and the FCR ulnarly. The radial border of the RRFF can be centered over the radial artery as shown here. Alternatively, the flap can be designed with its radial margin over the radial artery. The LABC and cephalic vein are optional structures that can be included in the flap design.

- The lateral antebrachial cutaneous nerve (LABC) can be harvested with the flap and coapted to a sensory nerve at the defect site to innervate the flap.
  - Alternatively, the LABC can be left in situ during flap harvest, preserving the sensation to the radial forearm.[6]
- The palmaris longus can be elevated with the flap for use as a vascularized tendon graft. For example, it can be used for an extensor tendon defect or to create a flexor pollicis longus during osteoplastic thumb reconstruction with an iliac crest bone graft and a RRFF.[7] The BR can also be included as a vascularized tendon graft or part of the radius as a vascularized bone graft.[8]
- The pivot point for the RRFF is the radial styloid.

PATIENT HISTORY AND PHYSICAL FINDINGS

- The patient is assessed for suitability for regional flap reconstruction following a wrist or hand injury.
  - Important history includes the patient's age, handedness, and occupation and avocations.
  - The patient's past medical history, medications, allergies, and social history are noted. In particular, risk factors for flap loss, poor wound healing, and additional postoperative complications are discussed.
  - Comorbidities associated with poor wound healing include smoking, diabetes mellitus, end-stage renal disease, cardiac disease, peripheral vascular disease, vasculitis, malnutrition, immunosuppression, and hypercoagulable states.
- Details of previous trauma or surgeries to the forearm are gathered. History of any previous radial artery cannulation for invasive blood pressure monitoring is also important.
  - If there is concern of damage to the radial artery or its perforators, angiography can be performed to evaluate the vascularity of the arm.
- The patient's defect is examined. The size of the wound is measured. Exposed structures, necrotic tissues, and any signs of infection are documented.
- Wounds with exposed tendon and bone are best covered using flaps. The radial forearm flap is a pedicled regional flap that can be safely performed in most patients. It alleviates the need for a two-stage flap reconstruction such as a groin flap or microvascular reconstruction with a free flap.
- The vascularity of the hand must be carefully assessed. If the radial artery is harvested for the RRFF, the patient must have an intact palmar arch with arterial inflow from the ulnar artery to prevent hand and finger ischemia.
  - The modified Allen test is used to clinically assess the integrity of the palmar arch (**FIG 2**). The examiner compresses the patient's ulnar and radial arteries at the volar wrist and then instructs the patient to open and close the hand into a tight fist until the palm is blanched. The examiner then releases the ulnar artery and looks for arterial flow from the ulnar artery through the palmar arch to the radial side of the hand within 6 seconds. The test is repeated to assess the radial artery.
- The motor and sensory nerves of the hand and forearm are tested. Any pre-existing abnormalities are noted.

IMAGING

- Plain radiographs are performed for patients with traumatic wounds. Any fractures, foreign bodies, and abnormal joint intervals secondary to ligamentous injuries are noted.

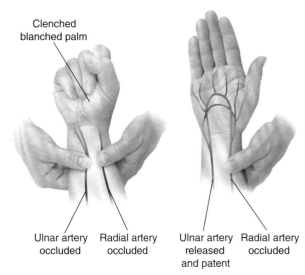

FIG 2 • The modified Allen test is used to confirm retrograde flow into the radial artery from the ulnar artery across the palmar arch prior to division of the radial artery for a RRFF. If the palmar arch is not patent, a reverse radial artery *perforator* flap or alternate flap should be used instead.

- The authors do not routinely perform angiography prior to RRFF harvest. If the patient has sustained previous trauma to the forearm or has undergone previous surgery to the forearm, angiography can be used to evaluate the integrity of the vascular system of the arm and the patency of the radial artery, ulnar artery, and palmar arch.
- An ultrasound (US) can be performed to do a Doppler Allen test if the patient is unable to participate in a clinical Allen test or to confirm clinical findings.[9] This is not necessary for most patients.

NONOPERATIVE MANAGEMENT

- Prior to flap coverage, the wound is debrided to ensure it is clean with no necrotic tissue.
- Antimicrobial dressings are used prior to RRFF coverage to minimize the bacterial load of the wound.

SURGICAL MANAGEMENT

- The size of the patient's wound and the presence of exposed bone and tendon help to guide the selection of an appropriate flap for reconstruction.
  - Local flaps can be used for small defects.
  - Regional flaps, such as the RRFF, are excellent options for moderate- to large-sized defects of the volar and dorsal hand and fingers.
  - Free flaps are an alternative but require a longer operative time, a distant donor site, and microsurgical expertise.

Preoperative Planning

- The risks and benefits of flap reconstruction are discussed in detail with the patient.
- The benefits of the RRFF include a supple, durable, and thin flap for reconstruction. The color match is excellent for dorsal hand defects. In dark-skinned patients, the color match for volar defects may be poor.
- The risk of partial or complete flap loss is discussed.

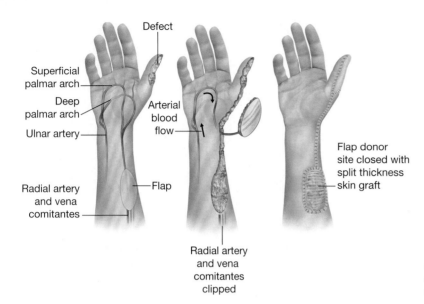

Defect

Superficial palmar arch

Deep palmar arch

Ulnar artery

Radial artery and vena comitantes

Flap

Arterial blood flow

Radial artery and vena comitantes clipped

Flap donor site closed with split thickness skin graft

FIG 3 • The RRFF is harvested over the proximal and/ or middle third of the forearm, depending on the required size and arc of rotation. For RRRFs harvested with a width over 6 cm, closure with an STSG is required.

- The patient is counseled about the donor-site defect of the RRFF. The donor site is visible over the proximal volar forearm.
  - For flaps over 6 cm in width, a split-thickness skin graft (STSG) is typically used to close the donor site (**FIG 3**).
  - The appearance of the STSG at the recipient site, the appearance of the STSG donor site (typically the anterior upper thigh), and the risk of the STSG failure are explained to the patient.
- If the LABC is harvested, the patient must be counseled about the sensory loss he or she will experience over the radial forearm postoperatively. This may improve with time due to collateral sprouting of adjacent nerves, but full sensory recovery is unlikely.
- The most feared complication of RRFF harvest is ischemia of the hand following division of the radial artery. If this occurs, a vein graft is typically used to restore the radial artery and thus the arterial inflow of the hand. The patient is counseled about this rare complication and the need for possible vein graft harvest, either the cephalic vein or the saphenous vein.

Positioning

- The patient is positioned supine with the arm supinated on a hand table for RRFF harvest.
- A tourniquet is applied over the upper arm.
  - After the flap incisions are designed, the tourniquet is inflated to permit safe flap elevation in a bloodless field.
  - Once the flap has been elevated with its pedicle, the tourniquet is deflated and the vascularity of the flap and the hand are assessed. Hemostasis is achieved prior to flap inset and donor-site closure to minimize the chance of hematoma and subsequent flap compromise.

Approach

- The flap is typically designed over the middle third of the volar forearm using a template of the wound to mark the flap dimensions. The arc of rotation of the flap is tested to ensure the inset will be tension-free. If the flap must reach further distally, it can be designed over the proximal third of the forearm.
- Loupes are worn to facilitate flap elevation.

■ Reverse Flow Radial Forearm Flap

- The flap can be designed with its radial margin over the radial artery or centered over the radial artery (**TECH FIG 1A–C**).
  - When centered over the radial artery, the flap is harvested around the radial border of the forearm that results in a more visible donor site.
- The radial artery can be palpated over the volar, radial wrist in the interval between the FCR and BR tendons, and then followed proximally using a Doppler US. The course of the radial artery is marked, starting from the volar, radial wrist to the middle of the antecubital fossa.
- An incision is designed from the distal margin of the flap skin paddle to the flap pivot point at the radial styloid. This permits elevation of the pedicle and rotation of the flap distally into the defect.

- When designed as a fasciocutaneous flap, the RRFF skin paddle is marked over the proximal and middle forearm. When used as an adipofascial or fascial flap, an incision is made over the radial proximal forearm centered over the radial artery. Thin skin flaps are lifted radially and ulnarly to expose the adipofascial tissue below.
- The RRFF is raised from ulnar to radial to the FCR and from radial to ulnar to the BR.
- The flap is elevated in either the suprafascial or the subfascial plane, depending on the tissues required for reconstruction of the defect. For both flap types, the fascia must be incised and harvested with the flap radially over the BR and ulnarly over the FCR to include the pedicle (**TECH FIG 1D**); the flap cannot be raised entirely in the suprafascial plane.

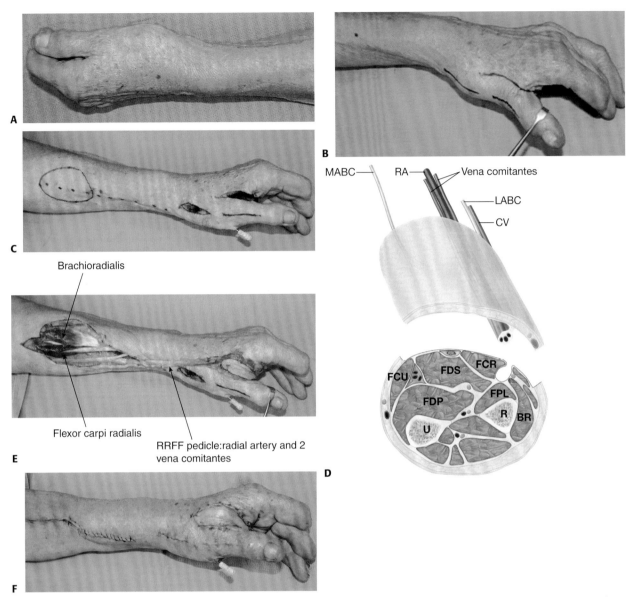

TECH FIG 1 • A. This patient presented with a first web space adduction contracture secondary to long-standing thumb carpometacarpal joint osteoarthritis. To alleviate the patient's basilar joint pain and to restore her first web space, a trapeziectomy was planned along with pinning of the first metacarpal in an abducted position and first web space contracture release with interposition of a RRFF. **B.** The surgical incisions are marked. A longitudinal incision was marked over the first web space, extending from the dorsal to the volar surface of the hand to permit the release of the contracted skin, subcutaneous tissues, and adductor pollicis. The metacarpophalangeal joint of the thumb was marked as a reference point. The carpometacarpal joint of the thumb was marked proximally; this incision was used for the trapeziectomy. **C.** An RRFF was designed using a template of the first web space defect site. A 6 cm long × 4 cm wide flap was marked over the middle of the volar forearm, centered over the radial artery. The radial artery can be palpated distally between the FCR and BR and followed proximally using a Doppler US. Its course is marked by the dotted line. The radial styloid is the flap pivot point. **D.** The fascia must be raised over the BR radially and over the FCR ulnarly to ensure that the radial artery and its vena comitantes are raised with the flap. The LABC and cephalic vein can be included in the flap design if desired. **E.** Prior to tunneling the flap through a wide subcutaneous tunnel over the dorsoradial wrist to the first web space, the arc of rotation of the flap is tested to ensure the flap reaches the first web space defect without tension on it or its pedicle. Care is taken to avoid kinking and compression of the pedicle during inset. The tendons of the BR and the FCR are visible at the flap donor site. **F.** RRFFs less than 6 cm in width can be closely primarily, as shown here. Wider flap donor sites are closed with a STSG. In this case, the RRFF was tunneled distally into the first web space defect. Alternatively, a skin incision can be used to allow flap rotation distally. A percutaneous pin is placed to maintain thumb metacarpal abduction following first web space contracture release for 4 weeks.

- Perforators from the radial artery to the overlying fascia and skin are identified in the lateral intermuscular septum between the BR and the FCR and are protected. To facilitate the identification of the lateral intermuscular septum, particularly in the proximal arm, the BR is retracted radially and the FCR is retracted ulnarly.
- The paratenon is preserved over all tendons during dissection; this permits STSG take when a wide flap is harvested. The superficial sensory branch of the radial nerve is protected throughout.
- The flap's proximal margin is incised. The radial artery and its vena comitantes are identified and ligated. Microclips or sutures can be used.
- If the LABC is harvested with the flap, it is divided at the proximal flap margin. If it is left in situ, it is identified and protected throughout the dissection as flap elevation continues.
- The dermis of the distal margin of the flap is incised sharply, taking care not to penetrate into the soft tissues below to prevent injury to the radial artery and vena comitantes.
- The skin incision is made from the distal flap margin to the flap pivot point. The flap is elevated from proximal to distal with its pedicle. The pedicle includes the radial artery and its vena comitantes as well as the cephalic vein and LABC when desired.
- When a fasciocutaneous flap is raised, the RRFF skin is secured to the underlying fascia using absorbable sutures to prevent shearing of the cutaneous perforators.

- Vascular branches from the radial artery to the flexor pollicis longus and to the radius are divided using microclips and bipolar cautery to permit pedicle elevation to proceed distally.
- The flap is inset into the defect site using sutures.
  - The flap can be inset through a wide tunnel (**TECH FIG 1E**) or using a skin incision from the flap pivot point at the radial styloid to the defect.
  - Care is taken to avoid kinking or compression of the pedicle and any flap tension.
- The RRFF donor site is closed primarily if the flap is adipofascial, fascial, or a narrow fasciocutaneous flap (**TECH FIG 1F**). Donor-site skin defects over 6 cm in width are closed with a STSG; a sheet STSG is preferred over a meshed STSG for improved appearance.
- The skin incision between the flap donor site to the radial styloid is closed primarily following pedicle dissection in this area.
- The flap vascularity is assessed after closure of all incisions. Color, capillary refill, temperature, and turgor are noted.
- The vascularity of the hand is confirmed, and arterial inflow to all digits is documented.
- Antibiotic-impregnated gauze is applied to all incisions and covered with sterile gauze. The skin paddle of the flap is left visible to facilitate postoperative flap checks.
- If used, the STSG is carefully padded to prevent shear and to optimize take.
- A well-padded forearm splint is applied.
- The arm is elevated postoperatively to minimize edema.

PEARLS AND PITFALLS

Physical findings	■ Previous trauma to the volar radial forearm precludes the use of the RRFF. In these cases, the small perforators to the overlying fascia and skin may have been injured.
Technique	■ For patients with recurrent or persistent carpal tunnel syndrome, an adipofascial RRFF can be used to wrap the median nerve.[10]
Postoperative	■ No anticoagulation is used for pedicled flaps. Prophylactic low molecular weight heparin injections are given daily to prevent deep vein thrombosis until the patient is mobilizing well postoperatively. ■ A Doppler US can be used after flap inset to identify audible arterial and venous perforators to the skin paddle. The location of these perforators can be marked with a 6-0 polypropylene suture. This is not critical for pedicled flaps, but can be a helpful adjunct for postoperative monitoring.
Therapy	■ Scar massage and desensitization exercises can be started under the guidance of a hand therapist once the incisions are healed, approximately 3 weeks postoperatively.

POSTOPERATIVE CARE

- Flap checks are performed every 2 hours postoperatively. The flap and hand are assessed. If there is a lack of arterial inflow or venous outflow noted for the flap, the patient is taken back to the operating room urgently for flap exploration. A kink in the pedicle, hematoma, or compression from a tight closure can result in flap compromise.
- The patient is discharged home on postoperative day 3.
- The patient returns to the clinic on postoperative day 5 for a wound check and dressing change. If an STSG was used, its take over the donor site is assessed.
- Early range-of-motion (ROM) exercises are performed for all uninvolved joints of the upper extremity. If the flap

crosses the wrist, gentle wrist ROM exercises are initiated on postoperative day 5 to 7 as long as no flap compromise occurs.
- For flaps crossing the wrist, a resting wrist splint is worn to maintain the wrist in neutral alignment to 20 degrees of extension for 2 weeks postoperatively. The splint is removed multiple times during the day for ROM exercises during the 2nd postoperative week. After 2 weeks, the splint is weaned.

OUTCOMES

- The fasciocutaneous RRFF provides excellent resurfacing for palmar defects. Adipofascial or fascia-only RRFFs with STSG coverage provide a thin reconstruction for the thinner dorsal skin of the hand; these flaps are less durable but minimize donor-site morbidity compared to fasciocutaneous RRFFs.

- The RRFF can be harvested with the LABC. This is particularly helpful for thumb reconstruction. The LABC is coapted to a digital nerve of the thumb to innervate the flap. Static two-point discrimination has been reported as 11 mm for these patients.[7] If the RRFF is used for wrist coverage, the LABC can be coapted to a branch of the superficial sensory branch of the radial nerve.[5]

COMPLICATIONS

- Flap loss is unusual with a pedicled RRFF.
- If the patient is bothered by the appearance of the RRFF donor site over the proximal arm following closure with an STSG, serial excision of the STSG can be performed.

REFERENCES

1. Masser MR. The preexpanded radial free flap. *Plast Reconstr Surg.* 1990;86(2):295-301.
2. Weinzweig N, Chen L, Chen ZW. The distally based radial forearm fasciosubcutaneous flap with preservation of the radial artery: an anatomic and clinical approach. *Plast Reconstr Surg.* 1994;94(5):675-684.
3. Hansen AJ, Duncan SF, Smith AA, et al. Reverse radial forearm fascial flap with radial artery preservation. *Hand.* 2007;2(3):159-163.
4. Ho AM, Chang J. Radial artery perforator flap. *J Hand Surg [Am].* 2010;35(2):308-311.
5. Chang SM, Hou CL, Zhang F, et al. Distally based radial forearm flap with preservation of the radial artery: anatomic, experimental, and clinical studies. *Microsurgery.* 2003;23(4):328-337.
6. Kaufman MR, Jones NF. The reverse radial forearm flap for soft tissue reconstruction of the wrist and hand. *Tech Hand Up Extrem Surg.* 2005;9(1):47-51.
7. Anani RAA-L, El-Sadek AN. Sensate reversed radial forearm flap for posttraumatic missing thumb reconstruction: long-term results. *Egypt J Plast Reconstr Surg.* 2009;33(1):25-30.
8. Cheema SA, Talaat N. Reverse radial artery flap for soft tissue defects of hand in pediatric age group. *J Ayub Med Coll Abbottabad.* 2009;21(1):35-38.
9. Habib J, Baetz L, Satiani B. Assessment of collateral circulation to the hand prior to radial artery harvest. *Vasc Med.* 2012;17(5):352-361.
10. Luchetti R, Riccio M, Papini Zorli I, Fairplay T. Protective coverage of the median nerve using fascial, fasciocutaneous or island flaps. *Handchir Mikrochir Plast Chir.* 2006;38(5):317-330.

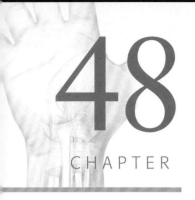

48

CHAPTER

Ulnar Artery Perforator Flap

Kate Elzinga and Kevin C. Chung

DEFINITION

- The ulnar artery perforator flap was first described by Becker as a pedicled flap based on the dorsal branch of the ulnar artery (**FIG 1**).[1] The mobility of this flap is limited by its short pedicle.
  - The ulnar artery perforator flap can also be designed based on the ascending branch of the dorsal branch of the ulnar artery, increasing its reach to distal hand defects (**FIG 2**).[2]
- The ulnar artery perforator flap is most commonly used as a pedicled flap. Alternatively, it can be harvested as a free flap.
- A major advantage of perforator flaps is the preservation of the major vessels of the forearm; the ulnar and radial arteries are not sacrificed.
- The ulnar artery perforator flap can be used for coverage of defects of the ulnar hand and wrist, both dorsal and volar, typically up to 10 × 5 cm in size.[1]
  - Larger flaps, up to 20 × 9 cm, can be harvested, but venous congestion can result.[3]
  - Supercharging a larger flap by anastomosing a subcutaneous flap vein to a nearby vein of the dorsal hand can improve venous outflow.[4]
- The flap can be raised as a fasciocutaneous or adipofascial flap.

ANATOMY

- The hand is supplied by the radial and ulnar arteries that branch from the brachial artery over the antecubital fossa, 1 cm distal to the elbow joint. The ulnar artery travels distally beneath the flexor carpi ulnaris (FCU), volar to the flexor digitorum profundus. Perforators from the ulnar artery travel to the overlying fascia and skin between the FCU and the flexor digitorum superficialis. The superficial and deep palmar arches are located in the palm, formed by the radial and ulnar arteries.
- Sacrifice of the radial or ulnar artery for flap elevation risks hand ischemia if the patient does not have an intact palmar arch. Perforator flaps may be safely used in these cases.
- The ulnar artery gives off seven ± two perforators to the skin over the ulnar forearm with a diameter of 0.5 mm or greater.[5]
  - The pedicle length for propeller or free flaps based on these perforators is 3.3 mm on average, ranging from 2.5 to 4.0 mm.[5]
- About 69% of the perforators of the ulnar artery are musculocutaneous, traveling through the FCU or flexor digitorum superficialis to reach the skin.[5]
  - The remaining perforators are septocutaneous.
- The ulnar artery perforator flap can be designed as a propeller flap based on the dorsal branch of the ulnar artery. It can be harvested up to 15 cm in length, to the mid-forearm, depending on the location of the perforator.
- Greater pedicle length can be obtained when the flap is based on the ascending branch of the dorsal branch of the ulnar artery.

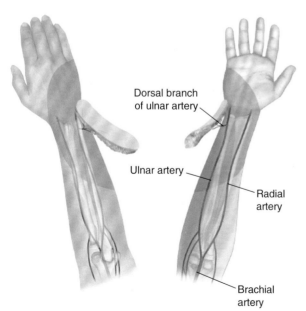

Dorsal branch
of ulnar artery

Ulnar artery

Radial
artery

Brachial
artery

FIG 1 • The ulnar artery perforator flap is shown here based on the dorsal branch of the ulnar artery. It can be used for coverage of defects over the ulnar dorsal and volar wrist and hand (*shaded area*).

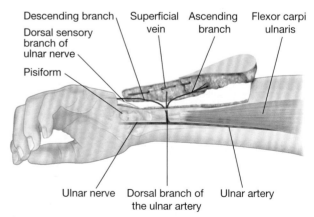

Descending branch   Superficial   Ascending   Flexor carpi
                      vein   branch   ulnaris
Dorsal sensory
branch of
ulnar nerve

Pisiform

Ulnar nerve   Dorsal branch of   Ulnar artery
                the ulnar artery

FIG 2 • The ulnar artery perforator flap has a longer pedicle and a greater arc of rotation when based on the ascending branch of the dorsal branch of the ulnar artery. The ascending branch travels proximally to the medial epicondyle. It supplies the overlying fascia and skin along its course.

- The dorsal branch of the ulnar artery arises from the ulnar artery 2 to 5 cm proximal to the pisiform.[6]
    - Infrequently, in 2 of 26 cadaver dissections, the dorsal branch arises from the anterior interosseous artery rather than from the ulnar artery.[7]
- The dorsal branch of the ulnar artery has a diameter of 1.0 to 1.3 mm.[2] It travels from the volar distal forearm from radial to ulnar, under the FCU, to give off three branches:
    - The proximal branch enters the FCU 4 to 6 cm proximal to the pisiform.
    - The distal branch supplies the pisiform. It is called the pisiform artery.
    - The middle branch divides into an ascending and a descending branch over the dorsoulnar forearm to supply the forearm and hand, respectively. The ascending branch travels proximally to the medial epicondyle. The descending branch joins the dorsal carpal arch over the dorsal hand. An ulnar artery perforator flap can be designed based on the ascending branch of the dorsal branch of the ulnar artery and its two vena comitantes.[2]
- The ulnar artery perforator flap can be designed from the palmaris longus tendon volarly to the extensor digitorum communis tendon of the fourth finger dorsally.[8]
- The ulnar artery perforator flap is approximately 3 mm thick, providing thin soft tissue coverage.[5]
- The ulnar artery perforator flap is designed along the flap axis between the medial epicondyle and the pisiform (**FIG 3**). Proximally, the perforators are larger and more consistent and primary donor-site closure is easier.
    - When used as a free flap, the ulnar artery perforator flap is typically designed over the proximal forearm.
- The dorsal sensory branch of the ulnar nerve passes beneath the FCU 5 to 8 cm proximal to the pisiform to travel to the dorsal forearm. It is protected during dissection of the dorsal branch of the ulnar artery.
- Flaps widths up to 6 cm can be closed primarily over the ulnar forearm. Wider flaps require closure with a split-thickness skin graft (STSG).
- Bone defects of the small finger metacarpal can be reconstructed by harvesting vascularized cortical bone of the ulna with the ulnar artery perforator flap.[9]
    - Bone is harvested from the ulna 10 to 15 cm proximal to the pisiform between the FCU and extensor carpi ulnaris (**FIG 4**).

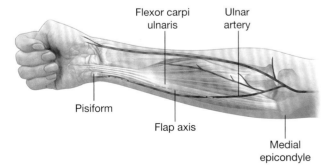

FIG 3 • To design an ulnar artery perforator flap, the medial epicondyle, pisiform, and FCU are marked. Next, the axis of the ulnar artery perforator flap is marked from the medial epicondyle to the pisiform. Ulnar artery perforators are identified along this line using a Doppler ultrasound. The flap is designed to include as mainly audible perforators as possible.

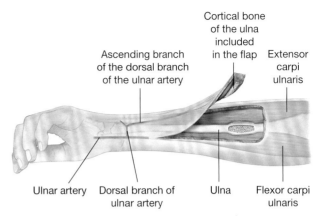

FIG 4 • The ulnar artery perforator flap can be used as an osteocutaneous flap for reconstruction of bone defects of the small finger metacarpal. Cortical bone of the ulna can be harvested in the flap 10 to 15 cm proximal to the pisiform, between the flexor carpi ulnaris and the extensor carpi ulnaris. The flap is elevated on the ascending branch of the dorsal branch of the ulnar artery.

PATIENT HISTORY AND PHYSICAL FINDINGS

- Important factors from the patient's history include the patient's age, sex, hand dominance, occupation and avocations, past medical history, medications, allergies, and social history.
- The timing and mechanism of the patient's injury are recorded. Traumatic injuries result from sharp, crush, and burn mechanisms. Oncologic defects result from sharp tissue resection.
- The patient's wound is explored, noting the size of the wound, contamination and tissue necrosis, and signs of infections.
    - Exposed structures are documented, in particular tendon and bone devoid of paratenon and periosteum; in these cases, flap coverage is required, graft take will not occur.
- Donor sites are assessed during wound reconstruction planning. Forearm local and regional flap donor sites are examined.
- Injuries to ulnar forearm preclude the use of the ulnar artery perforator flap. Ulna fractures often result in damage to the perforators, along with lacerations and crush injuries.

IMAGING

- Plain radiographs are used to assess for fractures, dislocations, and foreign bodies.
- Angiography is not typically performed unless there are specific concerns of the patency of the ulnar artery and its perforators.

NONOPERATIVE MANAGEMENT

- Prior to flap coverage, wound debridement is performed to prepare the wound bed for closure.
- Antibacterial dressings can be used prior to flap closure to decrease the wound's bacterial load.

SURGICAL MANAGEMENT

- The pedicled ulnar artery perforator flap is used for closure of ulnar wrist and hand defects.
    - It has a smaller arc of rotation than does the radial artery forearm flap.
    - It cannot reach the fingers.

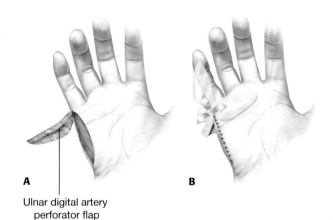

A

Ulnar digital artery
perforator flap

FIG 5 • A. An ulnar artery *digital* perforator flap can be raised over the ulnar hand. The largest perforators are found near the metacarpophalangeal joint. **B.** The flap can be rotated distally up to 180 degrees to cover defects of the small finger and volar and dorsal distal hand.

- The ulnar artery perforator flap can be raised as a free flap to cover a variety of defects, including finger injuries. Sizes of 3.5 × 2 cm to 24 × 4 cm have been reported.[5]
  - To cover finger injuries, the flap's arterial pedicle can be anastomosed to the digital arteries and the vena comitantes can be anastomosed to superficial dorsal veins of the finger.
  - The medial antebrachial cutaneous (MABC) nerve of the forearm can be harvested with the flap and coapted to a digital nerve for sensate flap reconstruction.
- For injuries of the small finger or distal dorsal or volar hand, an ulnar *digital* artery perforator flap can be elevated from the ulnar aspect of the hand and rotated distally as a propeller flap for closure (**FIG 5**).
  - Three or four perforators arise over the palmar aspect of the hypothenar eminence over the abductor digiti minimi from the ulnar artery to supply this flap.[10] The largest

perforators are found near the metacarpophalangeal joint. The flap can be raised as a subfascial or suprafascial flap.

Preoperative Planning

- The patient is counseled about flap reconstruction using the ulnar artery perforator flap. Benefits include thin, supple soft tissue coverage. The flap is durable and reliable.
  - Risks included partial or complete flap loss, wound dehiscence, sensitive scars, and a visible donor site over the ulnar volar forearm.
- To permit ulnar artery perforator flap elevation, the dorsal sensory branch of the ulnar nerve must be divided in some cases. The dorsal sensory branch of the ulnar nerve branches from the ulnar nerve 5 to 8 cm proximal to the pisiform.
  - Patients are counseled about the risk of sensory loss over the dorsal ulnar hand if the nerve is divided during flap elevation.
  - Primary nerve repair should be performed to aid sensory recovery and to prevent a painful neuroma.

Positioning

- The patient is positioned supine with the arm out on a hand table.
- A tourniquet is placed on the upper arm.

Approach

- Loupes facilitate safe elevation of the flap and pedicle.
- The ulnar artery can be palpated over the volar ulnar wrist. Ulnar artery perforators can be identified using a Doppler ultrasound.
  - The flap design is marked to maximize inclusion of audible perforators.
- Incisions are planned prior to inflation of the tourniquet. The tourniquet is inflated during flap elevation to permit bloodless dissection. Once the flap and its pedicle are raised, the tourniquet is deflated to assess the flap's vascularity. Hemostasis is achieved prior to flap inset and closure.

T E C H N I Q U E S

■ Ulnar Artery Perforator Flap

- The medial epicondyle, pisiform, and flexor carpi ulnaris (FCU) are marked. The axis of the flap is marked from the medial epicondyle to the pisiform, ulnar to the FCU. The approximate position of the dorsal branch of the ulnar artery is marked 4 cm proximal to the pisiform, ulnar to the FCU.
- The ulnar artery is palpated over the distal volar forearm. It is followed proximally using a Doppler ultrasound to identify and mark perforators of the ulnar artery on the overlying skin. The largest and most constant perforators are found over the volar ulnar forearm, at the junction of the proximal and middle third of the forearm.[5] Perforators are also consistently found at the junction of the middle and distal thirds of the forearm.
- A template of the defect is used to mark the flap dimensions.

Pedicled Flap

- The flap is designed over the junction of the proximal and middle thirds of the forearm, including as many perforators as possible from the ascending branch of the dorsal branch of the ulnar artery.
- The flap is incised proximally and elevated from proximal to distal in a subfascial plane. It can be raised as a fasciocutaneous or adipofascial flap.
- The skin between the flap and the pivot point is incised using a lazy S-shaped incision. Thin skins flaps are lifted radially and ulnarly exposing the subcutaneous tissue below containing the dorsal branch of the ulnar artery and its accompanying veins. The pedicle is raised with a 4-cm-wide strip of adipofascial tissue to prevent injury to the pedicle. The flap and pedicle are raised from proximal to distal until the dorsal branch of the ulnar artery is seen entering the undersurface of the pedicle. This marks the pivot point of the flap, 4 cm proximal to the pisiform.[11]

- The flap is tunneled into the defect, or a skin bridge is incised between the flap pivot point and the defect for flap inset.
- The flap donor site is closed primarily for fasciocutaneous flaps with a width less than 6 cm or using a STSG if wider. The STSG is typically harvested from the ipsilateral anterior thigh.
- Adipofascial flaps require coverage with a STSG after inset. Their donor sites can be closed primarily.
- Antibiotic-impregnated gauze and sterile dry gauze are placed over all incisions. The flap is left uncovered to facilitate.
- Postoperative flap monitoring. A well-padded splint is applied. Pressure on the flap is avoided.

Propeller Flap

- When used as a distally based propeller flap for hand and wrist coverage, the flap is designed over one dominant perforator from the dorsal branch of the ulnar artery; including additional perforators can prevent adequate rotation of the flap.
  - The largest caliber perforator or the most optimally located perforator is used.
  - Distal perforators facilitate flap rotation distally and thus are often selected when multiple perforators are available.
  - All perforators are preserved during initial flap dissection. The desired perforator is selected. All additional perforators are clamped to ensure that flap vascularity will be maintained based on the main perforator prior their division.
- The width of the flap is designed to match that of the defect (**TECH FIG 1A**).
- The length of flap is designed so that the distance between the perforator and the distal edge of the defect matches the distance between the perforator and the proximal edge of the flap.
- The skin distal to the flap is incised to confirm the location of the ulnar artery and its perforators prior to elevation of the flap. The skin is incised radial to the FCU.
  - The FCU is retracted ulnarly, exposing the ulnar artery and nerve below.

- The perforators of the ulnar artery are identified and followed to the overlying skin to confirm that the flap is properly centered over the perforators.
- The flap is elevated subfascially from ulnar to radial to the radial border of FCU.
- The radial aspect of the flap is then incised.
  - The flap is elevated in a subfascial plane from radial to ulnar to the ulnar aspect of FCU, where the dorsal branch of the ulnar artery is seen entering the flap.
- The basilic vein is typically elevated with the flap. The basilic vein can be followed 2 or 3 cm proximal to the proximal flap edge and harvested to permit venous supercharging if poor venous outflow is noted after inset.[4]
- The MABC nerve can be elevated with the flap or left in situ. The ulnar artery and nerve must be protected.
- The main perforator is skeletonized as necessary to permit adequate rotation of the flap and to prevent pedicle kinking.[12]
- Additional perforators are clamped, and flap vascularity is assessed.
  - If perfusion is maintained, the additional perforators are divided.
  - If not, the additional perforators are maintained to ensure flap viability.
- The flap is inset into the defect. It can be rotated up to 180 degrees (**TECH FIG 1B,C**).
- If used as a sensory flap, the MABC is coapted to a sensory nerve located within or adjacent to the defect.
- The flap donor site is closed primarily for flaps up to 6 cm in width (**TECH FIG 1D**) or using a STSG if a wider flap is harvested.
- A drain can be placed under the flap or the donor site.
- Antibiotic-impregnated gauze is placed over all incisions and covered with sterile gauze. The flap is left uncovered to facilitate postoperative flap monitoring.
- A well-padded splint is applied to protect the flap and to decrease tension on the flap.
  - When the flap is used for coverage of palmar defects, the wrist is splinted in mild flexion to decrease flap tension.
  - When used for dorsal defects, the wrist is splinted in extension.

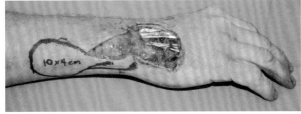

A

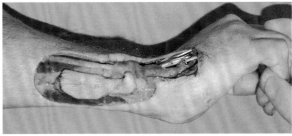

B

TECH FIG 1 • A. Following debridement of a traumatic wound, this patient had a 9 × 4 cm defect over the dorsal ulnar hand with exposed extensor tendons. An ulnar artery perforator flap was designed as a propeller flap for coverage. The width of the flap is designed to match the width of the defect. The length of the flap is marked so that when the flap is rotated 180 degrees around the perforator, the proximal edge of the flap will reach the distal edge of the defect. An umbilical tape, vessel loop, or surgical sponge can be used to visualize the arc of rotation of the proximal flap into the distal defect during flap marking. **B.** The ulnar artery perforator flap is elevated.

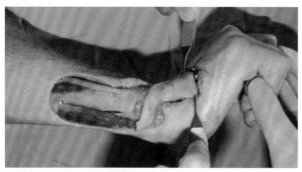

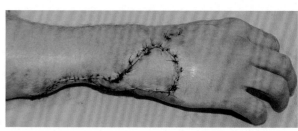

C **D**

TECH FIG 1 (Continued) • **C.** The flap can be rotated up to 180 degrees into the distal defect. **D.** Here, the donor site was closed primarily. The flap width was 4 cm. Flaps widths up to 6 cm can generally be closed with sutures directly. Wider flaps require closure with an STSG.

PEARLS AND PITFALLS

Physical findings	■ A modified Allen test is performed to assess the patency of the palmar arch. An intact palmar arch is not required for the ulnar artery perforator flap but provides valuable information about the arterial supply of the hand.
Technique	■ During ulnar artery perforator flap elevation, the dorsal sensory branch of the ulnar nerve may require division. In these cases, the nerve should be repaired using 9-0 nylon suture or fibrin glue.
	■ Dissection of the dorsal branch of the ulnar artery to its origin from the ulnar artery facilitates rotation of the flap up to 180 degrees.[8]
Postoperative	■ The patient is instructed to keep the hand elevated following flap coverage. This decreases flap edema, which lessens the risk of pedicle compression and venous congestion.
Therapy	■ The fingers, wrist, and forearm can be passively mobilized in the operating room to assess for flap tension with movement. Immediate range of motion exercises are performed for uninvolved joints that do not cause strain on the repair with motion.

POSTOPERATIVE CARE

■ The patient is monitored in hospital for signs of flap compromise.
  ■ Poor arterial inflow or venous congestion should prompt removal of the dressings, flap assessment, and urgent return to the operating room to assess for pedicle compromise due to hematoma, kinking, or compression.
■ The patient is discharged on postoperative day 3.
■ The patient returns to clinic 1 week postoperatively for a dressing change.
■ A thermoplastic splint can be worn for an additional week if range of motion causes tension on the flap.

■ Range of motion exercises are started under the guidance of a hand therapist 1 week postoperatively and advanced weekly.

OUTCOMES

■ The ulnar artery perforator flap provides thin, durable soft tissue coverage in a single-stage operation (**FIG 6**).
■ Compared to the radial forearm flap, the ulnar artery perforator flap donor site is less visible on the forearm and the skin paddle contains less hair.
■ The ulnar artery perforator flap provides an excellent color match for dorsal wrist and hand defects.
  ■ In dark-skinned patients, the color is not as well matched for palmar defects.

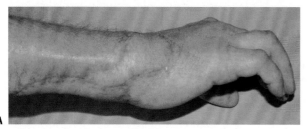

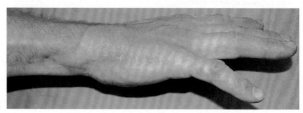

A **B**

FIG 6 • The ulnar artery perforator flap at 1 **(A)** and 10 **(B)** months postoperatively. Supple, durable, thin soft tissue coverage is provided for defects of the hand. The donor site heals well with minimal morbidity.

COMPLICATIONS

- The MABC can be harvested with the flap to restore sensation at the defect site. The donor-site sensory deficit is minimal because of existing sensory overlap and subsequent sensory axon ingrowth from neighboring nerves to the denervated skin.[13]
- The risk of venous congestion is lower for the ulnar artery perforator flap compared to reverse flow flaps, such as the reverse radial forearm flap or the reverse posterior interosseous flap. The ulnar artery perforator flap is a distally based island flap, not a reverse flow flap.
- Incisions over the ulnar forearm, wrist, and hand can be sensitive. Scar massage is recommended once the incisions are healed, starting approximately 3 weeks postoperatively.

REFERENCES

1. Becker C, Gilbert A. [The ulnar flap]. *Handchir Mikrochir Plast Chir*. 1988;20(4):180-183.
2. Karacalar A, Ozcan M. Use of a subcutaneous pedicle ulnar flap to cover skin defects around the wrist. *J Hand Surg Am*. 1998;23(3):551-555.
3. Ignatiadis IA, Mavrogenis AF, Avram AM, et al. Treatment of complex hand trauma using the distal ulnar and radial artery perforator-based flaps. *Injury*. 2008;39(suppl 3):S116-S124.
4. Gomez M, Casal D. The turbocharged Becker flap: a simple variation that allows coverage of most of the dorsum of the hand. *Eur J Plast Surg*. 2011;34:211-213.
5. Wei Y, Shi X, Yu Y, et al. Vascular anatomy and clinical application of the free proximal ulnar artery perforator flaps. *Plast Reconstr Surg Glob Open*. 2014;2(7):e179.
6. Antonopoulos D, Kang NV, Debono R. Our experience with the use of the dorsal ulnar artery flap in hand and wrist tissue cover. *J Hand Surg Br*. 1997;22(6):739-744.
7. Bertelli JA, Pagliei A. The neurocutaneous flap based on the dorsal branches of the ulnar artery and nerve: a new flap for extensive reconstruction of the hand. *Plast Reconstr Surg*. 1998;101(6):1537-1543.
8. Khan MM, Yaseen M, Bariar LM, Khan SM. Clinical study of dorsal ulnar artery flap in hand reconstruction. *Indian J Plast Surg*. 2009;42(1):52-57.
9. Choupina M, Malheiro E, Guimarães I, et al. Osteofasciocutaneous flap based on the dorsal ulnar artery: a new option for reconstruction of composite hand defects. *Br J Plast Surg*. 2004;57(5):465-468.
10. Panse N, Sahasrabudhe P. The ulnar digital artery perforator flap: a new flap for little finger reconstruction: a preliminary report. *Indian J Plast Surg*. 2010;43:190-194.
11. Unal C, Ozdemir J, Hasdemir M. Clinical application of distal ulnar artery perforator flap in hand trauma. *J Reconstr Microsurg*. 2011;27(9):559-565.
12. Karki D, Singh A. The distally-based island ulnar artery perforator flap for wrist defects. *Indian J Plast Surg*. 2007;40(1):12-17.
13. Bertelli JA, Kaleli T. Retrograde-flow neurocutaneous island flaps in the forearm: anatomic basis and clinical results. *Plast Reconstr Surg*. 1995;95(5):851-859.

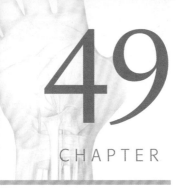

49 CHAPTER

Posterior Interosseous Artery Flap

Kate Elzinga and Kevin C. Chung

DEFINITION

- The posterior interosseous artery (PIA) flap is a perforator flap used for coverage of upper extremity defects. Its harvest avoids the sacrifice of a major artery, such as that of the radial artery during harvest of the radial artery flap.
  - It is available in patients without an intact palmar arterial arch.
- The PIA flap is typically used as a pedicled flap. It can also be harvested as a free flap.[1]
- The PIA flap is most commonly used as a retrograde regional flap based on the anteroposterior interosseous artery system to cover defects of the first web space, dorsal wrist, dorsal and volar hand, and dorsal thumb up to the proximal interphalangeal joint.
  - The PIA flap can also be used as an antegrade flap for defects of the elbow, antecubital fossa, and proximal volar forearm.
- The dimensions of the PIA flap are designed based on the defect size.
  - One case series of 53 patients, from whom two-thirds of the circumference of the forearm skin was harvested, reported the use of PIA flaps from 5 × 2.5 cm to 21 × 10 cm in size.[2]
- The PIA flap provides a good color match for defects of the forearm, wrist, and hand, particularly dorsally.
  - In dark-skinned patients, resurfacing of the palmar skin with a PIA flap leads to a color mismatch.

ANATOMY

- The PIA flap is classified as a Mathes and Nahai type B flap; it is supplied by a septocutaneous perforator.
  - Most commonly, the flap is harvested subfascially as a fasciocutaneous island flap.
  - It can also be harvested with a skin bridge or as an adipofascial flap, which permits primary closure of the donor site; the subcutaneous tissue and fascia are harvested; the dermis is preserved at the donor site.[3]
  - When used as an adipofascial flap, the flap is covered with a split-thickness skin graft (STSG) after inset.
- The flap pedicle is composed of the PIA and its two adjacent vena comitantes.
  - Proximally, the artery is 1.2 to 2.1 mm in diameter and the vena comitantes are 1.0 mm.
  - Over the middle third of the forearm, the PIA has its narrowest caliber, measuring 0.5 mm.
  - Distally, it measures 0.9 to 1.1 mm.[4]
- The PIA arises 4 cm from the lateral epicondyle from the common interosseous artery in 80% of cases and directly from the ulnar artery in 20% of cases.[5]

- The anterior interosseous artery (AIA) also arises from the common interosseous artery, or less commonly, directly from the ulnar artery. It runs along the volar surface of the interosseous membrane (IOM), deep to the flexor digitorum profundus and flexor pollicis longus.
- The PIA passes through the IOM from the volar forearm to the dorsal forearm 8 cm distal to the lateral epicondyle and 14.5 cm proximal to the ulnar styloid.[5]
  - In most cases, it gives origin to three fasciocutaneous perforators to the overlying skin in the proximal forearm and six to eight perforators in the distal forearm.[4]
  - The PIA runs with the posterior interosseous nerve (PIN) along the dorsal IOM to the hand in the septum between the extensor digiti minimi (EDM) and extensor carpi ulnaris (ECU).
- After passing under the supinator in the proximal forearm, the PIA runs over the abductor pollicis longus, extensor pollicis longus, extensor pollicis brevis, and extensor indicis proprius (FIG 1).
- Two centimeters proximal to the distal radioulnar joint (DRUJ), just proximal and radial to the head of the ulna, a branch of the PIA travels volarly through the IOM and anastomoses with the dorsal branch of the AIA.
  - This anastomotic connection is the basis for the retrograde PIA flap.
- The PIA continues distally and joins the dorsal carpal arch. The retrograde PIA flap also receives some flow through this arch.
- The axis of the flap is marked from the lateral epicondyle of the elbow to the head of the ulna.[5]
  - The flap design is centered on the septum between the EDM and ECU to maximize the number of perforators entering the flap from the PIA between the dorsal margins of the ulna and radius (FIG 2).
  - The flap is typically designed up to 18 × 8 cm in size.
- A segment of the proximal third of the ulna, with a cuff of the extensor pollicis longus, can be included in the PIA flap for use as an osteocutaneous flap.[6]

PATIENT HISTORY AND PHYSICAL FINDINGS

- Important aspects of the patient history include age, sex, handedness, occupation and avocations, past medical history, medications, allergies, smoking and recreational drug use, and previous injury to the affected arm.
- The wound is evaluated for
  - Exposed and damaged structures—skin, tendons, neurovascular structures, bone
  - Health of remaining structures—tissue necrosis, contamination, signs of infection
  - Local and regional donor sites

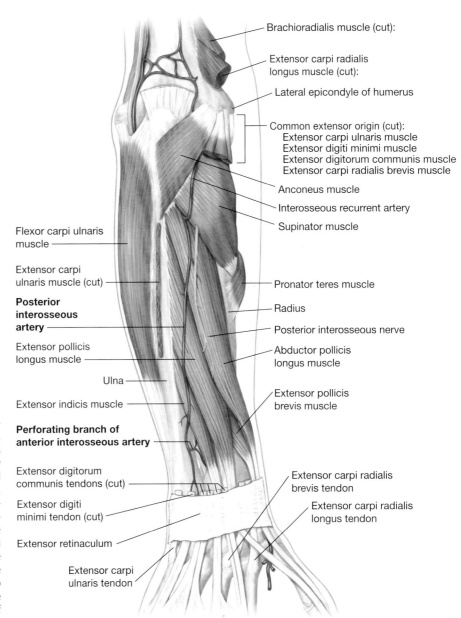

Brachioradialis muscle (cut):

Extensor carpi radialis longus muscle (cut):

Lateral epicondyle of humerus

Common extensor origin (cut):
Extensor carpi ulnaris muscle
Extensor digiti minimi muscle
Extensor digitorum communis muscle
Extensor carpi radialis brevis muscle

Anconeus muscle

Interosseous recurrent artery

Supinator muscle

Flexor carpi ulnaris muscle

Extensor carpi ulnaris muscle (cut)

Posterior interosseous artery

Extensor pollicis longus muscle

Pronator teres muscle

Radius

Posterior interosseous nerve

Abductor pollicis longus muscle

Ulna

Extensor indicis muscle

Extensor pollicis brevis muscle

Perforating branch of anterior interosseous artery

Extensor digitorum communis tendons (cut)

Extensor digiti minimi tendon (cut)

Extensor retinaculum

Extensor carpi ulnaris tendon

Extensor carpi radialis brevis tendon

Extensor carpi radialis longus tendon

FIG 1 • The course of the posterior interosseous artery is shown in the dorsal forearm. It originates from the common interosseous artery, or less commonly, from the ulnar artery directly. It passes under the supinator and then travels over the abductor pollicis longus, extensor pollicis longus, extensor pollicis brevis, and extensor indicis proprius. Two centimeter proximal to the DRUJ, a branch of the PIA travels volarly through the IOM to form an anastomosis with the dorsal branch of the AIA. The PIA continues distally to contribute to the dorsal carpal arch. The axis of the flap is marked from the lateral epicondyle to the head of the ulna to maximize the capture of PIA perforators into the flap.

- Radiographic imaging is used in conjunction with physical examination to determine the presence and extent of bone injuries.
- Skin and soft tissue defects can be adequately reconstructed using soft tissue flaps.
  - When the defect size is too large for local flap coverage, the PIA flap is a useful regional flap that can be performed. It alleviates the need for a microsurgical free flap from a distant donor site.
- Many tendon and bony defects can be reconstructed in the hand and then covered with a PIA flap during the same operation. This fasciocutaneous flap provides reliable, durable soft tissue coverage of exposed structures and a smooth gliding surface for underlying tendons.
- Skin laxity is assessed over the dorsal forearm using a pinch test.

- Flaps larger than 4 to 6 cm in width typically require donor site closure with a skin graft.
- If desired, the skin graft can be excised later using serial excision; the patient must be appropriately counseled prior to flap reconstruction regarding the expected appearance of the donor site given its visible location over the dorsal forearm.

IMAGING

- Radiographs are performed of the injured extremity to assess for fractures or foreign bodies.
- Angiography is not routinely performed prior to PIA flap reconstruction.
  - If there is concern of the integrity of the PIA or AIA-PIA anastomotic arch, angiography can be considered to evaluate the vessels or a different flap can be selected.

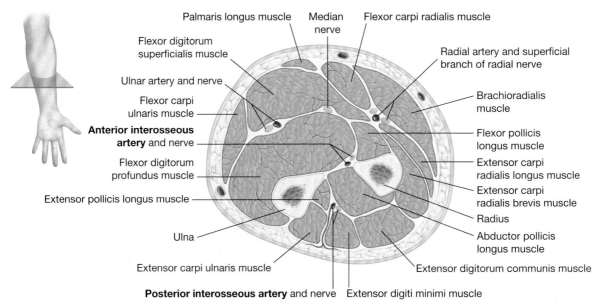

FIG 2 • The PIA perforators run in the interval between the EDM and ECU to supply the overlying skin. The AIA runs volar to the IOM in the forearm. Distally, 2 cm proximal to the DRUJ, the AIA gives off a dorsal branch that forms an anastomosis with the PIA.

NONOPERATIVE MANAGEMENT

- The wound must be adequately debrided and cleansed prior to flap reconstruction. Following traumatic injury, the wound is explored, injured structures are assessed, and necrotic tissue is debrided. Once the wound is clean and the tissues have demarcated, flap reconstruction can proceed.
- For the reconstruction of oncologic defects, final tumor pathology and negative margins are established prior to flap closure.
  - Moist, antibacterial dressings can be used in the interim to minimize tissue desiccation and bacterial load.

SURGICAL MANAGEMENT

- Local flaps are limited to coverage of small defects of the upper extremity.
- Larger regional flaps, such as the PIA flap, provide coverage of forearm, wrist, and hand defects without the need for free flap microsurgical reconstruction (**FIG 3**).
- Compared with free flaps, pedicled flaps require less general anesthesia time, avoid the need for flap harvest from an uninjured limb or the trunk, and are options when microsurgical equipment or expertise is unavailable.

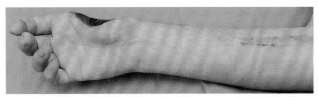

FIG 3 • This patient underwent a ray resection of the thumb for treatment of squamous cell carcinoma. In-transit metastases were resected from the volar radial forearm. Following pathological confirmation of negative margins at both locations, a PIA flap was used for coverage of the exposed trapezium at the base of the radial hand wound. (Courtesy of Steven Haase, MD.)

Preoperative Planning

- The risks and benefits of flap reconstruction with a PIA flap are reviewed with the patient.
  - The benefits include provision of durable, supple soft tissue coverage, a donor site limited to the affected upper extremity, and a single-stage procedure.
  - The risks include partial or complete flap failure and injury to the PIN. The patient is counseled that the PIA flap has a visible donor site.
- When used as a retrograde flap, the PIA flap is insensate.
  - For antegrade or free PIA flaps, the posterior antebrachial cutaneous nerve of the forearm can be included for sensory restoration.
- Previous injury to the PIA flap donor site is a contraindication to its use.
  - The PIA perforators are small and thin-walled, so crush or shear injury to dorsal forearm makes flap harvest unreliable.
- Injury to the DRUJ and possible damage to the AIA-PIA anastomosis precludes retrograde PIA flap use.
- Some authors have reported the absence of the AIA-PIA anastomosis or a hypoplastic or absent PIA in the middle third of the forearm. Penteado reported 5 such cases in 110 cadavers, Angrigiani reported 1 case in 80 patients, and Buchler reported 2 cases in 36 patients.[7–9]
  - Anatomic dissections have confirmed the reliability of the AIA-PIA system and presence of the PIA throughout the dorsal forearm.[5,7] Studies have noted that the PIA is more superficial and narrowest in caliber over the dorsal third of the forearm, measuring 0.5 mm.
  - If there are doubts of the integrity of the PIA, the incision can be closed and another flap can be used.
  - In rare cases, if the PIA is absent or hypoplastic, the AIA is dominant and an AIA perforator flap can be harvested instead.[10,11]

Positioning

- The patient is positioned supine with the arm out on a hand table.
- A tourniquet is placed on the upper arm of the affected limb.
- If the PIA flap is harvested with a width over 4 to 6 cm, closure with a skin graft is typically required. Most commonly, the patient's ipsilateral thigh is used for STSG harvest.

Approach

- Loupes are worn for flap harvest and inset. An operating microscope is not routinely required; in rare cases, it may be employed if there is difficulty visualizing the vascular anatomy or concern of pedicle injury during flap harvest.
- The flap incisions are designed, most commonly as a longitudinal ellipse.
- The arm is then elevated and the tourniquet is inflated.
- Exsanguination with an Esmarch bandage is avoided to maintain visibility of the PIA and its perforators.

- The axis of the flap is marked with the forearm in full pronation from the lateral epicondyle to the ulnar head. This marks the course of the PIA.
- A Doppler ultrasound is used to identify perforators running along this axis to the overlying skin. Typically, there is a large perforator found at the midpoint of the dorsal forearm, along the flap axis. The skin flap is designed to include this perforator and as many additional perforators as possible.
- To raise a fascia-only flap, the dorsal forearm fascia is exposed by incising the skin above the flap and elevating thin dermal flaps bilaterally.
- To raise a fasciocutaneous flap, the skin, subcutaneous tissue, and fascia are raised en bloc. Once elevated, it is recommended that the dermis is sutured to the underlying fascia using absorbable sutures to prevent shearing of the perforators to the skin.

■ Retrograde PIA Flap

- The pivot point of the flap is marked 2 cm proximal to the DRUJ, proximal to the edge of the extensor retinaculum, at the site of the AIA-PIA anastomosis (**TECH FIG 1A**).
- The rotation of the flap into the defect is tested using a sponge, umbilical tape, or vessel loop.
- The flap is typically designed at the junction of the proximal and middle thirds or over the middle third of the dorsal forearm to include the skin perforators arising distal to the supinator while permitting tension-free rotation into the distal defect of the wrist, hand, or first web space (**TECH FIG 1B**).
- The proximal flap limit is marked 3 cm distal to the lateral epicondyle. Proximally, there are no PIA perforators to the overlying skin.[12]

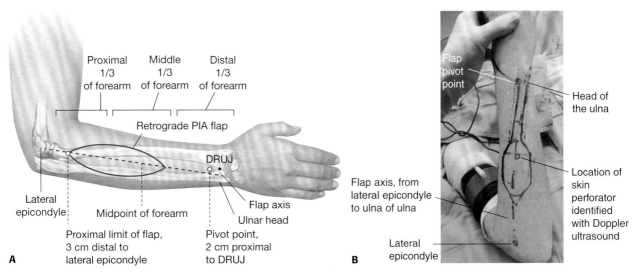

TECH FIG 1 • **A.** The axis of the PIA flap runs from the lateral epicondyle to the head of the ulna. The retrograde PIA flap is centered over the junction of the proximal and middle thirds of the forearm or over the middle third of the forearm based on the arc of rotation required to reach the defect. The flap pivot point is marked 2 cm proximal to the DRUJ. A large perforator is typically found near the midpoint of the dorsal forearm from the PIA to the overlying skin. The proximal flap limit is marked 3 cm distal to the lateral epicondyle. **B.** The flap axis is marked from the lateral epicondyle to the ulnar head with the forearm in full pronation. The pivot point is marked 2 cm proximal to the DRUJ. A Doppler ultrasound is used to mark skin perforators. The flap is designed as an ellipse over the proximal and middle thirds of the forearm to include audible skin perforators. The flap can be elevated as an island flap or with a skin bridge as shown here. The skin bridge overlies the pedicle and is elevated by incising a 1-cm strip of dermis (marked here in *solid lines*). An additional 0.75 cm of subcutaneous fat and fascia is included on either side of the dermis to protect the PIA and its vena comitantes (marked here with *dotted lines*). An incision is marked from the flap pivot point to the defect for inset of the flap (marked here with a *solid line* from the pivot point in a radial oblique direction to the thumb defect).

- A template of the defect is made using Telfa and used to mark the appropriate flap dimensions, up to 18 × 8 cm in size.
- The interval between the fifth and sixth extensor compartments can be palpated; the PIA is found in the septum between the EDM and ECU.
  - The flap is centered over this interval.
- The flap can be elevated as an island flap, or with a 1-cm skin bridge that can be closed primarily.
  - The skin bridge protects the pedicle, prevents kinking of the vessels on inset, and makes flap harvest safer.

Retrograde PIA Island Flap Harvest

- To raise the flap as an island flap, dissection is typically started distally by incising through the skin and subcutaneous tissue and identifying the PIA in the septum between the fifth and sixth extensor compartments (**TECH FIG 2A**).
  - The pedicle can be followed proximally to the distal edge of the flap. The flap markings are adjusted if needed to ensure that the flap is centered over the pedicle.
  - This is a most reliable way to ensure that the flap has been properly designed prior to elevation.

- The flap is raised subfascially from its ulnar border to the intermuscular septum (IMS) between the EDM and ECU (**TECH FIG 2B**).
- Next, elevation proceeds from the radial border of the flap, again toward the IMS between the EDM and ECU.
- Distal to the supinator, the PIN gives a branch to the ECU that crosses superficial to the PIA (**TECH FIG 2C**). The PIA is divided just distal to this nerve branch.
- Flap elevation proceeds from proximal to distal. The PIN runs with the PIA along the dorsal forearm and is protected throughout flap elevation.
- The pedicle is raised as a fascial strip between EDM and ECU containing the PIA and its vena comitantes.
- The PIA gives off multiple braches to the surrounding musculature; these are divided using microclips and bipolar cautery.

Retrograde PIA Flap Harvest With a Skin Bridge

- To raise a flap with a skin bridge, the flap is elevated first from its ulnar border in a subfascial plane toward the IMS between the EDM and ECU.
  - Gentle proximal traction on the muscle bellies confirms the anatomy; traction on the EDM will extend the small finger while traction on the ECU will extend the wrist.

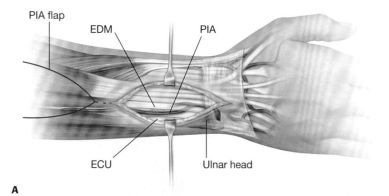

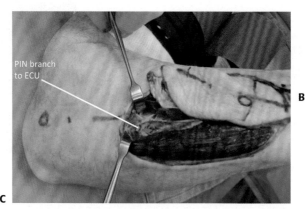

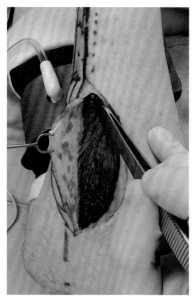

TECH FIG 2 • A. To confirm the flap is properly centered over the PIA, dissection starts distally. The PIA is identified in the interval between the EDM and ECU over the dorsal wrist. The flap design is confirmed over the proximal-middle forearm to ensure the PIA will be centered within it and then the flap is elevated. **B.** The PIA flap is raised subfascially, here shown from ulnar to radial. Perforators can be seen entering the flap in the interval between the EDM and ECU from the PIA below. **C.** The PIN gives a motor branch to the ECU distal to the supinator (shown here on top of the blue background material). This branch crosses superficial to the PIA. It is protected. The PIA and its vena comitantes are divided just distal to this nerve branch and then the flap is elevated from proximal to distal for retrograde use.

- Next, the radial border of the flap is raised toward the IMS between the EDM and ECU. The IMS between the extensor digitorum communis (EDC) and EDM will be encountered. The EDM is much smaller in size compared to the EDC that is found one interval radially. To elevate the flap subfascially above the EDC, the flap fascia is divided from the IMS between the EDC and EDM.
- Proximal retraction of the EDM radially and the ECU ulnarly with a self-retaining retractor facilitates exposure of the PIA (**TECH FIG 3A,B**).
- The skin bridge is incised from proximal to distal, a few centimeters at a time.
  - The pedicle location is confirmed sequentially.
  - The course of the skin bridge can be modified if needed to ensure the pedicle is maintained within it.

- A 1-cm dermal bridge is used. An additional 0.75 cm cuff of subcutaneous fat and fascia is harvested on each side of the skin bridge to protect the pedicle.
  - Restricting the width of the dermis elevation to 1 cm facilitates primary closure of this area.
- Distally, the pedicle is closely associated with the periosteum of the ulna. Ulnar retraction of the ECU tendon exposes the PIA (**TECH FIG 3C**).

Retrograde PIA Flap Inset

- Once flap elevation has reached the pivot point, 2 cm proximal to the DRUJ, dissection stops.
- The tourniquet is deflated and flap color, capillary refill, temperature, and turgor are assessed.
  - Arterial bleeding is noted from the flap edges.

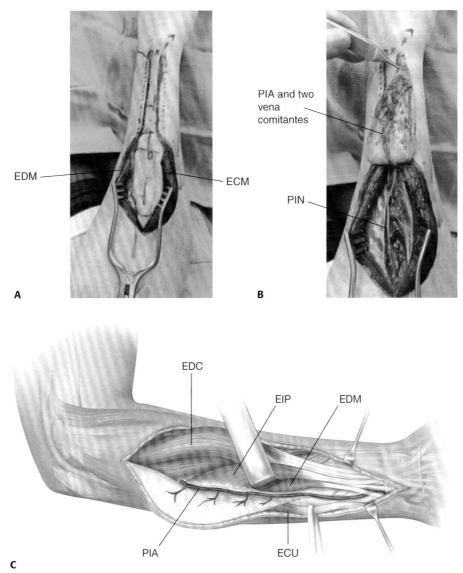

TECH FIG 3 • A. Radial retraction of the EDM and ulnar retraction of the ECU proximally facilitates exposure of the PIA and PIN in the septum between these muscles. **B.** The PIA and its vena comitantes are shown running centrally on the undersurface of the flap. The PIN is protected and left in situ between the EDM and ECU. Branches of the PIA to the surrounding musculature are divided as the flap is elevated. **C.** The PIA is closely associated with the periosteum of the ulna distally. The ECU tendon is retracted ulnarly to facilitate elevation of the flap pedicle.

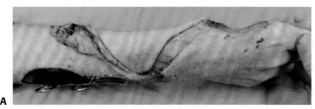 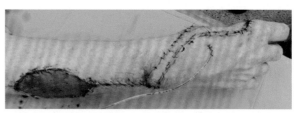

A **B**

TECH FIG 4 • A. An incision is made from the flap pivot point to the thumb defect to permit inset of the flap. Dorsal veins and branches of the radial sensory nerve are protected. Alternatively, a wide subcutaneous tunnel could have been used to pass the flap into the defect. The flap is shown with its pedicle centered on the undersurface. The donor-site extensor musculature offers a well-vascularized wound bed for reliable STSG graft take. The skin bridge defect is shown here tacked closed with towel clips; primarily closure will be performed. **B.** The flap is inset without tension into the defect. Release of the dermis over the skin bridge at the flap pivot point facilitates flap rotation and skin inset. The donor site is closed with an STSG from the ipsilateral thigh. A small drain can be placed under the flap, away from the pedicle.

- The AIA-PIA anastomotic connection is reliable and does not need to be skeletonized to confirm its presence unless there are concerns with flap perfusion.
- The flap is rotated into the defect. It can be tunneled into the wound.
  - To minimize the risk of pedicle compression and vascular compromise, we typically prefer to make an incision between the flap pivot point and the defect for inset (**TECH FIG 4A**). Skin flaps are elevated along this incision to achieve sufficient mobility to permit tension-free closure over the pedicle.
  - Alternatively, the pedicle can be covered with a skin graft.
  - For volar palm defects, the flap can be passed around the ulnar border of the hand or through the IOM using a wide tunnel.[13]
- The flap is inset into the defect and secured with sutures; it can be rotated up to 180 degrees.

- The pedicle is carefully rotated at the pivot point to avoid kinking.
  - If a skin bridge has been used, release of the dermis at the pivot point can facilitate inset.
  - A small-caliber drain can be placed under the flap, away from the pedicle, if desired (**TECH FIG 4B**).
- Narrow flap donor sites are closed primarily.
  - For flap donors site over 4 to 6 cm in width, a split-thickness skin graft (STSG) is used for closure.
- Antibiotic-impregnated gauze is applied to the flap incisions and covered with sterile gauze.
  - The flap skin paddle is left exposed for monitoring in the postoperative period.
- Antibiotic-impregnated gauze is placed over the STSG at the flap donor site and covered with sterile gauze and an elastic bandage to apply gentle compression and to avoid shear of the STSG.
- The wrist and hand are immobilized with a well-padded splint.

■ Antegrade PIA Flap

- The axis of the flap is marked from the lateral epicondyle to the head of the ulna. The flap is designed at the junction of the middle and distal thirds of the dorsal forearm.
  - The distal edge of the flap is marked 4 cm proximal to the wrist to avoid injury to the dorsal sensory branch of the ulnar nerve.
- The radial aspect of the flap is incised.
- The flap is raised from radial to ulnar in the subfascial plane toward the IMS between the EDM and ECU.
  - The PIA and its perforators are visualized.
- The flap design is confirmed, ensuring the perforators enter the center of the flap, and then the ulnar incision is made.
  - The flap is raised to the IMS between the EDM and ECU in an ulnar to radial direction.
- Distal to the flap, the anastomotic branch of the PIA to the AIA is identified and ligated.

- The flap is elevated from distal to proximal, following the pedicle in the septum between the EDM and ECU.
  - The flap is typically raised as an island flap.
  - The dorsal sensory branch of the ulnar nerve and the PIN are protected at all times.
- The flap is inset into the defect; it can be rotated up to 180 degrees.
  - Care is taken to avoid pedicle kinking and compression as the flap is sutured.
- The flap donor site is closed primarily or with an STSG.
- The incisions are covered with antibiotic-impregnated gauze and dry sterile gauze.
  - The visibility of the flap skin paddle is necessary for flap monitoring.
- If used, the STSG is dressed with antibiotic-impregnated gauze and covered with sterile gauze and an elastic bandage.
- The elbow is immobilized with a well-padded splint, avoiding pressure on the flap and pedicle.

PEARLS AND PITFALLS

Physical findings	■ The PIN must be protected throughout flap elevation. The PIA pedicle is dissected away from the PIN. If branches of the PIN cross superficial to the PIA and impede flap elevation, the flap can be converted to a free flap. ■ The PIA flap offers a better skin color match than the radial forearm flap for defects of the dorsal hand and first web space.
Technique	■ The vena comitantes of the PIA are small. To optimize the chances of flap survival, a cutaneous vein is raised with the flap to permit venous supercharging if venous congestion is noted after flap inset. ■ When harvesting a retrograde PIA flap, it is wise to harvest the PIA and its vena comitantes at least 1 cm proximal to the proximal flap edge. This also permits supercharging of the flap if there is poor arterial inflow through the PIA-AIA anastomosis or venous congestion. Conversion to a free flap is also possible. ■ Often the proximal and distal margins of the flap can be closed primarily. If the central flap width is over 4–6 cm, depending on the skin laxity, a skin graft may be required for closure. A sheet STSG is preferred rather than a meshed STSG for improved donor-site appearance.[4] ■ For large defects, the PIA flap can be harvested simultaneously with an ipsilateral lateral arm flap.[14] The two skin paddles are elevated together.
Postoperative care	■ Partial or complete flap necrosis is uncommon.[5,12] However, the patient must be counseled preoperatively of the risk of flap necrosis and the need for a second flap.
Therapy	■ After flap inset, the elbow, wrist, and fingers are moved passively to evaluate the effect of joint range of motion on the flap. Tension-free inset is ideal; this permits early range of motion exercises starting 5 days postoperatively after the donor site graft has taken.

POSTOPERATIVE CARE

■ Flap checks are performed every 2 hours for the first 24 hours postoperatively and then every 4 hours.
   ▪ Tissue turgor, color, capillary refill, and temperature are monitored.
   ▪ Any change in flap status, indicating possible arterial or venous insufficiency, should prompt a return to the operating room for flap assessment.
   ▪ Compression by a hematoma or pedicle kinking is a common cause of flap insufficiency.
■ The patient is typically discharged home on postoperative day 3.
■ The patient returns to clinic on postoperative day 5 to assess the skin graft take and replace the dressings.
   ▪ The splint is discontinued following this dressing change after confirming that the flap does not experience undue tension with elbow, wrist, and hand range of motion.
   ▪ If there are concerns, the splint can be continued for an additional week.

OUTCOMES

■ The PIA flap provides reliable soft tissue coverage for upper extremity defects.
■ Along with the radial forearm flap, it is a valuable option for pedicled flap coverage of the wrist and hand.

COMPLICATIONS

■ Most of the lymphatic drainage from the hand runs over the volar forearm. Compared with the radial forearm free flap, the PIA flap disrupts less lymphatic outflow that results in less edema postoperatively.
■ PIN palsy is rare following PIA flap harvest. Motor functions of the muscles of the extensor compartment of the forearm are tested postoperatively to confirm PIN innervation.

REFERENCES

1. Tonkin MA, Stern H. The posterior interosseous artery free flap. *J Hand Surg Br.* 1989;14(2):215-217.
2. Balakrishnan G, Kumar BS, Hussain SA. Reverse-flow posterior interosseous artery flap revisited. *Plast Reconstr Surg.* 2003;111(7):2364-2369.
3. Kim KS. Distally based dorsal forearm fasciosubcutaneous flap. *Plast Reconstr Surg.* 2004;114(2):389-396.
4. Hsu C, Chang J. The posterior interosseous artery flap revisited. *Operat Techn Plast Reconstr Surg.* 2003;9(4):173-180.
5. Costa H, Gracia ML, Vranchx J, et al. The posterior interosseous flap: a review of 81 clinical cases and 100 anatomical dissections—assessment of its indications in reconstruction of hand defects. *Br J Plast Surg.* 2001;54(1):28-33.
6. Costa H, Smith R, McGrouther DA. Thumb reconstruction by the posterior interosseous osteocutaneous flap. *Br J Plast Surg.* 1988;41(3):228-233.
7. Angrigiani C, Grilli D, Dominikow D, Zancolli EA. Posterior interosseous reverse forearm flap: experience with 80 consecutive cases. *Plast Reconstr Surg.* 1993;92(2):285-293.
8. Penteado CV, Masquelet AC, Chevrel JP. The anatomic basis of the fascio-cutaneous flap of the posterior interosseous artery. *Surg Radiol Anat.* 1986;8(4):209-215.
9. Büchler U, Frey HP. Retrograde posterior interosseous flap. *J Hand Surg [Am].* 1991;16(2):283-292.
10. Giunta R, Lukas B. Impossible harvest of the posterior interosseous artery flap: a report of an individualised salvage procedure. *Br J Plast Surg.* 1998;51(8):642-645.
11. Hu W, Martin D, Foucher G, Baudet J. Le lambeau interosseux anterieur. *Ann Chir Esthet.* 1994;39(3):290-300.
12. Fujiwara M, Kawakatsu M, Yoshida Y, Sumiya A. Modified posterior interosseous flap in hand reconstruction. *Tech Hand Up Extrem Surg.* 2003;7(3):102-109.
13. Gupta A, Wang A, Baylis W, Breidenbach W. Anterior transposition of the posterior interosseous artery flap through the interosseous membrane. *J Hand Surg Br.* 1997;22(1):32-33.
14. Shibata M, Hatano Y, Iwabuchi Y, Matsuzaki H. Combined dorsal forearm and lateral arm flap. *Plast Reconstr Surg.* 1995;96(6):1423-1429.

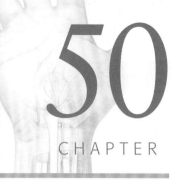

50
CHAPTER

Free Lateral Arm Flap

John R. Lien and Kevin C. Chung

DEFINITION

- The lateral arm flap is a reliable septofasciocutaneous flap for local and free tissue transfer.
- Originally described for reconstructive head and neck coverage,[1] the free lateral arm flap is useful for small to medium-sized defects of the hand and wrist.

ANATOMY

- The arm is composed of anterior and posterior compartments.
  - Anterior compartment includes the biceps, brachialis, and coracobrachialis muscles.
  - Posterior compartment includes the triceps muscle.
  - The lateral intermuscular septum divides the anterior and posterior compartments laterally.
- At the midpoint of the humeral shaft, the profunda brachii artery and radial nerve are located within the spiral groove of the humerus.
- The profunda brachii divides into two main branches within the spiral groove: the radial collateral artery (RCA) and middle collateral artery (MCA).
- The RCA accompanies the radial nerve and branches into the anterior and posterior radial collateral arteries (ARCA and PRCA) (**FIG 1**).
  - The PRCA is the nutrient artery for the lateral arm flap, feeding septocutaneous perforators along the lateral intermuscular septum.
  - The PRCA is accompanied by one or two venae comitantes.
- The posterior antebrachial cutaneous nerve (PACN) branches from the radial nerve and accompanies the PRCA.

PATIENT HISTORY AND PHYSICAL FINDINGS

- Assess for prior trauma or surgery at the potential donor site.
- Ensure adequate recipient site debridement.

IMAGING

- Doppler sonography can be used to ensure intact vascular pedicle and perforators in cases with prior trauma/surgery, but we generally avoid this flap in this situation.

SURGICAL MANAGEMENT

- Lateral arm flap is indicated for coverage of small to medium-sized defects of the volar and dorsal wrist and hand.
- Maximum skin island size is 8 × 25 cm, as the flap can be extended distal to the lateral epicondyle along the lateral forearm. Primary donor-site closure is dependent on body habitus, but generally 6 cm width can be closed primarily.
- Obese patients will have a bulky lateral arm flap that may be cosmetically unappealing in the hand and wrist.
- The PRCA pedicle is generally limited to 6 cm in length.
- For extremity reconstruction with bone defect, a vascularized segment of distal humerus may be included in the flap.[2]
- Doppler examination is used to center the skin paddle over the vascular pedicle.
- The patient is placed supine with the hand on a hand table.

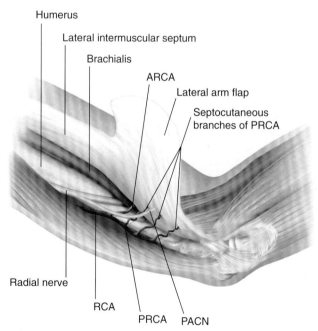

FIG 1 • Anatomy of the lateral arm flap.

Flap Design

- A line is drawn from the mid-deltoid to the lateral epicondyle, representing the lateral intermuscular septum (**TECH FIG 1**).
- Identify the PRCA with Doppler probe, and center the flap over this pedicle.
- Measure the dimensions of the flap and recipient site to ensure adequate coverage.

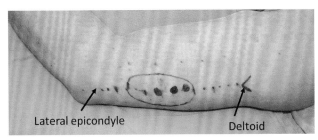

Lateral epicondyle · Deltoid

TECH FIG 1 • Lateral arm flap incision.

Flap Harvest

- This flap is harvested without the tourniquet because the flap is located at the mid-humerus.
- Perform the posterior flap incision along the posterolateral triceps.
- Expose and incise the deep fascia of the triceps in line with the posterior incision.
  - The PACN enters the flap proximally; take care to preserve the nerve if a neurosensory flap is desired.
- Elevate the triceps fascial layer from posterior to anterior until the lateral intermuscular septum is encountered.
  - Use tagging sutures to secure posterior skin border to underlying triceps fascia.
- Once the intermuscular septum is encountered, retract the lateral head of the triceps posteriorly, and identify the septocutaneous perforators arising from the PRCA proximally (**TECH FIG 2A**).
- Perform the anterior flap incision and elevate the deep fascia of the brachialis from anterior to posterior.
  - A smaller oblique septum will be encountered between the brachialis and brachioradialis muscles. This contains the ARCA perforators, which are ligated.

- Take care to flip the flap and look back from the posterior dissection to prevent accidental division of PRCA perforators.
- If the cephalic vein is within the anterior flap and one wishes to include it for additional venous outflow, dissect the vein proximally.
- Once the anterior dissection is complete, the flap should only be tethered to the intermuscular septum.
- Carefully dissect the PRCA and PACN proximally.
  - Dissect the PRCA proximally to the RCA and ligate the ARCA branch. Proceed to dissect the RCA proximally as necessary to obtain adequate pedicle length.
  - The proximal limit of dissection of the PACN is its origin from the radial nerve.
- Subperiosteally elevate the lateral intermuscular septum from the underlying humerus, taking care to preserve the PRCA perforators (**TECH FIG 2B**).
- Once the recipient site is prepared for microsurgical anastomosis, ligate the pedicle.
- The donor site is closed primarily with a subcutaneous drain.
  - If primary closure is not possible, skin grafting can be performed.

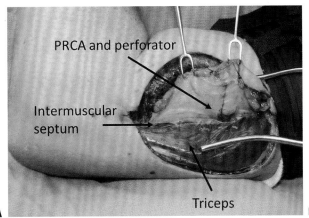

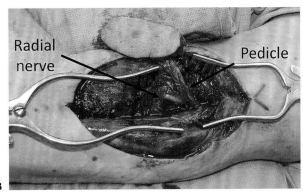

A — PRCA and perforator · Intermuscular septum · Triceps

B — Radial nerve · Pedicle

TECH FIG 2 • **A.** Posterior flap elevation. Note the septocutaneous perforators of the posterior radial collateral artery (PRCA). **B.** Flap after elevation of intermuscular septum from humerus. Note proximity of radial nerve to pedicle during proximal dissection.

PEARLS AND PITFALLS

Flap harvest technique	■ Do not detach the intermuscular septum until after pedicle dissection; the septum stabilizes the flap, allowing easier manipulation. ■ Dissect the vascular pedicle proximal to the PRCA and ARCA bifurcation to increase pedicle length and diameter.
Hemostasis	■ Donor-site hematoma can be minimized with meticulous hemostasis and suction drain placement.

POSTOPERATIVE CARE

- Early donor elbow range of motion is encouraged to prevent stiffness, as long as it does not compromise recipient site care.
- Drain is removed once output is appropriate, typically less than 30 mL/d.
- The free flap is monitored hourly with a Doppler probe for the first 48 hours, followed by Doppler checks every 4 hours for 48 hours.
- The patient is kept hydrated with intravenous fluids and kept on thrombosis prophylaxis therapy (low molecular weight heparin) while hospitalized.

OUTCOMES

- Overall success rate is 97% in a large retrospective series, with 16% of patients eventually requiring debulking.[3]

COMPLICATIONS

- Flap failure secondary to arterial or venous thrombosis is possible but uncommon.
- Unsatisfactory appearance of the donor site was noted in 27% of patients (**FIG 2**).[4] This was associated with female patients and with cases that required split-thickness skin grafting:
  - 59% with forearm numbness
  - 17% with hypersensitivity of donor site
  - 78% with hair formation at recipient site
  - 83% of patients found the flap to be bulky

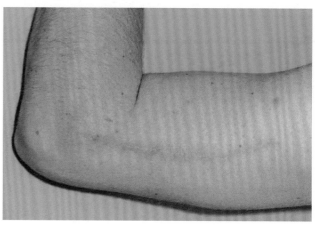

FIG 2 • Donor-site appearance.

REFERENCES

1. Song R, Song Y, Yu Y. The upper arm free flap. *Clin Plast Surg.* 1982;9:27-35.
2. Hennerbichler A, Etzer C, Gruber S, et al. Lateral arm flap: analysis of its anatomy and modification using a vascularized fragment of the distal humerus. *Clin Anat.* 2003;16(3):204-214.
3. Ulusal BG, Lin YT, Ulusal AE, Lin CH. Free lateral arm flap for one stage reconstruction of soft tissue and composite defects of the hand: a retrospective analysis of 118 cases. *Ann Plast Surg.* 2007;58:173-178.
4. Graham B, Adkins P, Scheker LR. Complications and morbidity of the donor and recipient sites in 123 lateral arm flaps. *J Hand Surg Br.* 1992;17(2): 189-192.

Pedicled and Free Groin Flap

Mark Morris and Kevin C. Chung

51
CHAPTER

DEFINITION

- A free flap requires the transfer of tissue from one body site to another, with anastomosis of arterial and venous systems to the recipient site using microsurgical techniques.
- A pedicled flap transposes tissue from a donor site to a recipient site while keeping the tissue partially attached to the donor site. The donor vascular pedicle is left intact to supply the flap. Pedicled flaps are reliable and do not require microsurgery.
- The groin flap was described in 1972 by McGregor and Jackson[1] for reconstruction of soft tissue defects of the hand. This was once a "workhorse" flap for hand reconstruction; however, with the introduction and advancement of microsurgery, it has fallen out of favor for many indications. Nevertheless, there are still many indications for its use.
- When a pedicled groin flap is used, patients must be counseled that they will require multiple operations (average 4.6 operations per patient), including flap division, debulking, and tissue rearrangement for contouring.[2]

ANATOMY

- The groin flap is based on the superficial circumflex iliac artery (SCIA).
  - The SCIA arises approximately 2 to 3 cm distal to the inguinal ligament, either directly from the femoral artery (70%) or from the superficial inferior epigastric artery (**FIG 1**).
  - The SCIA passes laterally from its origin and gives a deep branch at the medial border of the sartorius.
  - The superficial branch then pierces the fascia at the lateral border of the sartorius and runs 2 to 3 cm distal and parallel to the inguinal ligament, toward the anterior superior iliac spine (ASIS). This superficial branch supplies the skin to be used for the flap.
- After reaching the ASIS, the superficial branch of the SCIA branches further and anastomoses with branches of the superior gluteal, deep circumflex iliac, and ascending lateral femoral circumflex arteries.
- The SCIA pedicle is generally between 0.8 and 1.8 mm in diameter.[3]

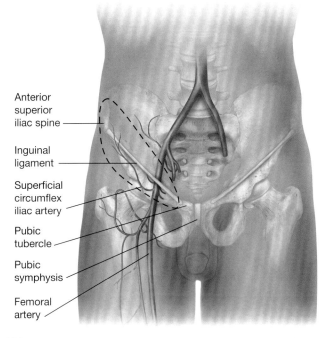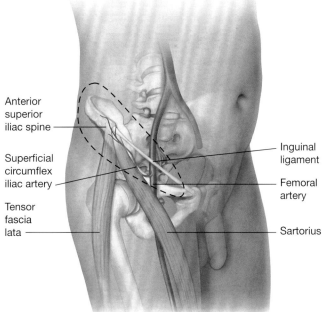

FIG 1 • Vascular and regional anatomy of the groin flap, which follows the axis of the superficial circumflex iliac artery.

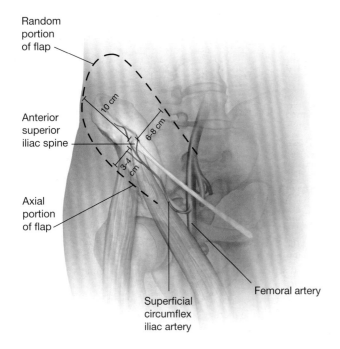

FIG 2 • Limits of the groin flap.

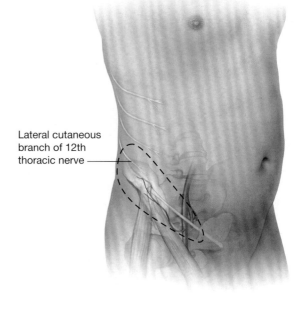

FIG 3 • The lateral cutaneous branch of the 12th thoracic nerve enters the graft opposite the vascular pedicle.

- Venous drainage of the flap is split between the superficial circumflex iliac vein and the venae comitantes of the SCIA. Both of these eventually drain into the femoral vein, either directly or via the saphenous vein.
- Flap size is limited to about 13 × 10 cm (**FIG 2**). The axis of the SCIA is marked by palpating the femoral pulse, marking the origin 2 to 3 cm distal to the inguinal ligament and then drawing a line to the ASIS. The flap will follow this axis.
  - The medial boundary of the flap is about 3 to 4 cm lateral to the femoral artery (2–3 cm medial to the medial border of the sartorius).
  - The maximum width of the flap that can be primarily closed in most patients is 10 cm. The flap should be positioned two-thirds superior to the vascular axis and one-third below the axis. This translates to up to 6 to 7 cm superior to the axis and 3 to 4 cm inferior to the axis.
  - The lateral portion of the flap should be designed with a 1:1 length-to-width ratio. This is because the portion of the flap lateral to the ASIS has a random pattern of vascularization. Therefore, because the width of the flap is limited to 10 cm, the lateral limit of the flap is then 10 cm lateral to the ASIS.
- Sensation to the lateral portion of the groin flap is supplied by the lateral cutaneous branches of the 12th thoracic subcostal nerve (**FIG 3**).[4] This nerve can be harvested with the flap to provide sensation to the hand, but a sensate nerve is infrequently used.
  - The 12th thoracic nerve pierces the internal and external oblique muscles and courses distally over the iliac crest, 5 cm posterior to the ASIS. Do not confuse the lateral femoral cutaneous nerve, which supplies sensation to the lateral thigh, for the 12th thoracic nerve.

PATIENT HISTORY AND PHYSICAL FINDINGS

- History must include the mechanism of injury.
  - Crush and blast injuries can lead to a much larger zone of injury than expected by initial examination (**FIG 4A,B**).
  - In the case of a crush injury, the physician must also assess the patient for signs of compartment syndrome.
- Contaminated wounds may require multiple irrigation and debridement procedures (**FIG 4C–E**).
- Medical and social history—such as diabetes mellitus, peripheral vascular disease, or smoking—does not contraindicate surgery but will affect the healing potential of the flap and must be discussed with the patient.
- Assess the vascular status of the remaining limb.
- Motor and sensory evaluation to assess damage to nerves, tendons, or muscles.

IMAGING

- Standard radiographs of the hand are done to evaluate for bony injury.

SURGICAL MANAGEMENT

- Free flaps are generally considered superior to the pedicled groin flap with today's microsurgical techniques. However, there are still many good indications for doing a pedicled groin flap:
  - Complex hand injuries in young children (less than 2 years). Microsurgery in infants is technically challenging because of the small size of the vessels.
  - In preparation for a toe-to-thumb transfer following thumb or finger loss. This preserves the recipient vessels for later microsurgery during transfer and also saves as much stump tissue as possible by providing coverage.

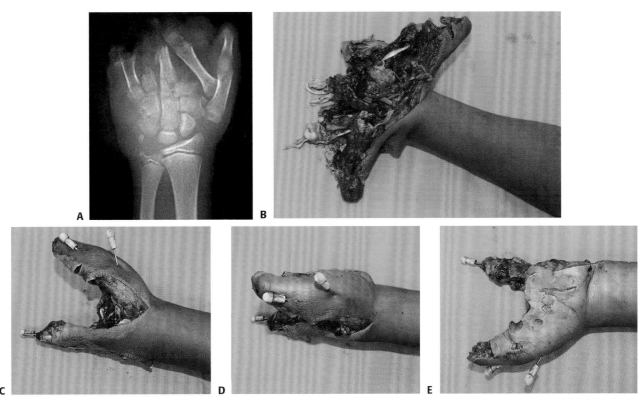

FIG 4 • A,B. Preoperative radiograph and clinical photograph, respectively, of a 12-year-old boy who sustained a bomb-blast injury to the left upper extremity. **C–E.** Images after left hand radical debridement, open reduction and internal fixation of the left thumb metacarpal using K-wires, and left index finger metacarpal transposition to the small finger and fixation with K-wires.

- Dorsal or palmar soft tissue defects involving multiple digits
- Degloving injury to all fingers
- Circumferential thumb soft tissue defect
- First stage of an osteoplastic thumb reconstruction
- High-voltage electrical burns with a hand surviving on collateral circulation. In some cases, a hand may survive based on collateral blood supply when both ulnar and radial arteries have thrombosed in the forearm. The extensive zone of injury affects available recipient vessels, and dissection of these vessels may inadvertently lead to hand necrosis.[5]

- Advantages to the pedicled groin flap are that it is thin and nearly hairless, it is reliable, flap elevation is quick, and the donor site can be closed primarily in most cases.
- Disadvantages of the pedicled groin flap are that it is a mandatory two-stage operation, the patient's hand is connected to his or her groin for 3 to 4 weeks (which leads to stiffness in the shoulder, elbow, and wrist, especially in older patients), and there is a high risk of injury to the lateral femoral cutaneous nerve with subsequent loss of sensation in the lateral thigh or a painful neuroma.

Preoperative Planning

- The following is a rough guideline for skin requirements for reconstruction in an adult male:
  - Thumb (circumferential)
    - Distal to the metacarpophalangeal joint: 9 × 8 cm
    - Distal to the thenar crease: 13 × 12 cm
  - Palmar hand: 12 × 10 cm
  - Dorsal hand: 12 × 10 cm
  - Finger (circumferential): 7 × 10 cm
- Assess for any scars in the groin.
- Use a Doppler probe to confirm the location of the SCIA.

Positioning

- The patient is positioned supine on the operating table with a hand table in place.
- A bump is placed under the ipsilateral hip to better visualize the elevation of the random portion of the flap lateral to the ASIS.
- The operative extremity and ipsilateral groin are prepped and draped widely.
- A tourniquet is placed on the upper extremity.

Approach

- The wound must be thoroughly debrided back to healthy tissue.
- Keep in mind the above-mentioned limits of the flap when designing the groin flap.
- Bone fixation and nerve reconstruction can be performed at the same time as the groin flap; however, tendon reconstruction should be delayed until passive joint range of motion is re-established for rehabilitation purposes.
- The surgeon must decide on whether or not to attempt an innervated flap prior to elevating the flap, as the lateral cutaneous branch of the 12th thoracic nerve will have to be harvested if this is desired.

■ Pedicled Groin Flap

Flap Design

- Mark the inguinal ligament from the pubic tubercle to the anterior superior iliac spine (ASIS).
- Palpate the femoral pulse.
  - Mark the origin of the superficial circumflex iliac artery (SCIA) off of the femoral artery, 2 to 3 cm distal to the inguinal ligament (**TECH FIG 1**).
  - Draw another line perpendicular to the first line, 2 to 3 cm inferior to the inguinal ligament. This marks the axis of the SCIA. This can be confirmed with a Doppler probe.
- Make a template of the defect and transfer it to the groin within the limits of the graft discussed earlier.

Flap Harvest

- Elevate the flap starting at the superolateral margin.
  - The incision is taken down to the level of the external oblique aponeurosis. The flap is elevated in this plane from lateral to medial (**TECH FIG 2A**).
  - If an innervated flap is desired, the surgeon must identify the lateral cutaneous branch of the 12th thoracic nerve. This nerve pierces the internal and external oblique muscles and descends 5 cm posterior to the ASIS. Harvest the nerve at this time as it enters the lateral portion of the flap.
- Elevate the lateral and inferior margins of the flap.
  - The inferior portion of the flap is elevated superficial to the fascia lata.
- The random portion of the flap is elevated to the ASIS.
  - The lateral borders of the sartorius and fascia lata are identified inferior to the ASIS.

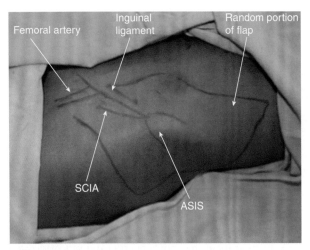

TECH FIG 1 • Markings for a pedicled groin flap.

- Elevate the axial portion of the flap.
  - An incision is made longitudinally over the fascia lata and sartorius fascia. The flap is now elevated in this deeper plane to include this layer of sartorial fascia medial to the ASIS (**TECH FIG 2B**). This is critical because the SCIA is superficial to the fascia over the sartorius. Elevating the sartorial fascia protects the SCIA. This also prevents the fascia from tethering and kinking the vessel, which could cause flap necrosis. The SCIA does not need to be isolated for the pedicled flap.
  - Identify and ligate the deep branch of the SCIA. It will arise at the medial border of the sartorius. The deep branch is very short and should be ligated within the substance of the sartorius to avoid injury to the SCIA.
  - Identify and protect the lateral femoral cutaneous nerve as it arises beneath the inguinal ligament, near the medial border of the sartorius.
  - Divide any connections between the inguinal ligament and fascia lata.
  - The flap can be elevated 2 to 3 cm medial to the medial border of the sartorius.
- Close the flap donor site.
  - Close from medial to lateral in layers.
  - A drain is not usually required if adequate hemostasis was attained. The closure is tight and should compress the bed sufficiently, so fluid collection under the flap is not a concern.
  - Undermining skin flaps and hip flexion will assist with closure. The bump can also be removed from under the hip.

Flap Placement and Division

- Thin the flap to match the thickness of the recipient site.
  - The random portion of the flap lateral to the ASIS can be made thin safely because the flap relies on the subdermal plexus in this location.
  - Leaving excess fat increases vascular demands of the flap.
- The 12th thoracic nerve can now be repaired to an available digital nerve from the recipient hand if an innervated flap is planned.
- Inset the flap to the recipient site using 3-0 nylon interrupted sutures (**TECH FIG 3A,B**).
- Flap division generally occurs after 3 weeks (**TECH FIG 3C–F**).
- The surgeon can passively move the patient's shoulder, elbow, and hand while still under anesthesia after division.
  - This will break up adhesions and facilitate recovery of motion postoperatively.

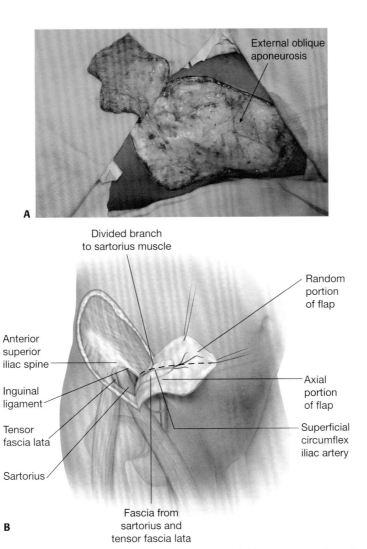

External oblique
aponeurosis

A

Divided branch
to sartorius muscle

Random
portion
of flap

Anterior
superior
iliac spine

Axial
portion
of flap

Inguinal
ligament

Tensor
fascia lata

Superficial
circumflex
iliac artery

Sartorius

Fascia from
sartorius and
tensor fascia lata

B

TECH FIG 2 • A. The flap is elevated from lateral to medial, superficial to the external oblique aponeurosis. **B.** The sartorius fascia is raised with the SCIA pedicle as the flap is elevated from lateral to medial.

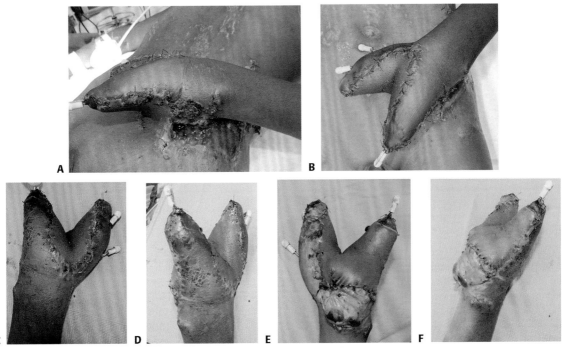

A   **B**

C   **D**   **E**   **F**

TECH FIG 3 • A,B. Images after the groin flap has been inset to the left hand. **C–F.** Postoperative images after flap division.

■ Free Groin Flap

Flap Design

- Follow the same steps as for a pedicled flap to plan and elevate the free flap, except that the medial portion of the flap must also be elevated.
- The free flap can be harvested from the contralateral or ipsilateral groin.
- Free groin flap is seldom performed because of the short pedicle and variability of the pedicle origin.
- Identify and dissect out the SCIA and concomitant vein. Cutaneous veins may have to be used if there is no concomitant vein.
- Identify suitable arterial and venous sites of anastomosis in the hand, depending on the location of injury.

Flap Harvest

- Divide the vascular pedicle.
- Anastomose the SCIA to the appropriate vessels, depending on the location of the defect. An end-to-side anastomosis is recommended for the artery in order to not devascularize the recipient site. End-to-end anastomosis of veins is performed.
- The 12th thoracic nerve can now be repaired to an available nerve from the recipient hand if an innervated flap is planned (**TECH FIG 4**).
- Inset the flap to the recipient site using 3-0 nylon interrupted sutures.

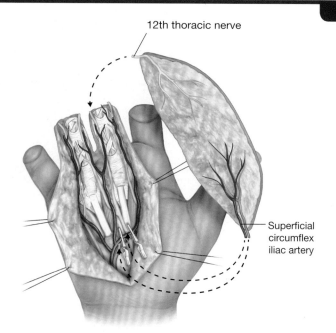

TECH FIG 4 • The SCIA and vein are anastomosed proximally, while a digital nerve or two can be repaired to a branch or branches of the 12th thoracic nerve.

PEARLS AND PITFALLS

Positioning	■ Place a bump under the ipsilateral hip to allow better visualization.
Technique	■ A full-thickness flap is raised. Thinning is done before inset. Leaving fat on the abdominal wall will make closure more difficult. ■ If the lateral femoral cutaneous nerve prohibits flap elevation, the surgeon can divide it to elevate the flap further and then repair the nerve. This nerve is usually not in the way when harvesting a pedicle flap because one does not need to skeletonize the pedicle medial to the sartorius fascia.
Postoperative care	■ The upper limb should be immobilized for 2 or 3 days, until the patient is comfortable with the position of the extremity and the flap. This is important to do prior to waking the patient up from anesthesia so the patient does not inadvertently reach for the endotracheal tube and damage the flap. ■ If the groin closure is very tight, patients may need to be immobilized with the hip in flexion. This can be done by placing pillows under the knee for a few days. ■ If there is marginal necrosis of the flap, wait for 2 to 3 days to let the necrosis demarcate as the initial postoperative swelling subsides. The patient should then return to the operating room for excision of necrotic portions and flap advancement and reinset. Waiting longer than 2 or 3 days risks further complications and failure of the flap. ■ The groin scar is closed under tension and will spread. Leave sutures in place until it is time for flap division, 3 to 4 weeks later.

POSTOPERATIVE CARE

- The open area near the pedicle is kept moist with bacitracin ointment twice daily and is covered with Xeroform gauze.
- Passive and active range of motion should start early under the supervision of a hand therapist.
- Compression bandages should be applied for bulky flaps.
- Surgery for thinning the flap should be delayed for at least 3 to 6 months.

OUTCOMES

- Arner and Moller[6] retrospectively studied 44 pedicled groin flaps for coverage of hand and forearm soft tissue defects.
  - Local complications (partial flap necrosis, infection, and seroma) occurred in 11 patients (25%).
  - Defatting was subsequently required in 38 (86%) patients, and 4 patients (9%) required secondary revisions of donor sites.

- Goertz et al.[2] treated 85 patients with pedicled groin flaps and prospectively collected data on these patients. Forty-nine patients were later interviewed and examined, with mean follow-up of 9 years. Mean hospital stay was 29 days. Patients each required a mean of 4.6 operations (including thinning of the flap, deepening of the interdigital fold, stump, and flap revisions).
  - One flap loss occurred.
  - Of the 49 patients interviewed, 82% would undergo the procedure again.
  - Mean Disabilities of the Arm, Shoulder, and Hand score was 23.
  - The Vancouver Scar Scale showed close to normal height and vascularity of the flap (0.2 and 0.3, respectively), but pigmentation was slightly abnormal (0.8) and pliability was rated between "supple" and "yielding" (1.5).

COMPLICATIONS

- Flap necrosis
- Infection
- Shoulder and elbow stiffness
- Scarring

REFERENCES

1. McGregor IA, Jackson IT. The groin flap. *Br J Plast Surg.* 1972;25: 3-16.
2. Goertz O, Kapalschinski N, Daigeler A, et al. The effectiveness of pedicled groin flaps in the treatment of hand defects: results of 49 patients. *J Hand Surg Am.* 2012;37(10):2088-2094.
3. Hsu W, Chao W, Yang C, et al. Evolution of the free groin flap: the superficial circumflex iliac artery perforator flap. *Plast Reconstr Surg.* 2007;199(5):1491-1498.
4. Joshi BB. Neural repair for sensory restoration in a groin flap. *Hand.* 1977;9(3)221-225.
5. Al-Qattan MM, Al-Qattan AM. Defining the indications of pedicled groin and abdominal flaps in hand reconstruction in the current microsurgery era. *J Hand Surg [Am].* 2016;41(6):917-927.
6. Arner M, Moller K. Morbidity of the pedicled groin flap: a retrospective study of 44 cases. *Scand J Plast Reconstr Surg Hand Surg.* 1994;28(2):143-146.

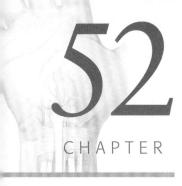

52

CHAPTER

Free Anterolateral Thigh Flap

John R. Lien and Kevin C. Chung

DEFINITION

- The anterolateral thigh flap is a versatile free flap that is often harvested as a fasciocutaneous flap, supplied by the descending branch of the lateral femoral circumflex artery (LFCA).
- It can be harvested also as a cutaneous or musculocutaneous flap with the vastus lateralis, with the option of an innervated flap with inclusion of the lateral femoral cutaneous nerve (LFCN).

ANATOMY

- The LFCA arises from the profunda femoris artery and divides into three branches (ascending, transverse, descending) deep to the sartorius and rectus femoris muscles (**FIG 1**).
- The descending branch of the LFCA courses distally along the medial border of the vastus lateralis, supplying perforators of the anterolateral thigh.
- Perforators supplying the anterolateral thigh are either of the following:
  - Musculocutaneous, which pass through the vastus lateralis muscle
  - Septocutaneous, which travel along the septum between the vastus lateralis and rectus femoris
- The LFCN passes under the inguinal ligament and pierces the deep fascia to innervate the skin of the anterolateral thigh.

PATIENT HISTORY AND PHYSICAL FINDINGS

- Patients with a history of peripheral vascular disease, active nicotine use, or generally poor health are not candidates for free tissue transfer.
- Obese patients may have a very thick flap and require primary thinning or secondary debulking procedures.
- Examine the donor site for scarring and obtain a thorough history to include previous injury or surgery to the thigh.
- We do not routinely obtain preoperative angiography.

SURGICAL MANAGEMENT

- Anterolateral thigh flap is indicated for large soft tissue defects, though it is versatile and can be used for smaller defects if needed.
- A two-team approach can be used to decrease surgical time.
- Flap vascular pedicle can be long (12 cm), allowing for anastomosis outside of zone of injury, if necessary.
- Flap dimensions are generally limited to 35 cm long and 15 cm wide on a single dominant perforator, though multiple perforators are preferred in large flaps.

- Limiting the width of the flap to 8 cm generally permits primary donor-site closure.

Preoperative Planning

- Preoperative Doppler exam is used to confirm the presence of a perforator.
- If one is not detectable, consider the contralateral thigh or a different type of flap.

Positioning

- Supine with a bump under the right hemipelvis, or lateral decubitus position
- Drape out the entire lower limb for leg manipulation.
- Ensure the anterior superior iliac spine (ASIS) and patella are included in the operative field.

Approach

- A suprafascial approach to flap harvest achieves a thinner flap design, though it is more technically challenging.
- Subfascial flap harvest is technically easier to identify the vascular anatomy but will result in a bulkier flap.

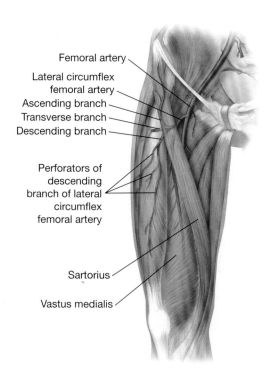

Femoral artery

Lateral circumflex femoral artery

Ascending branch

Transverse branch

Descending branch

Perforators of descending branch of lateral circumflex femoral artery

Sartorius

Vastus medialis

FIG 1 • Anterolateral thigh flap anatomy.

■ Flap Design

- Draw a line from the anterosuperior iliac spine (ASIS) to the superolateral border of the patella. This represents the intermuscular septum between the rectus femoris and vastus lateralis muscles (**TECH FIG 1**).
- Use a portable Doppler device to identify the perforator around the midpoint of this line.
  - 80% of perforators are found within 3 cm of this point.[1]
- Design the flap dimensions based on the recipient site defect.
  - We generally design the perforator to be centrally located in the flap.
  - For large flaps, we attempt to incorporate multiple perforators.

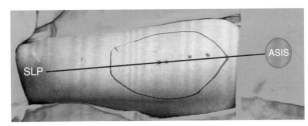

TECH FIG 1 • Flap design and identification of perforator. A line from the anterosuperior iliac spine (*ASIS*) to the superolateral patella (*SLP*) represents the intermuscular septum between rectus femoris and vastus lateralis. Perforators are identified with a Doppler ultrasound probe.

■ Flap Harvest

- Under loupe magnification, incise the medial margin of the designed flap.
- Suprafascial dissection
  - Deepen the medial incision to the deep fascia, and continue lateral dissection above the deep fascia.
  - Using tenotomy scissors, carefully separate the subcutaneous fat from underlying deep fascia. If possible, preserve cutaneous nerves overlying the fascia.
  - Continue dissection from medial to lateral and identify the marked perforator piercing though the fascia at the level of the intermuscular septum.
  - Incise the lateral margin of the flap and dissect from lateral to medial until the same perforator is visualized.
  - Leave a cuff of deep fascia around the perforator, and dissect retrograde toward its origin until adequate pedicle length and caliber is achieved.
  - Septocutaneous perforators allow for uneventful dissection along the intermuscular septum. However, the majority of the time perforators are musculocutaneous and pierce the muscle. To allow for safer dissection, the vastus lateralis is retracted laterally to visualize the descending LFCA, which can be dissected down to the perforator through the vastus lateralis muscle by separating the muscle fibers using scissors and bipolar cautery.

- Subfascial dissection (**TECH FIG 2A**)
  - Deepen the medial incision through the thigh fascia, exposing the rectus femoris muscle.
  - Continue dissection laterally under the deep fascia until the intermuscular septum between rectus femoris and vastus lateralis is visualized.
  - Retract the rectus femoris medially to visualize the descending branch of the lateral femoral circumflex artery (LFCA) and its perforating branches.
  - The perforators may be musculocutaneous, traveling through the vastus lateralis, or septocutaneous, passing directly through the intermuscular septum.
  - For septocutaneous vessels, dissection is performed from distal to proximal through the septum until adequate pedicle length and caliber is achieved. Leave a fascial cuff around the perforator (**TECH FIG 2B**).
  - For musculocutaneous skin perforators, expose the point of exit from the muscle. Spread transversely over the vessel and divide the overlying muscle fibers. Ligate any intramuscular branches of the perforator, and continue retrograde dissection up to the descending LFCA until adequate pedicle length and caliber is achieved.
- If additional pedicle length is needed, continue retrograde dissection up the descending LFCA. During proximal dissection of the descending LFCA, take care to preserve the motor branches of the femoral nerve to the vastus lateralis.

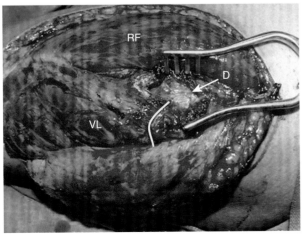

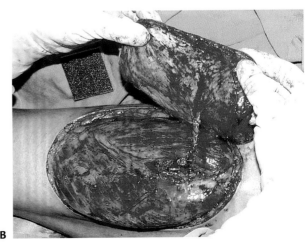

TECH FIG 2 • **A.** Elevation of flap. Subfascial elevation allows for identification of the descending branch of the LCFA (*D*). Perforator is highlighted in *yellow*. RF, rectus femoris; VL, vastus lateralis. **B.** Completion of flap elevation. The perforator is dissected proximally, and the pedicle is dissected up the descending LFCA.

■ Flap Thinning

- If the flap is too bulky for the recipient site (hand/wrist), one can perform flap thinning at the time of harvest, as opposed to debulking at a later date. For beginners, we do not recommend primary flap thinning as inadvertent perforator injury can result in flap necrosis.

- Perform flap thinning after elevation but prior to transection of the vascular pedicle.
- Preserve a 3-cm radius cuff of full-thickness adipose tissue around the perforator.
- Thin the flap by removing the deep fat tissue, which is characterized by wide and flat lobules.
- Removing this deep layer of fat should result in flap thickness of 5 to 6 mm.

■ Donor-Site Closure

- Obtain adequate hemostasis of the donor site.
- Reapproximate vastus lateralis muscle edges in cases of intramuscular dissection.
- Primary closure is usually possible when the flap width is limited to 8 cm.

- Place a suction drain to minimize risk of hematoma.
- If the donor-site width is more than 8 cm, the wound is unlikely to close primarily. Perform split-thickness skin grafting.

PEARLS AND PITFALLS

Flap dissection	■ Avoid unnecessary traction during flap elevation by dissecting around the perforator from the medial border and then lateral border, as opposed to elevating the entire flap from the medial border.
	■ If the skin perforators are too small to safely perform an intramuscular dissection, consider the use of the operating microscope, or elevate the flap in a myocutaneous fashion by incorporating a cuff of muscle around the intramuscular pedicle.
	■ Maintain the position of the flap during dissection. Traction on the perforator(s) from the weight of the flap may cause injury or vasospasm.
	■ If there is concern for vasospasm, bathe perforators in topical lidocaine.
Flap thinning	■ Inexperienced surgeons should avoid aggressive one-stage flap thinning due to the risk of perforator injury and flap necrosis.
Hemostasis	■ Meticulous dissection during flap harvest is necessary particularly with musculocutaneous perforator dissection, as hasty division of muscular perforator branches will retract and be difficult to ligate.
Flap inset	■ Avoid twisting of the pedicle by preserving a cuff of fascia and allowing the pedicle to fall into its normal orientation before final inset.

POSTOPERATIVE CARE

- Avoid compressive bandages on the flap.
- Flaps are checked hourly with Doppler ultrasound for the first 48 hours postoperatively and then every 4 hours for the next 48 hours.
- The patient is kept hydrated with intravenous fluids and kept on thrombosis prophylaxis therapy (low molecular weight heparin) while hospitalized.
- Drain is removed once output is appropriate, typically less than 30 mL/d.
- If a skin graft was applied to the donor site, bed rest is instituted until the graft takes.
- Secondary debulking of the flap is delayed until 6 to 9 months postoperatively.

OUTCOMES

- Good results are reported with 96% overall survival rate of 672 flaps.[2]

- Donor-site morbidity is generally minimal. Anterolateral thigh numbness may result from sensory nerve division but can be avoided by careful preservation of suprafascial nerve branches.

COMPLICATIONS

- General complications related to free tissue transfer such as flap necrosis and hematoma are possible.
- Flap necrosis can occur from overaggressive flap thinning and perforator injury.

REFERENCES

1. Kimata Y, Uchiyama K, Ebihara S, et al. Anatomic variations and technical problems of the anterolateral thigh flap: a report of 74 cases. *Plast Reconstr Surg.* 1998;102:1517-1523.
2. Wei FC, Jain V, Celik N, et al. Have we found an ideal soft tissue flap? An experience with 672 anterolateral thigh flaps. *Plast Reconstr Surg.* 2002;109:2219-2226.

Revascularization and Replantation of Digits

Mark Morris and Kevin C. Chung

DEFINITION

- Revascularization refers to the repair of injured structures and restoration of circulation to a digit that has been incompletely amputated. Restoration of vascularity to the incompletely severed digit is necessary to prevent necrosis.
- Replantation refers to the reattachment of a digit that has been completely amputated (**FIG 1**).
- Revision amputation refers to shortening a digit by debriding nonviable tissue and protruding bone in order to provide coverage of a digit that is not amenable to revascularization or replantation.

ANATOMY

- Each digit has a radial and ulnar proper digital artery. Each vessel is accompanied by a respective radial or ulnar proper digital nerve. Digital nerves are sensory only. In the digits, the artery is dorsal to the nerve (**FIG 2A**).
- There are three major palmar arches that arise from the digital arteries. The proximal, middle, and distal arches are located at the level of the C1 pulley, at the level of the C3 pulley, and just distal to the flexor digitorum profundus (FDP) insertion, respectively.

- Four palmar and four dorsal branches extend from each digital artery.
- The dorsal veins are larger than the palmar veins. Veins do not reliably travel with the arteries and nerves.
- Grayson ligament originates from the flexor tendon sheath and inserts on the skin. It lies palmar to the neurovascular bundle.
- Cleland ligament originates from the periosteum and inserts on the skin. It lies dorsal to the neurovascular bundle (**FIG 2B**).
- The flexor tendons travel within the flexor sheath. There is a series of five annular and three cruciform pulleys in which the flexor tendons pass through. The pulleys are discrete thickenings of the fibro-osseous sheath.
- Odd-numbered annular pulleys (A1, A3, A5) are located over the joints of the finger (metacarpophalangeal, proximal interphalangeal, and distal interphalangeal [DIP], respectively). Even-numbered annular pulleys (A2, A4) are located over the proximal and middle phalanges, respectively.
- The A2 and A4 pulleys are important in preventing bowstringing and should be preserved if possible.

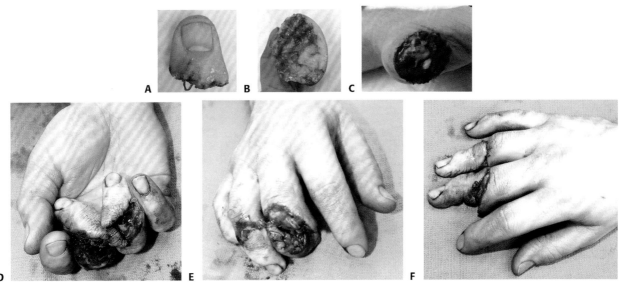

FIG 1 • A–C. Complete amputation of the thumb. This injury required replantation. **D–F.** Partially amputated long and ring fingers. This injury required revascularization.

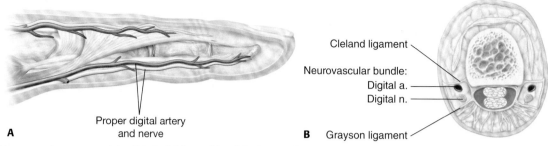

FIG 2 • A. Neurovascular anatomy of the digit. **B.** Axial cut of the digit, showing the relationship of Cleland and Grayson ligaments to the neurovascular bundle. The digital nerve is palmar to the artery.

- The flexor digitorum superficialis (FDS) splits into two slips at Camper chiasm and inserts as two slips into the midportion of the middle phalanx.
- The FDP tendon passes between the two slips of FDS at Camper chiasm and inserts at the proximal base of the distal phalanx.
- The extensor digitorum communis (EDC) sends a tendon to each digit. The index finger also contains the extensor indicis proprius (EIP), and the small finger also contains the extensor digiti minimi (EDM). The EIP and EDM tendons are ulnar to their respective EDC tendon.

PATHOGENESIS

- Amputation can be caused by sharp or blunt dissection, crush injury, or avulsion injury.
- Sharp amputations have a narrow zone of injury and are thus better suited for replantation or revascularization (**FIG 3A**).
- Crush and avulsion injuries have a larger zone of injury, which may preclude replantation or revascularization (**FIG 3B**).

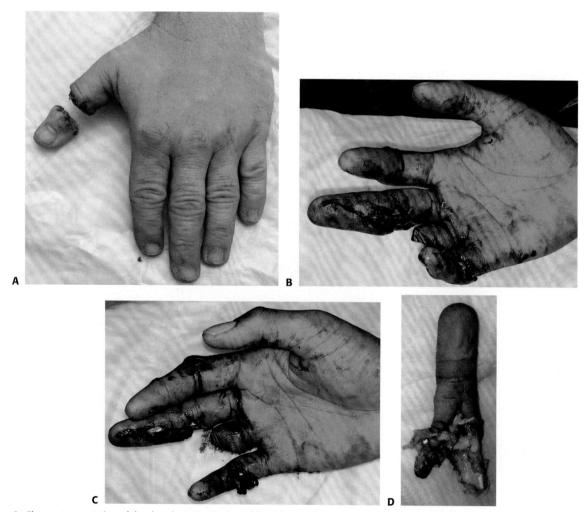

FIG 3 • A. Clean-cut amputation of the thumb. **B–D.** Crush-avulsion injury of the ring finger with a wide zone of injury secondary to the hand being caught in a gear mechanism, precluding successful replantation.

NATURAL HISTORY

- Mean survival rate after replantation is 86% reported by highly experienced surgeons and hospitals.[1]
- Clean-cut amputations have a better survival rate (92%) than crush-cut (80%) or crush-avulsion injuries (75%).
- Mean two-point discrimination after replantation is 7 mm.
- Ninety-eight percent of patients are able to return to work after digit replantation.[1]

PATIENT HISTORY AND PHYSICAL FINDINGS

- The history must include the mechanism and timing of injury. Crush injuries may preclude replantation depending on the degree of tissue damage.
- Ischemia time and method of transport must be evaluated. In general, warm ischemia time of less than 6 hours and cold ischemia time of less than 12 hours are desired for replantation.
  - Delayed replantation has been shown to have success, however. In a study of delayed and suspended replantation of digits and hands, Woo et al.[2] studied 28 digital and 4 hand amputations that underwent delayed or suspended amputation (mean cold ischemic time 15 hours 48 minutes). In this series, 24 of 28 digits and all 4 hands survived (88% survival rate). Case reports exist with successful replantation after warm ischemia times of 42 hours and cold ischemia times of 94 hours.[3,4]
- Transportation method of an amputated digit is important. The digit should not be placed directly on ice but should rather be wrapped in gauze moistened with normal saline or lactated Ringer's and placed into a plastic bag, which is then placed in an ice slush.
- A psychological and mental health history is important, as patients will require significant compliance with rehabilitation protocols.
- Medical history including diabetes mellitus, peripheral vascular disease, hypercoagulability, or smoking is not a contraindication to revascularization or replantation but will affect the healing potential of the digit(s) and must be discussed with the patient.
- The surgeon must examine the extremity to assess the number of digits injured, vascularity and sensation of partially amputated digits, wound contamination, and type of injury sustained.
- Several classifications exist for fingertip amputations. Two commonly used classifications are by Allen and Tamai.
  - Allen[5] (**FIG 4A**)
    - Type I: Only the pulp of the finger is involved. No suitable vessel for anastomosis.
    - Type II: Pulp and nail loss. Preserves half of the nail bed. No dorsal vein available for anastomosis.
    - Type III: Partial loss of the distal phalanx in addition to pulp and nail loss. High incidence of hook-nail deformity if nail bed is not ablated.
    - Type IV: Amputation proximal to nail fold. Dorsal vein usually available for anastomosis.
  - Tamai[6] (**FIG 4B**)
    - Zone 1: Fingertip to the base of the nail
    - Zone 2: Between the base of the nail and the DIP joint

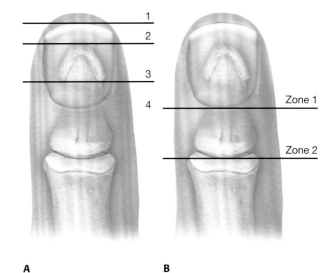

A   **B**

FIG 4 • Classification of fingertip amputations. **A.** Allen classification. **B.** Tamai classification.

- Red line sign—a red streak along the lateral border of a digit suggests hemorrhage from an avulsed branch of the digital artery after a traction injury.
- Ribbon sign—coiling of a digital artery at the amputation site. This also results from a traction injury (**FIG 5**). If replantation or revascularization is attempted, vein grafting will be required.

IMAGING

- Standard radiographs of the injured extremity and the amputated parts should be performed, in order to better understand the extent of injury and to plan fixation (**FIG 6**).

NONOPERATIVE MANAGEMENT

- There is no role for nonoperative management in digit amputations or dysvascular partial amputations.
- Occasionally, revision amputation can be performed in the emergency department, but this is often better done in the operating room with appropriate anesthesia, sterile conditions, lighting, and equipment.

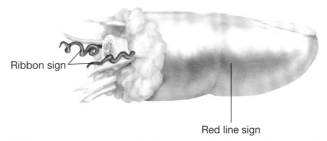

Ribbon sign

Red line sign

FIG 5 • The red line sign and ribbon sign are both signs of artery avulsion from a traction injury. If these signs are present, a vein graft should be attempted rather than direct repair, as the vessel walls have been injured.

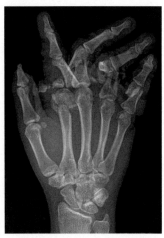
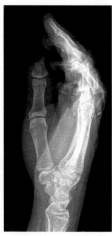

FIG 6 • A,B. Radiographs of a patient who sustained a crush injury to the right hand, with multiple devascularized digits.

SURGICAL MANAGEMENT

- Patients undergoing revascularization or replantation should also be consented for possible revision amputation, as a final decision to revascularize or replant a digit will be made after all structures are carefully evaluated in the operating room.
- Indications for replantation:
  - Thumb
  - Multiple digits
  - Partial hand (through-palm amputation)
  - Through wrist or forearm
  - Almost any part in a child
  - Individual digit distal to the FDS tendon
- Contraindications to replantation:
  - Severely crushed or mangled digit
  - Multilevel amputation
  - Concomitant life-threatening injuries
  - Severely atherosclerotic vessels
  - Patients who are unable to comply with a postoperative rehabilitation program
  - Prolonged warm ischemia time (relative; see discussion in history and physical section)
  - Individual finger amputation in an adult at a level proximal to the FDS insertion (controversial; limited function in a replanted digit at this level may negatively affect overall hand function)
- The sequence of repair is as follows:
  - Debridement and identification of injured and intact structures. Place vascular clips on the arteries. This will help with later identification. In addition, if the tourniquet needs to be let down prior to arterial repair, the field will remain dry.
  - Bone shortening and/or fixation
  - Extensor tendon repair
  - Flexor tendon repair
  - Vein repair while still under tourniquet. This is a deviation from the classic teaching (arteries before veins), because many surgeons find it easier to repair veins in a bloodless field.
  - Arterial repair
  - Nerve repair
  - Skin closure/coverage

Preoperative Planning

- Antibiotics and tetanus prophylaxis are given as soon as possible upon presentation to the emergency department.
- Regional anesthesia provides increased peripheral vasodilation.
- Amputated digits are transported to the operating room, and initial preparation begins as soon as possible.
  - This can be done while the anesthesia team is evaluating the patient and inducing anesthesia.
  - The surgical team can use a back table to start dissecting the amputated part to identify all the parts that will be connected.

Positioning

- The patient is placed supine on the operating table.
- The operative extremity is placed on a hand table.
- A brachial tourniquet is applied.

Approach

- Debridement and careful identification of structures is the key first step.
  - Keep track of each structure as it is identified by writing a count sheet or having the circulating nurse do so.
  - Each structure is tagged with a suture or a clip for future identification.
- Duration of surgery is decreased by repairing "structure by structure" rather than "digit by digit." Repair the same structure on each digit rather than completing all aspects of replantation on one digit at a time.
- A two-team approach can be used to save time. One team prepares the amputated digit(s) while the other team prepares the patient.
- Vein, artery, and nerve repairs are performed under the operating microscope. Microsurgical instruments are used.
- Never discard amputated parts until the surgery is over. Amputated parts are a useful source of autologous materials when needed such as nerve grafts, vascularized skin flap, tendons, bone, and vessels.

TECHNIQUES

■ Preparation of Amputated Digits and Stumps

- The amputated digits are brought to the operating room as soon as possible. One team will prepare the amputated digits while the other team prepares the patient.
- The parts are cleaned on a sterile prep table.
- Contaminated edges of the amputated digits and stumps are debrided, and arteries, nerves, and veins are identified.
  - Vascular clamps can be placed on arteries at this time for identification and later hemostasis.
- Midaxial incisions are made on the radial and ulnar sides of the digit to further expose neurovascular structures (**TECH FIG 1**).
- Flexor and extensor tendons are identified.
- Bone is shortened with a rongeur or a microsagittal saw to facilitate the vessel repair to obviate the use of vein graft and nerve graft. Bone should be shortened if much tissue debridement was required. Shortening will facilitate tension-free anastomosis and skin closure.
- Amputated digits should be kept cool until they are ready to be replanted.

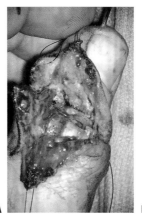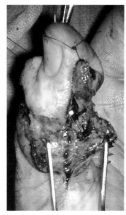

TECH FIG 1 • **A,B.** Midlateral incisions are made on either side of the amputation to assist in visualization, identification, and repair of neurovascular structures.

■ Bone Fixation

- Bone fixation can be accomplished using many different methods, including longitudinal K-wires, crossed K-wires, intraosseous wiring, tension band, intramedullary screws, and plate and screws.
  - Parallel longitudinal K-wires are fast and easy and have good success rates.
- In the amputated digit, two 0.045 K-wires are placed longitudinally into the bone in retrograde fashion.

- The wire should exit the tip of the digit just palmar to the nail.
- Advance the wire until just the tip is showing through the proximal end of the bone, ready to be advanced into the bone from the stump.
- Align the bones from the amputated part of the digit and its stump.
  - Take care to restore proper rotational alignment.
  - Advance the K-wires into the proximal bone and confirm location with radiographs (**TECH FIG 2**).

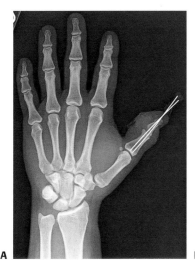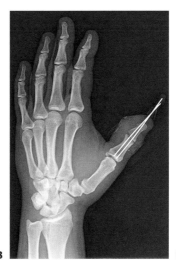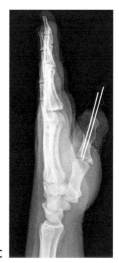

TECH FIG 2 • **A–C.** Parallel K-wire fixation was used in this case of thumb replantation.

■ Tendon Repair

- Extensor tendons are repaired with two 4-0 nonabsorbable sutures in horizontal mattress fashion.
- In-depth discussion of flexor tendon repair can be found in a separate chapter in this text.
  - We typically use a looped 4-0 Supramid suture to complete a six-strand repair of flexor tendons, followed by a running epitendinous 6-0 Prolene suture.
- Both flexor digitorum superficialis (FDS) and flexor digitorum profundus (FDP) can be repaired; however, it is not necessary to repair the FDS if this will impede tendon gliding if the FDS is shredded and too traumatized.
- If the amputation is distal to the FDS insertion, extensor and flexor tendon repair can be disregarded and the distal interphalangeal (DIP) joint can be fused.

■ Vein Repair

- Ideally, two veins are repaired for each artery that is repaired.
  - Research has shown a significantly better survival rate after two venous anastomoses per digit compared with one. However, there was no difference in this study between none and one vein repaired.[7]
  - Another study also showed no difference in survival rates between distal digit replantations with and without venous anastomosis.[8]
  - We recommend venous repair whenever possible, despite the findings of the later study.
- Venous repair prior to arterial repair allows for this most difficult task to be performed in a bloodless field and perhaps doing this critical procedure when the surgeon is still fresh, rather than at the end of the case when fatigue sets in.
- Because the veins are thin, the surgeon needs to take minimal bites of the vessel wall to prevent folding in of the adventitia. Side branches can be clipped to lengthen the vein so that it can reach to the other end.
- Irrigate the lumen of the vein with heparinized saline using a 30-gauge blunt-tipped needle to keep it open.
- Fewer sutures are required for venous repair than arterial repair because of the low-pressure flow.
- If vein grafts are required, appropriate-sized donor grafts (1–2 mm) can be harvested from the volar wrist.

■ Artery Repair

- Arteries have been previously clamped when structures were identified earlier. The tourniquet can be let down at this time. Vascular clamps will control bleeding.
- Both digital arteries should be repaired when possible, to maximize survival rates.
- Damaged ends of arteries are sharply debrided back to normal intima until one gets a robust spurt from the artery, which indicates suitable resection of the traumatized vessel.
- Vein grafts are used if there is any defect after debridement.
  - Vein grafts must be rotated 180 degrees with respect to flow, because of the valves that are present.
  - For proper size match, vein graft from the volar wrist is used.
  - For vein grafting in the palm, vein graft from the forearm has suitable size match.
- Artery ends are approximated in a tension-free manner, but without redundancy of the vein graft. This can be done with vascular approximating clamps (**TECH FIG 3**).
- A microsurgical dilator is used to dilate the arterial lumen and assess blood flow by transiently releasing the vascular clamp on the stump side.
- If there is inadequate blood flow, evaluate for reversible causes such as vasospasm, cold, acidosis, hypotension/hypovolemia, or mechanical constriction.
- Vasospasm can be treated by irrigating with papaverine solution (diluted 1:20 with normal saline).
- Irrigate the lumen with heparinized saline using a 30-gauge blunt-tipped needle.
- We recommend the use of a background to help with visualization.
- A bolus of 5000 units of intravenous heparin is given prior to anastomosis. A heparin drip is then initiated at 1000 units per hour.
- Suture size depends on the size of the vessel being repaired. In general, 11-0 nylon suture is used in the distal digit, 10-0 nylon suture is used in the proximal digit, and 9-0 nylon suture can be used in the palm.
- Interrupted sutures are placed circumferentially, with care to avoid capturing the back wall with the needle.
- Each bite of the needle should be 1 to 2 times the thickness of the arterial wall.
- Leave one limb of each of the initial sutures long. The suture ends can be used later to manipulate the vessel in a minimally traumatic manner.
- Release the vascular clamps and observe for pulsations and a water-tight seal.

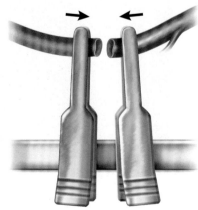

TECH FIG 3 • A vascular approximating clamp is used to bring the arterial ends together in a tension-free manner.

Nerve Repair

- The severed ends of the nerve are sharply cut using microsurgical scissors or a no. 11 blade against a wooden tongue depressor.
- Nerve ends are approximated in a tension-free manner.
  - If tension-free repair is not possible, primary nerve grafting is performed. The medial or lateral antebrachial cutaneous nerves can be harvested from the ipsilateral extremity.
    - Alternatively, other amputated digits that are not candidates for replantation can be used to provide nerve graft of appropriate caliber.
- Fascicles are aligned and epineural repair is performed using three or four 9-0 or 10-0 nylon sutures.

Closure

- Obtain hemostasis prior to skin closure. Hematoma will place pressure on vascular repairs and can result in failure of the replant.
- Interrupted 4-0 nylon sutures are used to close the skin (**TECH FIG 4**). Take care to avoid constriction of underlying structures.
- Skin grafts or flaps are used as needed.

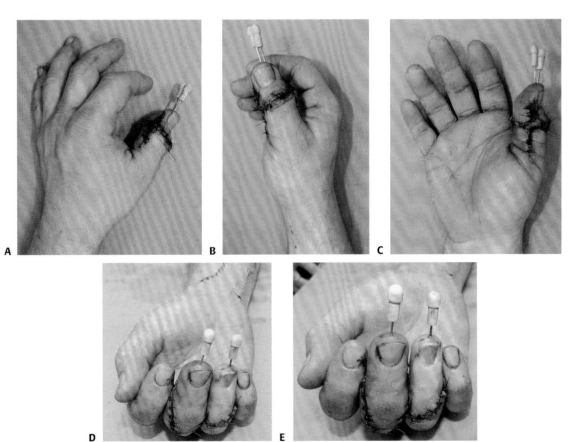

TECH FIG 4 • Same patient as in **FIG 1**. Postoperative images after thumb replantation **(A-C)** and long and ring finger revascularization **(D,E)**.

PEARLS AND PITFALLS

Preparation	■ Make a tally sheet for the structures that are injured in each digit as you debride and identify structures. This will help the case go smoother and will help with dictation postoperatively. ■ Prioritize the functional goals of the patient for replantation. If multiple digits are amputated and some are not replantable, the salvageable digits should be placed in the most functional position—ie, if the thumb is not salvageable, replant a finger in the thumb's position.
Technique	■ Duration of surgery is decreased by repairing "structure by structure" rather than "digit by digit." Repair the same structure on each digit rather than completing all aspects of replantation on one digit at a time. ■ All anastomoses should be tension-free. Bone shortening or vein grafting should be performed to accomplish this.
Treatment of venous congestion with leeches	■ If an inadequate number or quality of venous anastomoses are performed, venous congestion may occur in the digit. If this occurs, the nail can be removed and medical leeches (*Hirudo medicinalis*) can be placed postoperatively. They should be changed every few hours and continued for 7 days. ■ Patients should be treated with a third-generation cephalosporin while leeches are in use as prophylaxis against *Aeromonas hydrophila*, which is a symbiotic gram-negative rod in the leech gut.

POSTOPERATIVE CARE

■ The postoperative dressing should not be circumferential or constricting.
  ▫ Xeroform gauze is applied to the incisions.
  ▫ A well-padded plaster splint is applied, with the tips of the digits exposed to monitor for vascular status.
  ▫ Temperature probes or pulse oximeters can be applied to the fingertips for monitoring.
■ The splint is changed after 1 or 2 days in case a blood cast forms. If there is excessive bleeding, the clotted blood on the dressings and splint will solidify and cause circumferential constriction.
■ Color, warmth, and capillary refill are monitored by the surgeon and nursing staff.
■ The patient's room should be kept above 72°F (22°C). We alternatively use a Bair hugger to cover the extremity and keep it warm.
■ Bed rest is maintained for at least 2 or 3 days, or longer if the vascular status is tenuous.
■ No caffeine, chocolate, or nicotine is permitted.

■ A bolus of 50 mL Dextran 40 is given in the operating room, followed by a maintained rate of 20 mL/h while the patient is still hospitalized.
■ The patient is maintained on low molecular weight heparin or unfractionated heparin for 5 days. Low molecular weight heparin has been reported to be as effective as unfractionated heparin but with fewer adverse effects.[9]
■ Aspirin 325 mg daily is started postoperatively and continued for 6 weeks.
■ Anxiolytics can be provided to the patient so he or she does not unintentionally harm the repair secondary to anxiety.
  ▫ Thorazine 25 mg orally every 8 hours can be used as both an anxiolytic and a peripheral vasodilator.

OUTCOMES

■ Sebastin and Chung[1] performed a systematic review of the outcomes of replantation of distal digital amputation (**FIG 7**). Thirty studies were included in the review.
  ▫ Mean survival rate after replantation was 86%.

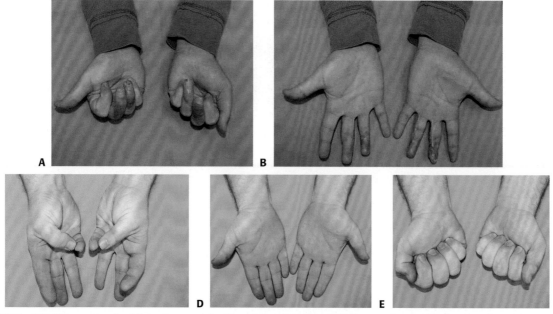

FIG 7 • **A,B.** Five months after bilateral long and ring finger revascularization. **C–E.** Ten months after left thumb replantation.

- There was no difference in survival of replanted digits based on Tamai classification of zone I or zone II.
- Clean-cut amputations had significantly better survival rates than crushed amputations (92% for clean-cut, 80% for crush-cut, and 75% for crush-avulsion).
- Repairing a vein improved survival in both zone I and II replantation (zone I with venous repair 92% survival vs 83% without repair. Zone II with venous repair 88% survival vs 78% without repair).
- Mean two-point discrimination after replantation was 7 mm.
- Ninety-eight percent of patients were able to return to work.
- Yu et al.[10] performed a meta-analysis to investigate non-surgical factors associated with survival rates of digital replantation.
  - Ischemia time (over or under 12 hours) had no significant correlation with survival rate.
  - Clean-cut injuries had better outcomes than crush and avulsion injuries.
  - The thumb had a better chance of survival than did the small finger (OR 2.09), while there were no significant differences between other digits.
  - The chance of survival was higher in digits that were transported cold when compared to those transported at room temperature (OR 4.89).

COMPLICATIONS

- Pulp atrophy (14%)
- Nail deformity (24%)
- Failure of replant (14%)
- Venous congestion
- Infection

- Cold intolerance—Almost all patients experience this. Cold intolerance is expected to improve over the first 2 years but may never resolve.
- Stiffness—Tenolysis should be delayed for at minimum 3 months postreplantation.
- Malunion
- Nonunion

REFERENCES

1. Sebastin SJ, Chung KC. A systematic review of the outcomes of replantation of distal digital amputation. *Plast Reconstr Surg.* 2011;128:723-737.
2. Woo SH, Cheon HJ, Kim YW, et al. Delayed and suspended replantation for complete amputation of digits and hands. *J Hand Surg Am.* 2015;40(5):883-889.
3. Baek SM, Kim SS. Successful digital replantation after 42 hours of warm ischemia. *J Reconstr Microsurg.* 1992;8:455-458.
4. Wei FC, Chang YL, Chen HC, Chuang CC. Three successful digital replantations in a patient after 84, 86, and 94 hours of cold ischemia time. *Plast Reconstr Surg.* 1988;82(2):346-350.
5. Allen MJ. Conservative management of finger tip injuries in adults. *Hand.* 1980:12(3):157-165.
6. Tamai S. Twenty years' experience of limb replantation: review of 293 upper extremity replants. *J Hand Surg Am.* 1982;7(6):549-556.
7. Efanov JI, Rizis D, Landes G, et al. Impact of the number of veins repaired in short-term digital replantation survival rate. *J Plast Reconstr Aestht Surg.* 2016;69:640-645.
8. Huang H, Yeong E. Surgical treatment of distal digit amputation: success in distal digit replantation is not dependent on venous anastomosis. *Plast Reconstr Surg.* 2015;135:174-178.
9. Chen Y, Chi C, Chan FC, Wen Y. Low molecular weight heparin for prevention of microvascular occlusion in digital replantation. *Cochrane Database Syst Rev.* 2013;7:CD009894.
10. Yu H, Wei L, Liang B, et al. Nonsurgical factors of digital replantation and survival rate. *Indian J Orthop.* 2015;49(3):265-271.

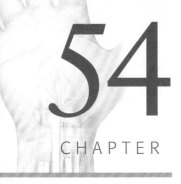

54
CHAPTER

Digital Artery Sympathectomy

John R. Lien and Kevin C. Chung

DEFINITION

- Raynaud disease (RD) is characterized by cold hypersensitivity and color changes to digits secondary to an exaggerated vasoconstrictive response to cold temperature, emotional stress, or trauma.
  - There is no underlying associated cause for these vasospastic events in RD.
- Raynaud phenomenon (RP) occurs in patients with a diagnosis of underlying collagen vascular disease such as scleroderma.

ANATOMY

- The superficial palmar arch is the continuation of the ulnar artery in the palm. The common digital arteries arise from this palmar arch (**FIG 1**).
- The common digital nerves course alongside the common digital arteries, supplying sympathetic fibers to the adventitial layer of the arteries.

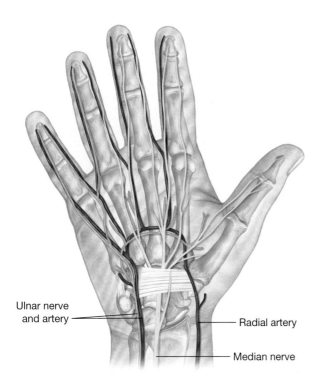

FIG 1 • Palmar neurovascular anatomy. The ulnar artery provides dominant flow to the superficial palmar arch (deep palmar arch not shown).

Ulnar nerve and artery

Radial artery

Median nerve

PATHOGENESIS

- The function of arterial smooth muscle is to constrict and decrease blood flow.
- Vasospastic disorders are characterized by reversible changes in flow, whereas occlusive disorders involve decreased flow unrelated to vasoconstriction.
- In occlusive disorders such as scleroderma, ischemia of the digit may result from inadequate collateral vessels or inadequate flow through collaterals secondary to vasospasm.

NATURAL HISTORY

- Natural history of the digital ischemia is largely dictated by the underlying cause.
- Patients with underlying mixed connective tissue disorder often have worsening digital symptoms/ischemia as their disease progresses. This can lead to trophic changes such as ulcers and gangrene.

PATIENT HISTORY AND PHYSICAL FINDINGS

- Patients typically report a triphasic color change (white, blue, red) in both RD and RP.
- Obtain a thorough rheumatologic history. Patients with suspected primary RD may have unrecognized mixed connective tissue disorders.
- Frequency and severity of ischemic episodes, extent of cold sensitivity, numbness, pain
- Association of symptoms with emotional changes
- Active nicotine use is a contraindication to surgical intervention.
- Allen testing should be performed to assess patency of palmar arches.
- Note trophic changes such as ulcers and gangrene.
- Assess for laterality; focal unilateral symptoms may be concerning for embolic disease.

IMAGING

- Angiography provides excellent anatomic detail and structural information. Vasospastic contribution to ischemia can be enhanced by the use of intra-arterial vasodilators. If the patient fails medical management, we obtain this study as part of our preoperative evaluation.
- Noninvasive vascular studies
  - Digital brachial index (DBI) values assess total flow to the digit. DBI less than 0.7 indicates abnormal flow.

- Doppler sonography
- Digital plethysmography (pulse volume recordings) can differentiate vasospastic from vaso-occlusive disease, particularly with cold stress testing.

DIFFERENTIAL DIAGNOSIS

- Primary Raynaud disease
- Secondary Raynaud phenomenon
  - Rheumatic disease, eg, scleroderma, systemic lupus erythematosus
  - Hematologic disorder
  - Atherosclerotic disease
  - Embolic disease

NONOPERATIVE MANAGEMENT

- Lifestyle modification
  - Tobacco cessation
  - Avoidance of cold environment (gloves, warmer climate in winter)
- Biofeedback therapy
- Medical management[1]
  - Calcium channel blocker such as nifedipine is a first-line treatment.
  - Phosphodiesterase-5 inhibitors (sildenafil, tadalafil, vardenafil), topical nitroglycerin, angiotensin-receptor antagonist (losartan), and selective serotonin reuptake inhibitors (fluoxetine) are other among second-line medications.
- There may be a role for botulinum toxin type A injection, but larger controlled trials are necessary to establish its effectiveness.[2]

SURGICAL MANAGEMENT

- Indications for digital sympathectomy include digital ischemic pain and/or trophic changes refractory to medical management. This commonly includes patients with autoimmune disorders such as scleroderma. Often, this is a surgery of last resort in patients with persistent and unrelenting ischemic pain.

- Patients with primary RD often respond to medical management. We rarely offer surgical sympathectomy to these patients.
- We do not offer this surgery to active smokers.
- Contraindication to sympathectomy includes severe primary atherosclerotic occlusive disease.
  - For the sympathectomy to produce increased flow to the digit, there must be a reversible vasospastic component to either the digital artery or its distal collaterals.

Preoperative Planning

- If preoperative studies demonstrate vasospastic disease with secondary occlusion of the radial/ulnar artery or palmar arch, we consider arterial reconstruction with vein grafting.

Positioning

- Supine with hand table and arm tourniquet

Approach

- For single-digit sympathectomy, we perform an extensile Bruner zigzag incision over the ray of the digit in the distal palm.
- In the setting of multiple-digit sympathectomies, we perform a transverse oblique incision at the palmar crease (**FIG 2**).

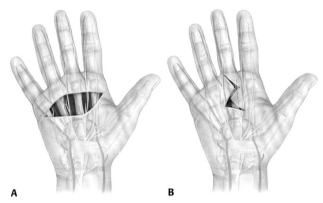

A   B

FIG 2 • Incision for multiple-digit artery sympathectomy (**A**) and single-digit sympathectomy (**B**).

■ **Exposure**

- Under tourniquet control, perform a Bruner incision overlying the appropriate ray in the distal half of the palm (or transverse oblique incision for multiple-digit sympathectomies; **TECH FIG 1A**).
- Elevate full-thickness skin flaps and expose the superficial palmar arch proximally.

- Identify the origins of the common digital arteries supplying the radial and ulnar aspects of the appropriate finger.
- Dissect the common digital arteries and nerves from proximal to distal, ensuring exposure of 2 to 3 cm of vessel length (**TECH FIG 1B**).

TECHNIQUES

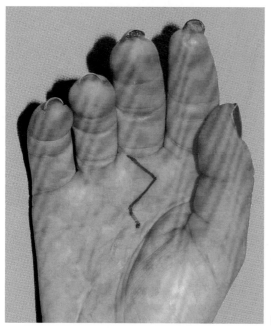
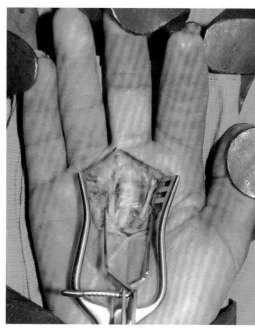

TECH FIG 1 • A. Brunner incision is marked. Trophic changes to the index and middle fingertips can be seen in this patient with scleroderma and persistent middle finger pain. **B.** Exposure of radial and ulnar digital neurovascular bundles to middle finger.

■ Sympathectomy

- Under microscope magnification, systematically strip the common digital artery adventitia for 2 to 3 cm.
- While doing this, any communicating sympathetic nerve branches from the digital nerve to the artery should be divided (**TECH FIG 2**).
- Take care to avoid injury to the digital artery. Small arterial branches should be tied off using microsurgical technique.
- Release the tourniquet and ensure hemostasis.
- Loosely close the wound.

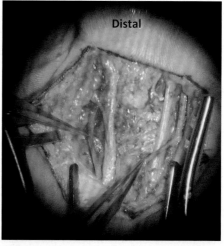

TECH FIG 2 • Microscope view of neurovascular bundles after sympathectomy.

PEARLS AND PITFALLS

Technique	■ Avoid iatrogenic arterial injury or vasospasm by minimizing trauma to the digital artery. Use microsurgical technique during adventitial stripping.
Arterial reconstruction	■ When possible, consider arterial reconstruction if there is inadequate collateral circulation with proximal occlusion. Sympathectomy alone can be performed as a palliative salvage procedure if occlusive disease is nonreconstructible.

TECHNIQUES

POSTOPERATIVE CARE

- Patient is placed in a volar forearm-based splint postoperatively.
- At the first 2-week postoperative visit, sutures are removed and range of motion is encouraged.

OUTCOMES

- Reported outcomes on ulcer healing and pain improvement are heterogeneous due to small case volume and lack of controlled studies.[3]
- In general, better outcomes in terms of ulcer healing are noted in patients who have underlying autoimmune disease as compared to severe atherosclerotic disease.[4]
  - Twenty-eight of forty-two digits in patients with autoimmune disease had complete ulcer healing or decrease in number of ulcers. Two of seventeen digits had healing in the atherosclerotic group.
  - At a minimum of 23 months of follow-up, 26% (11 of 42) of digits in the autoimmune disease group ultimately required amputation, whereas 59% (10 of 17) in the atherosclerotic group ultimately required amputation.

COMPLICATIONS

- Persistent ischemic pain
- Persistent wound/ulcers necessitating amputation
- Iatrogenic arterial injury/thrombosis

REFERENCES

1. Wigley FM, Flavahan NA. Raynaud's phenomenon. *N Engl J Med.* 2016;375:556-565.
2. Iorio ML, Masden DL, Higgins JP. Botulinum toxin A treatment of Raynaud's phenomenon: a review. *Semin Arthritis Rheum.* 2012;41:599-603.
3. Kotsis SV, Chung KC. A systematic review of the outcomes of digital sympathectomy for treatment of chronic digital ischemia. *J Rheumatol.* 2003;30:1788-1792.
4. Hartzell TL, Makhni EC, Sampson C. Long-term results of periarterial sympathectomy. *J Hand Surg [Am].* 2009;34A:1454-1460.

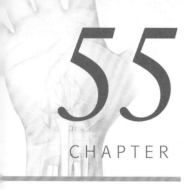

55 CHAPTER

Ulnar Artery to Superficial Arch Bypass With a Vein Graft for Ulnar Artery Thrombosis

Mark Morris and Kevin C. Chung

DEFINITION

- Hypothenar hammer syndrome refers to post-traumatic digital ischemia secondary to thrombosis of the ulnar artery.
- The ulnar artery at Guyon canal and the proximal superficial arch are the most common sites of occlusion.
- "Critical" vascular injuries result in tissue death without intervention.
- "Noncritical" vascular injuries occur when an artery is damaged, but collateral circulation is adequate and prevents tissue necrosis.
- A "complete" superficial or deep palmar arch is defined as having a significant connection to a branch from another independent arterial limb such that it provides branches to all digits. The superficial arch is complete in 78.5% of extremities, and the deep arch is complete in 98.5% of extremities.[1]

ANATOMY

- The major blood supply to the hand is from the superficial palmar arch, which is a continuation of the ulnar artery, and the deep palmar arch, which is a continuation of the radial artery (**FIG 1**).
- A median artery may also be present.
- The radial artery bifurcates into dorsal and volar branches at the level of the radial styloid. The dorsal branch traverses the floor of the snuffbox and passes through the first dorsal interosseous muscle, diving volar and becoming the primary contributor to the deep palmar arch. The volar branch contributes to the superficial arch.
- The ulnar artery bifurcates into deep and superficial branches at the level of the wrist. The deep branch anastomoses with the deep palmar arch, whereas the superficial branch terminates as the superficial palmar arch.

- The radial artery and deep palmar arch provide the dominant blood flow to three or more digits in 57% of normal extremities, whereas the ulnar artery and superficial arch provide dominant flow to three or more digits in 21.5%, and there is equal contribution from radial and ulnar arteries in 21.5% of extremities.[2]
- Deep palmar arch runs deep to the flexor tendons at the level of the base of the metacarpals, 1 cm proximal to the superficial arch.
- Superficial palmar arch is located at Kaplan line (line drawn across the palm from the first web space parallel to the proximal palmar crease toward the hook of the hamate), 1 cm distal to the deep palmar arch.
- The deep and superficial arches provide common digital arteries to the second, third, and fourth web spaces at the mid-metacarpal level. These then divide into proper digital arteries at the level of the MCP joint.
- A less significant dorsal circulation also exists, receiving contributions from dorsal carpal branches of the radial and ulnar arteries.

PATHOGENESIS

- A single or more likely repetitive impact to the hypothenar eminence leads to ulnar artery thrombosis or aneurysm (**FIG 2**).
- Ulnar artery thrombosis has been reported in patients participating in baseball, golf, weight lifting, karate, mountain biking, volleyball, and overenthusiastic clapping by fans. At-risk occupations are those requiring vibrating tools such as carpentry, construction, machine operators, and mechanics.
- The hook of the hamate acts as an anvil against which the ulnar artery is crushed.

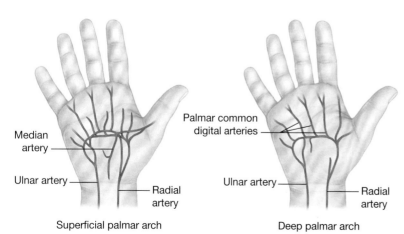

FIG 1 • Vascular anatomy of the hand. The superficial palmar arch is supplied by the ulnar artery. The deep palmar arch is supplied by the radial artery.

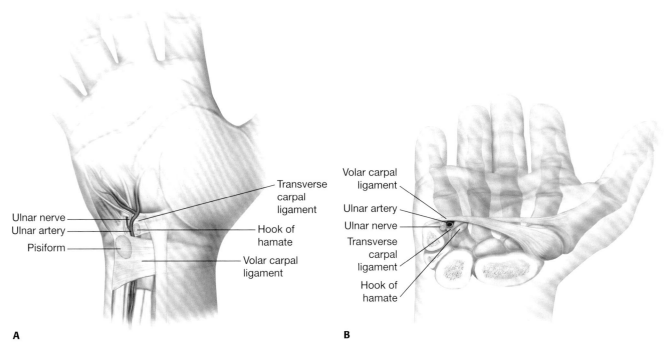

A   **B**

FIG 2 • The ulnar artery travels in Guyon canal with the ulnar nerve. **A,B.** The floor of the canal is made by the transverse carpal ligament, and the roof is made by the volar carpal ligament. The close proximity of the artery leaves it susceptible to impact into the hook of the hamate.

- Repetitive trauma can lead to direct intimal damage, which leads to thrombosis, or periadventitial thickening of the artery that constricts the vessel and obstructs flow.
- Disruption of the internal elastic lamina of the artery leads to aneurysm, which predisposes to mural thrombosis, complete occlusion, and distal thrombotic emboli (**FIG 3**).
- Arterial occlusion or distal emboli can lead to ulceration, gangrene, and necrosis of digits.

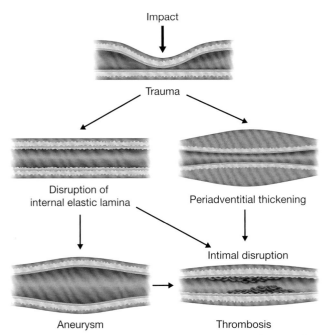

FIG 3 • Repetitive impact to the ulnar artery leads to either periadventitial thickening or disruption of internal elastic lamina. Both conditions leave the artery prone to thrombosis.

NATURAL HISTORY

- Depending on the severity of occlusion and quality of flow from the deep arch, the natural history will vary.
- The long, ring, and small fingers may develop cyanosis, pallor, splinter hemorrhages, ulcerations, atrophy of distal finger pads, or even necrosis of digits.
- Most patients will develop cold intolerance.
- Most patients will have persistent symptoms even after revascularization, although with decreased frequency and severity.

PATIENT HISTORY AND PHYSICAL FINDINGS

- Patients with post-traumatic ulnar artery thrombosis are predominantly male and present with unilateral hand and digit ischemia.
- The dominant hand is most commonly affected, although bilateral cases have been reported.
- History of interest includes vascular disease, smoking, manual labor, use of palm as a hammer, use of vibrating tools.
- Symptoms include pain, numbness or tingling, cold intolerance, and weakness in the ulnar nerve distribution.
- Signs on physical exam include pallor, cyanosis/mottling, a palpable hypothenar mass (if an aneurysm is present), atrophy of distal finger pads, splinter hemorrhages, ulcerations, and gangrene of the long, ring, and small fingers (**FIG 4**).
- Ischemic problems of the thumb have never been described with post-traumatic ulnar artery thrombosis. If present, a different diagnosis should be considered.
- Radial and ulnar pulses are palpated and examined by Doppler probe if not palpable.
- Doppler can also be used to assess the palmar arch and radial and ulnar digital arteries to each finger.

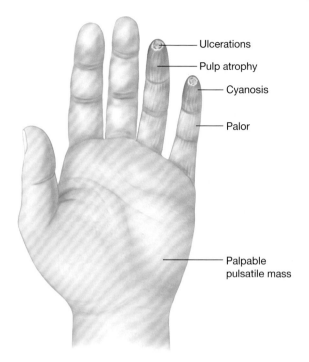

FIG 4 • Signs of ulnar artery thrombosis—pulp atrophy, ulcerations, cyanosis, pallor, palpable pulsatile mass in the hypothenar eminence. The thumb should appear normal. The number of affected digits will vary depending on perfusion from the radial artery and deep arch.

- A modified Allen test should be performed to assess blood flow to the hand from the radial and ulnar arteries independently (**FIG 5**):
  - One hand is examined at a time.
  - The patient is asked to clench the fist tightly for one minute.
  - Pressure is applied over the radial and ulnar arteries so as to occlude both.

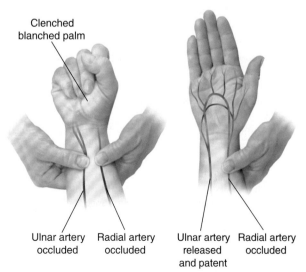

FIG 5 • Allen test in a patient with ulnar artery thrombosis. The examiner occludes both the ulnar and radial arteries and the hand is white as a result of a lack of perfusion. When pressure is released from the ulnar artery, the hand remains white because of an occluded ulnar artery.

- The patient opens the fingers. Pallor should be observed at this time.
- Pressure is released from the ulnar artery, and color should return if ulnar artery supply to the hand is sufficient. Pallor will remain if there is insufficient ulnar flow. The radial artery is then released and color should return to the entire hand if the deep arch is complete.
- The test is repeated, but with pressure being released from the radial artery first.
- Several questionnaires exist to assess symptoms and disability related to ischemia of the hand:
  - The Levine-Katz questionnaire assesses pain, symptoms of dysesthesia, and hand function.[3]
  - The McCabe Cold Sensitivity Test assesses cold sensitivity and associated symptoms.[4]
  - The Cold Intolerance Symptom Severity questionnaire adds questions and assessments that are not addressed by the McCabe test.[5]

IMAGING

- Noninvasive studies are done first.
  - Standard PA, lateral, and oblique radiography of the hand are performed to evaluate bony architecture as well as vascular calcifications.
  - Pulse volume recording measures the volume of arterial blood flow. Inadequate flow to the hand and digits can be detected by comparing proximal and distal blood flow. The severity and general location of occlusive disease can be determined by pulse volume recording.
  - Digital brachial index (DBI) compares digital blood pressure to contralateral brachial blood pressure in order to quantify perfusion to the hand and digits. The normal range for DBI is 0.75 to 0.97. Values equal or less than 0.7 signify inadequate perfusion.
  - Doppler or vascular duplex ultrasound can be used to evaluate flow. This provides audible and color-coded visual information about flow. Duplex can provide information about flow abnormalities, structural abnormalities of vessels, presence of thrombus, and aneurysm. The weakness of this study is the lack of standardization and operator-dependent nature of the study.
- Invasive tests can be performed if noninvasive tests are abnormal.
  - Computed tomographic angiography (CTA) and magnetic resonance angiography (MRA) are minimally invasive tests that require venous access for the administration of contrast dye. Both hands can be evaluated simultaneously for comparative assessment. Anatomic details provided by both tests are similar, but both have advantages and disadvantages. MRA contrast is less nephrotoxic than CTA contrast. MRA is susceptible to motion artifact and cannot be used in patients with certain metallic implants or claustrophobia. MRA is significantly more expensive than CTA, although both are cheaper than conventional angiography.
  - Conventional angiography/arteriography is the standard for evaluation of ulnar artery thrombosis (**FIG 6**). Angiography shows the surgeon the features of ulnar artery thrombosis including a corkscrew appearance of the ulnar artery, alternation of stenosis and dilation, aneurysm formation, occlusion of the ulnar artery at

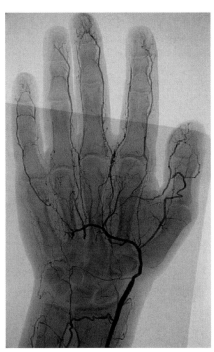

FIG 6 • Arteriogram demonstrating absent flow from the ulnar artery into the hand.

the hook of the hamate, or occlusion of the superficial palmar arch or digital arteries with a normal proximal ulnar artery. Conventional angiography requires arterial access and contrast dye administration and has risks of bleeding, hematoma, thrombosis, pseudoaneurysm, allergic reaction, renal toxicity, and a fourfold higher dose of radiation than CTA. Conventional angiography is contraindicated in patients with renal insufficiency.

DIFFERENTIAL DIAGNOSIS

- Hypothenar hammer syndrome (post-traumatic ulnar artery thrombosis)
- Raynaud disease
- Malignancy, vascular tumors
- Pseudoaneurysm
- Trauma, iatrogenic injury
- Buerger disease
- Arteritis
- Peripheral vascular disease (atherosclerosis)
- Connective tissue disorders (scleroderma, systemic lupus erythematosus)

NONOPERATIVE MANAGEMENT

- Nonoperative treatment can be considered for patients without impending digital loss.
- Smoking cessation
- Medications can be used to decrease sympathetic tone and vasospasm—calcium channel blockers, α-blockers, β-blockers, steroids, prostaglandins, and prostacyclin have been described.

- Antiplatelet or anticoagulant agents can be used in patients with thrombosis and embolic disease.
- Intra-arterial thrombolytics can be percutaneously directed to the site of ulnar artery thrombosis. Success of this procedure is limited, with a high complication rate.
- Digital sympathectomy with botulinum toxin A can be performed, with low morbidity.

SURGICAL MANAGEMENT

- Surgical intervention is indicated in patients who have failed medical management or those with impending digital necrosis.
- Surgical options include open sympathectomy, exploration and ligation of the diseased segment of artery, exploration and primary repair of the ulnar artery, or exploration and revascularization by arterial bypass.

Preoperative Planning

- Preoperative imaging (eg, CTA, MRA, angiogram) is reviewed to determine the site of bypass.
- Donor vessels are identified and marked.
- Venous or arterial grafts can be used.
  - Vein interpositional grafts must be reversed because of the presence of valves.
  - Veins are typically more expendable than arteries and provide longer grafts.
  - Arterial grafts are easier to match in size. They are less flimsy and do not need to be reversed.
  - Table 1 covers donor grafts available for ulnar artery bypass.
- An operating microscope and microsurgical instruments are used for microvascular anastomosis.

Table 1 Donor Grafts for Ulnar Artery Bypass

Graft	Length (cm)	Comments
Vein		
Greater saphenous	50–85	Found superficially, easier dissection, but decreased long-term patency rates compared to arterial grafts. Greater saphenous and basilic have poor size match to the ulnar artery at the wrist.
Lesser saphenous	35–60	
Forearm	14–20	
Basilic/cephalic	15–30	
Dorsum of foot	5–8	
Artery		
Subscapular	2–4	Short pedicle length
Superficial inferior epigastric	6–10	Abdominal bulge
Deep inferior epigastric	10–12	Abdominal bulge
Thoracodorsal	11–14	Dissection in axilla
Lateral circumflex femoral	10–18	Deep, variable anatomy

Positioning

- The patient is placed supine on the operating table with a hand table for the operative extremity.
- A brachial tourniquet is placed.
- Depending on the graft to be used, another extremity (usually a lower extremity) may need to be prepped and another tourniquet placed.

Approach

- The affected segment of artery will be excised. The surgeon must first obtain proximal and distal control of the ulnar artery and superficial arch.
- Palmar arches are exposed via zigzag incisions extending proximally from the phalanges or through an inverted J-shaped incision in the palm. The ulnar artery is exposed using a zigzag incision more proximally in the palm. The wrist crease is crossed in an oblique fashion.

T E C H N I Q U E S

■ Approach

- An incision is made that parallels the thenar crease, zigzags in the palm, and extends proximally into the forearm between the flexor carpi ulnaris and palmaris longus (**TECH FIG 1**).
  - Alternatively, two separate incisions can be made and the graft is tunneled under the skin, depending on the location of ulnar artery to be resected.
- The ulnar artery and nerve are identified 3 to 5 cm proximal to the wrist crease, and vessel loops are placed around each structure.
  - The artery is radial to the nerve at the wrist. The ulnar artery enters the hand through the Guyon canal. It runs deep to the volar carpal ligament and superficial to the transverse carpal ligament.

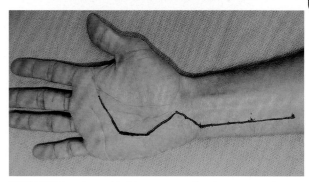

TECH FIG 1 • Planned incision to access the ulnar artery and superficial palmar arch. The wrist crease is crossed with an oblique incision. A zigzag incision is made in the palm. If the entire superficial arch needs to be accessed, continue the incision along the proximal palmar crease. The extent of the forearm incision depends on the length of bypass required.

■ Dissection of the Ulnar Artery

- Dissect from proximal to distal, following the ulnar artery. First identify the patent portion of the ulnar artery proximal to the wrist crease (**TECH FIG 2A**).
- Identify the arterial branch or branches that accompany the deep motor branch of the ulnar nerve. Identify the origin of the proper digital artery to the small finger and the origins of the common digital arteries from the superficial arch.
- Mobilize the ulnar artery and superficial arch (**TECH FIG 2B**). Spread the artery away from surrounding tissue and venae comitantes using scissors. Venae comitantes are cauterized with bipolar electrocautery.

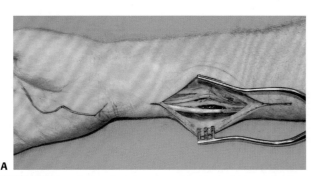
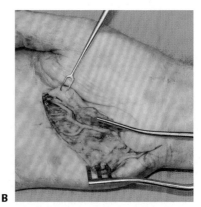

TECH FIG 2 • **A.** The ulnar artery is exposed in the forearm. **B.** The superficial palmar arch is exposed in the hand.

Resection of Affected Segment of Ulnar Artery and Superficial Arch

- All abnormal segments are resected to normal vessel.
- Once all damaged vessels are resected, distal outflow can be assessed by transiently deflating the tourniquet and observing backflow (**TECH FIG 3**).
- Measure the size of the defect.

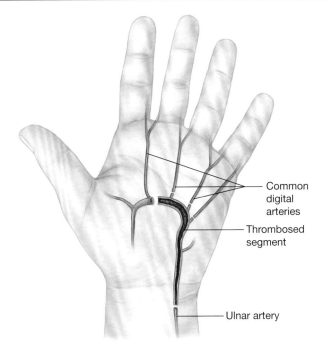

Common digital arteries

Thrombosed segment

Ulnar artery

TECH FIG 3 • The thrombosed section of ulnar artery and superficial arch is resected back to normal artery. Measure the segment that is resected in preparation for vein harvest.

Harvesting of Vein Graft

- Select the appropriate donor graft depending on the length and diameter needed (see Table 1).
- A vein graft is harvested through a longitudinal incision under tourniquet.
- Adequate length is mobilized (harvest 10%–30% longer than estimated to perform the bypass).
- Draw an axial line down the length of the vein to be harvested while it is still in situ. This will help the surgeon prevent inadvertent twisting of the graft during the anastomosis.
- Occasionally, branches are desired for anastomosis. All other branches are ligated or coagulated with bipolar electrocautery.

- Harvest the graft (**TECH FIG 4**).
- Reverse the vein graft and prepare for anastomosis.
- The vein is distended with heparinized saline, and veins are dilated.

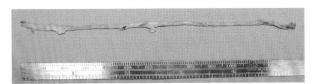

TECH FIG 4 • The vein graft is harvested and reversed. A saphenous vein graft is pictured here.

Microvascular Anastomoses

- The proximal anastomosis is done first. End-to-side or end-to-end anastomosis of the graft to the ulnar artery stump is performed (**TECH FIG 5A**).
- End-to-end or end-to-side anastomoses are performed to the superficial arch or the common digital arteries, as indicated by the amount of resected artery (**TECH FIG 5B**).

- Size discrepancy is managed by making a closing V in the vein graft, an opening V in the artery, a sleeve anastomosis, or a 30-degree oblique cut in the artery (**TECH FIG 5C**).
- If multiple anastomoses are required, end-to-end and end-to-side repairs can be performed serially.
- Intravenous heparin 2000 units is given prior to tourniquet release. Dextran 40 is started at 20 mL/h in the operating room and continued postoperatively.

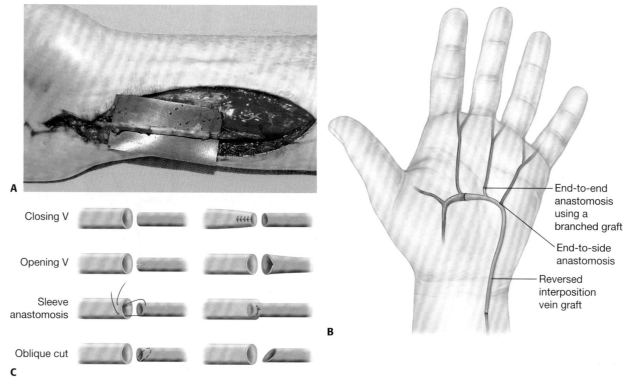

TECH FIG 5 • A. The vein graft is anastomosed into place. **B.** A branched graft is used in order to perform an end-to-end anastomosis to one common digital artery and end-to-side anastomoses to the remaining common digital arteries. **C.** Several methods of addressing an oversized vein graft are shown.

■ Assessing Flow and Closure

- Vascular clamps are released (or the tourniquet is deflated if this has not been done previously) after all anastomoses have been completed.
- Compress the radial artery manually for a few minutes to maximize flow across the anastomoses.
- Any leaks are repaired.

- A Doppler probe is used to assess distal arterial flow.
- Hemostasis is achieved.
- The wrist incision and vein donor sites are closed using 4-0 nylon sutures.
- Splint is placed to immobilize the operative site, with care to avoid any pressure on the underlying anastomosis.

PEARLS AND PITFALLS

Preoperative planning	▪ Adequate arterial inflow and distal runoff is essential.
Technique	▪ Resecting to normal intima is critical to success. ▪ Use an extensile incision. ▪ Close over a drain if indicated.
Vein grafting	▪ A vein graft with a larger diameter than the artery does not usually pose a problem, but a vein graft that is significantly smaller than the artery leads to higher rates of thrombosis. ▪ Anastomoses must be performed in a tension-free manner. ▪ Set the tension to prevent kinking. ▪ Avoid rotation of the graft. ▪ For the proximal anastomosis, end-to-end anastomosis is easier, but end-to-side anastomosis will help to maintain any remaining circulation to the hand from the ulnar artery.
Postoperative expectations	▪ Cold sensitivity is expected. ▪ Recurrent thrombosis is possible and has been reported up to 10 years postoperatively.

POSTOPERATIVE CARE

- The operative extremity is splinted from fingertips to elbow, with care to avoid pressure on the anastomosis.
- No nicotine, caffeine, or chocolate
- The patient's room is kept warm, or alternatively, we use a Bair Hugger over the operative extremity. The room should also remain quiet and free of unnecessary stimuli.
- Dextran 40 is continued at 20 mL/h for 2 to 5 days.
- The patient is given aspirin 81 mg daily for 3 months.
- Anxiolytics can be used to protect the patient from damaging the repair inadvertently.
- Sutures are removed at 10 to 14 days postoperative.
- The patient is kept off of work for at least 4 to 6 weeks, or potentially longer depending on the nature of his or her occupation.
- The patient is forever forbidden from using the hand as a hammer.

OUTCOMES

- Most patients have continued symptoms, but with decreased frequency and severity.
- In a series of 47 patients, Marie et al.[6] found that digital necrosis healed, and there was no recurrence of hypothenar hammer syndrome after surgical intervention.
  - Recurrence of hypothenar hammer syndrome was 27.7% after medical management. Of the patients in this study, 69.2% continued to smoke.
- Long-term patency rates of arterial grafts are higher than venous grafts. Venous graft patency ranges from 77% to 88%.[7]
- Chloros et al.[8] studied 13 patients who underwent reverse interpositional vein grafting for post-traumatic ulnar artery thrombosis with a minimum of 2-year follow-up.
  - Ten of 13 grafts (77%) were patent at final follow-up.

- Patients with patent grafts all significantly improved on the Levine symptom scale, McGill visual analog pain scale, McCabe cold sensitivity severity scale, and isolated cold stress testing.
- Patients with nonpatent grafts were more likely to complain of pain, numbness, and cold sensitivity.

COMPLICATIONS

- Persistent cold intolerance
- Thrombosis of the graft
- Donor site complications (neuroma)
- Wound healing complications
- Hand stiffness

REFERENCES

1. Coleman SS, Anson BJ. Arterial patterns in the hand based upon a study of 650 specimens. *Surg Gynecol Obstet*. 1961;4:409-424.
2. Kleinert JM, Fleming SG, Abel CS, et al. Radial and ulnar dominance in normal digits. *J Hand Surg Am*. 1989;14:504-508.
3. Levine DW, Simmons BP, Koris MJ, et al. A self-administered questionnaire for the assessment of severity of symptoms and functional status in carpal tunnel syndrome. *J Bone Joint Surg Am*. 1993;75A(11): 1585-1592.
4. McCabe SJ, Mizgala C, Glickman L. The measurement of cold sensitivity of the hand. *J Hand Surg Am*. 1991;16A(6):1037-1040.
5. Ruijs AC, Jaquet JB, Daanen HA, et al. Cold intolerance of the hand measured by the CISS questionnaire in a normative study population. *J Hand Surg Br*. 2006;31(5):533-536.
6. Marie I, Herve F, Primard E, et al. Long-term follow-up of hypothenar hammer syndrome: a series of 47 patients. *Medicine*. 2007;86(6): 334-343.
7. Hui-Chou HG, McClinton MA. Current options for treatment of hypothenar hammer syndrome. *Hand Clin*. 2015;31:53-62.
8. Chloros GD, Lucas RM, Li Z, et al. Post-traumatic ulnar artery thrombosis: outcome of arterial reconstruction using reverse interpositional vein grafting at 2 years minimum follow-up. *J Hand Surg Am*. 2008;33A:932-940.

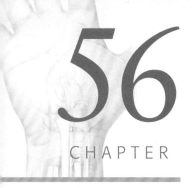

56 CHAPTER

Second Toe to Thumb Transfer

John R. Lien and Kevin C. Chung

DEFINITION

- The thumb is critical for hand function.
- Toe to thumb transfer is a composite tissue microsurgical reconstructive option for patients with loss of significant thumb length.

ANATOMY

- Great toe
  - Wider pulp and nail plate than native thumb and lesser toes; "thumblike" appearance
  - Significant aesthetic and functional morbidity at donor site; difficulty with push-off during gait
- Second toe
  - Pulp is bulbous and more rectangular in appearance than the native thumb or fingers.
  - Interphalangeal joints tend to claw.
  - Superior cosmetic and functional results on donor foot
- Arterial anatomy of the foot
  - The anterior tibial artery becomes the dorsalis pedis artery (DPA) distal to the ankle extensor retinaculum. The DPA courses along the dorsal foot lateral to the extensor hallucis longus tendon.
  - At the first intermetatarsal space, the DPA terminally divides into the first dorsal metatarsal artery (FDMA) and the deep plantar artery. The deep plantar artery communicates with the deep plantar arch of the foot, connecting the dorsal and plantar arches (**FIG 1**).
  - The FDMA generally travels deep to the extensor hallucis brevis tendon and usually dorsal to the first dorsal interosseous muscle. It then communicates (through the distal communicating artery) with the first plantar metatarsal artery (FPMA) distal to the deep intermetatarsal ligament. The FDMA also terminally branches into the lateral dorsal digital artery of the great toe and medial dorsal digital artery of the second toe, which are of small caliber and clinically insignificant[1] (see **FIG 1**).
  - **FIG 2** shows variants of FDMA anatomy in relation to the first dorsal interosseous muscle, as well as a variant unfavorable for vascular anastomosis.
  - The plantar digital arteries are the effective blood source to the great and second toes. Their origin is the distal communicating artery connecting the FDMA and FPDA distally (**FIG 3**).
- Venous anatomy of foot
  - The superficial dorsal venous system is utilized for venous anastomosis.
  - The dorsal veins of the toes join the dorsal venous arch in the forefoot, which supplies the greater and lesser saphenous veins.

- Sensory nerve anatomy of foot
  - The superficial peroneal nerve innervates the dorsal foot while the deep peroneal nerve innervates the first dorsal web space.
  - Branches from the posterior tibial nerve innervate the plantar foot and toe pulps. Coaptation of plantar digital nerves are important for pulp sensation.

PATIENT HISTORY AND PHYSICAL FINDINGS

- Advanced age is not a contraindication to surgery, but the patient must be in generally good health to tolerate a prolonged surgery.
- Active nicotine use and a history of atherosclerotic disease are contraindications to toe transfer.
- Assess whether there is adequate, supple skin coverage. If not, consider a staged procedure (groin flap) to increase pliable tissue at the recipient site. Harvesting too much soft tissue from the foot will lead to foot deformity and marked donor-site morbidity.

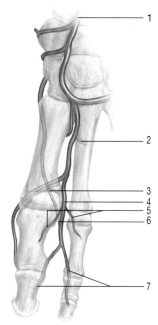

FIG 1 • Dorsal foot arterial anatomy: (*1*) dorsalis pedis artery (DPA), (*2*) deep plantar artery, (*3*) first plantar metatarsal artery (FPMA), (*4*) first dorsal metatarsal artery (FDMA), (*5*) dorsal digital arteries, (*6*) distal communicating branch (intersection of the FDMA and FPMA), (*7*) plantar digital arteries.

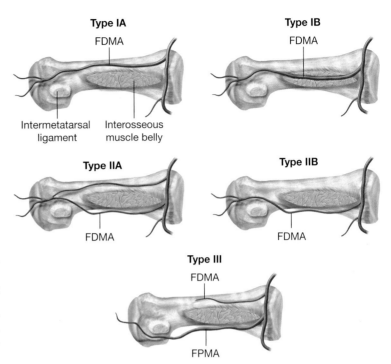

FIG 2 • Variants of first dorsal metatarsal artery (*FDMA*) anatomy. In type I, the FDMA passes superficial (IA) or within (IA) the interosseous muscle belly. In type II, the FDMA passes at the deep aspect of the interosseous muscle belly but superficial to the intermetatarsal ligament. Type IIA includes a fine accessory branch superficial to the interosseous muscle, whereas IIB does not have an accessory branch. In type III, the FDMA is miniscule or absent with plantar-dominant (*FPMA*) flow.

- The level of thumb amputation will dictate harvest length.
- Assess the donor foot (contralateral foot for second toe transfer) to ensure no prior trauma or surgery that would alter vascular anatomy to the second toe. Doppler ultrasound examination can be used to confirm presence of DPA and FDMA.

IMAGING

- Review preoperative radiographs of the recipient site to prepare for bone fixation and length requirement of donor toe (**FIG 4**).
- We do not routinely obtain preoperative angiography of the foot, but this is an option if there is concern for altered vascular anatomy on physical and Doppler exam.

SURGICAL MANAGEMENT

- Toe to thumb transfer is generally performed after the acute traumatic injury has healed and adequate soft tissue coverage is obtained.
- Ensure adequate soft tissue coverage and pliability prior to transfer.
- Amputations through the thumb metacarpal (with preserved carpometacarpal joint) or proximal half of the proximal phalanx are good candidates for toe transfer. We prefer the second toe transfer to minimize donor-site morbidity. Other options for toe transfer include great toe and trimmed great toe. Alternatives to toe transfer include metacarpal bone lengthening and on-top plasty. Osteoplastic reconstruction of the thumb using iliac crest bone graft and groin flap is of historical significance only.

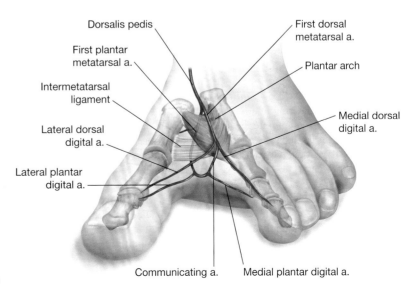

FIG 3 • First web space arterial anatomy.

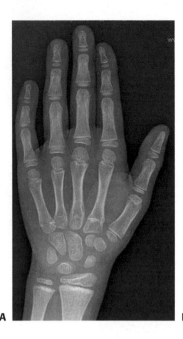
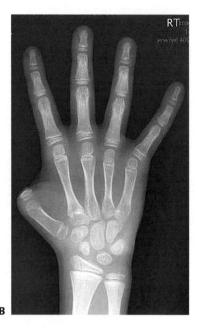

FIG 4 • Preoperative radiograph of recipient hand. Amputation level is at the proximal phalanx base. Contralateral radiographs help estimate defect length.

- Amputations at the distal proximal phalanx or distal phalanx often retain enough length for thumb function. Web space deepening may be performed as needed.
- Amputations through the base of the metacarpal or though the carpometacarpal joint require index finger pollicization to recreate a basilar thumb joint.

Preoperative Planning

- The contralateral toe vascular pedicle is in a better position for radial artery anastomosis at the snuffbox.
- The length of the transferred toe should be based on the length of the contralateral uninjured thumb (see **FIG 4**).
- A two-team approach is preferable to minimize operative time. One team prepares the recipient site while the other harvests the contralateral toe.

- Good communication between teams is necessary to harvest tendons, nerves, and vessels of adequate length and caliber for primary repair.

Positioning

- Supine
- General anesthesia
- Thigh and arm tourniquets
- The recipient upper extremity and contralateral donor lower extremity are prepped.

Approach

- For second toe transfer as well as great toe transfer, the FDMA is the preferred arterial supply.
  - However, one may need to alter the approach and harvest the FPMA if it is dominant (about 20% of cases).

■ Foot Exposure and Second Toe Harvest

- Identify and mark the DPA and FDMA using Doppler ultrasound probe.
- Identify the course of the dorsal forefoot veins to the greater saphenous vein on the dorsomedial foot.
- Design dorsal and plantar curvilinear incisions on the dorsal and plantar foot (**TECH FIG 1A,B**).
  - Avoid incision over the thick plantar skin overlying the weight-bearing first metatarsal head.
- Gravity exsanguinate the limb and inflate the tourniquet.
- Perform an incision over the first web space and identify the vascular pattern of the FDMA using retrograde dissection (**TECH FIG 1C**). Be sure to visualize the proper palmar digital artery to the second toe.
  - A dorsal-dominant system is present in most cases. In this case, continue proximal dissection along the FDMA and DPA after ligating the communicating branch to the proximal FPMA. If necessary, perform intramuscular dissection through the first dorsal interosseous muscle. If planning an osteotomy of the second metacarpal shaft to restore length of significant metacarpal thumb

defects, preserve the vascular connections between the FDMA and second metatarsal. This is performed by preserving the interposed interosseous muscle.
  - If the patient has a plantar-dominant system, divide the deep intermetatarsal ligament and dissect the FPMA proximally. We often do dissect out the more inaccessible FPMA in case the dorsal circulation is insufficient to perfuse the toe, which may require anastomosis of the FPMA.
- Extend the dorsal incision proximally and identify the dorsal vein to the second toe, and extensor digitorum longus. The extensor digitorum brevis is divided (**TECH FIG 1D,E**).
- Perform the plantar curvilinear incision and identify the flexor digitorum profundus tendon and both plantar digital nerves (**TECH FIG 1F**).
- Perform the osteotomy at the planned level with a microsagittal saw while protecting identified structures.
  - Alternatively, a metatarsophalangeal disarticulation is an option depending on length needs. Detach the collateral ligaments and volar plate from the metatarsal head.

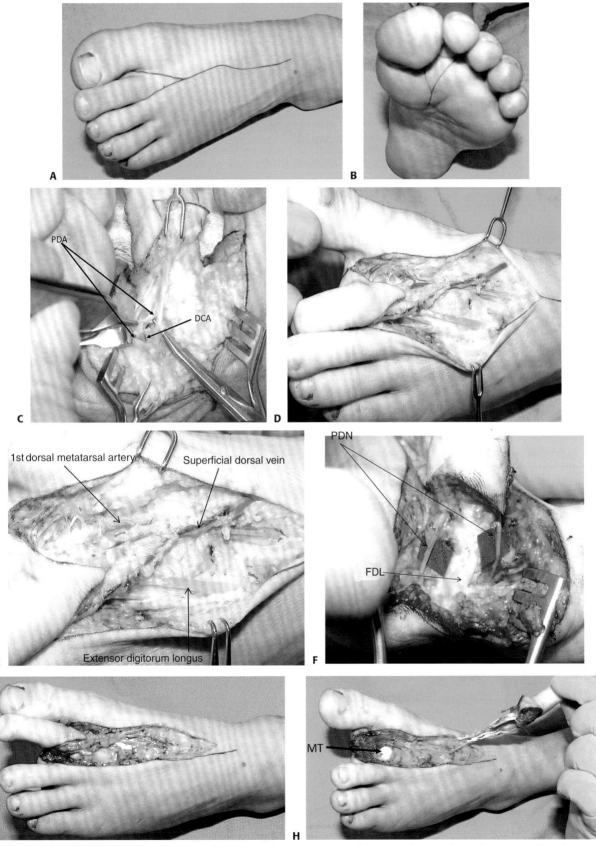

TECH FIG 1 • **A,B.** Donor foot incisions. Dorsal and plantar curvilinear incisions avoid the weight-bearing plantar first metatarsal head. **C.** First web space dissection. Note the palmar digital arteries (*PDA*) and the distal communicating artery (*DCA*) to the FPMA. The forceps is overlying the FDMA. **D,E.** Dorsal exposure of second toe. **F.** Plantar foot dissection. Note the plantar digital nerves (*PDN*) and flexor digitorum longus (*FDL*). **G,H.** Completion of second toe harvest. In this case, a metatarsophalangeal disarticulation was performed. Note the metatarsal head (*MT*) in the wound.

TECHNIQUES

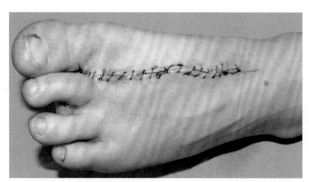
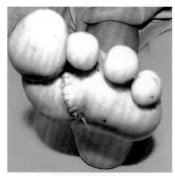

TECH FIG 1 (Continued) • **I,J.** Donor foot closure. Note preservation of the longitudinal and transverse arches of the foot.

- Determine the proper length of appropriate structures in the toe. Divide the nerves and tendons, taking care to tag the nerves with fine suture (6-0 Prolene) for easy identification. Leave the vessels intact.
- Deflate the tourniquet and check perfusion of the toe. It may take 5 minutes of warming the toe before adequate perfusion is seen.

- Once adequate perfusion is appreciated and the recipient site is ready, detach the dorsalis pedis artery and dorsal vein (**TECH FIG 1G,H**).
- Use nonabsorbable suture to repair the deep intermetatarsal ligament if transected.
- Obtain hemostasis and then close the wound primarily (**TECH FIG 1I,J**).

■ Recipient Site Preparation

- Create an incision at the thumb amputation stump and extend it proximally with a dorsal zigzag incision toward the anatomical snuffbox (**TECH FIG 2A,B**).
  - If previous soft tissue transfer was performed, elevate the margin of the tissue flap dorsally.
- Identify the radial artery at the snuffbox, cephalic vein, and dorsal branch of superficial radial nerve (**TECH FIG 2C,D**).
- Identify the residual extensor pollicis longus (EPL) tendon and perform a tenolysis to ensure free gliding. If the

EPL is not salvageable, transfer the extensor indicis proprius (EIP) tendon.
- Extend the incision on the palmar residual thumb to identify the digital nerves of the thumb and flexor pollicis longus (FPL) tendon. A counterincision may be necessary at the carpal tunnel to retrieve the FPL tendon.
- Debride the residual metacarpal or proximal phalangeal bone of any fibrous scar or articular remnants. Preserve thenar muscle attachments to the metacarpal.

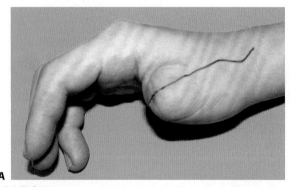
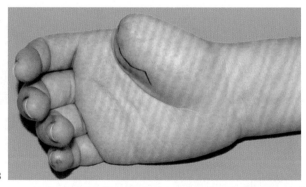

TECH FIG 2 • **A,B.** Dorsal and palmar thumb incisions. The dorsal incision must extend proximally to the anatomical snuffbox to allow for arterial anastomosis to the radial artery.

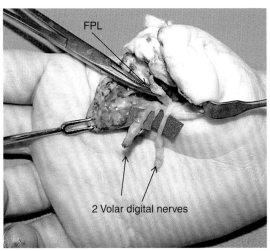
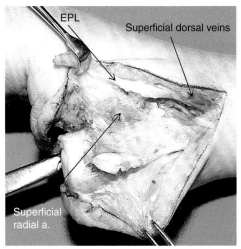

TECH FIG 2 (Continued) • **C,D.** Recipient site preparation. FPL, flexor pollicis longus; EPL, extensor pollicis longus.

▪ Transfer of Second Toe

- Kirschner wire, 90-90 intraosseous wiring, and rigid plate fixation are options for bone fixation.
  - We prefer two longitudinal Kirschner wires for ease of fixation and less soft tissue dissection inherent with plate fixation.
    - However, using plate fixation does have the advantage of initiating more aggressive tendon gliding exercises.
- After bone fixation, the flexor digitorum profundus tendon of the toe is transferred to the FPL tendon using four- or six-core strand repair technique.
- The extensor digitorum longus is weaved to the EPL or EIP tendon using Pulvertaft technique. Tension this weave tightly.

- Using microsurgical technique, the radial and ulnar digital arteries are coapted as distally as possible to promote early sensory recovery.
- Repair any branches of the superficial radial nerve to the superficial and deep peroneal nerves dorsally.
- The arterial anastomosis is performed in an end-to-side fashion to the radial artery at the snuffbox. The venous anastomosis is then performed to a dorsal hand vein, feeding into the cephalic vein.
- The transferred toe is warmed, and perfusion is assessed.
- The wounds are then closed loosely to avoid compression of the dorsal anastomoses (**TECH FIG 3**).

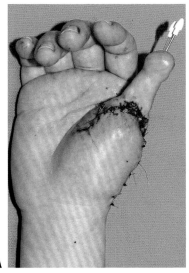
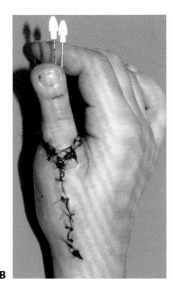

TECH FIG 3 • **A,B.** Thumb closure.

PEARLS AND PITFALLS

Preoperative evaluation	▪ Ensure adequate soft tissue coverage and pliability prior to transfer. Otherwise, wound closure will be difficult and cause potential compression of the vascular anastomosis.
FDMA dissection	▪ Retrograde dissection of the first web space facilitates efficient identification of the variations in FDMA anatomy. Identify the FDMA, the distal communicating artery to the FPMA, and the medial and lateral plantar digital arteries to the great and second toe, respectively.
FPMA dominant pedicle harvest	▪ If there is only one sizeable vessel that is plantar to the deep intermetatarsal ligament, the toe pedicle should be harvested based on the FPMA through the plantar incision. The dissection is challenging proximal to the metatarsal neck, and for this reason, we avoid more proximal dissection and use an interpositional vein graft to augment our arterial pedicle length.
Claw deformity of the transferred toe	▪ The lesser toes tend to form claw deformities at the interphalangeal joint. If this causes a functional problem for the patient in subsequent follow-up, consider interphalangeal joint arthrodesis.

POSTOPERATIVE CARE

- The hand is placed in a well-padded volar forearm-based thumb spica splint with dorsal window and elevated at heart level in a warm room.
- Transferred digit skin color, capillary refill, and Doppler ultrasound checks are performed hourly for the first 48 hours.
- Oral aspirin is administered daily for 2 weeks.
- Prophylactic heparin or low molecular weight heparin anticoagulation per inpatient hospital protocol is performed.

- Patient is kept non–weight bearing to the donor foot for two weeks until sutures are removed.
- At 4 to 6 weeks postoperatively, we remove the Kirschner wires and begin tendon motion protocol.

OUTCOMES

- Toe to hand transfer is a safe procedure, with approximately 95% success rate in experienced centers (**FIG 5**).

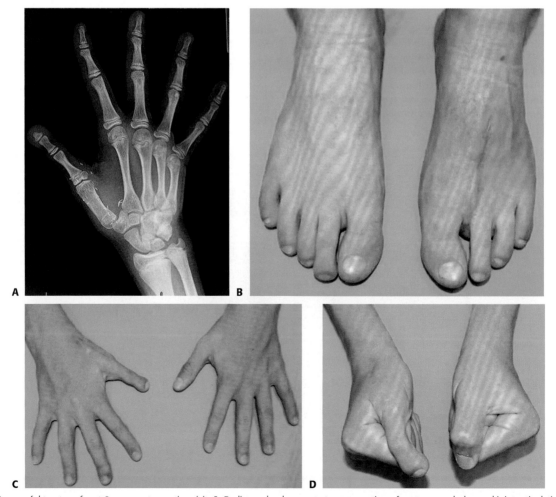

FIG 5 • Successful toe transfer at 6-year postoperative visit. **A.** Radiographs demonstrate preservation of metacarpophalangeal joint articulation. **B.** Donor site with mild hypertrophic scar but overall good aesthetic appearance. **C,D.** Clinical photographs of hand.

- Toe transfer patients have superior outcomes in overall hand function, activities of daily living, work performance, aesthetics, and satisfaction compared to patients with thumb MCP level amputations without reconstruction.[2]
- Average static two-point discrimination is approximately 8 mm at long-term follow-up.[3]
- Average digit mobility was 33 degrees of flexion with extensor lag of 34.5 degrees at long-term follow-up for second toe to long finger transfer.[3]

COMPLICATIONS

- Arterial vasospasm is a potential complication and may occur within the first three days postoperatively.
  - If spasm occurs, consider loosening the dorsal sutures, placing the hand in a more dependent position, and use a warming lamp or warming blanket.
  - Papaverine or lidocaine can be injected.
  - Regional nerve block with a continuous flow catheter can be attempted.
  - If there is no improvement, return to the operative room and explore the anastomosis for thrombosis or compressive hematoma.
- If there is development of significant vascular congestion, loosen dorsal sutures and any potentially compressive dressings.
  - Consider venous exploration if there is no clinical improvement.

REFERENCES

1. May JW Jr, Chait LA, Cohen BE, O'Brien BM. Free neurovascular flap from the first web of the foot in hand reconstruction. *J Hand Surg [Am]*. 1977;2(5):387-393.
2. Chung KC, Wei FC. An outcome study of thumb reconstruction using microvascular toe transfer. *J Hand Surg [Am]*. 2000;25:651-658.
3. Foucher G, Moss AL. Microvascular second toe to finger transfer: a statistical analysis of 55 transfers. *Br J Plast Surg*. 1991;44(2):87-90.

57
CHAPTER

Dupuytren Contracture

John R. Lien and Kevin C. Chung

DEFINITION

- Dupuytren disease is a benign fibroproliferative disorder affecting the palmar and digital fascia of the hand.
- Dupuytren disease can result in progressive contracture of the metacarpophalangeal (MCP) and proximal interphalangeal (PIP) joints.

ANATOMY

- The palmar fascia consists of thenar, hypothenar, and central palmar aponeuroses.
- The palmar aponeurosis (PA) is usually involved with Dupuytren disease.
  - It is triangular with a proximal apex confluent with the palmaris longus tendon.
- The PA is a three-dimensional structure consisting of longitudinal, transverse, and vertical fibers (**FIG 1A**).
  - Longitudinal fibers fan out as pretendinous bands that bifurcate and divide into three layers extending to the distal palm (**FIG 1B**).
    - The first layer inserts into the dermis of the distal palm.
    - The second layer continues toward the digit as the spiral band, which lies deep to the natatory ligament and neurovascular bundle at the level of the palmodigital crease.

- The third, deepest layer passes vertically toward the flexor tendon sheath.
  - Transverse fibers form the natatory ligament in the distal palm and the superficial transverse palmar ligament more proximally.
  - Vertical fibers form the septa of Legueu and Juvara, which lie deep to the palmar fascia (**FIG 1C**). These eight septa form seven fibro-osseous compartments separating the flexor tendons from the lumbricals and neurovascular bundles. Superficial vertical bands of Grapow insert into the dermis of the palmar skin.
- Digital fascia
  - Grayson ligament is palmar to the neurovascular bundle.
  - Cleland ligament is dorsal to the neurovascular bundle.
  - The lateral digital sheet receives contributions from the natatory ligament and spiral band (**FIG 2**).
- PIP joint
  - The proximal attachment of the volar plate tapers into separate radial and ulnar bands, termed the checkrein ligaments (**FIG 3**).
  - The accessory collateral ligament arises from the head of the proximal phalanx and inserts on the volar plate.
    - The accessory collateral ligaments become lax in flexion and taut in extension.

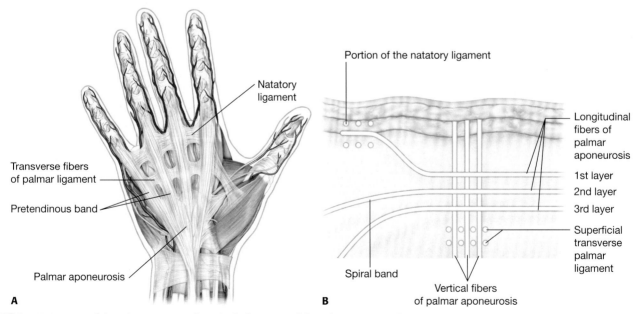

Natatory ligament

Transverse fibers of palmar ligament

Pretendinous band

Palmar aponeurosis

Portion of the natatory ligament

Longitudinal fibers of palmar aponeurosis

1st layer

2nd layer

3rd layer

Superficial transverse palmar ligament

Spiral band

Vertical fibers of palmar aponeurosis

A

B

FIG 1 • **A.** Anatomy of the palmar aponeurosis. **B.** Sagittal anatomy of the palmar aponeurosis.

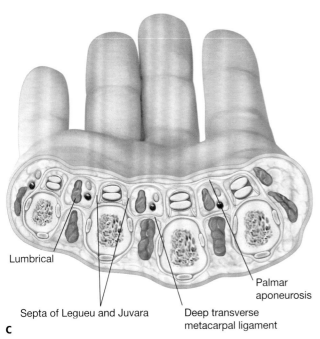

FIG 1 (Continued) • **C.** Septa of Legueu and Juvara are formed from the vertical deep extensions of the palmar aponeurosis.

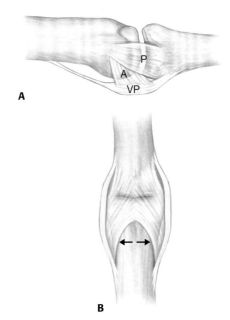

FIG 3 • Lateral **(A)** and volar **(B)** representations of the soft tissue support at the PIP joint. *Arrows* indicate the radial and ulnar checkrein ligaments. A, accessory collateral ligament; P, proper collateral ligament; VP, volar plate.

PATHOGENESIS

- Nodules are often the first sign of Dupuytren disease. They are found superficially in the palm or finger, adherent to the dermis and underlying fascia.
- Normal fascial bands become pathologic cords.
- The pretendinous cord develops from the pretendinous band.
  - Cords are pathologic structures, whereas bands are normal structures.

- Isolated pretendinous cords can result in MCP joint contracture.
- The spiral cord is composed of pathologic pretendinous band, spiral band, lateral digital sheet, and Grayson ligament.
  - The spiral course of this cord around the neurovascular bundle causes proximal, superficial, and central displacement of the bundle as it contracts (**FIG 4**).
- Spiral cords can cause MCP and PIP joint contracture.

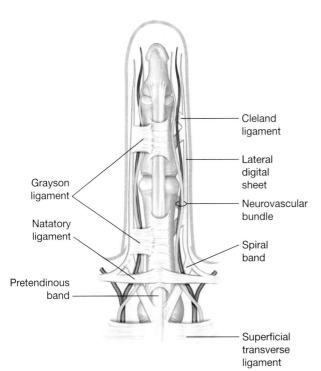

FIG 2 • Digital fascia. Note the contributions of the natatory ligament and spiral band to the lateral digital sheet.

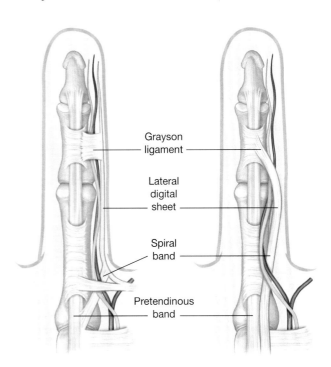

FIG 4 • In contrast to normal spiral cord anatomy (*left*), pathologic spiral cord anatomy (*right*) can displace the neurovascular bundle.

- The natatory cord can cause web space contracture.
- The central cord is a distal extension of the pretendinous cord in the palm but does not cause neurovascular bundle displacement.
- The lateral cord is diseased lateral digital sheet and can cause PIP joint contracture.
- The abductor digiti minimi cord runs from the abductor digiti minimi fascia to the base of the middle phalanx and can displace the neurovascular bundle toward the midline.
- The retrovascular cord causes flexion contracture of the distal interphalangeal joint.

NATURAL HISTORY

- Early presentation of Dupuytren disease causes isolated nodules and skin pitting.
- With progression of disease, pathologic cords will form.
- As cords contract, the MCP and PIP joints may be drawn into flexion.
- Fixed PIP joint contractures may develop over time.

PATIENT HISTORY AND PHYSICAL FINDINGS

- Patients with Dupuytren disease are commonly older men with northern European ancestry but can present in all ethnic groups and both genders.
- Dupuytren diathesis describes a predisposition toward aggressive disease and increased recurrence after surgical treatment. Five factors[1]:
  - Male gender
  - Age of onset younger than 50 years
  - Family history with one or more affected siblings/parents
  - Ectopic lesions in the dorsal hand (Garrod pads)
  - Bilateral disease
- Palpate for thick, diffuse disease in the palm and finger, compared to discrete well-defined cords.
- Document the degree of MCP and PIP joint contracture.
  - If the cord spans the MCP and PIP joints, assess for fixed PIP contracture by testing passive PIP extension with the MP joint in maximal flexion.
- Examine for web space contracture.
- Carefully document the sensory examination, particularly if the patient has had previous surgery.

IMAGING

- Radiographs are obtained if there is a significant PIP joint flexion contracture.
  - Assess for articular congruency or arthritic change.

NONOPERATIVE MANAGEMENT

- Observation is appropriate for mild disease without compromise of function and minimal contracture.
- Percutaneous needle aponeurotomy (PNA) is mechanical division of a Dupuytren cord with the bevel of a hypodermic needle.
- Collagenase *Clostridium histolyticum* (CCH; Xiaflex, Auxilium Pharmaceuticals, Inc., Malvern, PA) is an enzyme used for nonsurgical chemical division of Dupuytren cords. CCH therapy received Food and Drug Administration approval in 2010.[2]

- Consider CCH and PNA as a minimally invasive option for patients with discrete cords who meet indications for surgery. Patients may:
  - Wish to avoid the recovery associated with surgery
  - Have significant medical comorbidities precluding surgery
- We offer these minimally invasive options to patients with discrete palpable cords.

SURGICAL MANAGEMENT

- Limited fasciectomy excises diseased palmar and digital fascia. This is the most widely used surgical technique for Dupuytren contracture.
  - We prefer limited fasciectomy for patients with diffuse disease and severe PIP joint contractures or those who have failed PNA and/or CCH therapy.
- Indications for limited fasciectomy include the following:
  - Palpable disease with flexion contracture of the MCP joint greater than 30 degrees
  - Palpable disease with flexion contracture of the PIP joint greater than 15 degrees
- The "surgical techniques" discussed in this chapter include minimally invasive techniques discussed in nonoperative management (CCH and PNA).

Preoperative Planning

- Long-standing PIP joint contractures may persist after cord division or excision.
  - Consider PIP joint capsulotomy and checkrein release if residual contracture is present.
  - Review hand radiographs if the patient has significant contractures of the PIP joint. Consider arthrodesis in the setting of severe contracture or articular degeneration.

Positioning

- PNA
  - This procedure can be performed in an office procedure room or in the operating room.
  - Explain the procedure to the patient so that he/she will be prepared to participate.
  - Supine positioning with a hand table or padded Mayo stand.
- CCH
  - The patient is positioned sitting upright with the affected hand on the examination table.
  - Alternatively, position the patient supine with the hand on a Mayo stand.
- Limited fasciectomy
  - Upper arm tourniquet
  - Regional or general anesthesia
  - Supine positioning with a hand table

Approach

- PNA
  - The importance of reporting paresthesias or numbness to the fingertips is reviewed with the patient. Establish a baseline "normal sensation" to light touch of the radial and ulnar finger pulp.

- Have the patient demonstrate short arc motion of the PIP and DIP joints; this will be useful to rule out intratendinous needle placement.
  - Cords are approached from distal to proximal for nerve monitoring.
  - Anesthetic is injected intradermally to avoid digital nerve anesthesia.
- CCH
  - Initial on-label use involved the injection of one cord at a time, and finger extension manipulation was recommended post injection day one. Recent studies broadened this approach.
  - Coleman et al.[3] concluded that two affected joint contractures can be effectively and safely treated with concurrent injections. The incidence of multiple adverse events was higher, but the incidence of severe adverse events was not greater than single cord injection.
  - Compared to 1-day postinjection manipulation, 7-day postinjection manipulation had no significant differences in correction, pain, or skin tears.[4] This suggests manipulation can be scheduled within the first 7 days after injection.
- Limited fasciectomy
  - Surgical incisions are variable and depend on the location of the cord (**FIG 5**).
  - Hand: For extensive palmar disease, make a transverse incision at the distal palmar crease.

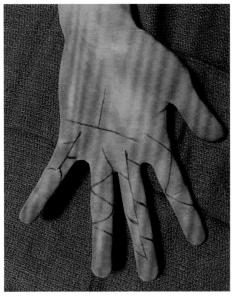

FIG 5 • Skin incisions for palmar fasciectomy.

- If there is significant MCP contracture, the distal palmar crease is left open to heal by secondary intention.
- Consider PIP joint volar capsulotomy if there is residual joint contracture after fasciectomy.

Percutaneous Needle Aponeurotomy

- Prepare the hand with antiseptic solution.
- Plan and mark fasciotomy portals in areas with supple skin overlying a discrete linear cord (**TECH FIG 1A**). The cord should change from soft to firm with joint extension.
  - Portals are placed directly over the cord or along each side of the cord if it is broad.
  - Space portals out at least 5 mm.
- Avoid portals over nodules.
- Avoid portals in skin creases because of:
  - Risk of skin tears
  - Proximity to flexor tendons
- Use a small probe to evaluate portals near skin dimples. To avoid entering a pit, avoid making the portal too close to the dimple sinus.
- Use a 30-gauge needle and inject 0.05 to 0.10 mL of anesthetic at the most distal portal site (**TECH FIG 1B**).
  - Penetrate into the dermis and then inject as the needle is withdrawn.
  - Do not inject subcutaneously.
- Place a 5/8-in. 25-gauge needle into the portal, with the needle bevel perpendicular to the cord fibers (**TECH FIG 1C**).
  - Nerve assessment: Ask the patient if he or she feels pain, paresthesia, or electric shocks along the finger. Reassess sensation to light touch along the side of the digit.
  - Tendon assessment: Have the patient slightly flex and extend the PIP and DIP joints. The needle should be withdrawn more superficial if there is needle bowing with flexor tendon excursion.

- Repeatedly check nerve and tendon proximity to ensure the safety of the current portal.[5]
  - If the fingertip is numb, remove needle from current portal and move to a proximal portal.
  - If it is not, and the finger AROM does not catch the needle, continue with the current portal.
  - However, if the fingertip is not numb and the finger AROM *does* catch the needle, remove needle from current portal and move to a proximal portal.
- Hold tension on the cord by pulling adjacent skin or nodules.
  - Tension allows the needle to cut and moves the cord away from underlying structures.
- The cutting edge of the needle is used as a scalpel to divide the cord fibers deep to the dermis. Three maneuvers are performed (**TECH FIG 1D**)[5]:
  - Clear: Use a side-to-side motion to clear a plane between the dermis and cord.
  - Perforate.
    - Orient the needle vertically with the bevel transverse, and perforate the needle through the cord.
    - Pull the needle back superficial to the cord but still deep to dermis.
    - Using this up-and-down motion, move the needle radially and ulnarly to make multiple perforations at the level of the portal along the width of the cord.
    - Tactile feedback is important during this procedure, as one should feel a crackly or grating sensation as the bevel cuts the fascia.

TECHNIQUES

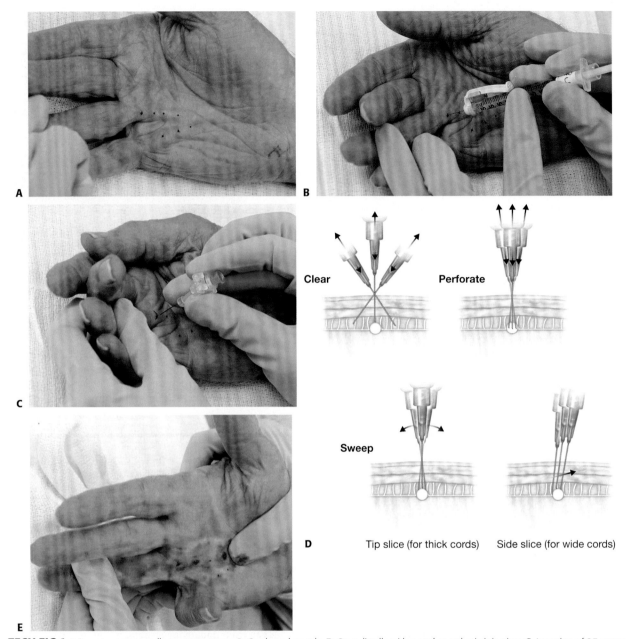

TECH FIG 1 • Percutaneous needle aponeurotomy. **A.** Cords and portals. **B.** Start distally with portal anesthetic injection. **C.** Insertion of 25-gauge needle with bevel perpendicular to cord. Left thumb is used to hold tension on the cord without extending the digit. **D.** Needle maneuvers. **E.** Ring finger manipulation to rupture cord.

- Sweep
  - Once the cord is defined and perforated, use the needle bevel to transversely sweep across the width of the cord, from superficial to deep.
  - Tactile feedback should include a scraping sensation with the needle.
  - Avoid being overaggressive to avoid neurovascular or tendon injury deep to the cord.
  - Rupture can be achieved without complete needle transection of the cord.
- If the patient reports shooting or electric pain along the finger at any time, reposition the needle to avoid nerve injury.

- Move from distal to proximal portals and repeat the anesthetic injection and needle process.
  - Passively stretch after each portal release to attempt to rupture the cord (**TECH FIG 1D**).
  - If a portal looks concerning for skin tear, avoid manipulation until more proximal portals are established.
- When the cord ruptures, an audible "pop" may be heard.
- Reassess for residual flexion contracture.
  - If there is still palpable cord proximally, reassess for more portal placement and further fasciotomy.
  - Remember to monitor the nerve and tendon.
- Once the procedure is complete, apply a Band-Aid on the portal sites. If a skin tear occurs, apply a soft bandage.

■ Collagenase Therapy[6]

- Before use, allow the vial containing the powder form of collagenase and the vial containing the diluent for reconstitution to stand at room temperature for 15 to 60 minutes. Remove the flip-off caps and clean the surface of the vials with alcohol (**TECH FIG 2A**).
- Using a 1-mL syringe with a 27-gauge 0.5-in. needle, withdraw the appropriate volume of diluent from the diluent vial (see package insert):
  - 0.39 mL for cords affecting the MCP joint
  - 0.31 mL for cords affecting the PIP joint
- Inject the diluent slowly into the sides of the vial containing the powder form of Xiaflex.
- Slowly swirl the vial to ensure the powder is in solution. The reconstituted solution should be clear.
- Using a new 1-mL syringe with a 27-gauge 0.5-in. needle, withdraw the appropriate volume of reconstituted solution (containing 0.58 mg of Xiaflex):
  - 0.25 mL for cords affecting the MCP joint
  - 0.20 mL for cords affecting the PIP joint
- Do not inject local anesthetic as the tumescence may interfere with proper placement of the Xiaflex injection.
- Confirm the cord to be injected. The ideal site should be where the cord is maximally separated from the underlying flexor tendon and where the skin is not intimately adhered to the cord (**TECH FIG 2B**).
- Clean the injection site with an antiseptic.
- With the nondominant hand, secure the patient's hand and apply tension to the cord.
- With the dominant hand, place the needle into the cord, taking care to keep the needle within the cord.

- If there is concern that the needle is in the flexor tendon, passively move the distal interphalangeal joint to assess for tension on the needle.
  - Reposition the needle as necessary.
- Once you are satisfied with needle placement, inject one-third of the dose into the cord (**TECH FIG 2C**).
- Next, withdraw the needle and reposition it slightly more distally in the cord (2–3 mm) and inject another one-third of the dose.
- Finally, withdraw the needle and position it in the cord proximal to the initial site of injection (2–3 mm) and inject the remaining dose into the cord.
- When administering two concurrent injections, use separate vials and syringes for each cord.
  - For multiple digit injections, begin with the more ulnar digit.
  - For multiple cords in one digit, begin injections in the proximal cord and move to the more distal cord (move from the MCP joint to the PIP joint).
- Place the treated hand in a soft bulky dressing.
- Patient should follow up 1 to 7 days post injection.
- Assess the cord for autorupture.
- Assess the involved joint range of motion.
- Apply local anesthetic to the area of manipulation.
- For MCP joint cords, apply extension force to the MCP joint while the wrist is held in a flexed position.
- For PIP joint cords, perform the finger extension maneuver with the MCP joint in a flexed position.
- Hold moderate extension pressure for 10 to 20 seconds.
- If the cord is not disrupted, second and third manipulation attempts are performed at 5- to 10-minute intervals.
- If the cord does not disrupt after three attempts, additional collagenase injections and manipulation are performed after 4 weeks.

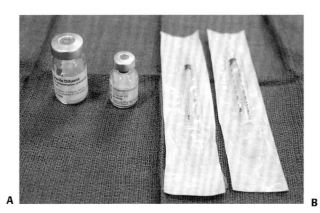

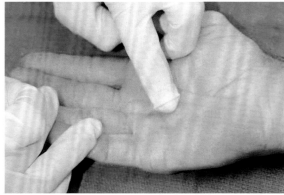

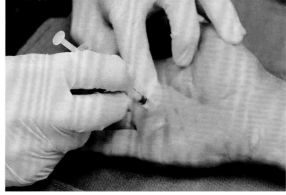

TECH FIG 2 • Collagenase therapy. **A.** Powder, diluent, and needles for reconstitution and injection. **B.** Palpation of a pretendinous ring finger cord. **C.** Collagenase injection. Note multiple sites of injection along the cord.

T E C H N I Q U E S

■ Limited Fasciectomy

- If there is widespread disease in the palm, make a transverse incision in the distal palmar crease to allow access (see **FIG 5**).
- Make an oblique longitudinal incision proximally toward the apex of the palmar aponeurosis.
- Make an incision from the distal palmar crease to the palmodigital crease.
  - This incision can be extended distally in the digit if there is digital involvement.
- If there is digital extension of disease, we prefer to extend the incision using modified Bruner incisions or a longitudinal midline incision with V-shaped extension (**TECH FIG 3A,B**).
- Raise skin flaps off the diseased fascia, taking care not to buttonhole through the dermis.
- Identify the neurovascular bundles proximally.
- Release the pretendinous cord proximally (**TECH FIG 3C**).
  - The MCP joint should extend, allowing better access and visualization distally.

- In the digit, raise full-thickness skin flaps and identify the neurovascular bundle proximally.
- Carefully dissect the neurovascular bundle from the cord from proximal to distal.
  - If the pretendinous cord extends into a spiral cord, the neurovascular bundle will be displaced proximal, toward the midline of the ray, and superficial. The cord will spiral deep and from central to lateral to the neurovascular bundle as it extends into the lateral digital sheet (**TECH FIG 3C**; see **FIG 4**).
- Once the neurovascular structures are identified and protected along the involved cord (**TECH FIG 3D**), separate and excise the diseased cord from the surrounding tissue.
- Reassess for residual joint contracture.
  - If there is a persistent PIP joint contracture after fasciectomy, consider volar capsulotomy.
- After fasciectomy and any other concurrent procedures, release the tourniquet.
  - Hemostasis is critical to prevent hematoma formation.
- If a longitudinal incision is made, make a Z-plasty at the flexion creases to prevent scar contracture (**TECH FIG 3E**).

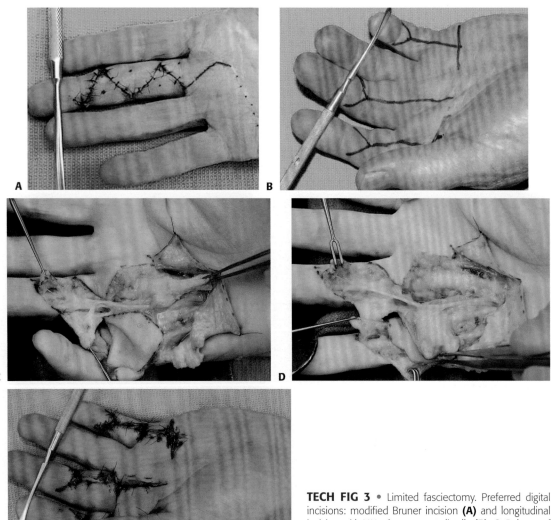

TECH FIG 3 • Limited fasciectomy. Preferred digital incisions: modified Bruner incision **(A)** and longitudinal incision with V-Y advancement distally **(B)**. **C.** Release of pretendinous cord proximally. Note course of ulnar spiral cord (*blue*, dorsal to nerve) and digital nerve (*yellow*, superficial). **D.** After excision of spiral cord. **E.** Closure of incision after Z-plasty across flexion creases.

- Close the skin loosely.
  - Leave the transverse palm incision open to heal with secondary intention if there is significant tension with MCP joint extension.
  - The open palm technique will also decrease the risk of hematoma formation.

- Apply a volar forearm-based extension splint.
  - If digital perfusion is compromised in full extension, allow the digit to remain slightly flexed. This can occur after correction of severe contractures.

PIP Joint Volar Capsulotomy

- If there is persistent PIP joint flexion contracture after fasciectomy, consider volar plate release.
- Identify and release the A3 pulley.
- Retract the flexor tendons with a Ragnell retractor.
- Identify the proximal volar plate, and release the check-rein ligaments (**TECH FIG 4**).
- If necessary, release the accessory collateral ligaments, which course from the condyle to the lateral edge of the volar plate.
- Gentle passive extension of the PIP joint should be achieved after sufficient release.
  - Reassess the vascularity of the digit with the joint fully extended. Splint in as much flexion as necessary to preserve perfusion to the digit.

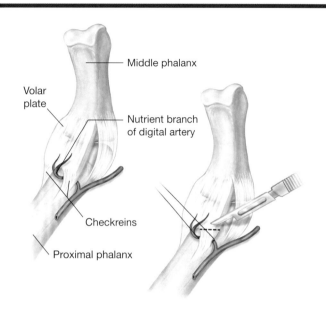

Middle phalanx

Volar plate

Nutrient branch of digital artery

Checkreins

Proximal phalanx

TECH FIG 4 • Checkrein ligament release.

PEARLS AND PITFALLS

Indications	▪ Consider PNA or CCH in patients with discrete cords who will accept a higher recurrence rate in order to avoid surgery. ▪ Diffuse, matted disease without a defined cord is better suited for surgical fasciectomy.
PNA portal placement	▪ Avoid portals over flexion creases, nodules, and matted skin.
PNA nerve monitoring	▪ Use anesthetic sparingly to avoid nerve blockade. A sensate nerve with a cooperative patient will help avoid digital nerve injury.
PNA technique	▪ Do not pull on the fingertips to gain tension on the cord. This will place the flexor tendons under tension, increasing risk of tendon injury during needling. ▪ Replace needles regularly, as a dull bevel impairs tactile feedback and will not cut cord fibers.
CCH injection technique	▪ Avoid injection into the flexor tendon; injection should be superficial within the involved cord. ▪ Slight resistance to injection is normal.
PNA and CCH finger extension technique	▪ Isolate and extend each involved joint individually to minimize risk of skin tears. ▪ Hold other joints in a flexed position to minimize skin tension.
Limited fasciectomy	▪ Neurovascular bundles can be displaced to the midline by spiral cords. ▪ Take care to dissect the nerve from proximal to distal prior to excision of diseased tissue. ▪ Meticulous hemostasis and loose wound closure (or open palm technique) minimizes hematoma formation. ▪ Hematoma formation can cause painful swelling and skin flap ischemia.

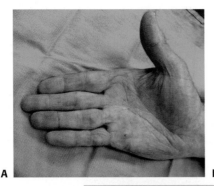
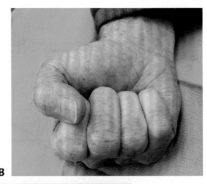
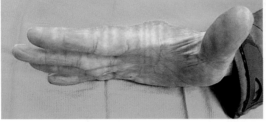

FIG 6 • A–C. Two-week postoperative visit after percutaneous needle aponeurotomy of ring and small fingers, showing full active range of motion.

POSTOPERATIVE CARE

- PNA and CCH
  - Immediate active digital flexion and extension is encouraged (**FIG 6**).
  - No formal therapy is prescribed.
  - Skin tears are managed with local wound care.
  - Patients perform activities as tolerated.
- Limited fasciectomy
  - Remove the splint one week postoperatively.
  - Begin range of motion exercises.
  - For open palm wounds, local wound care with nonadherent gauze is initiated after splint removal.
  - For contractures involving the PIP joint, night extension splints are worn for 6 months postoperatively.

OUTCOMES

- PNA has a high rate of immediate contracture correction (less than 5-degree residual contracture).[7]
  - 98% success of MCP joint correction
  - 67% success of PIP joint correction
- PNA contracture recurrence rate is higher and occurs sooner compared to open fasciectomy.[8]
- With CCH, the overall rate of clinical success (residual contracture 0–5 degrees) ranges from 44% to 64%.[2,9,10]
  - Higher success is reported for treatment of MCP contractures (65%–77%) compared to PIP contractures (28%–40%).
- CCH disease recurrence (20 degree or greater increase of joint contracture in the presence of a palpable cord) after 5 years is reported at 39% for MCP joints and 66% for PIP joints.[11]
  - 16% of recurrent contractures underwent additional procedures, most commonly fasciectomy or repeated CCH therapy.
- 94% of MCP and 47% of PIP joints achieved clinical success with limited fasciectomy, with deformity correction to within 0 to 5 degrees of full extension.[8]
- 6 months postoperatively after limited fasciectomy, 73% of patients are satisfied with their hand function.[12]

- Volar capsulotomy is controversial, as combined volar capsulotomy and fasciectomy does not have better results than fasciectomy alone.[13]
- Recurrence rates vary due to inconsistent definitions, but a recent study demonstrates a 20.9% recurrence rate (defined as worsening of total passive extension deficit of 30 degrees or more in a ray) at 5 years postoperatively after limited fasciectomy, which is significantly lower than recurrence after PNA (85%).[8]

COMPLICATIONS

- PNA: Overall complication rate is low.[7]
  - 3.4% skin tear
  - 1.2% transient neuropraxia
  - 0.1% nerve laceration
- CCH[14]:
  - Skin tear
  - Peripheral edema
  - Contusion
  - Drug ineffective
  - Injection-site hematoma
  - Lymphadenopathy
  - Pain in extremity
  - Blood blister
  - Injection-site pain
  - Tenderness
  - Localized rash/pruritus
  - Flexor pulley injury
  - Flexor tendon rupture can occur with injection into the flexor tendon; care must be taken when treating the small finger.
- Limited fasciectomy
  - Hematoma
  - Infection
  - Skin flap necrosis
  - Postoperative stiffness
  - Subjective paresthesias
  - Digital nerve injury
  - Digital ischemia
  - Tendon injury

REFERENCES

1. Hindocha S, Stanley JK, Watson S, et al. Dupuytren's diathesis revisited: evaluation of prognostic indicators for risk of disease recurrence. *J Hand Surg [Am]*. 2006;31(10):1626-1634.

2. Hurst LC, Badalamente MA, Hentz VR, et al. Injectable collagenase *Clostridium histolyticum* for Dupuytren's contracture. *N Engl J Med*. 2009;361:968-979.

3. Coleman S, Gilpin D, Kaplan FT, et al. Efficacy and safety of concurrent collagenase *Clostridium histolyticum* injections for multiple Dupuytren contractures. *J Hand Surg [Am]*. 2014;39(1):57-64.

4. Mickelson DT, Noland SS, Watt AJ, et al. Prospective randomized controlled trial comparing 1- versus 7-day manipulation following collagenase injection for Dupuytren contracture. *J Hand Surg [Am]*. 2014;39(10):1933-1941.

5. Eaton C. Percutaneous fasciotomy for Dupuytren's contracture. *J Hand Surg [Am]*. 2011;36(5):910-915.

6. Auxilium Pharma. *Xiaflex: Prescribing information and medication guide*. Retrieved from: https://www.xiaflex.com/wp-content/themes/xiaflex/assets/pdf//PI-and-MedGuide-Combined.pdf

7. Pess GM, Pess RM, Pess RA. Results of needle aponeurotomy for Dupuytren contracture in over 1,000 fingers. *J Hand Surg [Am]*. 2012;37A:651-656.

8. van Rijssen AL, Linden HT, Werker PM. Five-year results of a randomized clinical trial on treatment in Dupuytren's disease: percutaneous needle fasciotomy versus limited fasciectomy. *Plast Reconstr Surg*. 2012;129(2):469-477.

9. Gilpin D, Coleman S, Hall S, Houston A, et al. Injectable collagenase *Clostridium histolyticum*: a new nonsurgical treatment for Dupuytren's disease. *J Hand Surg [Am]*. 2010;35A:2027-2038.

10. Witthout J, Jones G, Skrepnik N, et al. Efficacy and safety of collagenase *Clostridium histolyticum* injection for Dupuytren contracture: short-term results from 2 open-label studies. *J Hand Surg [Am]*. 2013;38(1):2-11.

11. Peimer CA, Blazar P, Coleman S, et al. Dupuytren contracture recurrence following treatment with collagenase *Clostridium histolyticum* (CORDLESS study): 5-year data. *J Hand Surg [Am]*. 2015;40(8):1597-1605.

12. Engstrand C, Krevers B, Nylander G, et al. Hand function and quality of life before and after fasciectomy for Dupuytren contracture. *J Hand Surg [Am]*. 2014;39(7):1333-1343.

13. Weinzweig N, Culver JE, Fleegler EJ. Severe contractures of the proximal interphalangeal joint in Dupuytren's disease: combined fasciectomy with capsuloligamentous release fasciectomy alone. *Plast Reconstr Surg*. 1996;97(3):560-566.

14. Peimer CA, McGoldrick CA, Fiore GJ. Nonsurgical treatment of Dupuytren's contracture: 1-year US post-marketing safety data for collagenase clostridium histolyticum. *Hand*. 2012;7:143-146.

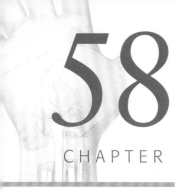

58
CHAPTER

Section XII: Spastic Conditions

Elbow Extension Procedures

Paymon Rahgozar and Kevin C. Chung

DEFINITION

- The impairment suffered by patients with spastic conditions can be quite debilitating, robbing them of their ability to perform basic activities of daily living and independence.
- Depending on the level of spinal cord injury, the deficits, and, in turn, the options for reconstruction, can vary. Spinal segments C5 through T1 innervate the upper extremity.
- The International Classification for Surgery of the Hand in Tetraplegia (ICT)[1] is a useful way to group tetraplegic patients based on functioning muscles with strength of grade 4 or higher to determine the potential donors for tendon transfer:
  - Group 1: Brachioradialis (BR)
  - Group 2: Extensor carpi radialis longus (ECRL)
  - Group 3: Extensor carpi radialis brevis (ECRB)
  - Group 4: Pronator teres (PT)
  - Group 5: Flexor carpi radialis (FCR)
  - Group 6: Extensor digitorum communis (EDC) and finger extensors
  - Group 7: Extensor pollicis longus (EPL) and thumb extensors
  - Group 8: Finger flexors
  - Group 9: All except intrinsic muscles
- With spinal cord injury at the C5/C6 level, patients will maintain shoulder function through an innervated deltoid muscle and maintain elbow flexion through innervated biceps and brachialis muscles.
- The role of the shoulder and elbow is to move the hands in a functional "workspace." The forearm and wrist then position the hand in preparation for specific tasks of daily living.
- In spinal cord injury, a spastic elbow flexion contracture may develop from spasticity of the elbow flexors and an absence of elbow extension. The patient becomes entirely dependent on the weight of the forearm for stability, limiting the effective "workspace." The ability to extend the hand an additional 12 in. from the body will provide an additional 800% of workspace.[2]
- An elbow extension deficit severely interferes with performing activities of daily living and with wheelchair propulsion. Active elbow extension gives the patient the ability to transfer and to provide pressure relief, reducing the risk of developing ischial or sacral pressure ulcers.
- In cases of cerebral palsy, stroke, or traumatic injury, an elbow extension deficit may also result from a fixed elbow flexion contracture from biceps, brachialis, or brachioradialis muscle contracture.
- The first priority in patients with spasticity and/or tetraplegia is to improve elbow extension. The outcome of any other reconstruction for improvement of wrist or hand function

will be entirely dependent on the patient having a usable workspace to perform new functions.

ANATOMY

- The deltoid originates from the scapula and inserts on the lateral shaft of the humerus.
  - The axillary nerve and the posterior circumflex humeral artery supply the deltoid posteriorly after passing through the quadrangular space (**FIG 1**).
  - The average fiber length is nearly twice that of the triceps muscle giving it a large amount of excursion and a good potential donor for transfer.
- The biceps originates from the coracoid process and the supraglenoid tubercle inserting on the radial tuberosity and the bicipital aponeurosis.
  - It is innervated by the musculocutaneous nerve that travels between the biceps and the brachialis.
  - The boundaries of the cubital fossa are the pronator teres medially and the brachioradialis laterally. The brachial artery and the median nerve are medial to the biceps brachii tendon. Lateral to it is the lateral cutaneous nerve of the forearm (**FIG 2**).
  - The biceps muscle has a large physiologic cross-sectional area and long fibers empowering it to exert large amplitudes of force.
  - Transfer requires the biceps tendon to curve around the humerus either laterally across the radial nerve or medially across the ulnar nerve.
- The triceps originates from the infraglenoid tubercle of the scapula and the posterior superior humerus.
  - It has three heads that converge to form the central tendon of the triceps inserting on the posterior olecranon (**FIG 3**).
  - The radial nerve passes through the triangular space and travels posterior to the lateral head of the triceps from a medial to lateral direction in the radial groove of the humerus.

PATIENT HISTORY AND PHYSICAL FINDINGS

- Factors that influence functional ability must be considered during the examination:
  - Whether the injury is neurologically complete
  - Cognitive impairment from brain injury
  - Age of the patient
  - Concomitant upper extremity injuries
  - Presence of uncontrolled spasticity
  - Contractures limiting mobility
  - Patient depression

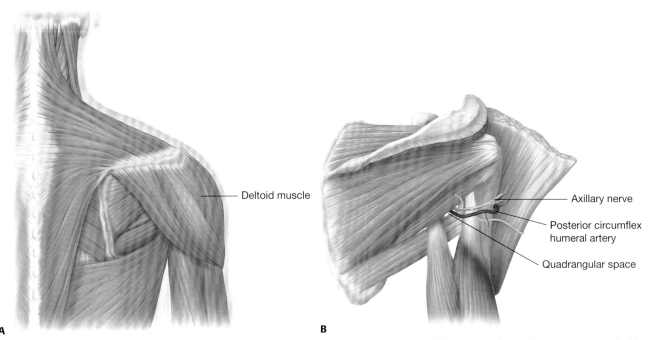

FIG 1 • **A.** Posterior view of the deltoid. It originates from the scapula and inserts on the anterolateral humerus to abduct the arm. **B.** It is supplied by the axillary nerve and the posterior circumflex humeral artery emerging from the quadrangular space.

- Patients with motor levels of C5 or higher (ICT ≥ 1) will have deltoid, biceps, and brachialis function.
- The exam should include an accurate assessment of the range of motion of the elbow, including the strength of the deltoid and biceps muscles. Supple joints and a Medical Research Council (MRC) grade of 4 or higher are a prerequisite for tendon transfer.

- To test the posterior deltoid, the examiner places one palm on the patient's posterior humerus with the patient's arm in 90 degrees of abduction and the elbow in flexion. The patient is asked to push as hard as possible against the examiner's palm while the examiner places the other hand against the posterior half of the deltoid assessing its tension and mass.

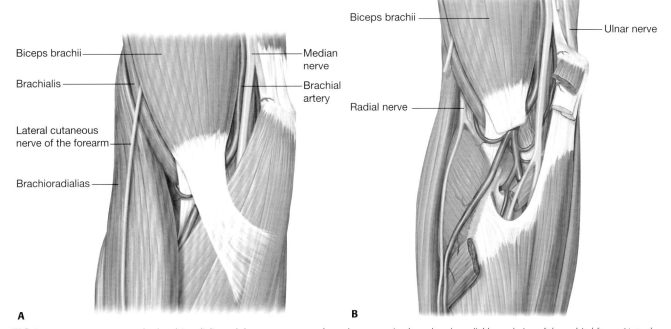

FIG 2 • Biceps anatomy. **A.** The brachioradialis and the pronator teres form the respective lateral and medial boundaries of the cubital fossa. Note the relationship of the biceps with the median nerve and brachial artery. **B.** Transfer of the biceps tendon can be done laterally crossing the radial nerve or medially crossing the ulnar nerve. Medial transfer is more often performed, particularly if the patient does not have ulnar nerve function.

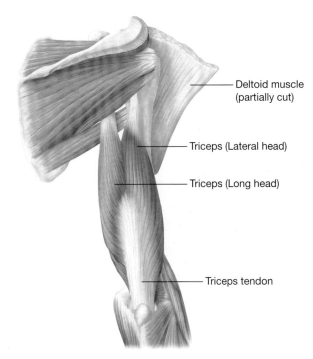

FIG 3 • Triceps anatomy. The triceps tendon is identified and used for the deltoid and biceps transfers.

- If the examiner can easily push the patient's arm out of this position, the posterior deltoid likely does not have sufficient strength for transfer.[2]
- The role of the biceps muscle is to flex the elbow and supinate the forearm. Therefore, prior to consideration of the biceps as a donor muscle, examination of the supinator and brachialis muscles are imperative to ensure adequate postoperative flexion and supination.
- Forearm supination without resistance activates the supinator, which can be palpated along the proximal radius. Similarly, elbow flexion without resistance will activate the brachialis, and it is palpable along the anterior humerus.
  - If the exam is equivocal, the biceps may be paralyzed with injection of local anesthetic around the musculocutaneous nerve, facilitating an independent evaluation of the supinator and brachialis.[3]
- The patient's overall psychosocial and mental state must be evaluated.
  - This includes consideration of the patient's social support network and personal motivation for improvement of function.
  - There will be a long period of postoperative rehabilitation, and without long-term cooperation from the patient and adequate assistance, a successful outcome is unlikely.

IMAGING

- Plain radiography can identify the presence of heterotopic ossification, a potential cause of joint contracture that must be ruled out or treated before any tendon lengthening or transfer.
- If, despite clinical examination, the examiner is still uncertain of whether a muscle is under volitional control, electromyography focusing on the muscle of interest can help identify spastic and flaccid muscles and determine phasic activity.

NONOPERATIVE MANAGEMENT

- Attempts to control the position of the elbow can be done with serial splinting or casting. Phenol motor blocks have been used to alleviate spasticity.
- Patients who are many years from their injury may be well adapted to their deficits. For example, some will learn to substitute the biceps to propel themselves in a wheelchair and do not wish any surgical intervention.
  - It is important to thoroughly question each individual patient to determine what the postoperative goal is and whether surgery can realistically attain that goal.

SURGICAL MANAGEMENT

- The primary goal of surgical intervention in spasticity is to achieve, maintain, or maximize the patient's physical independence. Any treatment that can improve a level of function will have a dramatic effect on the patient's independence.
- The goals of reconstructing elbow extension are to provide improvement in the following activities[4]:
  - Reaching for an object above shoulder level
  - Driving
  - Handwriting
  - Wheelchair propulsion
  - Pressure relief when seated
  - Using the hand while supine
- In patients with multiple levels of deficits, the reconstitution of active elbow extension should be performed first. It not only will stabilize the elbow and facilitate the transfer of other muscles in the future, such as the brachioradialis, but also gives the patient confidence in the rest of his or her treatment.[5]
- The following principles of tendon transfers apply in reconstruction of spastic conditions:
  - Supple joints with a functional arc of motion
  - Sufficient strength of donor muscle for its new function
    - Although an MRC ≥ 4 is recommended, a muscle will lose one grade of strength after transfer, and therefore, an MRC of 5 is preferable.
  - Comparable force of contraction and excursion between the donor muscle and the muscle to be replaced
  - Synergy—motions that are synchronized during functional activity (finger flexion with wrist extension)
  - Transfer should occur across a healthy bed of tissue with minimal inflammation or scarring
  - Stabilization of a joint whenever a transfer spans multiple joints
  - Straight line of pull for the transfer whenever possible
  - Minimal morbidity from loss of the donor muscle
- Elbow extension can be restored with a posterior deltoid or biceps transfer to the triceps. In cases of contracture as a result of spasticity, tendon lengthening is another treatment option.
- Deltoid to triceps transfer
  - The deltoid transfer uses the posterior half of the deltoid muscle. There is minimal to no functional loss of the donor muscle, as arm abduction is preserved postoperatively.
  - The deltoid and the triceps are synergistic muscles. Reaching for an object overhead involves abduction of the arm (deltoid) and extension of the elbow (triceps).
  - One significant disadvantage of the posterior deltoid muscle is that it does not have sufficient length to be directly inserted into the triceps tendon. Therefore, the gap must be bridged with a free tendon graft.

- The deltoid transfer is also prone to stretching, particularly at the proximal suture repair between the deltoid and the tendon graft. The tendon elongation most commonly occurs during the first 4 to 6 weeks after surgery but has been found to occur months after surgery. Tendon elongation will result in a loss of strength and excursion for elbow extension. Thus, a strict and rigorous postoperative rehabilitation program is essential to optimize results.[6]
- Absolute contraindications include a fixed elbow contracture or inadequate posterior deltoid strength on clinical examination.
- Biceps to triceps transfer
  - A biceps to triceps transfer can be considered in cases where there is less than grade 4 strength of the posterior deltoid but biceps with strength of 4 or greater.
  - Patients with elbow contracture less than 20 degrees may benefit from biceps transfer over a deltoid transfer, because biceps lengthening would likely be necessary to correct the elbow contracture.
  - Although there is a postoperative reduction in elbow flexion power of up to 47% after biceps transfer, patients report that the significant functional improvement with added elbow extension far outweighs the decrease in flexion strength.[7,8] Again, it is important to confirm that the patient has active supinator and brachialis muscles to minimize the elbow flexion deficits after biceps transfer.
  - Advantages of the biceps transfer over the deltoid transfer include a shorter operation, ability to use a tourniquet for a portion of the operation, avoiding the need for a tendon interposition graft, and the need to heal only one tendon junction to permit earlier mobilization.
  - Biceps transfer is not without its disadvantages. The transfer requires routing the biceps tendon around the humerus resulting in a drop in power across the transfer.
  - Furthermore, the biceps and triceps are antagonist muscles. Normally, with triceps contraction and elbow extension, the biceps muscle relaxes. However, after biceps to triceps transfer, biceps contraction is necessary to activate elbow extension. The patient will require a longer period of rehabilitation to train the biceps to function as an elbow extensor.
- Tendon lengthening procedures for contracture
  - Patients with volitional control of the elbow and hand and with more than 40 degrees of contracture are candidates. Additionally, those without volitional control and more than 100 degrees of contracture would also benefit for help with personal hygiene.
  - Patients recovering from strokes are typically older with weaker muscles, resulting in poor recovery of motor function regardless of the surgical procedure. Stroke patients with contractures will likely have some benefit in correction of the contracture, but less likely to have a significant improvement in function.
  - For biceps or brachialis lengthening procedures, a fractional lengthening can be performed for mild contractures, whereas a Z-lengthening (step cut) is indicated for more severe contractures.

Preoperative Planning

- A local nerve block is a useful preoperative tool differentiating muscle spasticity from muscle contracture. In the case of contractures, movement will not improve with neuromuscular blockade.

- The underlying cause of the spasticity will guide preoperative preparation.
  - Cerebral palsy
    - Voluntary hand use, sensibility, intelligence quotient, and presence of athetosis must be measured. An uncooperative patient with limited preoperative function is unlikely to have significant postoperative functional improvement.
    - The examiner must confirm the cause of contracture: joint contracture, muscle contracture, or muscle spasticity. Unlike muscle or joint contractures, muscle spasticity presents with full range of motion of the affected joint. The contractures should be treated with either therapy or surgery before a tendon transfer.
    - Older patients may have learned to compensate for their disability, and reconstruction in those cases must be considered carefully.
  - Stroke
    - Patients often present with hemiplegia of the upper extremity and less spasticity than younger patients.
    - Surgery should be delayed until there is maximal neurologic recovery, typically around 12 to 18 months.
  - Traumatic brain injury
    - On average, patients are younger than stroke patients and will present with a greater degree of spasticity.
    - Trauma patients may also have concomitant injuries, heterotopic ossification, deformities from other fractures, and possible quadriplegic involvement that can complicate postoperative functional improvement. Each patient must be considered individually.
    - Similar to cerebral palsy, patient cognition and cooperation is variable and must be carefully assessed preoperatively to predict likelihood of patient cooperation and a successful postoperative outcome.
- If the patient has had a contracture treated preoperatively, it is important to repeat examination of the range of motion on the day of surgery to confirm there is no contracture recurrence.

Positioning

- The patient is placed in a lateral decubitus position for the deltoid to triceps transfer.
  - Alternatively, the patient can be supine with a surgical "bump" placed beneath the torso to elevate the shoulder anteriorly.
- The supine position is appropriate for the biceps to triceps transfer and the biceps/brachialis lengthening.
- A high proximal tourniquet can be applied for the biceps and brachialis lengthening, as well as for a portion of the biceps to triceps transfer.

Approach

- A variety of tendon grafts can be used for the deltoid to triceps transfer, including toe extensors, tensor fascia lata, tibialis anterior, extensor carpi ulnaris, or the central third of the triceps tendon.
- The deltoid to triceps incision can be made as two separate incisions, one overlying the posterior deltoid and one over the triceps, or it can be made as one continuous incision.
- The biceps to triceps transfer can be performed by tunneling the biceps tendon either laterally or medially, though medially is the preferred method to avoid compression of the radial nerve.[8,9]

■ Posterior Deltoid to Triceps Transfer

- To reach the triceps, the posterior deltoid must be lengthened with a free tendon graft harvested from the surgeon's preferred donor site. A free tensor fascia lata graft has sufficient length and strength and leaves minimal donor-site morbidity (**TECH FIG 1A,B**).
- Make an S-shaped incision from the posterior tip of the acromion to the deltoid insertion on the humerus (**TECH FIG 1C**).
- Dissect along the posterior edge of the deltoid from proximal to distal. Identify the tendinous band marking the separation between the middle and posterior parts of the deltoid.
- Sharply dissect the posterior muscle fibers from their insertion on the humerus. This measures an area of approximately 1 × 6 cm (**TECH FIG 1D**). Include the periosteum and a small rectangular strip of fascia to include tissue with sufficient strength to hold suture for the tendon repair and to provide as much length as possible.
  - ▪ Take care to avoid dissection too far distal. The radial nerve emerges several centimeters distal to the deltoid insertion and can be injured with overzealous dissection.
- Completely separate the posterior deltoid muscle fibers from the remainder of the muscle, providing approximately 3 cm of excursion (**TECH FIG 1E**).
  - ▪ Avoid injury to the axillary nerve and the posterior circumflex pedicle, located approximately 10 cm proximal to the insertion on the humerus.
- To expose the triceps tendon and fascia, make a separate lazy-S incision along the distal third of the humerus lateral to the olecranon process (see **TECH FIG 1A,B**).
- Create a subcutaneous tunnel connecting the proximal and distal incisions (see **TECH FIG 1E**).
- First, interweave the graft proximally to the deltoid. Then, secure the tendon graft to the triceps tendon under moderate tension with the elbow fully extended and the shoulder slightly abducted. Secure the repair with two double rows of 4-0 nonabsorbable, running suture (**TECH FIG 1F**).
- Ensure adequate hemostasis and close the incisions primarily.
- Apply a splint with the elbow in 5 to 10 degrees of flexion.

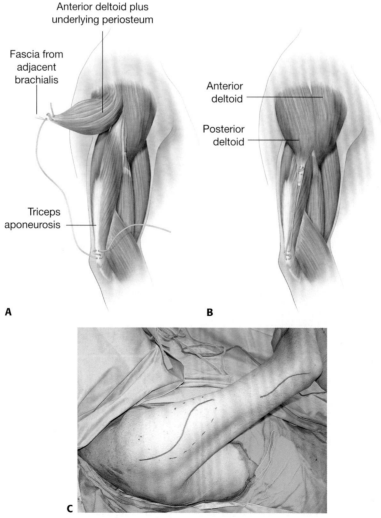

TECH FIG 1 • A,B. The gap between the deltoid tendon and the triceps tendon must be bridged with a tendon graft. **C.** The deltoid is palpated and marked out with a dashed line. The incision is a lazy-S, spanning from the proximal extent of the muscle to near its insertion. The triceps incision is similarly S-shaped and is placed lateral to the lateral epicondyle to avoid potential pressure necrosis.

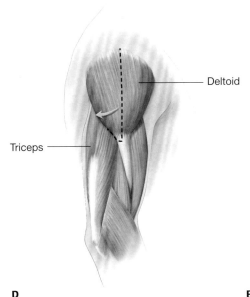

Deltoid

Triceps

D

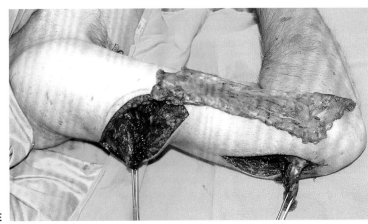

E

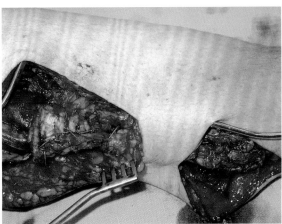

F

TECH FIG 1 (Continued) • **D.** The posterior deltoid is freed from its attachments to the humerus and will be transferred posteriorly toward the triceps tendon. **E.** The posterior deltoid (held by left clamp) after dissection has an approximate 3-cm excursion. The triceps tendon (held in right clamp) is prepared for the transfer. The free tensor fascia lata graft has sufficient length and strength for transfer. **F.** Suture repair of the tendon graft to the deltoid proximally (*left*) and the triceps distally (*right*).

■ Biceps to Triceps Transfer

- Make an anterior longitudinal incision over the medial biceps muscle belly. Extend the incision obliquely across the antecubital fossa (**TECH FIG 2A**).
- Dissect and expose the biceps muscle. Identify and protect the musculocutaneous nerve.
- Divide the lacertus fibrosus while avoiding injury to the brachial artery and the median nerve lying deep to it. If the lacertus fibrosus has a substantial antebrachial fascia, preserve to use as an additional tail for subsequent tendon weaving (**TECH FIG 2B**).
- Identify the biceps tendon and trace it distally to its insertion on the radial tuberosity. To identify the radial tuberosity, flex the elbow and supinate the forearm.
- Detach the biceps tendon from its insertion as far distally as possible. Avoid injury to the recurrent radial vessels,

as they are the main blood supply to the brachioradialis and the extensor carpi radialis, which may be donor muscles for potential future transfers.
- Place a braided, nonabsorbable suture through the substance of the biceps tendon.
- Make a second incision overlying the distal triceps aponeurosis. Ensure that the incision is lateral to the olecranon to avoid pressure ulceration and a narrow medial skin bridge.
- After exposing the triceps tendon, split it over the tip of the olecranon. Drill a unicortical hole into the medullary canal from the olecranon tip. This hole can be sequentially drilled to an appropriate size to receive the biceps tendon (**TECH FIG 2C**).
- From the posterior incision, create a generous subcutaneous tunnel medial to the humerus and deep to the ulnar nerve, traveling toward the anterior incision. The medial

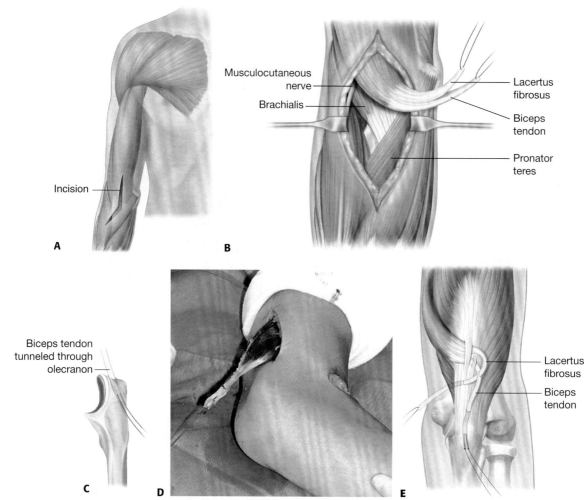

TECH FIG 2 • A. Anterior incision for exposure of the biceps. **B.** Elevation of the biceps tendon and the lacertus fibrosus. If the lacertus fibrosus is of substantial thickness, it can be preserved and used for the tendon weave. **C.** The biceps tendon is brought from the medial incision to the lateral incision through a subcutaneous tunnel. Sufficient proximal dissection of the biceps is necessary. **D.** The biceps tendon is brought through a slit in the triceps (posterior view). A unicortical hole is drilled in the proximal olecranon large enough to fit the biceps tendon. Two smaller distal holes are drilled in continuity with the proximal hole large enough to pass through a Keith needle with each end of the suture holding the biceps tendon. The two ends of the suture are secured and tied over the olecranon.

intermuscular septum may need to be resected to create the tunnel.

- Free the biceps muscle as far proximally as possible to provide the straightest line of pull possible toward the olecranon. The tourniquet must be removed for this portion to permit adequate proximal exposure. Avoid injury to the vascular pedicle to the biceps, which enters the deep surface of the proximal third of the muscle. Proximal dissection should stop once the distal motor branches of the musculocutaneous nerve entering the biceps are identified.[10]

- Transfer the biceps tendon from the anterior incision medially toward the posterior incision (**TECH FIG 2D**).

- Pull the biceps tendon through the slit in the triceps tendon and secure with a Pulvertaft weave with a braided nonabsorbable suture. The tail of the biceps tendon should remain free to be brought through the olecranon.

- Drill two small holes through the opposite cortex of the olecranon to permit passage of a Keith needle. Secure

a suture in the tail of the biceps and bring each end of the suture through each of the distal olecranon holes with a Keith needle. With the elbow in full extension, tie the two ends of the suture together over bone (**TECH FIG 2E**).[9]

- Place additional braided nonabsorbable sutures between the biceps and triceps tendon to further secure the transfer. If a tail of lacertus fibrosus was preserved, it can be secured at this time, either to the biceps tendon or to the triceps tendon.

- Set the tension maximally with the elbow held in full extension, such that the elbow cannot be passively flexed beyond 30 degrees when the arm is abducted about 30 to 40 degrees.[8]

- Achieve hemostasis, and close all skin incisions primarily. A suction drain can be placed at the surgeon's discretion.

- Place a splint holding the arm in 10 degrees of elbow flexion and the wrist in 30 degrees of extension. The shoulder is not immobilized.

Biceps and Brachialis Lengthening

- Make a 15-cm S-shaped incision across the antecubital fossa beginning laterally above the elbow and curving distally in an anteromedial direction (**TECH FIG 3A**).
- Dissect from medial to lateral, exposing the lacertus fibrosus, biceps brachii tendon, median nerve, brachial artery, and the lateral antebrachial cutaneous nerve (see **FIG 2**).
- Identify the bicipital aponeurosis medial to the biceps brachii tendon, and resect it completely (**TECH FIG 3B**).
- Identify the lateral antebrachial cutaneous nerve between the biceps and brachialis lateral to the biceps tendon and retract it laterally. Expose the biceps completely and dissect distal to its insertion.
- For a fractional lengthening, make two cuts in a slightly oblique direction, spaced approximately 1 to 2 cm apart. One cut is made on the lateral side of the tendon, and the other is made on the medial side. The cuts should be no more than halfway through the tendinous portion of

the musculotendinous junction, leaving the muscle fibers intact (**TECH FIG 3C**). Gently extend the elbow facilitating separation of the tenotomy sites, keeping the muscle in continuity.

- After release of the biceps, the brachialis can be visualized. Similarly, perform a fractional lengthening. Again, if two releasing incisions, space them approximately 1 to 2 cm apart and perform the proximal incision first. If the distal incision is made first, proximal migration of the brachialis will make it challenging to make the second incision (**TECH FIG 3D**).
- To perform a Z-lengthening of the biceps, make a transverse cut halfway through the tendon on the proximal side. Make a second distal transverse cut halfway through the opposite side of the tendon. The two cuts are connected longitudinally completely releasing the tendon with each end representing half the Z limbs (**TECH FIG 3E**).

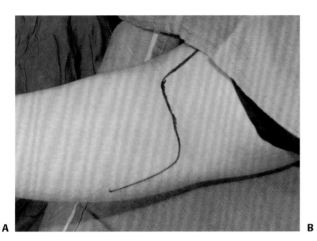

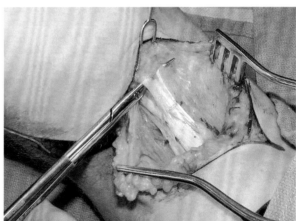

A   B

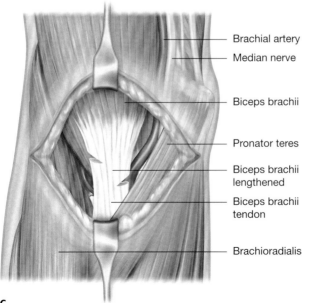

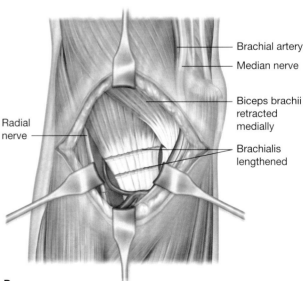

C   D

TECH FIG 3 • **A.** Incision for biceps and brachialis lengthening. An S-shaped incision starts on the lateral arm and crosses the cubital fossa transversely to the medial forearm. **B.** Exposure of the bicipital aponeurosis. **C.** Fractional lengthening of the biceps tendon. **D.** Fractional lengthening of the brachialis.

TECHNIQUES

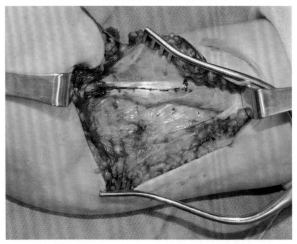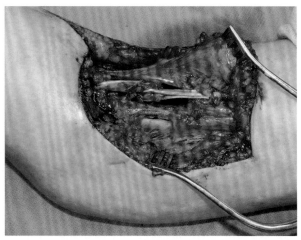

E   F

TECH FIG 3 (Continued) • **E.** Markings for Z-lengthening of the biceps tendon. **F.** Repair of the two ends of the biceps following Z-tenotomy and lengthening of the biceps.

- The elbow is extended to 30 degrees of flexion lengthening the tendon to the appropriate length. The two ends are sutured together where they remain overlapping using a Pulvertaft weave with 3-0 braided, nonabsorbable sutures (**TECH FIG 3F**).
- Be certain to perform the Z-lengthening over as much of the tendon length as possible to maximize the amount of tendon available for reattachment.
- If adequate lengthening of the brachialis cannot be obtained with fractional lengthening or Z-lengthening, the muscle can be completely transected.

- If preoperative evaluation revealed a spastic brachioradialis, it can be assessed for partial or complete release at this time. Dissect between the brachialis and brachioradialis to identify the origin of the brachioradialis. Perform the release (partial or complete) at the origin, permitting the muscle to slide distally. Be certain to identify and protect the radial nerve before performing a brachioradialis release.
- Release the tourniquet, achieve hemostasis, and close the wound primarily.
- Place the arm in a splint with the elbow at 30 degrees of flexion.

PEARLS AND PITFALLS

Incision	■ Avoid making incisions directly over the olecranon to prevent pressure ulceration. ■ Make a longitudinal incision on the lateral elbow for patients with contractures greater than 100 degrees facilitating skin closure with multiple Z-plasties if necessary.
Deltoid to triceps transfer	■ A tendinous band in the intermediate part of the deltoid can be used to help demarcate the separation between the middle and posterior portions of the deltoid. ■ Include the periosteum when dissecting the deltoid insertion from the humerus to better hold sutures for repair. ■ The axillary nerve is approximately 10 cm proximal to the humeral insertion of the deltoid and must be avoided.
Biceps to triceps transfer	■ Identify and protect the lateral cutaneous nerve of the forearm. ■ If using a tourniquet, release will be necessary to achieve adequate proximal dissection of the biceps. ■ Create a generous subcutaneous tunnel to avoid any compression or loss of strength of the transferred biceps tendon. ■ If the lacertus fibrosus has substantial fascia, it can be preserved and used as a second tail to further strengthen tendon weaving. ■ Medial routing of the biceps tendon avoids the potential for radial nerve palsy. ■ Avoid injury to the recurrent radial vessels so that the blood supply to potential donor muscles for future transfers is not compromised.
Biceps and brachialis lengthening	■ Perform a fractional lengthening in cases of mild contractures and a Z-lengthening for more severe contractures. ■ When performing a double incision release of the brachialis, perform the proximal incision first. ■ Avoid placing the elbow in full extension in patients with volitional control, as this may result in postoperative problems with elbow flexion.

POSTOPERATIVE CARE

- Deltoid and the biceps to triceps transfer
  - Immobilization is continued for 4 weeks. The patient is then placed in an active exercise program gradually increasing elbow flexion at a rate of 15 to 20 degrees per week with a daytime dial-hinge brace and a nighttime splint in full extension.
  - Occupational therapy is used to train biceps activation for elbow extension and to incorporate functional activities of daily living.[8]
  - The dial-hinge brace is continued until the patient is at 90 degrees of elbow flexion. The nighttime splint is used for 12 weeks, after which strengthening can begin.
- Biceps and brachialis lengthening
  - The wound is inspected and sutures removed in 10 to 14 days.
  - If a fractional lengthening was performed, the patient can begin mobilization immediately.
  - For biceps Z-lengthening, the elbow is splinted in 30 degrees of flexion for 4 weeks to protect the tendon repair. Active and passive range of motion can then begin with nighttime splints worn for an additional 3 weeks for protection.

OUTCOMES

- The biceps comprises one of the two strong elbow flexors. Therefore, transfer does result in an approximate 47% reduction of preoperative strength.[4,8]
- The biceps is an antagonist to the triceps, leading to a longer rehabilitation period to learn to activate it as an elbow extensor. This learning curve can vary from 2 to 6 months.[4,8]
- Patients typically regain full or near full elbow extension against gravity with both tendon transfer techniques.[2,3] In cases where patients do not, myofeedback with electrical stimulation can be used with good success.[4]
- On average, fractional lengthening of the biceps leads to a 10- to 30-degree improvement in flexion contracture with minimal loss of flexion power.

- For patients with a Z-lengthening procedure, there is on average a 45- to 60-degree improvement of elbow flexion contracture albeit with a loss of flexion power.

COMPLICATIONS

- Wound breakdown, infection, iatrogenic nerve injury, or inappropriate tensioning of a tendon transfer are all uncommon but possible surgical complications.
- For tendon transfers, tendon rupture or stretching of the repair can occur postoperatively leading to ineffective elbow extension. This can best be avoided with a strict postoperative immobilization and rehabilitation regimen.
- Tendon pullout from the olecranon is another potential complication that can best be prevented with a secure fixation.
- Though rare, compartment syndrome is a potential complication and can easily be missed in a patient with lack of preoperative sensation.[3]

REFERENCES

1. McDowell CL, Moberg EA, House JH. The second International Conference on Surgical Rehabilitation of the Upper Limb in Tetraplegia (quadriplegia). *J Hand Surg [Am]*. 1986;11:604-608.
2. Leclercq C, Hentz VR, Kozin SH, Mulcahey MJ. Reconstruction of elbow extension. *Hand Clin*. 2008;24(2):185-201.
3. Kozin SH, D'Addesi L, Chafetz RS, et al. Biceps-to-triceps transfer for elbow extension in persons with tetraplegia. *J Hand Surg [Am]*. 2010;35(6):968-975.
4. Ejeskär A. Elbow extension. *Hand Clin*. 2002;18(3):449-459.
5. Allieu Y. General indications for functional surgery of the hand in tetraplegic patients. *Hand Clin*. 2002;18(3):413-421.
6. Friden J, Ejeskar A, Dahlgren A, Lieber R. Protection of the deltoid to triceps tendon transfer repair sites. *J Hand Surg [Am]*. 2000;25(1):144-149.
7. Mulcahey MJ, Lutz C, Kozin SH, Betz RR. Prospective evaluation of biceps to triceps and deltoid to triceps for elbow extension in tetraplegia. *J Hand Surg [Am]*. 2003;28(6):964-971.
8. Revol M, Briand E, Servant JM. Biceps-to-triceps transfer in tetraplegia: the medial route. *J Hand Surg Br*. 1999;24(2):235-237.
9. Kuz JE, Van Heest AE, House JH. Biceps-to-triceps transfer in tetraplegic patients: report of the medial routing technique and follow-up of three cases. *J Hand Surg [Am]*. 1999;24(1):161-172.
10. Endress RD, Hentz VR. Biceps-to-triceps transfer technique. *J Hand Surg [Am]*. 2011;36(4):716-721.

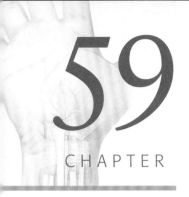

59
CHAPTER

Wrist Extension Procedures

Paymon Rahgozar and Kevin C. Chung

DEFINITION

- Patients with tetraplegia may have difficulty with wrist extension, constantly assuming a partially flexed posture.
- A flexed wrist position diminishes the tenodesis effect on the digital flexors, leading to a weakened grip, difficulty with hygiene, and obstructed visual feedback when grabbing objects.
- After elbow extension, the second priority in reconstruction for tetraplegia or spinal cord injury is the restoration of wrist extension. Augmentation of wrist extension can indirectly enable passive thumb and finger flexion by improving pinch and grasp. This tenodesis effect is valuable in patients who do not have enough donor muscles to reconstruct active grasp and pinch.
- Those patients with an International Classification for Surgery of the Hand in Tetraplegia (ICT) score of 1 have an active brachioradialis that can be used for tendon transfer to augment wrist extension (see Table 1 from Elbow Extension chapter).

ANATOMY

- Tetraplegic patients with an active brachioradialis typically have an innervated biceps and brachialis muscle. Therefore, there is minimal donor-site morbidity on elbow flexion with its use for tendon transfer, making it a versatile workhorse muscle in tetraplegia reconstruction.
- The brachioradialis originates from the lateral supracondylar ridge of the humerus and the lateral intermuscular septum and inserts on the lateral base of the radial styloid beneath the tendons of the abductor pollicis longus and extensor pollicis brevis.
- It is innervated by a branch from the radial nerve entering the deep portion of the muscle, proximal to the elbow.
- The superficial branch of the radial nerve (radial sensory nerve) runs deep and medial to the brachioradialis between it and the supinator muscle. In the mid to distal forearm, the radial artery can be found between the brachioradialis and the flexor carpi radialis tendon (**FIG 1**).
- The brachioradialis is a long muscle with good excursion and a large circumference, giving it a high force of contraction.[1] Its tendon is bound with fascial coverings and does not glide freely past the mid-forearm (**FIG 2**).
  - Releasing the tendon fascial attachments and freeing the muscle belly from the surrounding muscle significantly increases its excursion.[2]

- The extensor carpi radialis brevis (ECRB) attaches to the long finger metacarpal and is a more efficient wrist extensor than the extensor carpi radialis longus (ECRL), whose tendon attaches to the radial side of the second metacarpal, resulting in both extension and radial deviation of the wrist (**FIG 3**).

PATIENT HISTORY AND PHYSICAL FINDINGS

- As for all patients with spastic conditions considering surgical reconstruction, there are a variety of anatomic, functional, and psychosocial factors that must be examined (see Elbow Extension chapter).
- The strength of the brachioradialis must have a Medical Research Council grade 4 or higher. To test the brachioradialis, position the patient's elbow in a midprone position and have the patient flex against resistance contracting the brachioradialis. Palpate and attempt to move the belly of the muscle. If the muscle is tight, the brachioradialis has adequate strength for transfer (**FIG 4**).

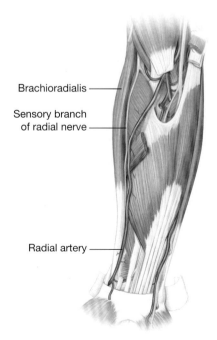

FIG 1 • Relevant volar anatomy. Note the relationship of the brachioradialis with the sensory branch of the radial nerve and the radial artery.

Labels on figure:
- Brachioradialis
- Sensory branch of radial nerve
- Radial artery

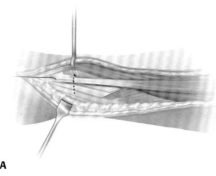

A

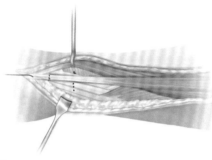

B

FIG 2 • Excursion from dissection of the brachioradialis. **A.** A mark is placed on the distal tendon of the brachioradialis and extended to the surrounding tissue as a reference point. **B.** After ligation of the distal tendon and freeing the tendon and muscle attachments, there is approximately 3 cm of advancement beyond the reference point.

■ Examination also includes the wrist and metacarpophalangeal joints to ensure a full passive range of motion with good passive tenodesis of the fingers with wrist flexion and extension.[3]

IMAGING

■ Electromyography can confirm volitional activity of the brachioradialis if the exam is equivocal. It will identify whether the muscle is spastic or flaccid and will determine its phasic activity.

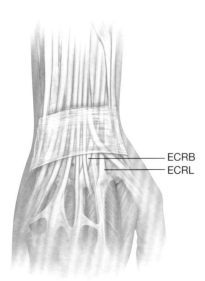

FIG 3 • Dorsal forearm anatomy. Note the location of the extensor carpi radialis longus (ECRL) and the extensor carpi radialis brevis (ECRB).

— ECRB
— ECRL

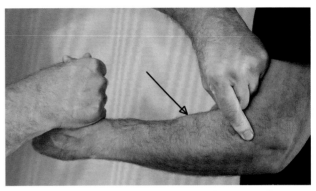

FIG 4 • To examine the brachioradialis, place the patient's forearm in neutral position and ask the patient to flex the elbow against resistance. The prominence of the muscle belly is evident along the proximal radial forearm (*arrow*). Difficulty to displace the muscle with the examiner's hand confirms adequate strength for transfer.

SURGICAL MANAGEMENT

■ The goal of surgery is to improve pinch and grasp by taking advantage of the tenodesis effect. Wrist extension effectively lengthens the palmar surface of the wrist by increasing tension on the digital flexors and reducing tension on the digital extensors. This results in bringing the thumb and fingers into passive flexion[4] (**FIG 5**).

■ With restoration or augmentation of active wrist extension, the patient can grasp light objects and pinch to hold and write with a pencil.

■ Prerequisites include an active brachioradialis muscle and full range of motion of the wrist and MCP joints.

■ The transfer can be performed with a number of other procedures as described by Moberg to maximize lateral pinch tenodesis[5]:
  ▪ Resection of the thumb annular ligament to release the flexor pollicis longus (FPL) tendon over the metacarpophalangeal joint, increasing its mechanical advantage
  ▪ Stabilization of the thumb interphalangeal joint with a buried Kirschner wire to prevent interphalangeal flexion with pinch (Froment sign)
  ▪ Tenodesis of the FPL by attaching it to the volar radius

■ It is best to delay tendon transfer for at least 1 year following injury to facilitate maximal recovery prior to surgical reconstruction.[6]

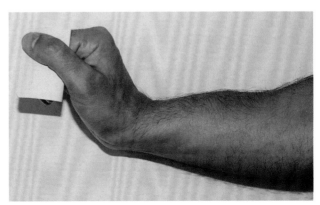

FIG 5 • Active wrist extension results in finger flexion and automatic pinch via the tenodesis effect.

Preoperative Planning

- The patient's underlying cause of spasticity and the current psychosocial state must be carefully assessed before proceeding with surgical reconstruction (see Elbow Extension chapter).
- Any preoperative contractures must be diagnosed and treated with tendon transfer. A local nerve block can differentiate spasticity from contractures. Paralysis of the muscle will have no effect on contractures but will improve range of motion with spasticity.
- Contractures can be treated with occupational therapy, progressive splinting, or surgery depending on the severity.

- On the day of surgery, full range of motion must be confirmed before proceeding with a tendon transfer, particularly in patients who were treated for preoperative contractures.

Positioning

- The patient is positioned in the supine position with the arm extended on an armboard. A nonsterile upper arm tourniquet is applied to provide a bloodless operative field.

Approach

- The brachioradialis can be transferred to the ECRB or to both the ECRB and ECRL. Transfer to the ECRL alone is not advised, as this can lead to more radial deviation than wrist extension.[3,6]

■ Brachioradialis to Extensor Carpi Radialis Brevis Tendon Transfer

- Make a longitudinal dorsoradial incision from the mid-forearm to the wrist (**TECH FIG 1A**).
- Identify the brachioradialis, ECRL, and ECRB tendons (**TECH FIG 1B**).
- Longitudinally incise the paratenon of the brachioradialis. Sharply divide the terminal tendon as distal as possible under the abductor pollicis longus and the extensor pollicis brevis.
- Dissect along the deep aspect of the brachioradialis freeing it from its fascial connections proximally to the mid-forearm (**TECH FIG 1C**).
  - Take care to identify and protect the superficial branch of the radial nerve and the radial vessels during the dissection.
- Continue proximal dissection until an approximate 3 cm of excursion is obtained. If necessary, dissection can continue proximally to just distal to the elbow crease. The radial recurrent vessels traveling transversely on the deep aspect of the muscle mark the extent of the proximal dissection.
- Dissect the ECRB tendon proximally and sharply divide it at the level of the mid-forearm (**TECH FIG 1D**).
- Avoiding compression of the radial sensory nerve, transfer the brachioradialis dorsally toward the ECRB superficial to the ECRL.

- In an end-to-end fashion, perform a Pulvertaft weave between the brachioradialis and the ECRB using multiple 2-0 nonabsorbable braided sutures.
- Place the elbow in 90 degrees of flexion, the forearm in neutral, and the wrist in 45 degrees of extension prior to suturing the tendons.[7] Do not pull up on the tendons when placing the first suture to avoid a lax repair once the tendon falls back to its natural position.
- Set the tension on the brachioradialis so that the normal resting length is re-established. To estimate this, passively stretch the muscle to its initial length relative to the radius. Place a mark on the brachioradialis tendon at its most proximal intersection with the ECRB tendon. Confirm that the mark remains in the same location after placement of all the sutures between the brachioradialis and ECRB.[4]
- **The tension should be set such that the wrist is in a neutral to slightly extended position but passive flexion is still possible (TECH FIG 1E).**
- Release the tourniquet, achieve hemostasis, and close the incision primarily.
- Place a splint holding the elbow in 90 degrees of flexion, the forearm in neutral rotation, and the wrist in 45 degrees of extension.

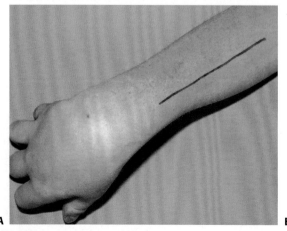
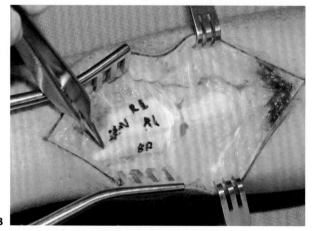

A   **B**

TECH FIG 1 • A. A longitudinal dorsoradial incision will provide exposure to the brachioradialis and the ECRB. The incision can be extended proximally, if necessary, for additional exposure of the brachioradialis. **B.** The brachioradialis, extensor carpi radialis longus, and extensor carpi radialis brevis in situ prior to dissection.

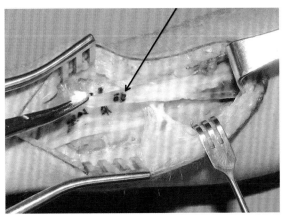
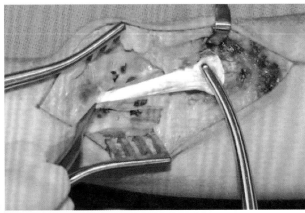
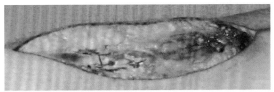

TECH FIG 1 (Continued) • **C.** After division of its distal tendon, dissection of the brachioradialis (*arrow*) proceeds proximally until there is approximately 3 cm of excursion. **D.** The ECRB is identified, and its tendon is incised proximally, permitting enough length for the transfer of the brachioradialis. **E.** The Pulvertaft weave completes the transfer. The weave is set with the elbow in 90 degrees of flexion, the forearm in neutral position, and the wrist in 45 degrees of extension. It is important to confirm that passive flexion of the wrist is possible at the completion of the transfer.

PEARLS AND PITFALLS

Tension	■ Elbow extension causes a tenodesis effect on the brachioradialis. The tension should be set with the elbow flexed in 90 degrees to eliminate this effect. ■ Postoperatively, the elbow should be immobilized in 90 degrees of flexion to minimize tension during tendon healing.
Neurovascular structures	■ Identify and protect the radial sensory nerve before commencing dissection and before dividing the brachioradialis tendon. ■ Do not injure the radial recurrent vessels when dissecting the BR proximally. They can be found on the deep surface of the muscle just distal to the elbow flexion crease signaling the extent of proximal dissection. ■ The neurovascular supply to the brachioradialis should not be at risk because it enters the muscle proximal to the elbow.
Tendon transfer	■ Free the brachioradialis until a 3-cm excursion is obtained. ■ Tension on the brachioradialis should be set to re-establish normal resting length.

POSTOPERATIVE CARE

■ After 4 weeks of immobilization, the patient can begin passive range of motion exercises with occupational therapy. The patient remains in a dorsal splint holding the wrist in 45 degrees of extension.

■ Active range of motion exercises and strength training can begin 6 weeks after surgery. For 12 weeks, the patient remains in a protective splint removing it only to participate in therapy.

OUTCOMES

■ The strength of wrist extension improves in almost all patients undergoing brachioradialis transfer without compromising strength in elbow flexion.[3,6]

■ The greater the preoperative strength of the brachioradialis and wrist extensors, the better the postoperative result.[6]

COMPLICATIONS

■ Failures from tendon ruptures or adhesions are rare but can occur. Tenolysis should be delayed until 9 to 12 months after surgery.

REFERENCES

1. Freehafer AA, Peckham PH, Keith MW, Mendelson LS. The brachioradialis: anatomy, properties, and value for tendon transfer in the tetraplegic. *J Hand Surg [Am]*. 1988;13(I):99-104.
2. Fridén J, Albrecht D, Lieber RL. Biomechanical analysis of the brachioradialis as a donor in tendon transfer. *Clin Orthop Relat Res*. 2001;(383):152-161.
3. Johnson DL, Gellman H, Waters RL, Tognella M. Brachioradialis transfer for wrist extension in tetraplegic patients who have fifth-cervical-level neurological function. *J Bone Joint Surg Am*. 1996;78(7):1063-1067.

4. Leclercq C. Surgical rehabilitation for the weaker patients (groups 1 and 2 of the International Classification). *Hand Clin.* 2002;18(3):461-479.
5. Moberg E. Surgical treatment for absent single-hand grip and elbow extension in quadriplegia: principles and preliminary experience. *J Bone Joint Surg Am.* 1975;57(2):196-206.
6. Freehafer AA, Mast WA. Transfer of the brachioradialis to improve wrist extension in high spinal-cord improve injury. *J Bone Joint Surg Am.* 1967;49(4):648-652.
7. Revol M, Cormerais A, Laffont I, et al. Tendon transfers as applied to tetraplegia. *Hand Clin.* 2002;18(3):423-439.

Finger Extension Procedures

Paymon Rahgozar and Kevin C. Chung

DEFINITION

- Patients with spastic conditions may develop a finger flexion deformity resulting in difficulty with passive finger extension, even with the wrist in full flexion.
- The deformity can be quite severe with fingers clasped into the palm resulting in skin maceration and breakdown from the digging of fingernails into palmar skin.
- This also results in problems for the patient with activities of daily living and personal hygiene.

ANATOMY

- The flexor digitorum superficialis (FDS) and the flexor digitorum profundus (FDP) are most often involved in flexion deformities.
- The surgeon must be familiar with the volar forearm muscle anatomy, including the location of critical neurovascular structures such as the median nerve, ulnar nerve, radial artery, and ulnar artery.
- The FDS originates from the medial epicondyle, the coronoid process of the ulna, and the anterior oblique line of the radial head before splitting into four bellies at the junction between the middle and distal thirds of the radius. It has a humeroulnar head and a radial head, with the median nerve and ulnar artery traveling between them.
  - Each muscle belly contributes a tendon that passes through the carpal tunnel and inserts on the middle phalanx of the corresponding digit (**FIG 1**).
  - The tendons of the middle and ring finger travel volar to the tendons of the index and small finger through the carpal tunnel.
- The FDP originates from the proximal ulna and the interosseous membrane and sends tendons through the carpal tunnel to insert on the distal phalanges of the medial four digits.
- The extensor digitorum communis (EDC) origin is on the lateral epicondyle as a single muscle eventually splitting into separate muscle bellies to insert on the extensor expansions of the corresponding digits.

PATIENT HISTORY AND PHYSICAL FINDINGS

- The exam must involve a full examination of all flexor muscles of the wrist, hand, and fingers.
- The patient typically presents with the fingers flexed into the palm. A thumb-in-palm deformity is also frequently present (**FIG 2**).

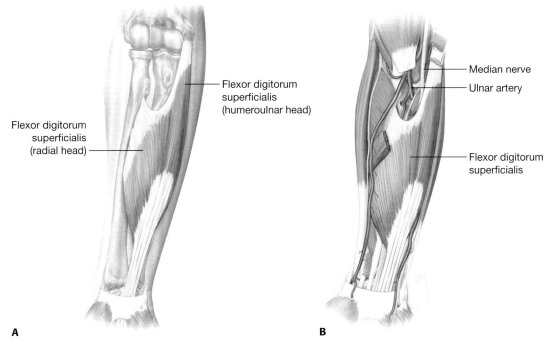

Flexor digitorum superficialis (humeroulnar head)

Flexor digitorum superficialis (radial head)

Median nerve

Ulnar artery

Flexor digitorum superficialis

A

B

FIG 1 • Volar forearm anatomy. **A.** The flexor digitorum superficialis has a humeroulnar and a radial origin with insertion on the proximal phalanges of the medial four digits. **B.** The median nerve and ulnar artery travel between the two heads.

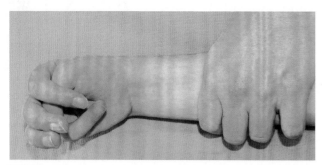

FIG 2 • Common clinical appearance of finger flexion deformity with flexed digits and a thumb in palm deformity.

- Any degree of active finger flexion or extension must be ascertained. The examiner can test active flexion by placing a finger in the patient's palm and asking the patient to grasp. Any increase in pressure indicates some degree of muscle control.
- Active extension can be tested by eliminating flexor tone with an anesthetic block of the median nerve in the antecubital space and the ulnar nerve in the cubital tunnel.
- Patients who have marked flexion of the proximal interphalangeal joints without flexion of the distal interphalangeal joints (DIP) likely have involvement of the FDS. On the other hand, flexion of the DIP suggests FDP involvement.
- To best differentiate between FDS and FDP involvement, examine the patient with the wrist flexed.
- It is imperative to examine the remainder of the hand for any other fixed contractures that could lead to a suboptimal postoperative outcome with a tendon transfer or fractional lengthening.

IMAGING

- Electromyography (EMG) may be helpful to evaluate which muscles are under volitional control prior to transfer.

SURGICAL MANAGEMENT

- Finger extension can be established with a tendon transfer or a fractional lengthening.
- The advantages of an FDS to EDC tendon transfer include a straight line of pull, sufficient power, and adequate excursion.[1]
- Fractional lengthening is best performed for functional hands where the fingers cannot be actively extended with the wrist in a neutral position but can be extended when the wrist is flexed.
- The maximum length of excursion that can be gained from fractional lengthening is 2.5 cm. If a greater degree of lengthening is necessary, a transfer may be more appropriate.[2]

Preoperative Planning

- In cases of spasticity as a result of neurologic injury, it is important to delay surgery until there is a plateau in neurologic recovery, as the degree of spasticity can change with recovery.
  - This period of recovery can range from 6 to 18 months.
- For flexor lengthening, the amount of preoperative active extension is measured and noted, as this will be used to measure the amount of lengthening required intraoperatively.

Positioning

- Position the patient supine with the arm on an armboard. A nonsterile tourniquet can be applied to the upper arm to provide a relatively bloodless field during the procedure.

Approach

- The superficialis tendon can be routed through a radial or ulnar subcutaneous route or through the interosseous membrane.
- Either the superficialis tendon to the ring or the long finger can be used for transfer to the EDC.
- A longitudinal volar incision in the distal third of the forearm is typically used for fractional lengthening of the flexor tendons.

TECHNIQUES

■ Flexor Digitorum Superficialis to Extensor Digitorum Communis Tendon Transfer

- Make an approximate 5-cm longitudinal incision along the border of the volar mid-forearm (**TECH FIG 1A**).
  - Dissect through the subcutaneous tissue to visualize the pronator quadratus and the interosseous membrane.
- Make a transverse incision at the base of the long or ring finger. Carry out dissection through the palm and identify the interval in the flexor sheath between the A1 pulley and the A2 pulley.
  - While protecting the flexor digitorum profundus (FDP) tendon, sharply divide the flexor digitorum superficialis (FDS) proximal to Camper chiasm, which should be adequate length for transfer to the extensor digitorum communis (EDC).
  - Deliver the FDS through the forearm wound with the wrist flexed (**TECH FIG 1B**).
- Make a longitudinal incision along the dorsal hand to identify the EDC tendons (**TECH FIG 1C**).

- Create a radial-based subcutaneous tunnel from the volar incision to the dorsal incision. Avoid injury to the radial neurovascular structures. Transfer the FDS tendon through this tunnel from a volar to dorsal direction (**TECH FIG 1D**).
- Perform a Pulvertaft weave with the FDS tendon to the EDC tendons in an end-to-end fashion distal to the extensor retinaculum (**TECH FIG 1E**). Set the tension with the wrist in 30 degrees of extension while the assistant clenches the fingers and the thumb into a fist to ensure that the repair is not too tight. Range the wrist from 30 degrees flexion to 30 degrees of extension and observe the finger cascade to confirm an appropriate tenodesis effect. The fingers should passively extend with wrist flexion and passively flex with wrist extension. If this does not occur, the tension of the repair may need to be adjusted.
- Release the tourniquet and achieve hemostasis. Close all the wounds primarily.
- Apply a splint with the wrist and digits in extension to the level of the proximal interphalangeal joints.

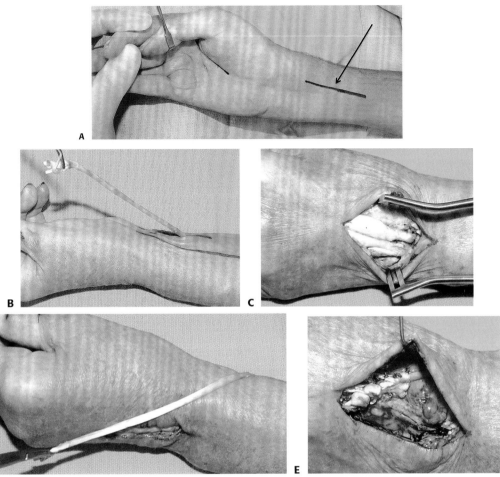

TECH FIG 1 • **A.** Volar mid-forearm incision (*arrow*) to approach the flexor tendons both for the FDS to EDC transfer and for flexor lengthening. **B.** FDS tendon divided distally and delivered through proximal forearm wound. **C.** Dorsal incision with exposure of the extensor digitorum communis tendons. **D.** Transfer of the FDS tendon from a volar to dorsal direction around the radial side of the wrist. **E.** Pulvertaft weave of FDS to EDC in an end-to-end fashion.

■ Step-Cut Fractional Lengthening of Flexor Tendons

- Make an approximate 5-cm longitudinal volar incision in the mid-distal forearm overlying the musculotendinous junctions of the flexor muscles.
- Carry out subcutaneous dissection to visualize the tendinous portions of the flexor muscles (**TECH FIG 2A**).
- Identify the musculotendinous junction (**TECH FIG 2B**).
- Measure the amount of lengthening necessary by placing the wrist and digits in the position of maximum active extension determined preoperatively. From this position, passively extend the fingers and measure the amount of tendon excursion. The tendons will need to be lengthened by a value half of that measured.
- Obliquely divide each of the FDS tendons at the musculotendinous junction without injuring the muscle fibers (**TECH FIG 2C**). The vascularity and support of the muscle will be necessary for postoperative tendon healing.
- Passively extend each digit just short of the desired length and observe as the tendon and muscle fibers slide distally creating a 2- to 3-cm gap.

- If the procedure is also being performed for wrist flexion, first divide the flexor carpi radialis and flexor carpi ulnaris myotendinous junctions before the finger flexors.
- Determine if FDP lengthening is necessary by examining the amount of extension attained after FDS lengthening.
  - If FDP lengthening is required, dissect the FDP tendons.
  - During the dissection, carefully ligate small ulnar artery perforators with bipolar cautery to prevent postoperative bleeding.
  - Divide the FDP tendons at the musculotendinous junction as described above.
- The flexor pollicis longus tendon can also be lengthened if necessary.
- If, after dividing all the FDS and FDP tendons, there is still inadequate lengthening, a second recession can then be made.
- Deflate the tourniquet and achieve hemostasis. Close the incision primarily (**TECH FIG 2D**).
- Provided there is no excess tension on the neurovascular structures, splint the patient with the wrist in neutral position and permitting mobilization of the fingers.

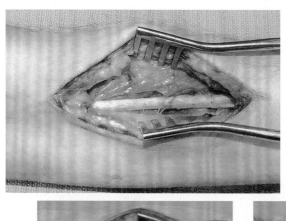
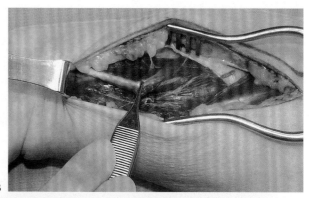
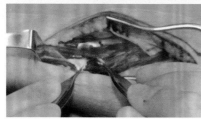
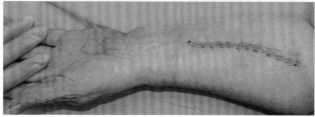

TECH FIG 2 • A. Volar incision with visualization of the FDS tendon. **B.** The musculotendinous junction is identified and will be the location of the lengthening. **C.** Recessions made in the FDS and FDP. Note the lengthening of the tendon between the two forceps. **D.** Wound closure with the fingers in extension. Care is taken to appreciate any tension on neurovascular structures before closing the wound and splinting the fingers in extension.

PEARLS AND PITFALLS

Flexor digitorum superficialis to extensor digitorum communis transfer	▪ Confirm that the extensor retinaculum does not impinge on the conjoined tendons. It can be incised if necessary. ▪ Perform a Pulvertaft weave and confirm that appropriate tension has been set by observing the finger cascade with tenodesis of the wrist. Wrist extension should result in passive finger flexion. Similarly wrist flexion should result in passive finger extension.
Flexor lengthening	▪ Be certain to identify the median nerve prior to dividing any of the flexor tendons. ▪ Incise the flexor tendons within the muscle to provide adequate lengthening. Do not cut the tendons too distally. ▪ Do not incise the muscle belly when dividing the tendons. ▪ Re-examine the neurovascular structures prior to postoperative positioning to ensure there is no excess tension with the wrist in neutral position. If there is tension, position the wrist as close to neutral as possible. ▪ Do not fully extend the digits intraoperatively to prevent overcorrection and excess weakening of the flexor tendons, which can lead to a swan-neck deformity.

POSTOPERATIVE CARE

- After the FDS to EDC transfer, the postoperative splint is maintained for 4 weeks. At that point, the splint can be removed for therapy but is to otherwise be worn for another 2 weeks.
  - At 6 weeks, the patient will no longer need external support.
- After flexor tendon lengthening, active and active-assisted exercises begin on the first postoperative day. The immediate active motion permits the flexor tendons to continue to lengthen as necessary given each individual patient's tone and control.
- Passive extension can begin after 4 weeks, and the patient wears a custom orthotic to maintain passive extension for an additional month.
  - The patient can then transition to a nighttime orthotic for an additional 3 months.

OUTCOMES

- After the FDS to EDC transfer, almost all patients have an improvement in function with the majority being excellent to good.[1]
- With flexor lengthening, improvement in function can be observed in up to 90% of patients.[2]

COMPLICATIONS

- With FDS to EDC transfer, patients may rarely develop postoperative extension contractures of the metacarpophalangeal joints necessitating a joint capsulectomy with extensor tenolysis.[1] Other possible complications include setting the tension too loosely or pulling out the tendon weave.

- Transfer of the FDS tendon can lead to proximal interphalangeal joint flexion contracture or hyperextension deformity. This can best be avoided by diving the FDS tendon proximal to the decussation, and not at the level of its insertion, to prevent disruption of the blood supply to the profundus tendon.[3,4]
- In flexor lengthening, it is possible to overlengthen the flexor tendons, leading to a loss of grip strength and a decrease in function.[2] Similarly, an inadequate lengthening can result in persistent postoperative flexion deformity.

REFERENCES

1. Chuinard RG, Boyes JH, Stark HH, Ashworth CR. Tendon transfers for radial nerve palsy: use of superficialis tendons for digital extension. *J Hand Surg [Am]*. 1978;3(6):560-570.
2. Keenan MAE, Abrams RA, Garland DE, Waters RL. Results of fractional lengthening of the finger flexors in adults with upper extremity spasticity. *J Hand Surg [Am]*. 1987;12(4):575-581.
3. North ER, Littler JW. Transferring the flexor superficialis tendon: technical considerations in the prevention of proximal interphalangeal joint disability. *J Hand Surg [Am]*. 1980;5(5):498-501.
4. Moussavi A, Saied A, Karbalaeikhani A. Outcome of tendon transfer for radial nerve paralysis: comparison of three methods. *Indian J Orthop*. 2011;45(6):558-562.

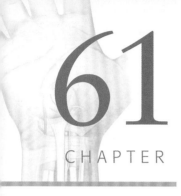

61
CHAPTER

Lateral Key Pinch Reconstruction

Paymon Rahgozar and Kevin C. Chung

DEFINITION

- Lateral key pinch is necessary to secure small objects for many activities of daily living including writing, feeding, drinking, and self-catheterization.
- The act of pinching involves four phases:
  - Object acquisition
  - Pinch/grasp
  - Holding/manipulation
  - Object release
- Patients with C5-C6 tetraplegia most often present with an International Classification for Surgery of the Hand in Tetraplegia (ICT) of 1 or higher. The only muscle available for transfer is the brachioradialis, which is typically used for wrist extension. Therefore, these patients are entirely dependent on tenodesis for passive lateral pinch, resulting in a weak pinch that often stretches with time.
- Patients with an ICT of 2 or more have active wrist extension and are candidates for augmentation of lateral pinch with a brachioradialis (BR) to flexor pollicis longus (FPL) transfer.
  - Those with ICT of 4 or higher are candidates for pronator teres (PT) transfer to the FPL, freeing up the BR for additional tendon transfers.

ANATOMY

- The surgeon must be familiar with the forearm anatomy, including the brachioradialis and its local neurovascular structures (**FIG 1**).
- Two-thirds of the pronator teres (PT) originates from the medial epicondyle inferior and lateral to the flexor carpi ulnaris. One-third originates from the anterior proximal ulna. The PT has very little free tendon distal to its muscle belly, measuring approximately 1 cm and often blending with the periosteum.[1]
- The FPL origin is the volar surface of the radius adjacent to the interosseous membrane, and it inserts on the base of the distal phalanx of the thumb. It runs in the same plane as the flexor digitorum profundus.

PATIENT HISTORY AND PHYSICAL FINDINGS

- The exam should include a complete motor and sensory assessment of the extremity. Patients with inadequate sensation are less likely to use the reconstruction, leading to suboptimal outcomes.
- The patient's ability to perform baseline lateral pinch should be assessed, with the wrist in 30 degrees of flexion, neutral position, and 30 degrees of extension.
- The brachioradialis or the pronator teres must be confirmed to have a MRC grade 4 or higher prior to transfer.

- The strength of the brachioradialis must have a Medical Research Council grade 4 or higher. To test the brachioradialis, position the patient's elbow in a midprone position and have the patient flex against resistance contracting the brachioradialis. Palpate and attempt to move the belly of the muscle. If the muscle is tight, the brachioradialis has adequate strength for transfer (**FIG 2**).
- The pronator teres can be palpated on the lateral forearm distal to the antecubital fossa with resisted pronation.
- The index finger strength should be evaluated to ensure stability to serve as a post for the reconstructed thumb.

IMAGING

- If the examination is equivocal, electromyography (EMG) may be used to confirm or verify that the brachioradialis or pronator teres is under volitional control prior to transfer.

SURGICAL MANAGEMENT

- The goal of surgery is to establish a strong key pinch between the pulp of the thumb and the radial side of the index finger, independent of wrist extension.

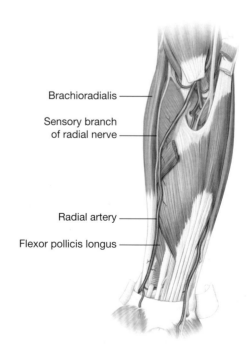

FIG 1 • Relevant volar anatomy. Note the relationship of the brachioradialis with the sensory branch of the radial nerve and the radial artery.

Brachioradialis

Sensory branch of radial nerve

Radial artery

Flexor pollicis longus

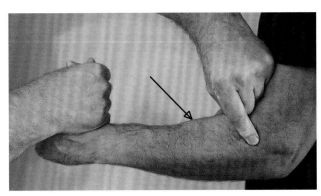

FIG 2 • To examine the brachioradialis, place the patient's forearm in neutral position and ask the patient to flex the elbow against resistance. The prominence of the muscle belly is evident along the proximal radial forearm (*arrow*). Difficulty to displace the muscle with the examiner's hand confirms adequate strength for transfer.

- Prerequisites to surgery include[2] the following:
  - Stability in a wheelchair. The patient must be able to sit for extended periods of time to use the reconstruction for meaningful tasks.
  - Control of the elbow. Control of the arm and hand position in space is imperative for key pinch.
  - Ability to pronate the arm. With pronation, gravity will enable wrist flexion to releasing the pinch.
  - Sufficient power in wrist extension to augment the power of the pinch
  - Normal passive range of motion of the thumb carpometacarpal (CMC) joint
  - Stability of the index finger to serve as a post against which the thumb can push during pinch
- Patients should have intact two-point discrimination of less than 1.5 cm at the thumb and index finger.[3]
- Patients with active wrist extensors and the ability to passively or actively flex the fingers are the ideal candidates for active key pinch reconstruction.

- In patients with tetraplegia, activation of the FPL alone will often interfere with the normal balance of the thumb. This will lead to unpredictable thumb positioning and instability. To help circumvent this problem, the following procedures can accompany the tendon transfer to the FPL:
  - Preposition the thumb ray through a fusion at the CMC joint. This helps to stabilize the normally complex movements of the CMC saddle joint.
  - Stabilize the interphalangeal (IP) joint of the thumb to prevent IP joint hyperflexion from unopposed FPL flexion across the IP joint (Froment sign).
  - Tenodesis of the extensor pollicis longus (EPL) extending the IP joint of the thumb with wrist flexion to aid in release of the pinch
- In cases of spinal cord injury, it is important to delay the surgical intervention until the patient's recovery has plateaued, typically 12 to 18 months.

Preoperative Planning

- The patient's underlying cause of spasticity and the current psychosocial state must be carefully assessed before proceeding with surgical reconstruction (see chapter on Elbow Extension Procedures).
- Any contractures preventing passive range of motion must be treated prior to tendon transfer. On the day of surgery, the range of motion must be assessed to rule out recurrence of the contracture.

Positioning

- Position the patient supine with the arm extended on an armboard.
- An upper arm tourniquet can provide a relatively bloodless field during the procedure.

Approach

- The brachioradialis or the pronator teres can be utilized for transfer to the FPL depending on the number of active muscles available with an MRC score of 4 or higher.

■ Brachioradialis/Pronator Teres to Flexor Pollicis Longus Transfer

- Make an 8- to 10-cm longitudinal incision on the dorsoradial wrist beginning at the radial styloid and extending proximally.
- If the brachioradialis will be used for transfer, begin subcutaneous dissection and identify the tendon of the brachioradialis, the superficial branch of the radial nerve, and the radial artery. Protect the neurovascular structures, longitudinally incise the paratenon, and dissect the brachioradialis.
- Sharply divide the terminal tendon as distal as possible under the abductor pollicis longus and the extensor pollicis brevis.
- Dissect along the deep aspect of the muscle by freeing it from its fascial and muscle connections proximally toward the elbow. As dissection proceeds proximally from the tendon insertion, the radial artery and the dorsal sensory branch of the radial nerve become more prominent. Ligate the small perforating vessels entering the muscle belly.

- Continue proximal dissection until the radial recurrent vessels are identified. The vessels will be traveling transversely on the deep aspect of the muscle just distal to the elbow flexion crease.
  - This marks the extent of the proximal dissection.
- An approximate 3 cm of excursion will be obtained if the muscle is completely freed.
- If the pronator teres is to be used for transfer, identify and incise it at its insertion on the radius. Similar to the brachioradialis, elevate the PT from the radial periosteum proximally for 4 to 5 cm (**TECH FIG 1A**).
- Identify the FPL tendon deep to the flexor carpi radialis (FCR) and radial to the flexor digitorum profundus. Take care to identify and protect the radial artery. Divide the FPL 1 cm proximal to the proximal edge of the pronator quadratus (**TECH FIG 1B**).
- Tunnel the brachioradialis under the radial neurovascular bundle so that it can reach the FPL. Suture the BR or the PT tendon to the FPL with 2-0 nonabsorbable braided sutures with a Pulvertaft weave (**TECH FIG 1C**).

T E C H N I Q U E S

- Set the tension so that passive wrist flexion causes thumb abduction and extension and so that wrist extension flexes the thumb metacarpophalangeal joint, positioning the pulp of the thumb against the radial side of the middle phalanx of the index finger (**TECH FIG 1D,E**).

- Release the tourniquet and achieve hemostasis. Close the incisions primarily.
- Place a long-arm splint with the elbow in midprone position and 90 degrees of flexion, the wrist in 10 to 20 degrees of flexion, and the thumb in abduction.

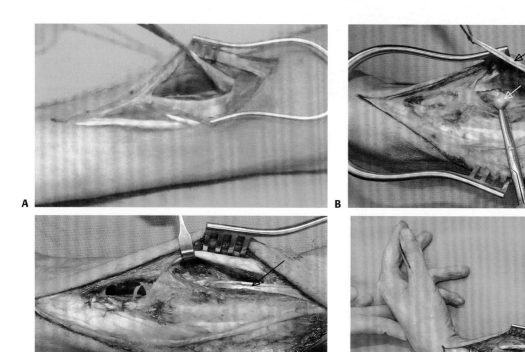

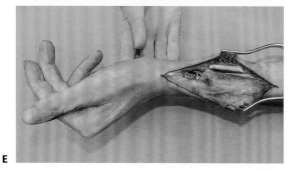

TECH FIG 1 • A. Dissection of the pronator teres muscle. An approximate 4 to 5 cm of elevation off the periosteum of the radius is necessary. **B.** The FPL (*white arrow*) is identified and ligated proximal to the pronator quadratus for transfer. The *black arrow* indicates the brachioradialis. **C.** The brachioradialis (*black arrow*) is tunneled deep to the radial neurovascular bundle and sutured to the FPL with a Pulvertaft weave. **D,E.** The tension is set so that passive wrist flexion causes thumb abduction and wrist extension positions the pulp of the thumb against the radial side of the middle phalanx of the index finger, effectively creating a pinch.

PEARLS AND PITFALLS

Patient selection	▪ Confirm that there is adequate index finger strength and stability to serve as a post for the thumb. ▪ Sensation is important for useful pinch function.
Surgical procedure	▪ Identify and protect the radial sensory nerve before dividing the brachioradialis tendon. ▪ Do not injure the radial recurrent vessels when dissecting the BR proximally. They can be found on the deep surface of the muscle just distal to the elbow flexion crease signaling the extent of proximal dissection. ▪ The neurovascular supply to the brachioradialis should not be at risk because it enters the muscle proximal to the elbow. ▪ Free the brachioradialis proximally to the level of the elbow (without injuring the vascular pedicle) to provide adequate excursion. ▪ Pass the brachioradialis deep (dorsal) to the radial artery before performing the tendon repair. ▪ Elevate the pronator teres off the radial periosteum for approximately 4–5 cm. ▪ Other procedures such as IP joint stabilization, CMC fusion, or EPL tenodesis may be necessary depending on the individual.

POSTOPERATIVE CARE

- The patient remains immobilized in a splint for 6 weeks followed by mobilization with occupational therapy.

OUTCOMES

- Patients can achieve an average postoperative key pinch strength of 2 kg, facilitating many activities of daily living including hygiene, grooming, mobility, and writing.[3] The longevity of the reconstruction is excellent with a minimal decrease in strength over time.[4]

COMPLICATIONS

- Tendon adhesions are a potential complication particularly if additional tendon transfers are being performed during the procedure.[5]
- Brachioradialis transfer to the FPL can result in hyperflexion of the interphalangeal joint resulting in a pinch posture

between the dorsal distal thumb phalanx and the volar index middle phalanx.[6] This can be addressed with stabilization of the IP joint.

REFERENCES

1. Lieber RL, Jacobson MD, Fazeli BM, et al. Architecture of selected muscles of the arm and forearm: anatomy and implications for tendon transfer. *J Hand Surg [Am]*. 1992;17(5):787-798.
2. Hentz VR. Surgical strategy: matching the patient with the procedure. *Hand Clin*. 2002;18(3):503-518.
3. Waters R, Moore KR, Graboff SR, Paris K. Brachioradialis to flexor pollicis longus tendon transfer for active lateral pinch in the tetraplegic. *J Hand Surg [Am]*. 1985;10(3):385-391.
4. Dunn JA, Rothwell AG, Mohammed KD, Sinnott KA. The effects of aging on upper limb tendon transfers in patients with tetraplegia. *J Hand Surg [Am]*. 2014;39(2):317-323.
5. Failla JM, Peimer CA, Sherwin FS. Brachioradialis transfer for digital palsy. *J Hand Surg Br*. 1990;15(3):312-316.
6. Leclercq C. Surgical rehabilitation for the weaker patients (groups 1 and 2 of the International Classification). *Hand Clin*. 2002;18(3):461-479.

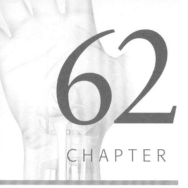

62
CHAPTER

Grasp Improvement Procedures

Paymon Rahgozar and Kevin C. Chung

DEFINITION

- The primary purpose of the hand is for gripping, feeling, and engaging in human contact. The capacity to pinch and grasp is key to productive gripping.
- With the ability to grasp objects in the palm, an individual can handle larger objects than would otherwise be possible with pinch alone. Manipulating cans, bottles, or a telephone becomes a reality, significantly expanding an individual's breadth and capacity to perform activities of daily living.
- Patients with a midlevel tetraplegia or International Classification for Surgery of the Hand in Tetraplegia (ICT) scores of 3 or higher have sufficient donor muscles for active grasp reconstruction (see chapter on Elbow Extension Procedures). The extensor carpi radialis longus (ECRL) can be used for tendon transfer while preserving the extensor carpi radials brevis (ECRB) for active wrist extension.
- The ECRL is a good potential donor for active finger flexion because it is synergistic with the finger flexors. Normally, finger flexion is paired with wrist extension, making postoperative rehabilitation much easier for the patient.
- Additionally, patients with spasticity may present with fixed finger flexion deformities.
- A fixed flexion deformity of the flexor digitorum superficialis (FDS) and the flexor digitorum profundus (FDP) can lead to difficulty with personal skin care and hand hygiene.
  - An FDS to FDP (superficialis to profundus, STP) transfer can alleviate such contractures.
- Performing grasp is also challenging in patients with an intrinsic minus hand position: metacarpophalangeal (MCP) hyperextension and interphalangeal (IP) flexion.
- A Zancolli lasso procedure using the FDS tendons can provide hand intrinsic balancing in patients with an intrinsic minus deformity via a dynamic tenodesis effect.

ANATOMY

- The surgeon must be familiar with the anatomy of the finger flexors including both the FDS and the FDP (see Finger Extension chapter).
- The ECRL originates from the distal supracondylar ridge and inserts on the base of the index metacarpal. It serves to extend and radially deviate the wrist.

PATIENT HISTORY AND PHYSICAL FINDINGS

- The entire upper extremity must be examined for both motor and sensory function including range of motion. The evaluation must also incorporate the resting position of the hand, as this will guide the surgical approach. Patients with a contracture and flexion posture of the fingers will benefit from an STP transfer, whereas those with clawing may require a lasso procedure.
- In patients with tetraplegia, the ICT score must be determined. Both the ECRL and the ECRB must be active with sufficient wrist extension if the ECRL is to be used as a donor muscle for active grasp reconstruction.
- To test the ECRB and ECRL, the patient attempts wrist extension against resistance. A palpable groove, or V sign, forms between the two proximal muscle bellies if both have an MRC grade of 5 (**FIG 1**).[1]
- For patients presenting with a contracture, it is important to specifically evaluate the contribution of the FDS and FDP muscles to the contracture. Examine finger extension both with the wrist in maximum flexion and in maximum extension.
  - In cases of FDS and FDP contracture, finger flexion deformity will be worse on examination with the wrist in maximum extension as compared to maximum flexion. This occurs because wrist extension tightens the flexor tendons exacerbating the deformity.
- The MCP, proximal IP, and distal IP joints should be examined to rule out joint contracture and intrinsic tightness.
  - An ulnar nerve lidocaine block during examination can help better determine the presence of intrinsic spasticity or contracture.[2] Spasticity will improve after a nerve block whereas a contracture will not.

IMAGING

- If despite clinical examination, the examiner is still uncertain of whether a muscle is under volitional control, electromyography focusing on the muscle of interest helps identify spastic and flaccid muscles and determine phasic activity.

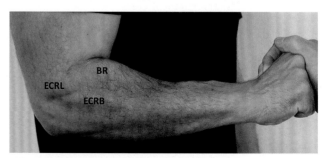

FIG 1 • Test to confirm active use of the ECRL and ECRB. A V sign forms between the two muscle bellies of the wrist extensors with resisted wrist extension.

NONOPERATIVE MANAGEMENT

- Modest attempts to control the position of the hand in contracture or spasticity can be performed with serial splinting or casting.
- Phenol motor blocks may alleviate spasticity to a degree.

SURGICAL MANAGEMENT

- ECRL to FDP transfer
  - For an effective grasp, the fingers must first be able to extend to wrap around an object and then flex to grab it.
  - Unlike lateral pinch where tenodesis of the EPL can be used to extend the thumb in preparation for pinch, for grasp, and for release, the reconstruction cannot rely solely on finger tenodesis for finger extension. The presence of active finger flexion without active finger extensors will create a tendon imbalance, leading to flexion contractures.
  - Finger extension and finger flexion reconstructions have competing postoperative rehabilitation protocols. Historically, a two-staged reconstruction has been described. The ECRL to FDP transfer is typically the second stage, whereas the extensor reconstruction is the first stage (see Finger Extension chapter). However, both stages are more frequently performed simultaneously, particularly in a more frail and elderly patient who may not tolerate multiple operations with multiple periods of immobilization.
  - Before active grasp reconstruction, the priority is to first ensure the patient has active elbow and wrist extension. Therefore, only patients with ICT grade 3 or higher have sufficient donor muscles for reconstruction.
  - ECRL to FDP transfer is indicated in patients who require active finger flexion and have good active wrist extension with supple wrist and PIP joints.
  - Wrist extension occurs synergistically with finger flexion, making the ECRL an ideal motor for transfer to the FDP. Postoperative learning and rehabilitation is simpler than with other nonsynergistic transfers. Additionally, active wrist extension will shorten the flexors via tenodesis. The ECRL to FDP transfer takes advantage of this biomechanical principle by enhancing FDP flexion with wrist extension and providing an additional 2 cm of tendon excursion.[3]
- STP transfer
  - The STP transfer is indicated in patients with severe spasticity or in patients with an established contracture of the forearm musculotendinous units, resulting in fixed finger flexion contracture.[4]
  - The patient typically has no functional use of the fingers and often suffers from hygiene problems with skin maceration and nonhealing palmar wounds.
  - The goal of the procedure is to position the hand in a more functional posture, facilitating hygiene and personal care, without leaving the patient with flaccid fingers.
  - The procedure alleviates contracture by transecting the finger flexors but still maintains wrist balance by transferring the FDS to the FDP tendons (**FIG 2**). The STP transfer can be performed with concomitant lengthening of wrist and thumb flexors when necessary, to achieve a position of balance between the wrist and digits.[4]
- Zancolli lasso procedure
  - The Zancolli lasso procedure is indicated in patients with clawing or an intrinsic minus deformity of the digits.

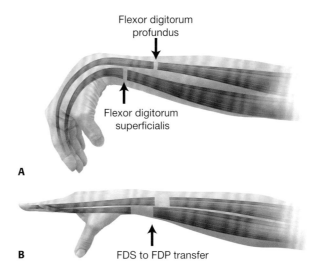

FIG 2 • FDS to FDP transfer. **A.** Finger flexion deformity involving both the FDS and FDP muscles. A transection is made in the proximal FDP and the distal FDS. **B.** The wrist is extended and the proximal end of the FDS is transferred to the distal end of the FDP to re-establish wrist balance and permit finger flexion.

  - As originally described by Zancolli, the lasso procedure results in a dynamic passive tenodesis causing MP flexion with active wrist extension. This augments grasp by initiating the first stage of grasping: MP flexion.
  - Patients with a concurrent PIP flexion deformity from FDS spasticity further benefit from the lasso procedure by releasing the FDS as the spastic deforming force and transferring it into an MP flexor.
  - The lasso procedure can also be performed prophylactically to prevent MP joint hyperextension and clawing with finger extension.
  - Taking advantage of the tenodesis effect, the lasso procedure is also effective in patients with a paralyzed FDS.

Preoperative Planning

- It is imperative to confirm that the patient is not entirely dependent on the ECRL for wrist extension prior to its use for transfer. The V sign confirming the presence of a strong ECRL and ECRB on physical exam is very reliable, but if there is any doubt, the surgeon should leave the ECRL intact (see **FIG 1**).
- Prior to an STP transfer, confirm that the MCP and IP joints are supple. If joint contracture is present, the transfer alone will do little to improve the flexion deformity. The patient may need additional procedures such as closed manipulation, capsulotomies, or joint fusions.
- Following an STP transfer, the patient will continue to have limited finger motion. The purpose of the operation is to improve finger position for better hygiene, not function. This should be clearly discussed with the patient and caregivers before surgery.
- If an anterior elbow release is also planned, perform the release prior to the FDS tendon transfer. This will facilitate positioning the forearm, simplifying exposure and visualization for STP transfer.

Positioning

- The patient is placed in the supine position with the arm extended on an arm board. A nonsterile upper arm tourniquet is applied to provide a bloodless operative field. General anesthesia can help provide maximum muscle relaxation.

Approach

- Various approaches are possible, and multiple incisions are often required.
- The ECRL can be transferred to the FDP around the radial border of the radius or through the interosseous membrane. An advantage of transfer around the radius is that the line of pull provides secondary forearm supination.
- The Zancolli lasso is an intrinsic reconstruction that is an adjunct to the extrinsic tendon reconstruction. It can be performed during either of the two stages of hand reconstruction (extensor or flexor stage).
- For the Zancolli lasso procedure, a single transverse incision or separate zigzag incisions can be made across the MP flexion creases. The lasso can be performed with the FDS of each individual finger used as a lasso or splitting the slips of the FDS of the middle and ring finger to lasso around the index/middle and the ring/small fingers, respectively. Another technique involves taking only the middle finger FDS tendon and splitting it into four slips to be used for all the fingers.[5]

■ Extensor Carpi Radialis Longus to Flexor Digitorum Profundus Transfer for Active Finger Flexion

- Make an 8- to 10-cm longitudinal dorsal incision (**TECH FIG 1A**).
- Identify the extensor carpi radialis longus (ECRL) and the extensor carpi radialis brevis tendons (ECRB). Identify and protect the superficial radial nerve (**TECH FIG 1B**).
- Sharply transect the ECRL tendon as distal as possible at the level of its insertion on the index metacarpal and deliver it proximal to the extensor retinaculum.
- Dissect the ECRL as far proximal as possible to maximize its excursion and to provide a straight line of pull for its new insertion.
- Make a volar incision to identify the FDP tendons at its musculotendinous junctions at the wrist crease (**TECH FIG 1C**).
- Pass the ECRL tendon under the radial vessels into the volar forearm and perform a Pulvertaft weave in an end-to-end fashion to the flexor digitorum profundus tendons with 2-0 nonabsorbable braided sutures (**TECH FIG 1D**).
  - Be certain to include the FDP tendon to the index finger. It often is separate from the remaining digital profundus tendons and can easily be missed in the transfer.[6]
- Set the tension with the wrist in maximal tension. The fingertips should touch the palm with the wrist in full passive extension after tendon transfer.[7]
- If a Zancolli lasso procedure is also part of the reconstruction plan, perform it before ECRL transfer (either as a first-stage procedure or just before the ECRL transfer). The tension can be better gauged in this manner.
  - After the lasso procedure is complete, set the ECRL tension with the finger MP joints at 0 degrees when the wrist is at neutral. With the wrist in extension, the MP joints should flex 30 to 40 degrees.
- Release the tourniquet and achieve hemostasis. Close the incisions primarily.

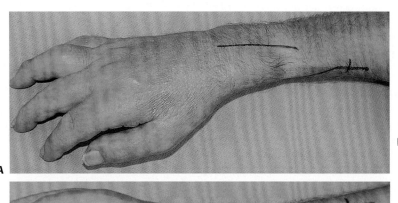

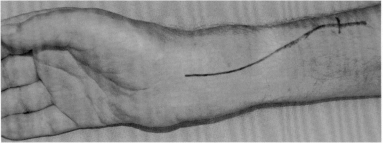

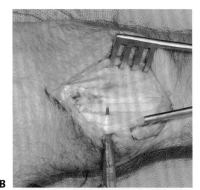

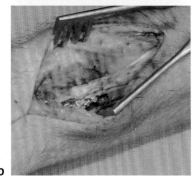

TECH FIG 1 • **A.** Dorsal incision for exposure of the extensor tendons. **B.** Identification of the ECRL tendon. **C.** Volar incision for exposure of the FDP tendons. **D.** Transfer of the ECRL tendon in the volar direction and completion of a Pulvertaft weave with the FDP tendons. Left, distal; right, proximal.

■ Flexor Digitorum Superficialis to Flexor Digitorum Profundus Transfer (Superficialis to Profundus Transfer)

- Identify the FDS and FDP tendons through a volar forearm incision (see **TECH FIG 1C**). Take care to avoid injury to the median nerve and the ulnar neurovascular bundle.
- Identify the palmaris longus, and perform a tenotomy proximally.
- Flex the wrist and identify the tendons of the FDS to the index, long, ring, and small fingers. Proximal to the transverse carpal ligament, suture all the FDS tendons together with a running, locking, nonabsorbable suture creating a single tendon unit.
- Sharply transect the FDS tendons at the level of the wrist distal to the suture line (**TECH FIG 2A**).
- Retract the FDS tendon unit proximally exposing the FDP tendons. In a similar fashion, create a single tendon unit across the most proximal convergence of the FDP tendons to the index, long, ring, and small fingers. This location is approximately 10 cm proximal to the wrist crease. Sharply transect the FDP tendons proximal to the suture line (**TECH FIG 2B**).
- Extend the wrist and fingers, and note that the distal ends of the cut FDP tendons migrate distally.
- Suture the proximal FDS tendon unit to the distal FDP tendon unit with a nonabsorbable braided suture. Set the tension with an assistant holding the wrist and the fingers in maximum extension (**TECH FIG 2C**).
- Confirm that there is corrected finger extension and presence of the normal finger cascade.
- Release the tourniquet and achieve hemostasis. Close the wound primarily.
- Place a postoperative splint with the wrist in 20 degrees of extension and fingers in 20 degrees of flexion at the metacarpophalangeal and interphalangeal joints.

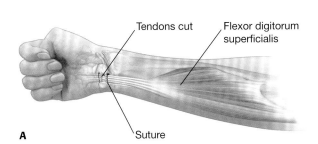

A

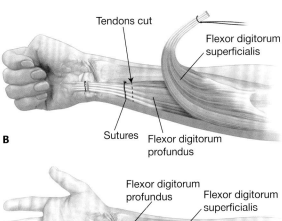

B

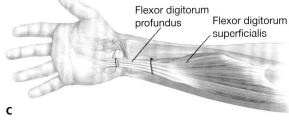

C

TECH FIG 2 • **A.** The tendons of the FDS are sutured together at the level of the wrist creating a single tendon unit. The tendons are ligated distal to the suture line. **B.** The sutured FDS unit is retracted proximally, and the FDP is identified. Approximately 10 cm proximal to the wrist crease, the FDP tendons are sutured together. The tendons are ligated proximal to the suture line. **C.** The hand is extended and the distal end of the FDP unit will migrate distally. The proximal end of the FDS is sutured to the distal end of the FDP.

■ Zancolli Lasso Procedure

- Make zigzag incisions on the palm and proximal digits to expose the flexor tendon sheaths from the middle of the metacarpal to the middle of the proximal phalanx. Take care to avoid injury to the neurovascular bundles.
- Identify the proximal and distal limits of the A1 pulley.
- Using a forceps, apply tension to the A1 pulley, simulating transfer, to determine whether the MP joint will be pulled into flexion.
  - If the MP joint cannot be pulled into flexion, include a portion of the A2 pulley in the transfer.
- Open the tendon sheath distal to the A1 pulley with an L-shaped incision.
- Flex the finger and identify the two slips of the FDS (**TECH FIG 3A**). Place a suture in the FDS to minimize proximal retraction with ligation.
- Divide both slips of the FDS tendon as far distally as possible. Use the suture in the FDS to help minimize handling of the FDP tendon and potential postoperative adhesions.
- Pull the FDS slips through the opening in the pulley sheath. Ensure that both slips of the FDS are free from all surrounding attachments, including the synovial sheath and vincula (**TECH FIG 3B**).
- Repeat the same procedure for each finger.
- Loop the FDS tendons back over the pulley sheath in a palmar and proximal direction. Suture the FDS tendon to itself using a 4-0 nonabsorbable suture in an interweave fashion (**TECH FIG 3C**).
- After inserting the first suture, confirm that there is appropriate tension by observing the MP motion to passive tenodesis.
  - When the wrist is extended, the MP joints should flex with a uniform cascade.
  - When the wrist is flexed, the MP joints should extend fully without hyperextending.
- Adjust the tension as necessary. Typically, the tension is increased gradually from the index to small fingers to restore a physiologic cascade.[3]

T
E
C
H
N
I
Q
U
E
S

- Confirm that the position of the index finger's MP joint will continue to permit key pinch with the thumb.
- Release the tourniquet and achieve hemostasis. Close the wounds primarily.

- Place the patient in postoperative immobilization with the wrist in 20 to 30 degrees of flexion, MP joints at 60 to 70 degrees of flexion, with the PIP and DIP joints free for 4 weeks.

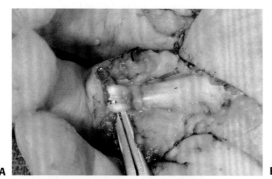
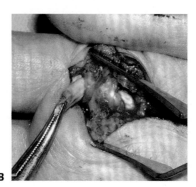
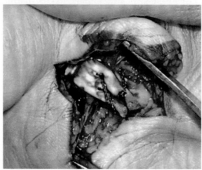

TECH FIG 3 • A. The two slips of the FDS tendon are identified distal to the A1 pulley. The slips are ligated as distal as possible. **B.** The FDS tendon is pulled through the opening in the flexor sheath after ensuring that it is not tethered by the synovial sheath or vincula. **C.** The FDS tendon is looped around the A1 pulley in a palmar and proximal direction. It is sutured to itself forming a lasso around the A1 pulley.

PEARLS AND PITFALLS

General	▪ Release the tourniquet and check for hemostasis prior to wound closure for the STP transfer. There are multiple perforators from the ulnar artery to the FDP that can easily be missed.
	▪ The median nerve can easily be mistaken for a flexor tendon under tourniquet control. A gentle exsanguination will preserve the longitudinal neural blood supply, making it easier to correctly identify and protect the nerve.
ECRL to FDP transfer	▪ Patients must have strong wrist extension and not be solely dependent on the ECRL for wrist extension.
	▪ Identify the tendons of both the ECRL and the ECRB prior to transection to avoid injury to the ECRB.
	▪ Be certain to identify and include the FDP tendon to the index finger.
FDS to FDP transfer	▪ Before closure, confirm that there is no excess tension on the neurovascular structures. This can limit the length of contracture release.
	▪ Create a single tendon unit of the FDS and FDP prior to transection to maintain the normal finger cascade.
	▪ Excursion of the median nerve may be a limiting factor for the amount of contracture release that can safely be attained.
Zancolli lasso procedure	▪ If the small finger FDS is vestigial, the ulnar slip of the ring finger FDS can be used for the lasso.

POSTOPERATIVE CARE

- Following the ECRL to FDP transfer, the patient remains immobilized for 4 weeks until the tendon junctures have healed.
  - At that point, the patient begins mobilization and training with occupational therapy.
- After the STP transfer, the wound is examined at 10 days and sutures are removed.
  - The patient remains immobilized for another 4 weeks. Active finger flexion and extension can then begin, but

the patient is to remain in a splint when not undergoing hand therapy or bathing.
  - After 4 weeks, the patient can transition to a nighttime splint for 3 to 6 more months.
- After the Zancolli lasso procedure, patients begin immediate daily therapy with passive range of motion of the IP joints.
- After 4 weeks, convert the patient to a nighttime resting splint in the same position and active range of motion can be initiated.

OUTCOMES

- The ECRL to FDP transfer typically has good results in establishing active finger flexion.
- Following STP transfer, the majority of patients have an open position of the hand and wrist with resolution of palmar hygiene problems.[2,4]
- Most patients have good to excellent results following the Zancolli lasso procedure with a significant improvement in grip strength.[8]

COMPLICATIONS

- In addition to typical surgical complications, rupture of the tendon repairs is a potential complication. This should be suspected if there is a sudden loss or drop of function during rehabilitation.
  - There should be a low threshold to return to the operating theater for exploration and the surgeon should be prepared to repair or revise the transfer with a tendon graft if necessary.
- If wrist extension is not properly assessed preoperatively and it is not properly established that the patient is dependent on the ECRL for wrist extension, its transfer can lead to postoperative difficulty with wrist extension.
- Following STP transfer, the risk of superficial wound infections is elevated, particularly in patients with macerated palmar skin at time of surgery.[2]

- In patients with intrinsic hypertonicity, a swan-neck deformity can result if the intrinsic spasticity is not also addressed.
- FDP adhesions in the metacarpophalangeal area are common in the Zancolli lasso procedure, occasionally requiring tenolysis.

REFERENCES

1. Mohammed K, Rothwell A, Sinclair W, et al. Upper-limb surgery for tetraplegia. *J Bone Joint Surg Br.* 1992;74(6):873-879.
2. Keenan MA, Korchek JI, Botte MJ, et al. Results of transfer of the flexor digitorum superficialis tendons to the flexor digitorum profundus tendons in adults with acquired spasticity of the hand. *J Bone Joint Surg Am.* 1987;69(8):1127-1132.
3. Revol M, Cormerais A, Laffont I, et al. Tendon transfers as applied to tetraplegia. *Hand Clin.* 2002;18(3):423-439.
4. Braun RM, Vise GT, Roper B. Preliminary experience with superficialis-to-profundus tendon transfer in the hemiplegic upper extremity. *J Bone Joint Surg Am.* 1974;56(3):466-472.
5. Gupta V, Consul A, Swamy MKS. Zancolli lasso procedure for correction of paralytic claw hands. *J Orthop Surg (Hong Kong).* 2015;23(1): 15-18.
6. Freehafer AA. Tendon transfers in tetraplegic patients: the Cleveland experience. *Spinal Cord.* 1998;36(5):315-319.
7. Zancolli EA. Midcervical tetraplegia with strong wrist extension: a two-stage synergistic reconstruction of the hand. *Hand Clin.* 2002;18(3):481-495.
8. Ozkan T, Ozer K, Yukse A, Gulgonen A. Surgical reconstruction of irreversible ulnar nerve paralysis in leprosy. *Lepr Rev.* 2003;74(1):53-62.

63

CHAPTER

Section XIII: Congenital Hand Disorders
Release of Finger Syndactyly Using Dorsal Rectangular Flap

Amir H. Taghinia

DEFINITION

- Syndactyly is fusion of adjacent digits (Gr. *syn* with or together + *dactylos* finger).
- Syndactyly can be congenital or acquired. This discussion focuses on congenital syndactyly.

ANATOMY

- Syndactyly can involve skin, nail, bone, nerves, vessels, and tendons.
  - It can be simple, involving only skin, or complex, involving bone and other tissues. It can also be complicated, wherein the delineation of structures belonging to different digits is difficult to differentiate (**FIG 1A**).
  - It can be complete (involving the entire finger) or incomplete (partial involvement).
  - It can also be wide or narrow (**FIG 1B**). Most authors do not discuss this issue, but it bears greatly on the operative plan for release.
- The normal interdigital web space has an hourglass appearance. It begins dorsally distal to the metacarpophalangeal joint and takes a 45-degree palmar angle. The web meets the palmar skin halfway between the metacarpal head and the proximal interphalangeal (PIP) joint (**FIG 2**).

PATHOGENESIS AND NATURAL HISTORY

- The exact etiology of syndactyly has not been elucidated. It is considered to be a malformation, based on the Oberg, Manske, and Tonkin classification, likely due to failure of apoptosis.[1]
- Syndactyly occurs in 1 out of 2000 to 3000 births. The natural history of untreated syndactyly is dependent on the degree of involvement.

PATIENT HISTORY AND PHYSICAL FINDINGS

- Patients are usually seen in infancy. The diagnosis is clear, but the involvement of deeper structures can be difficult to ascertain via physical examination alone.
- The surgeon should examine and record the web spaces involved, degree of involvement, deviation or angulation, nail involvement, and any deficits in range of motion. In most simple cases, range of motion is normal.
- The surgeon should elicit family history and determine if there are any associated medical conditions (syndromes).

IMAGING

- Plain radiographs are the study of choice, although they are rarely needed for simple syndactyly.

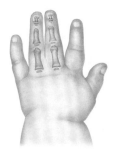
Simple, Incomplete

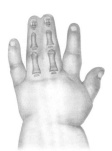
Simple, Complete

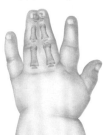
A Complex

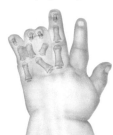
Complicated

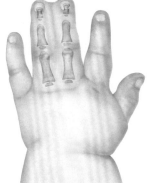
B Wide syndactyly

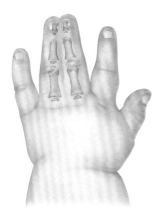
Narrow syndactyly

FIG 1 • A. Four types of syndactyly are shown. **B.** Syndactyly can be wide or narrow. Wide cases provide more skin for closure and allow easier interdigitation of flaps.

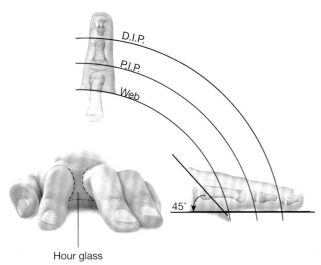

FIG 2 • The normal web space has an hourglass appearance with a 45-degree inclination. It meets the palmar skin halfway between the MP and PIP joints.

- Plain radiographs help delineate the degree of bone involvement and guide timing and technique of surgical release in complex and complicated cases (**FIG 3**).
- A few experts have advocated CT angiography to understand the vasculature when considering simultaneous release of neighboring web spaces,[2] but this is not routinely done.
- Even if simultaneous releases of adjacent digits are planned, the surgeon can make intraoperative judgment by dissecting the neurovascular bundles to preserve at least one artery to each digit.

SURGICAL MANAGEMENT

- The principles of syndactyly release are dorsal flap for commissure reconstruction, volar zigzag incisions to avoid contractures across flexion creases, and use of skin grafts as needed for coverage of open wounds.

- The author plans timing of syndactyly release based on the degree of involvement.
    - Patients with distal phalangeal coalition, especially between the small and ring fingers (with or without involvement of the middle finger), can develop significant deviation and flexion contractures of the longer fingers as the distal phalanges cause tethering (see **FIG 3**). Early intervention can help relieve this problem and allow improved directional growth.
- Simple syndactyly releases can be performed between 1 and 2 years of age. To relieve tethering and deviation, earlier release around 9 months is advocated. The decision to operate early has to be carefully weighed against possible long-term consequences of general anesthesia early on in childhood.
- The decision to use skin grafts, whether they should be split or full thickness, and the places from which to harvest them have been hotly debated in the literature.[3,4] A number of surgeons have presented different techniques for release without use of skin grafts.
    - The author prefers to use of full-thickness skin grafts in most syndactyly release procedures. Syndactyly is a problem of missing skin. Skin grafting provides the best possible release and widest web space.
- The author takes full-thickness grafts from the lower abdomen (not the groin). This area provides ample skin for subsequent releases if there is multiple web involvement and heals nicely.
- Bilateral syndactyly release procedures are performed routinely in infants and toddlers.
- Neighboring web space releases are not performed simultaneously; they are staged about 6 to 9 months apart.
    - Vascular insufficiency concerns alone do not inform this practice; rather, skin deficit on both sides of a finger makes closure more difficult.

Preoperative Planning

- Review radiographs again.
- Discuss risks, benefits, and expectations again with parents on the day of surgery. Specifically outline the risks of dense scarring, flap or graft loss (partial or complete), future web

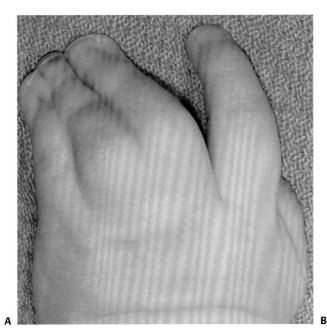
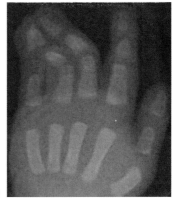

FIG 3 • Complex third and fourth web space syndactyly. Distal phalangeal coalition causes flexion and ulnar deviation of the longer digits.

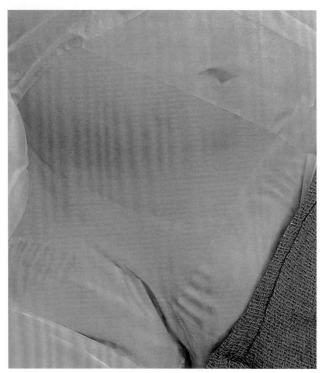

FIG 4 • Draping of lower abdominal donor site for skin graft.

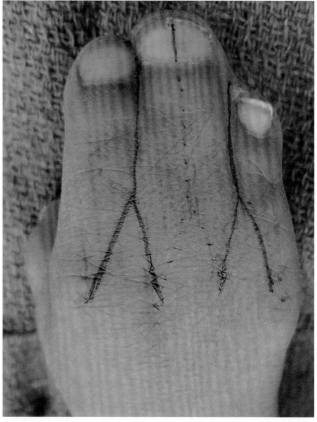

FIG 5 • When the syndactyly is very narrow (usually due to bone fusion) and/or multiple adjacent web spaces are involved—such as in this patient with type I Apert syndrome—there is not enough skin to allow the dorsal and volar triangular flaps to interdigitate. Accordingly, a straight-line dorsal release is planned. In the case shown, adjacent rectangular commissure flaps (for both third and fourth web spaces) would remove too much skin from the nonborder digits; accordingly, triangular flaps were planned.

creep, and hyperpigmentation of skin grafts (especially in those with Fitzpatrick skin type IV and above).

Positioning

- The patient is positioned supine with the arm out on a small hand table.
- The lower abdominal area for the skin graft is squared off with Steri-Drapes (**FIG 4**).

Approach

- Incisions are planned carefully prior to use of the tourniquet. The majority of the "case" is incision planning. The markings dictate where flaps will transpose and where skin grafting is needed.
- In cases where skin is deficient and dorsal and palmar flaps will not interdigitate, the author plans a dorsal straight-line

release (**FIG 5**) and zigzag volar incisions (if flexion creases are present) as outlined above. This approach creates more open wounds to skin graft.
- Dorsal and volar incisions are made for every syndactyly release. Conjoined bones and neurovascular bundles are best approached dorsally.

■ Dorsal Rectangular (Hourglass) Flap for Syndactyly Release

Dorsal Markings

- Mark the metacarpal head pit for each neighboring digit. Draw an hourglass-shaped flap with the distal straight-lined, transverse incision located two-thirds to three-fourths of the distance between the metacarpal head and proximal interphalangeal joint (**TECH FIG 1A**).
- The palmar border of the normal web space lies about halfway between these two anatomic landmarks (see **FIG 2**).
  - Planning the flap's distal extent beyond the halfway point allows it to rotate about its axis proximally

(at the metacarpal heads) and reach just proximal to the ideal location of the web space.
- Mark the extension creases with transverse or slightly oblique lines.
  - In complete and near-complete syndactyly cases, draw these lines from (just shy of) the midpoint of one finger to the other (**TECH FIG 1B**). In incomplete cases, these lines can be shorter (**TECH FIG 1C**).
  - Connect the lines via oblique lines that create the least acute angle to allow for optimal blood flow to the flap. The reason for longer flaps in narrower cases is not additional skin (the amount of skin remains fixed) but greater flexibility in maneuvering the flaps.

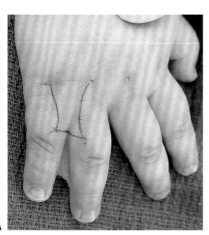 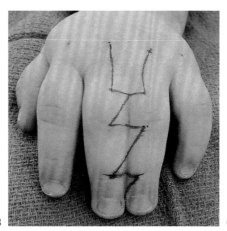 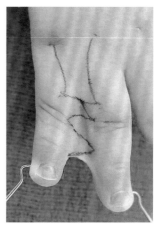

TECH FIG 1 • Dorsal hourglass commissural flap markings **(A)** with extensions for complete syndactyly **(B)** and incomplete syndactyly **(C)**.

Volar Markings

- Draw a transverse line 2 to 3 mm proximal to the mid-proximal phalanx flexion crease (**TECH FIG 2A**).
  - A small triangular dart in the middle of this line helps to break up the web scar.
- Mark the flexion creases similarly to the extension creases on the dorsum.
  - Similar to the dorsal markings, the extension of these transverse lines is dictated by the degree of involvement. These are then connected via oblique lines similar to the dorsal oblique markings (**TECH FIG 2B, C**).
  - Ensure that the dorsal and volar flaps are designed such that they will interdigitate once raised.

Flap Creation

- Exsanguinate the upper extremity.
  - In infants and toddlers, an Esmarch bandage is used as a tourniquet because it is more effective at providing a bloodless field in small arms (**TECH FIG 3**). The technique is controversial, as the pressure is not known; however, with experience, the surgeon can perform it predictably and safely in cases of short duration.
  - In older children, a standard pneumatic tourniquet is used.
- Raise the dorsal flap in the subcutaneous plane leaving 2 to 3 mm of fat on the flap (**TECH FIG 4A**).

- Raise the remaining dorsal and volar flaps. Raise the dorsal flaps on the extensor mechanism. Raise the volar flaps subcutaneously.
- Approach the web space with fine scissors and forceps. Spreading helps define the neurovascular structures (**TECH FIG 4B**).
  - Any interdigital bands/fascia should be excised.
  - Defat the fingers as needed, protecting the neurovascular bundles, to allow for the dorsal and palmar flaps to transpose.
- Split the dorsal flap down the midline to allow inset (**TECH FIG 4C**). The dorsal flap insets into the dart on the volar side (**TECH FIG 4D**).
  - By design, two volar flaps on either side of the web are created (see **TECH FIG 4D**), which are sutured to either edge of the dorsal flap thereby dividing the web scar even more.
- Mobilize, trim, and appropriately inset the dorsal and palmar flaps.

Grafting

- Use suture foil to create templates of the resultant defects for skin grafting (**TECH FIG 5A, B**).
- Release the tourniquet and obtain hemostasis. The author uses the bipolar electrocautery for bleeding in the skin graft bed only.

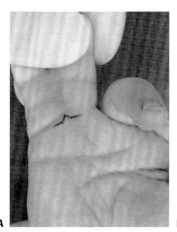 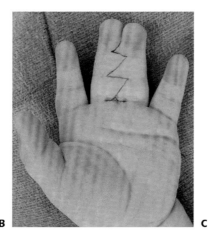 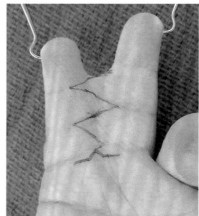

TECH FIG 2 • Volar markings with small dart to break up web scar **(A)** and for complete syndactyly **(B)** and incomplete syndactyly **(C)**.

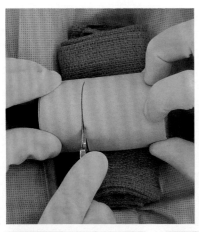
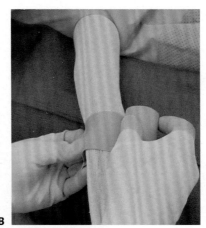
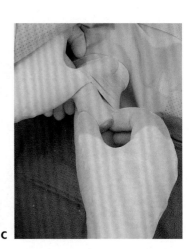
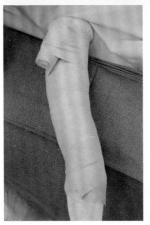
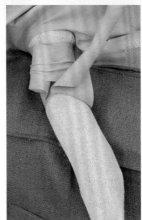

TECH FIG 3 • Technique of applying Esmarch bandage as tourniquet. In small children, the standard 3-in. Esmarch bandage is too wide. **A.** It is trimmed to about 2 in. long by using a no. 10 blade. It is then rolled out, and about one-third of its length is cut off and discarded to decrease its bulk (not shown). It is then wrapped around the extremity **(B)** and secured at the upper arm **(C–E)**. Tightness is gauged by using the thumb **(C)**.

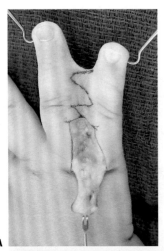
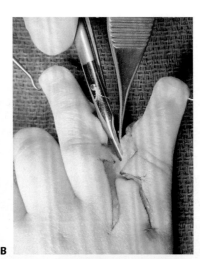
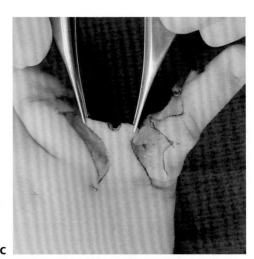
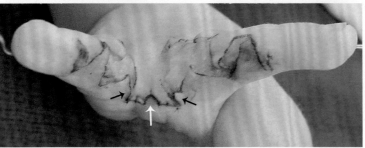

TECH FIG 4 • **A.** Dorsal flap raised in the subcutaneous plane. **B.** Spreading to divide soft tissue in the web with fine instruments. Dorsal flap split **(C)** and inset **(D)**. The dorsal flap insets into the previously created volar dart (*white arrow*). The two volar flaps on either side of the web (*black arrows*) are sutured to either edge of the dorsal flap thereby breaking up the web scar.

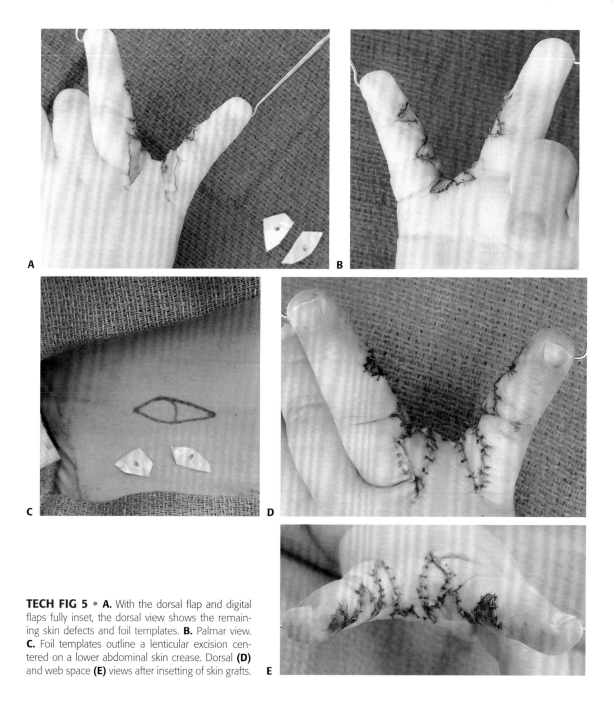

TECH FIG 5 • A. With the dorsal flap and digital flaps fully inset, the dorsal view shows the remaining skin defects and foil templates. **B.** Palmar view. **C.** Foil templates outline a lenticular excision centered on a lower abdominal skin crease. Dorsal **(D)** and web space **(E)** views after insetting of skin grafts.

- Skin edge bleeders usually stop when the skin grafts are applied.
- Mark a transverse crease in the lower abdomen for skin graft harvest. Avoid areas near the midline to prevent subsequent hair growth. A crease just below the anterior superior iliac spine provides ample skin, is well hidden, and heals beautifully.
  - Transpose the foil templates to this area and mark out a lenticular excision (**TECH FIG 5C**).
- With assistants holding traction, harvest a thin full-thickness skin graft. With enough traction, one can use the blade alone to harvest a graft that requires no defatting.
- Apply the skin grafts (**TECH FIG 5D,E**). The author uses 6-0 chromic sutures.

- The grafts have elasticity in multiple dimensions, so the surgeon must take care to apply them under appropriate tension and disallow pleating and redundancy of the graft.
- Running horizontal mattress sutures provide the best appearance on the dorsum.

Dressing and Immobilization

- Dressings and immobilization are critical to predictable healing (**TECH FIG 6**).
- Antibiotic-impregnated gauze is applied to incisions and grafts. Gauze wrap and cotton packing are used in the web space help to provide compression on the grafts.

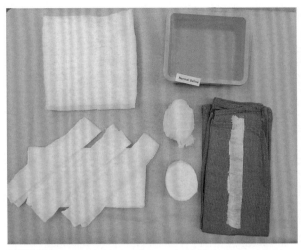

TECH FIG 6 • Dressing supplies needed include antibiotic-impregnated gauze (in *yellow*), 4 × 8 gauze sponges cut longitudinally into thirds for wrapping the digits, cotton for compression in the web, and cling and Webril wraps.

- The limb is immobilized in a well-padded long-arm mitten cast for 3 weeks.
  - Slip on a long 2-in. stockinette and apply the padding high up to the shoulder with the elbow at 90 degrees.
  - Apply the cast with the fingers buried but the thumb exposed.
- Infants between 9 and 15 months of age, especially those with significant subcutaneous fat, are notorious for slipping out of their casts. One can minimize this by taking several steps:
  - Extend the cast high up to the shoulder (but avoid compressing the vessels in the axilla).
  - Apply skin adhesive (such as Benzoin or Mastisol) to the arm and forearm prior to placing the stockinette.
  - Mold the cast to create a well-defined 90-degree angle on the posterior aspect of the elbow as the arm meets the forearm. Additionally, mold the cast to the contour of the underlying skeleton with a supracondylar and proximal forearm "squeeze."
  - Finally, leave the thumb out and instruct parents to call if the thumb slips into the cast.

PEARLS AND PITFALLS

Surgical management	■ Syndactyly can be narrow or wide. This bears on surgical planning because wide syndactyly has more skin for transposition. It is important to ascertain how much skin is available in the web preoperatively.
Exsanguination and tourniquet	■ Regular pneumatic tourniquets are not effective in small children—the Esmarch bandage works better. The surgeon must be careful not to make the tourniquet too tight.
Release	■ The most proximal extent of release is the bifurcation of the arteries. A distal nerve bifurcation can be teased apart with gentle intraneural dissection and splitting of the fascicles. Occasionally, one will encounter an arterial bifurcation that is too distal. In these instances, the smaller branch can usually be sacrificed depending on the blood supply to the other side of the digit. One can place a microvascular clamp, release the tourniquet, and assess vascularity before dividing any branches.
Postoperative	■ Adequate compression and immobilization is critical to successful skin graft take and predictable healing. Children between 9 and 12 months of age occasionally will slip out of long-arm casts; these should be reapplied promptly.

POSTOPERATIVE CARE

- Immobilize the arm for 3 weeks as noted previously. If the cast falls off, it should be replaced.
- Remove the cast in the office and assess healing of skin grafts. Sutures, old clots, and debris can be removed from the wounds at this time.
- Occupational therapy to make nighttime volar resting thermoplast splints with web space conformers at this time. The conformers put pressure on the scars and allow them to soften and settle more quickly. These should be worn for about a month after the cast is removed.

OUTCOMES

- Functional outcomes after syndactyly release depend mostly on the preoperative status of the digits and the hand.
- In simple cases where the joints are not involved, full range of motion of the involved digits should be expected postoperatively (**FIG 6**).

- In complex cases, reconstruction is difficult and common postsurgical functional issues include rotational and angular deformity and nail deformity.[5]

COMPLICATIONS

- Web creep (loss of initial depth of the web space) can occur over time, with incidence ranging from 2% to 24% (**FIG 7**).[4]
  - Web scars are best corrected right before the child starts school, around 5 or 6 years of age, after a significant growth spurt has occurred and the scars have had ample time to soften.
  - Most webs scars respond well to Z-plasty, but occasionally, skin grafting may be necessary.
- Skin graft loss or flap loss, partial or complete
- Vascular compromise—especially in complex and complicated cases
- Nail deformity
- Rotational and angular deformities
- Dense scars

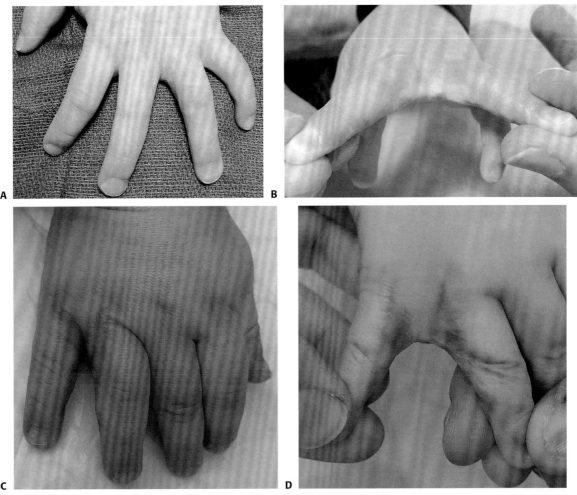

FIG 6 • Long-term postoperative dorsal **(A)** and web space **(B)** views of the patient with complete third web space syndactyly in TECH FIGS 1B and 2B. Patient has a pliable web space with no limitations in range of motion or function. Three-month postoperative dorsal **(C)** and web space **(D)** views of the patient with incomplete fourth web space syndactyly in TECH FIGS 1A and 2A. Early healing with good maintenance of web and normal function.

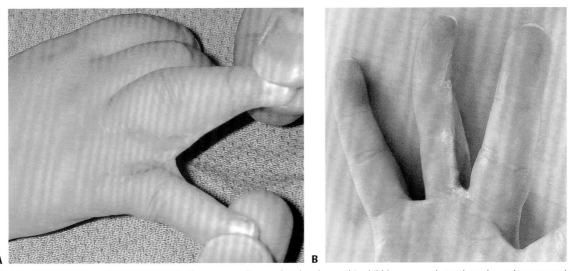

FIG 7 • Web space scar after syndactyly release. **A.** Three years after syndactyly release, this child has a scar that tethers the web space and prevents full extension of the ring finger. **B.** Twenty years after syndactyly release, this adult patient has a web scar that is bothersome but does not interfere with function. Note desquamation of scarred skin.

REFERENCES

1. Oberg KC, Feenstra JM, Manske PR, Tonkin MA. Developmental biology and classification of congenital anomalies of the hand and upper extremity. *J Hand Surg [Am]*. 2010;35:2066-2076.
2. Hynes SL, Harvey I, Thomas K, et al. CT angiography-guided single-stage release of adjacent webspaces in non-Apert syndactyly. *J Hand Surg Eur Vol*. 2015;40:625-632.
3. Deunk J, Nicolai JP, Hamburg SM. Long-term results of syndactyly correction: full-thickness versus split-thickness skin grafts. *J Hand Surg Br*. 2003;28:125-130.
4. McCarroll HR. Congenital anomalies: a 25-year overview. *J Hand Surg [Am]*. 2000;25:1007-1037.
5. Goldfarb CA, Steffen JA, Stutz CM. Complex syndactyly: aesthetic and objective outcomes. *J Hand Surg [Am]*. 2012;37:2068-2073.

Hypoplastic Thumb Reconstruction

Amir H. Taghinia

DEFINITION

- A thumb is considered hypoplastic if any of its osseous, musculotendinous, or articular components is deficient or missing or if the web space that it forms with the index finger is shallow.

ANATOMY

- The normal thumb is broad with osseous and articular structures that allow ample movement in multiple planes. Its intrinsic muscles provide a short moment arm, powering the motion enabled by the osseoarticular column. The normal first web space has a gentle curve spanning from the thumb metacarpophalangeal (MP) joint to the index finger MP joint.
- The modified Blauth classification system[1] provides a surgically useful basis for categorizing thumb hypoplasia.
  - Type I thumbs have minimal shortening and narrowing. No surgical intervention is needed.
  - Type II thumbs have narrowing of the first web space, hypoplastic intrinsic thenar muscles, and laxity of the MP joint. Reconstruction is recommended.
  - Type IIIA thumbs have features seen in type II thumbs, but they also have extrinsic tendon anomalies and a hypoplastic metacarpal. Reconstruction is recommended.
  - Type IIIB thumbs have features seen in type IIIA thumbs, but they also have an absent proximal metacarpal and instability of the carpometacarpal (CMC) joint. Pollicization is the treatment of choice.
  - Type IV (*pouce flottant*, floating thumb) and V (*aplasia*, complete absence) thumbs are also best treated with pollicization—these thumbs are discussed in the chapter on Index Finger Pollicization.
- Specific anatomic deficiencies in types II and III thumbs include the following[1-3]:
  - Laxity of the MP joint ulnar collateral ligament (UCL). The radial collateral ligament (RCL) may also be lax, as may the entire joint capsule (global laxity).
  - Hypoplasia or absence of the thenar muscles manifested as poor opposition
  - The flexor pollicis longus (FPL) tendon may be eccentrically attached to the distal phalanx. But it also may be absent, may follow an abnormal path (usually radially transposed), may have a very distal muscle belly, or may anomalously attach to the proximal phalanx.
  - The extensor pollicis longus (EPL) tendon may also be eccentrically attached to the distal phalanx. It may also be absent or follow an abnormal, more radial path.
  - Abnormal radial interconnections between the EPL and FPL lead to a characteristic radial deviation of the thumb termed pollex abductus. These connections are usually present at the MP joint and prevent active interphalangeal (IP) joint motion.
- The distinction between type II and IIIA may not bear strongly on the choice of surgical intervention, as there can be some overlap. If the thumb requires web space deepening, collateral ligament reconstruction, and opponensplasty, then there is usually some degree of extrinsic tendon abnormality present.[2] The surgeon should focus on treating the individual deficiencies that are present in a given thumb.

PATHOGENESIS

- Thumb hypoplasia occurs as a result of multiple potential factors—including genetic (associated syndromes), environmental, teratogenic (thalidomide), and idiopathic causes.
- It is considered to be a malformation, based on the Oberg, Manske, and Tonkin classification of 2010.[4]

NATURAL HISTORY

- Thumb hypoplasia occurs in 1 out of 100 000 live births. A large number of patients with thumb hypoplasia will have associated conditions such as cardiac or hematologic anomalies.

PATIENT HISTORY AND PHYSICAL FINDINGS

- Patients with type I to IIIA can present anytime in life. In milder cases, the differences can be so subtle that parents do not notice a mild deficiency (in function or appearance) until much later in life, especially if the nondominant side or both sides are involved.
- Physical findings:
  - Intrinsic thenar muscle hypoplasia (**FIG 1A**). This finding is usually evident early, especially if there is a comparative normal contralateral side. Patients lack strong opposition.
  - MP joint instability (**FIG 1B,C**). The stability of this joint is difficult to assess in an infant because of global joint laxity. However, as the child grows, the laxity becomes more evident on examination. Patients sometimes use a

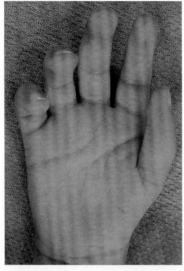
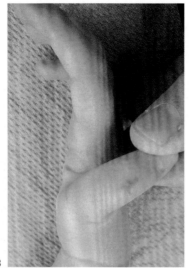
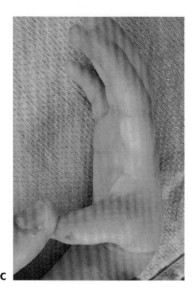

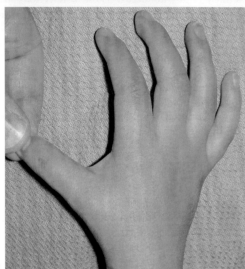

FIG 1 • A. Palmar view of hand with thumb hypoplasia. The thumb is short with flattening of the thenar eminence and lack of flexion or extension creases at the IP joint. The RCL **(B)** and UCL **(C)** are lax, allowing significant deviation of the joint. **D.** The first web space is shallow; radially deviating the thumb any more to widen the web space would result in deviation at the MP joint rather than splaying of the metacarpals.

"metacarpal grasp"—when an object is held between the fingers and the thumb metacarpal head, thus avoiding the distal thumb.

■ Shallow web space (**FIG 1D**). This finding is also evident early, though the degree of involvement is assessed subjectively. An incompetent UCL can sometimes mask a shallow web space. It is best to assess the web space by the angle achieved between the index and thumb metacarpals.

■ Extrinsic muscle abnormalities. These include abnormal size, length, strength, and insertion of the thumb flexor and extensors. These anomalies are typically manifested as joint deviations (MP joint) and/or lack of flexion or extension creases (IP joint).

■ The functional ability of the CMC joint is often not obvious on the infant's plain film radiograph. Functional differentiation can be made by allowing the child to grow and watching the toddler at play. If the thumb is bypassed in favor of the index finger, the joint is likely nonfunctional.

■ The hand surgeon should be aware of the conditions associated with thumb hypoplasia (eg, VACTERL, Fanconi anemia, and Holt-Oram syndrome) and have a low threshold to refer if suspicions arise.

■ In particular, Fanconi anemia is a fatal disease that occurs mainly in those with thumb hypoplasia and is easily diagnosed with a simple blood test.

IMAGING

■ Plain radiographs (**FIG 2**) help to determine the status of the metacarpal, CMC joint, any abnormalities of the index finger, and the status of the distal radius and ulna (presence of radial longitudinal deficiency).

NONOPERATIVE MANAGEMENT

■ Most patients with Blauth type I thumb hypoplasia do not need surgical intervention.

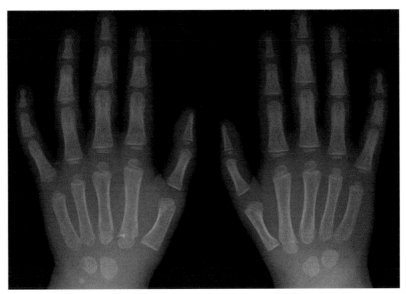

FIG 2 • Plain radiographs of both hands demonstrate a comparatively shorter right thumb with thinner first metacarpal.

SURGICAL MANAGEMENT

- The author performs hypoplastic thumb reconstruction around 2.5 to 3 years of age, particularly if MP joint ligament reconstruction is needed. The metacarpal head should be big enough to allow creation of a tunnel without fracturing. Key procedures are outlined below.
- Opponensplasty
  - In congenital cases, opponensplasty is done using the flexor digitorum superficialis (FDS) tendon to the ring finger or the abductor digiti minimi (ADM).
  - The FDS is advantageous because it provides simultaneous opponensplasty *and* ligament reconstruction.
  - The ADM is used in patients who have had previous pollicization procedures (and have weak opposition) or those with thumb hypoplasia who do not need ligament reconstruction.
- MP joint ligament reconstruction
  - This procedure is done with tightening of the existing capsular tissues or extrinsic reconstruction with either the FDS to the ring finger (in cases that need simultaneous opponensplasty) or the palmaris longus tendon. In cases of global laxity, chondrodesis or epiphyseal arthrodesis is advocated, though both of these procedures have significant downsides.
  - The author errs toward stability. Thus, for most cases, both UCL and RCL are reconstructed using a tendon graft. The tendon is split, and one-half is routed through a tunnel made in the metacarpal head to reconstruct the UCL. The tendon is then passed underneath the adductor aponeurosis and routed from dorsal to palmar through a tunnel in the periosteum in the proximal phalanx. It is then passed under the aponeurosis once again before being sutured back to itself at the metacarpal head. The RCL is reconstructed on the radial side using a similar method.

- Web space deepening.
  - This procedure is best done with a four-flap Z-plasty.
  - Multiple other procedures have been proposed, but the Z-plasty remains the workhorse for this condition.
- Other adjunct procedures include correction of MP and IP joint deviation by division of the tendinous attachments of the flexor to the extensor (pollex abductus), division of the musculus lumbricalis pollicis, step-lengthening of the extrinsic flexor tendon, and detachment and reinsertion of the EPL and/or FPL tendon.
  - Pin fixation is advocated after these procedures.
- Depending on the degree of involvement and interventions planned, it is important to establish a logical sequence for performing these procedures. For example, performing the web space release first releases the investing tight fascia of the intrinsic muscles, thus allowing better palmar abduction prior to opponensplasty.

Preoperative Planning

- Discuss risks, benefits, and expectations with parents on the day of surgery.

Positioning and Approach

- The patient is positioned supine with the arm out on a small hand table.
- Incisions are planned carefully prior to use of the tourniquet.
- Plan all incisions before exsanguinating the upper extremity.
- In toddlers, an Esmarch bandage is used as a tourniquet as it provides better hemostasis. In older children, a pneumatic tourniquet works best.

▪ Four-Flap Z-Plasty for First Web Space

- Splay the web with the help of an assistant and draw a transverse line across the tightest area of the web. On the thumb side, draw a perpendicular line dorsally. On the index finger side, draw a perpendicular line palmarly. Bisect these 90-degree angles with two additional lines at 45 degrees.
  - The five lines that are drawn should be the same length (**TECH FIG 1A–C**).
- Incise the limbs and raise the flaps with a few millimeters of fat to preserve the blood supply.

- Spread in the web space, and define and protect the neurovascular structures. Bluntly dissect the muscles and sharply divide their investing fascia to widen the distance between the index and thumb metacarpals (**TECH FIG 1D**).
  - Releasing the fascia of the adductor pollicis and first dorsal interosseous muscle is critical to obtaining a wide web space.
- If designed correctly, the flaps should transpose into their new respective positions.
- If performing a ligament reconstruction, extend the ulnar skin incision to fully expose the MP joint.

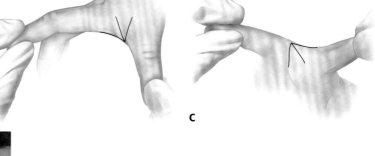

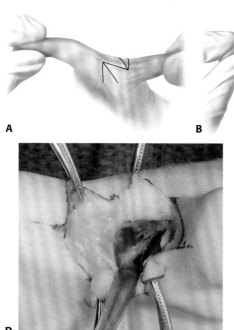

TECH FIG 1 • A–C. Designing the four-flap Z-plasty. The dorsal incision perpendicular to the web should be next to the thumb; the alternative approach would place the incision on the volar thumb and cause a flexion contracture. **D.** The investing fasciae of the adductor pollicis and first dorsal interosseous are seen in the first web space. These should be sharply divided or excised to allow optimal widening of the web.

▪ Opponensplasty and Ligament Reconstruction Using FDS

Markings

- Design a radial mid-lateral incision on the thumb MP joint, just dorsal to where the glabrous skin meets the nonglabrous skin.
- Design a transverse incision over the distal wrist flexion crease; this incision should be long enough to gain access to the flexor carpi ulnaris (FCU) tendon ulnarly and the ring finger flexor digitorum superficialis (FDS) tendon radially.
- Finally, design a longitudinal A1 pulley incision in the distal palm over the ring finger ray (**TECH FIG 2**).

Exposure and Tendon Harvest

- Incise the wrist crease incision. Find and isolate the FCU tendon while identifying and protecting the ulnar artery and nerve.

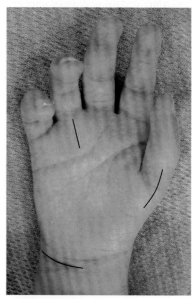

TECH FIG 2 • Design of the incisions, palmar view.

- Find and isolate the FDS tendon to the ring digit at the wrist. It is usually the most palmar and ulnar flexor tendon.
  - Retract the tendon and confirm that it flexes the ring proximal interphalangeal (PIP) joint. Free its distal attachments.
- Incise the A1 pulley incision over the ring finger, spread down to the tendon sheath, and sharply divide the A1 pulley. Using a small retractor, pull the FDS up into the wound with the finger in maximal flexion.
  - Obtain maximal exposure in the wound, and free the FDS from the FDP in both directions. Incise the two limbs of the FDS as distally as possible, leaving its insertion intact.
- Occasionally, the FDS tendons of the ring and little digits are joined proximally. If pulling on the ring FDS causes flexion of the little digit PIP joint, a separate incision to release the little finger FDS may be necessary (**TECH FIG 3A**).
- Deliver the FDS into the wrist wound, and wrap with moist gauze so it does not desiccate.
- Incise the radial thumb incision and dissect to the extensor mechanism.
- If present, release the pollex abductus and free the extensor from the flexor (**TECH FIG 3B,C**).

- It is crucial to divide these attachments, as they will otherwise act as a deforming force, stressing the MP ulnar collateral ligament (UCL) reconstruction.
  - Once released, pull the extensor and flexor proximally to ensure that the MP joint does not deviate radially.
- Correct any extrinsic tendon abnormalities. Depending on the anatomy, options include realignment of tendons with pulleys, step-lengthening, and/or reinsertion of eccentrically attached tendons. (None were performed in the example case.)

Tunnel Creation

- Retract the extensor dorsally and identify the metacarpal head on the radial side without entering the joint.
- Define the metacarpal head in the ulnar incision as well. Create a tunnel underneath the adductor aponeurosis in the proximal to distal direction. The tendon will be routed underneath the aponeurosis.
- To create the tunnel in the metacarpal head, incise the periosteum over the metacarpal head and strip off a small area. Clearly define the dorsal and palmar aspects of the metacarpal head and mark a spot exactly in the middle.

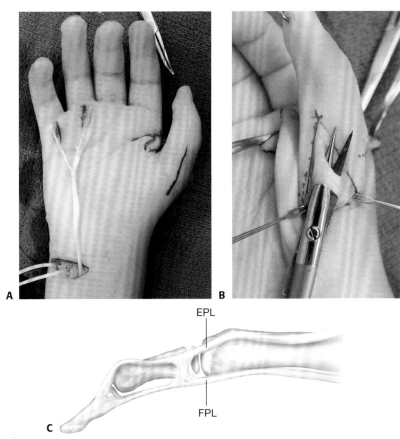

TECH FIG 3 • A. The first web space has been released and the FDS tendon has been isolated and delivered through the wrist wound. The fourth and fifth digit FDS tendons were joined up to the mid-palm, so a separate A1 pulley incision was needed on the fifth ray. **B.** Pollex abductus is radial deviation of the thumb caused by attachments of the extensor pollicis longus (EPL) tendon to the flexor pollicis longus (FPL) tendon present at the MP joint level. **C.** Extrinsic tendons can be radially transposed and attached to each other via tendinous bands. In addition, the extrinsic tendons can have eccentrically placed insertions (radially) on the distal phalanx.

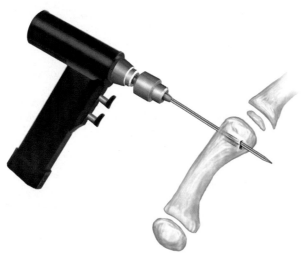

TECH FIG 4 • Multiple drill holes using a K-wire through the metacarpal head allow for creation of an elliptical tunnel through which the tendon can be passed for ligament reconstruction.

- Make one wide tunnel by drilling multiple holes side by side using a 0.035-in. Kirschner wire (**TECH FIG 4**), then drilling in between these holes.
  - The tunnel may also be created with a single pass of a drill, appropriately selected for size.
- Ensure that the tunnel is generous and visibly larger than the tendon. Pulling the tendon through a small tunnel causes it to fray.
- The thumb metacarpal's physis is located proximally, in contrast to the physes for the finger metacarpals, which are located distally. Therefore, there are no concerns about growth arrest when this bone tunnel is created.

- Create two vertical (dorsal to palmar) tunnels in the periosteum on the radial and ulnar aspects of the proximal phalanx just distal to the physis. These tunnels should be centered volarly to best mimic the normal collateral ligaments.
  - The author does not bore vertical bone tunnels in proximal phalanges of small children. This technique is technically difficult, threatens the physis, and has not been found to be necessary.

Passing the Tendon

- Create a subcutaneous tunnel from the distal wrist incision to the radial thumb incision.
  - Loop the FDS tendon around the FCU tendon and pass it through the tunnel into the radial thumb wound.
- Pass one limb of the distal FDS through the metacarpal head tunnel from radial to ulnar (**TECH FIG 5A**).
  - Split the FDS proximally and keep pulling the tendon limb through until palmar abduction reaches about 70 degrees.
  - Suture the tendon to the periosteum on the radial and ulnar sides of the metacarpal head to secure the opponensplasty.
- On the ulnar side, pass the tendon under the aponeurosis, then dorsal to palmar through the periosteal tunnel, and then under the aponeurosis again (**TECH FIG 5B**) and suture it to the tendon itself at the metacarpal head (**TECH FIG 5C**).
- Repeat this procedure on the radial side; there is more tendon length on this side and there is no aponeurosis in the way.
- Trim any excess tendon and place additional securing sutures if necessary (**TECH FIG 5D,E**).
- Test the integrity of the ligament reconstruction to assure there is no laxity. Usually, pins are not necessary.

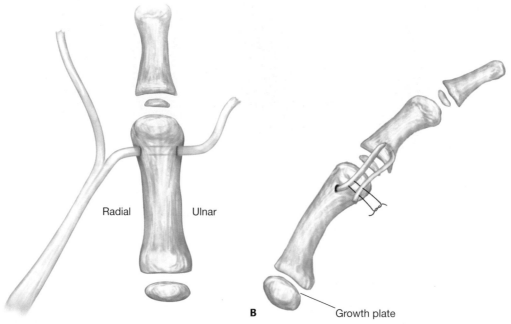

A   Radial   Ulnar

B   Growth plate

TECH FIG 5 • **A.** The FDS limbs are separated, and one is passed through the bone tunnel to create the UCL, while the other creates the RCL. **B.** The UCL is reconstructed in the shape of a triangle. The tendon is passed superior to inferior in the periosteal tunnel and sutured back to itself.

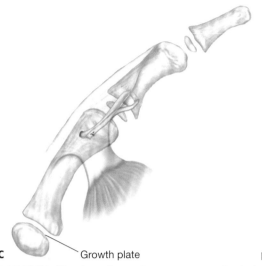

C | Growth plate

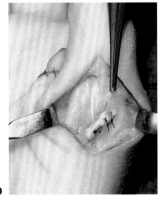

D

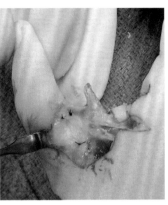

E

TECH FIG 5 (Continued) • **C.** The UCL reconstruction is done under the adductor aponeurosis. **D.** RCL reconstruction is demonstrated. **E.** UCL reconstruction performed under the adductor aponeurosis.

Completion

- Close the wrist wound using several deep dermal 4-0 Monocryl sutures followed by a running 5-0 Monocryl intracuticular suture. Close the palm and radial thumb wounds with interrupted simple or horizontal mattress 6-0 chromic gut sutures.

- Transpose the Z-plasty flaps, and close the web space wounds using simple interrupted 6-0 chromic gut sutures (**TECH FIG 6**).
- Place antibiotic-impregnated petroleum gauze (Xeroform) on the wounds and apply compression gauze.
- Deflate (or remove) the tourniquet and assess perfusion.
- Apply dressings and a well-padded long-arm cast for 3 to 4 weeks.

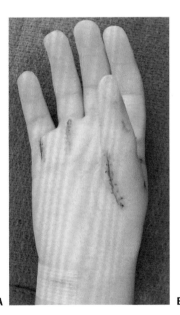

A

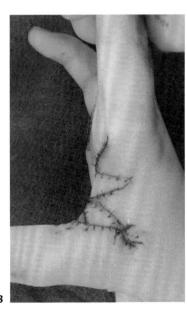

B

TECH FIG 6 • Immediate postoperative palmar view shows good opposition **(A)** and a wide web space after four-flap Z-plasty **(B)**.

■ Opponensplasty With Abductor Digiti Minimi (Huber)

- Design an L-shaped incision on the ulnar side of the hand (**TECH FIG 7A**).
  - The long limb of the incision should be a high mid-lateral ulnar incision extending from just distal to the fifth digit MP joint to the pisiform.

- The short limb is a transverse volar incision on the distal wrist crease just proximal to the pisiform. This second incision helps to free the proximal origin of the abductor digiti minimi (ADM) muscle *if needed* for additional mobilization of the muscle. Note: The transfer can also be raised as a myocutaneous flap thus avoiding tunneling and adding more bulk to the thenar area.[5]

- Incise the mid-lateral ulnar marking and dissect down to the ADM muscle. Isolate and protect any branches of the dorsal sensory ulnar nerve.
- Incise the fascia and dissect the muscle free (**TECH FIG 7B**), following it distally until its insertion is encountered on the fifth digit proximal phalanx.
- Disinsert the muscle, leaving a long cuff of periosteum attached to the muscle to facilitate subsequent reinsertion.
- Dissect the muscle proximally and identify and protect its neurovascular bundle. If additional length is needed on the muscle, the short limb of the L-incision can be made and the origin mobilized off the pisiform and flexor carpi ulnaris. The author does not transfer the origin.
- Make a high mid-axial incision on the radial aspect of the thumb MP joint and dissect down to the distal metacarpal.
- Create a generous subcutaneous tunnel between the thumb MP joint and the proximal aspect of the ulnar wound (**TECH FIG 7C**). Tunnel the muscle through.

- There are multiple sites where the muscle can now be attached: the extensor hood, the proximal aspect of the proximal phalanx, or the distal aspect of the metacarpal.
  - The author typically attaches the muscle to periosteum near the metacarpal head. This insertion site gives the most direct pull without taxing the MP joint UCL. It also avoids radial pull on the extensor mechanism, which may disrupt the learned prehensile patterns in postpollicization cases or translate the (already radially displaced) extensor tendon in hypoplastic cases.
- Attach the muscle and secure with several sutures to obtain maximal palmar abduction under moderate tension. Ensure that the pedicle is not kinked.
- Close the wounds with absorbable sutures (**TECH FIG 7D**). The ulnar incision is closed with a running intradermal suture.
- Place antibiotic-impregnated petroleum gauze (Xeroform) on the wounds and apply compression gauze.
- Deflate (or remove) the tourniquet and assess perfusion.
- Apply a well-padded long-arm cast for 3 weeks.

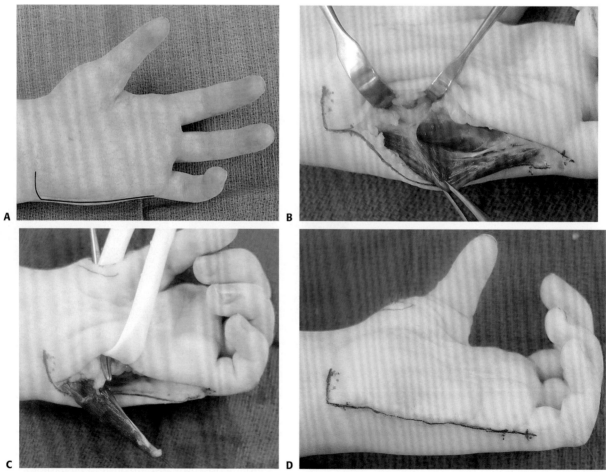

TECH FIG 7 • A. A 6-year-old boy who underwent left index finger pollicization for type IV thumb hypoplasia presented with weakness of palmar abduction and opposition. A high midlateral ulnar incision is planned with a transverse extension at the distal wrist crease, just proximal to the pisiform. **B.** The ADM muscle is seen as the most ulnar/palmar structure deep to the skin. **C.** The ADM muscle has been mobilized. A generous tunnel housing a Penrose drain connects the ulnar incision to the mid-lateral incision on the radial aspect of the neothumb "MP joint." **D.** The muscle has been tunneled and inset in maximal palmar abduction/opposition. The wounds have been closed.

PEARLS AND PITFALLS

Anatomy	▪ There are numerous variations of extrinsic and intrinsic muscle/tendon anatomy, including a lumbrical emanating from the flexor (so-called musculus lumbricalis pollicis), flexor that inserts partially on the proximal phalanx, joined flexor and extensor proximally, eccentric insertions, and various degrees of attachment of the FPL to the EPL. Not all of these abnormalities need to be surgically repaired.
Technique	▪ Radial deviation at the MP and IP joints can be improved by releasing the pollex abductus with or without step-lengthening of the flexor tendon and reinsertion of the EPL and/or FPL into a more ulnar position on the distal phalanx. Pin fixation may be necessary after this procedure to keep the joints straight.
Surgical management	▪ Although many parents ask the surgeon to restore active IP joint motion, this is possible only in a small subset of patients who have preoperative passive but not active IP joint motion. ▪ On occasion, the MP joint laxity is so severe (global) that one should consider MP joint chondrodesis or epiphyseal arthrodesis. Chondrodesis does not heal predictably, and epiphyseal arthrodesis is only possible if there is enough epiphysis to allow fusion. Both techniques shorten the thumb and stress the CMC joint.

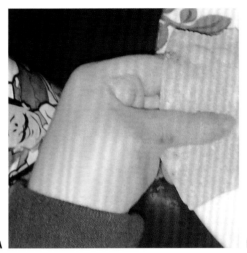 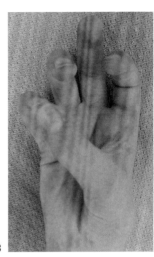 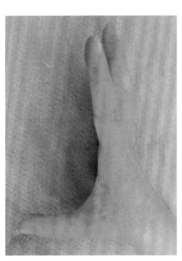

FIG 3 • A. Two months postoperatively, the patient was using the opposition transfer for grasping food. Three years postoperatively, he demonstrates a stable MP joint with strong opposition **(B)** and a wide first web space **(C)**.

POSTOPERATIVE CARE

▪ Remove the cast after 3 or 4 weeks of immobilization.
▪ Fashion a thumb spica thermoplast splint that can be worn for 2 or 3 weeks at night for protection.
▪ Start range of motion exercises with hand therapy.

OUTCOMES

▪ Functional outcomes for hypoplastic thumb reconstruction are satisfactory if the anatomic abnormalities are appropriately treated (**FIG 3**).
  ▪ There is a lack of good long-term data on functional outcomes, especially data that have been controlled for severity of involvement.
▪ The reconstructed thumb remains smaller and less powerful than the normal thumb.

COMPLICATIONS

▪ Immediate complications are rare. Long-term functional concerns relate to the degree of hypoplasia, correct preoperative diagnosis, and appropriate treatment.

▪ Persistent lack of active IP joint motion can be seen despite adequate release of the tendon adhesions.
▪ Inadequate release of pollex abductus attachments can cause a deforming radial force and weaken the MP joint UCL repair in the long term.
▪ If the collateral ligament is reconstructed dorsal to the axis of rotation, hyperextension of the MP joint may result. Ensure that the vertical tunnel on the proximal phalanx is centered volarly.

REFERENCES

1. Manske PR, McCarroll HR Jr, James M. Type III-A hypoplastic thumb. *J Hand Surg [Am]*. 1995;20:246-253.
2. Tonkin M. Surgical reconstruction of congenital thumb hypoplasia. *Indian J Plast Surg.* 2011;44:253-265.
3. Light TR, Gaffey JL. Reconstruction of the hypoplastic thumb. *J Hand Surg [Am]*. 2010;35:474-479.
4. Oberg KC, Feenstra JM, Manske PR, Tonkin MA. Developmental biology and classification of congenital anomalies of the hand and upper extremity. *J Hand Surg [Am]*. 2010;35:2066-2076.
5. Upton J, Taghinia AH. Abductor digiti minimi myocutaneous flap for opponensplasty in congenital hypoplastic thumbs. *Plast Reconstr Surg.* 2008;122:1807-1811.

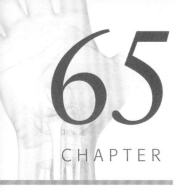

65 CHAPTER

Reconstruction of Radial Polydactyly

Amir H. Taghinia

DEFINITION

- Polydactyly refers to the presence of extra digits. Most surgeons prefer this term to duplication, as the latter implies that the partners are exactly identical, which is the exception rather than the rule.
- Radial polydactyly is the presence of extra digits involving the thumb ray. This terminology is preferable to preaxial polydactyly because the term preaxial encompasses the thumb through ring rays.

ANATOMY

- Radial polydactyly is most commonly classified using the Iowa classification system.[1] The system divides polydactyly based on longitudinal level of bone and/or joint arborization but does not account for soft tissue differences (**FIG 1**).
- Not considering small soft tissue–only (nubbin) polydactyly cases, type IV is the most common radial polydactyly (approximately 45% of cases) and type II is the second most common (approximately 20% of cases).
- Type VII radial polydactyly, which has a triphalangeal component, is further subdivided into six types.
- The Iowa classification does not include soft tissue differences and certain types of radial polydactyly. Accordingly, additional classification systems have been proposed.
- The Rotterdam system gives broader classification possibilities (including triplicate thumb) but introduces more complexity.[2]
- Although the thumb partners may be nearly identical, the ulnar partner is usually the more dominant one; it is larger and better developed and has greater range of motion and strength.
- Nevertheless, both partners may exhibit findings of thumb hypoplasia, including smaller stature, poorly developed joints and tendons with lack of flexion or extension creases,

joint deviations, eccentrically inserting extrinsic tendons, and abnormal or deficient intrinsic muscles.

PATHOGENESIS

- The exact etiology of radial polydactyly remains unknown. The literature suggests an imbalance between the apical ectodermal ridge (AER) and the underlying mesoderm as one cause.
- Based on the Oberg, Manske, and Tonkin classification,[3] polydactyly is considered to be a malformation with abnormal formation/differentiation of the hand plate in the radioulnar axis.

NATURAL HISTORY

- Radial polydactyly occurs more commonly in those with Caucasian and Asian descent, with an incidence of 1 in every 3000 live births.

PATIENT HISTORY AND PHYSICAL FINDINGS

- Patients are usually seen in infancy.
- Radial polydactyly may run in families.
- Associated conditions may occur, even Fanconi anemia, a rare condition that can be fatal if not diagnosed early.
- Examine the thumbs for flexion and extension creases, passive and active range of motion, joint stability, and strength.
- During late infancy, the child usually starts to use the more dominant thumb. It is worthwhile to see the child at play to better understand the developing prehensile patterns.

IMAGING

- Plain radiographs are the study of choice and should be obtained for most polydactyly cases involving bone.

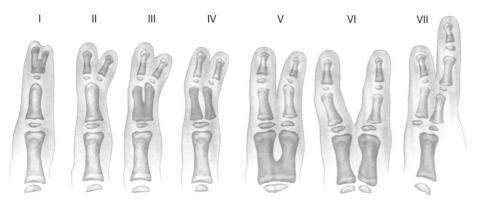

FIG 1 • Iowa classification of radial polydactyly. The distinctions are based on increasing levels of proximal divergence. The radial partner tends to be smaller and less developed.

- Radiography resolves all uncertainty about the level and involvement of a polydactyly that may not be clear on physical examination.

SURGICAL MANAGEMENT

- Small pedunculated ("nubbin") polydactyly is treated in the office before a month of age. Young infants are not strong enough to resist small procedures, and they can be soothed easily with a pacifier or sugar water.
    - Suture ligation can leave a small bump, so two alternatives are preferred, both using local anesthesia in the clinic treatment room: excision and suture closure or clipping at base with a hemoclip and excision. Both options are offered to the parents in this early age.
    - The advantage of the clipping is that it is quick, but the clip can stay several weeks and cause local skin irritation, and there is a small risk of ingestion (especially on the radial side) if not covered with a dressing at all times.
    - The excision and closure option takes more time but with likely fewer potential complications.
- For older infants or those in whom the polydactyly has a wide base, the author prefers excision in the operating room under general anesthesia at about 9 to 12 months of age.
- General anesthesia is also required in cases with more extensive involvement. No clear consensus exists regarding timing of repair. The risk of anesthesia in a small child should be weighed against early repair that takes advantage of brain plasticity. Other medical comorbidities should be taken into account.
- Small object grasp in the infant starts around 9 months of age; accordingly, the author prefers to correct polydactyly between 9 months and 1.5 years of age.
    - For very complex cases, it is worthwhile to delay repair until the structures are large enough to conduct a more technically precise operation. An example is a small trapezoidal or delta phalanx that requires a closing wedge osteotomy (eg, triphalangeal thumb).

Surgical Options

- There are three methods for repair of radial polydactyly: resection and reconstruction, the sharing technique, and acral transposition ("on-top plasty").
    - The surgeon should not apply one technique to one type of polydactyly based purely on algorithm.
    - Instead, a careful analysis of the clinical and radiographic findings, as well as expected functional outcome and patient factors, should dictate the choice of reconstruction.
- The main principles for repair are ablation of nonfunctional structures, creation of the best functional and aesthetic single digit from parts of both partners, and preservation of length, stability, and a wide first web space.

Resection and Reconstruction

- Resection and reconstruction involves resecting the more hypoplastic partner and augmenting the better developed one (see Technique section).
- This technique is indicated when the dominant partner alone is sufficient to be a thumb with good appearance and function.
- It is the easiest and the most favored approach. It can be applied to all types of polydactyly and is the most common operation for types IV to VI.
- The main sequence of this procedure is as follows:

- Disarticulation of the discarded partner but preservation of a ligamentoperiosteal flap and (if present) muscle insertion
- Shaving of redundant proximal articulation
- Osteotomies to correct angulation, if needed
- Reattachment of the ligamentoperiosteal flap and muscle insertions
- Rebalancing of eccentrically aligned extensor and flexor tendons, if needed

Sharing Technique

- The sharing technique uses parts from both partners to create a single digit. The most common expression of this technique is the Bilhaut operation, which removes central tissues and combines two digits into one.
- The procedure is indicated for nearly symmetrical but hypoplastic partners when removal of one partner only would leave a small thumb.
- The original Bilhaut technique removed equal parts from symmetrical partners but resulted in unsatisfactory outcomes including nail ridging, growth disturbance, and stiffness.
- The modified Bilhaut technique proposed by Baek[4] shows more promising results. It removes extra-articular unequal parts from symmetrical partners, thus avoiding articular reconstruction and creating a well-contoured distal phalanx for the nail.
    - The technique is typically performed for types II and III thumbs when the two partners are small but nearly equal in size.
    - It can also be applied to type IV thumbs, but because the phalanges are usually asymmetrical, articular step-offs and bony misalignment are more likely to occur, resulting in less satisfactory outcomes.[5]
    - Dorsal and volar incisions are made, the central soft tissue is excised, and the phalangeal components are identified. The dominant phalanx's articular surface is preserved. Similarly shaped extra-articular osteotomies are performed in each phalanx such that the defect in the dominant distal phalanx will be matched by a small nonarticular, soft tissue–bearing bone segment of the nondominant distal phalanx (**FIG 2**). The phalanges are then opposed and secured with Kirschner wires or sutures.

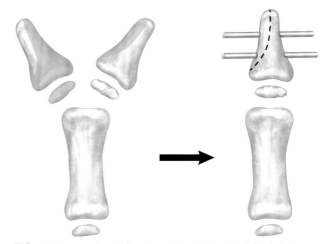

FIG 2 • In the modified Bilhaut operation for type II radial polydactyly, an extra-articular portion of each distal phalanx is shared to reconstruct one distal phalanx. Typically, a greater portion of the more dominant partner is preserved. Kirschner wires (shown) or sutures provide fixation for the osteotomy.

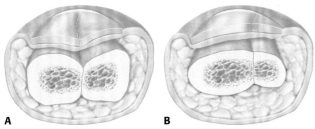

FIG 3 • In the original Bilhaut operation, half of each distal phalanx was used to reconstruct the thumb. **A.** The contour was suboptimal, leading to a groove in the nail. **B.** In the modified Bilhaut technique, slight volar axial rotation of the distal phalanges prior to fixation ensures a smoother nail contour.

- Slight volar axial rotation of the distal phalanges prior to fixation will ensure a smoother nail contour without a groove, avoiding the so-called seagull deformity (**FIG 3**).
- The nail bed and skin are then repaired using fine sutures.

Acral Transposition

- On-top plasty is performed when one digit has better proximal components and the other has better distal components.
- This reconstruction is more common for cases with metacarpal or carpometacarpal arborization such as in types V to VII radial polydactyly.
- The procedure involves moving the better distal component of one partner onto the better proximal component of the other.
  - The better distal component is isolated as a neurovascular island flap, and an osteotomy is performed at the desired

level of transfer. The lesser distal component is excised and an osteotomy of the better proximal component is done at the desired level of transfer (**FIG 4**).
- The transfer is then performed and fixed with pins or interosseous wires. The intrinsic muscles are rebalanced and the skin is closed.
- Joint and bone deviations should be corrected (to the greatest extent possible) in the first operation with osteotomies and tendon rebalancing as needed. Subsequent repairs may be needed with growth.[6]
- In more proximal cases (eg, type V and VI), the surgeon should carefully consider the first web space. Because the ulnar partner is the one that is most commonly preserved and it is usually ulnarly deviated, the surgeon should perform maneuvers necessary to make sure that the first web space will be sufficiently wide.

Preoperative Planning

- Discuss risks, benefits, and expectations with parents on the day of surgery.
- Specifically outline the risks of scarring, joint deviations, stiffness, and bulges.

Positioning

- The patient is positioned supine with the arm out on a small hand table.

Approach

- Incisions are planned carefully prior to use of the tourniquet. The author prefers mid-lateral incisions to dorsal incisions, since they produce the best appearance.
- In infants and toddlers, an Esmarch bandage is used as a tourniquet.

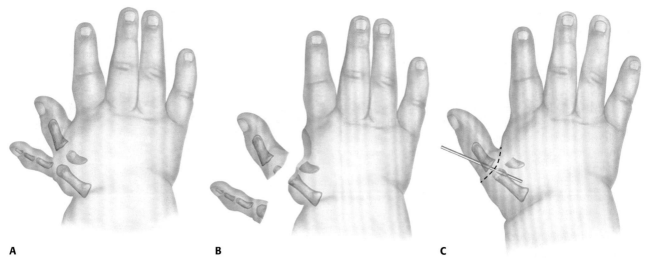

FIG 4 • Acral transposition ("on-top plasty") is usually indicated in more proximal radial polydactyly where one partner is dominant distally and the other is dominant proximally. **A.** In this case, the dominant ulnar distal partner will be transferred to the dominant proximal radial partner. Osteotomy sites are indicated in blue highlighting. The shaded portion of the ulnar partner's metacarpal will be discarded. The skin incisions are planned such that plenty of skin is preserved on the hand from the radial partner. The goal is to dissect the ulnar partner as a vascularized island flap and translate it into the soft tissue sleeve of the radial partner. The wound where the ulnar partner resided will then be closed linearly, thus constructing a wide first web space. **B.** During the operation, the distal radial partner is discarded while any intrinsic muscles that attach to it are preserved for subsequent attachment onto the transferred partner. **C.** After the ulnar partner is isolated as a vascularized island flap, osteotomy is performed, and it is transferred onto its new position and secured with interosseous wires or Kirschner wires. The intrinsic muscles are reattached, and the skin is closed, resulting in an improved web space.

■ Reconstruction of Type IV Radial Polydactyly

Markings and Exposure

- The case of a 9-month-old boy with type IV polydactyly is presented with step-by-step surgical treatment (**TECH FIG 1A–C**).
- Draw the markings for a mid-lateral closure. Leave excess skin on the preserved partner and trim the skin later to create a custom closure (**TECH FIG 1D,E**).
  - The closure takes extra time but improves appearance.
- Once the tourniquet is applied, incise the dorsal markings and dissect sharply to the extensor tendon (**TECH FIG 1F**).
- Develop a plane above the extensor mechanism to just beyond the metacarpophalangeal (MP) joint (**TECH FIG 1G**).
- Incise the extensor tendon distal to its bifurcation and dissect under the extensor above the MP joint capsule.
- Incise the palmar markings; dissect and divide the neurovascular bundle (**TECH FIG 1H**).

- Dissect a plane over the flexor mechanism and the intrinsic abductor of the thumb (**TECH FIG 1I**). The abductor usually inserts on the radial and volar aspects of the proximal phalanx, but the anatomy is quite variable.

Flap Creation

- Design a proximally based periosteal flap on the radial aspect of the proximal phalanx (**TECH FIG 2A**).
- Incise the markings and elevate this flap with the radial partner's MP joint radial collateral ligament and the abductor muscle (**TECH FIG 2B**).
  - This flap will be used for subsequent reconstruction of the retained partner.
- Isolate and divide the extrinsic flexor tendon (**TECH FIG 2C**).

Disarticulation, Osteotomy, and Fixation

- Disarticulate at the MP joint. A bifid metacarpal head will now be visible (**TECH FIG 3A**).
- Cut the metacarpal head that articulated with the discarded partner (see **TECH FIG 2B**).

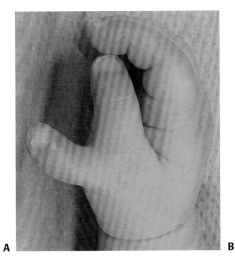
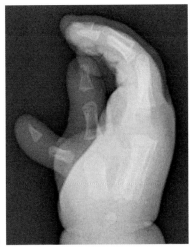

A   **B**

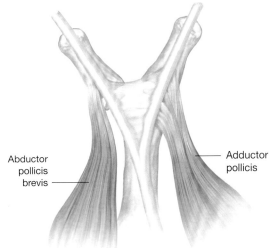

TECH FIG 1 • Type IV radial polydactyly in a 9-month-old boy. **A,B.** Anteroposterior clinical and radiographic views demonstrate a smaller, less developed radial partner. The ulnar partner is inline (parallel) to the metacarpal, and so an osteotomy of the metacarpal will not be needed. **C.** Simplified anatomy of radial polydactyly. The abductor pollicis brevis muscle can have variable, and potentially multiple, insertion sites, such as onto the extensor, the bone, and the flexor tendon. If on-top plasty is planned, the insertion of the adductor pollicis should be considered.

Abductor pollicis brevis

Adductor pollicis

C

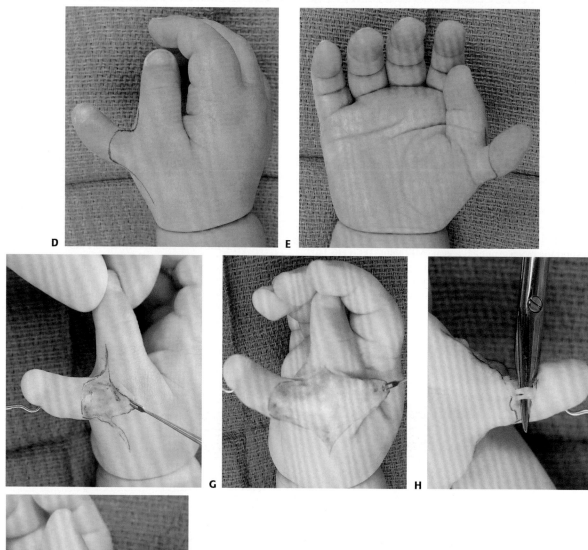

TECH FIG 1 (Continued) • **D,E.** Dorsal and palmar views of the operative markings for planned excision of radial partner. A mid-lateral closure is planned. Excess skin is left on the retained partner for subsequent closure. **F.** The dorsal skin incision has been incised, the dorsal veins are cauterized, and a plane is developed over the extensor mechanism. **G.** The dorsal skin flap is elevated proximal to the MP joint. **H.** The volar incision is made, and the neurovascular bundle to the radial partner has been identified. **I.** The volar skin flap is elevated to expose the flexor tendon and the intrinsic abductor musculature.

- If only cartilage is involved (in minor cases), a knife will be sufficient to complete this task (**TECH FIG 3B**).
- In most cases, however, a retrograde osteotomy with a saw or a fine bone cutter is needed (**TECH FIG 3C**).
- Assess the need for closing wedge metacarpal osteotomy. When MP joint ulnar angulation of the retained partner is prominent, a closing wedge osteotomy is needed (**TECH FIG 3D**).

- Pin fixation is necessary after osteotomy (**TECH FIG 4**). Insert a retrograde 0.028 in. Kirschner wire from the ulnar side.

Tendon Correction in Type IV Polydactyly

- In divergent-convergent (rhomboid) type IV polydactyly, the extensor and flexor tendons can have eccentric insertions onto the distal phalanges (**TECH FIG 5**).

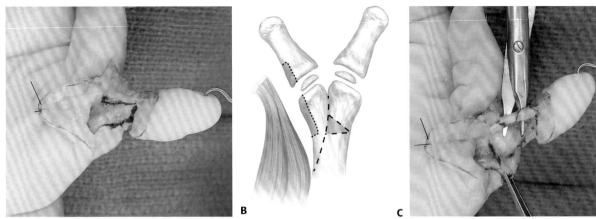

TECH FIG 2 • A. A proximally based periosteal flap is designed. The flap will include the radial collateral ligament and the abductor muscle insertion. Note that the muscle is inserting onto the bone (periosteum) and the flexor tendon. **B.** Technical maneuvers necessary for reconstruction of type IV radial polydactyly. The periosteal/muscle flap has been lifted, the dotted area showing the previous area of flap adherence. It is ideal to leave a long periosteal cuff on the flap to make subsequent repair easier. The radial head of the bifid metacarpal is cut, and a closing wedge osteotomy is performed if there is deviation of the ulnar partner. **C.** The flexor tendon is isolated. Note the periosteal/muscle flap reflected proximally and held with forceps.

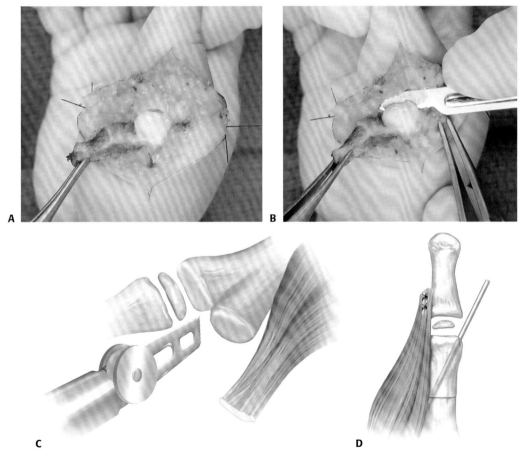

TECH FIG 3 • A. The radial partner has been disarticulated at the MP joint, and the bifid metacarpal head is noted. **B.** In minor cases, such as this one, the radial head of the metacarpal is mostly cartilaginous and can be excised using a blade. **C.** In most cases, the radial head of the metacarpal has an osseous component and a retrograde osteotomy with a saw is needed. **D.** Illustration demonstrates result after closing wedge osteotomy (secured with a pin) and reattachment of the periosteal/muscle flap.

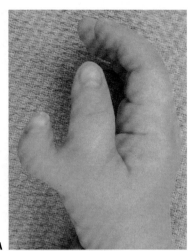
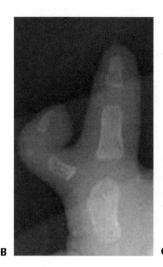
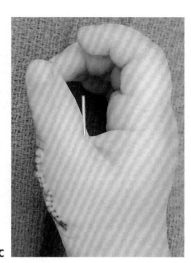
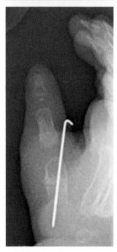

TECH FIG 4 • **A,B.** A different patient is demonstrated with type IV radial polydactyly and more significant ulnar angulation of the ulnar partner at the MP joint. Improvement in angulation is noted after closing wedge osteotomy and pin fixation intraoperatively **(C)** and 3.5 weeks postoperatively **(D)**.

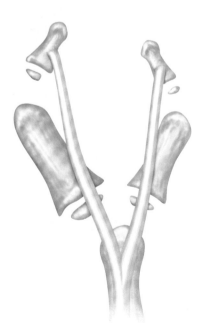

TECH FIG 5 • In rhomboid type IV polydactyly, the extrinsic tendons can attach eccentrically on the distal phalanges, thus exaggerating the deviation. If these abnormal insertions are not addressed, deviation can recur with growth.

- If left alone, these abnormal tendons can contribute to long-term misalignment and deviation of the thumb.
- They should be detached and reattached at the proper location on the distal phalanx.

Reattachment and Closure

- Reattach using sutures the flap of periosteum, collateral ligament, and muscle to the radial aspect of the retained proximal phalanx (**TECH FIG 6A**).
  - After removal of the radial metacarpal head, the radial aspect of the remaining metacarpal is bare and not attached to the collateral ligament; however, the collateral ligament heals well to the metacarpal.
  - Additional reinforcing sutures to the metacarpal may be necessary.
- There will be excess skin in multiple dimensions. In most cases, the excess skin can be trimmed and "cheated in" and a mid-lateral closure completed.
  - If there is abundant excess, a better approach is to make a separate palmar incision along the MP joint flexion crease to excise skin in an orthogonal dimension (**TECH FIG 6B,C**).
- Apply a soft dressing and a long-arm cast for 3 to 4 weeks.

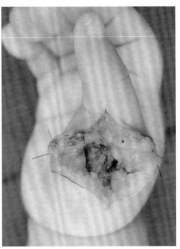 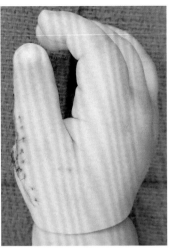 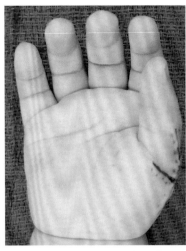

TECH FIG 6 • A. The periosteal, collateral ligament, and muscle flap have been reattached to the proximal phalanx with additional reinforcing sutures onto the radial aspect of the metacarpal. **B.** Final appearance after closure. **C.** Note that the "dog ear" has been ablated via a separate incision in the volar MP joint flexion crease.

PEARLS AND PITFALLS

Surgical management	■ It is the author's opinion that, when possible and especially in more proximal polydactyly cases, resection and reconstruction give a better aesthetic outcome than does the Bilhaut "sharing" technique. The downside is that the thumb is usually smaller. ■ The surgeon should have a well-defined stepwise approach for each case.
Technique	■ When developing muscle and/or collateral ligament flaps, leave a long periosteal sleeve to allow easier subsequent reattachment. ■ In polydactyly cases that have multiple levels of joint deviation (eg, rhomboid type IV), multiple simultaneous osteotomies should be undertaken.

POSTOPERATIVE CARE

- Immobilize the extremity with a long-arm cast with the elbow at 90 degrees of flexion for 3 or 4 weeks. The author immobilizes longer in those patients who have undergone osteotomies.
- Remove the cast (and pins) and refer to hand therapy for fabrication of a thermoplast thumb spica splint.
- Start range-of-motion exercises.
- Wear the splint for 2 or 3 weeks at night.
- See patients once every 1 to 2 years to assess function, growth, and joint deviation.

OUTCOMES

- Although multiple different outcome scoring systems have been proposed, reliability appears highest for the scoring system proposed by the Japanese Society for Surgery of the Hand.[7]
- The results after polydactyly repair are generally satisfactory but depend greatly on the initial deformity.
  - Results of type III, V, and VI repairs are less satisfactory.

- The affected side is weaker than the normal side and revisions are common, but patients have favorable scores on objective outcome measures.[6]
- Long-term unfavorable outcomes after repair include deviations and angulations (with associated pain), bony prominences, stiffness, and nail deformity. Deviations maybe the result of trapezoidal or delta phalanges, canted or unstable joints, or asymmetrical growth and can occur long term despite an adequate initial repair.
- The Bilhaut procedure has had unfavorable results including stiffness and nail deformity. Many prefer resection and reconstruction to this technique,[5] although the aforementioned modification of the Bilhaut technique for more distal polydactyly cases[4] has shown promising results and gained support.

COMPLICATIONS

- Immediate complications are rare and include bleeding, infection, and wound dehiscence.
- Wound dehiscence is almost always due to inadequate immobilization and can be prevented with a long-arm cast.

REFERENCES

1. Wassel HD. The results of surgery for polydactyly of the thumb. *Clin Orthop Relat Res.* 1969;64:175-193.
2. Zuidam JM, Selles RW, Ananta M, et al. A classification system of radial polydactyly: inclusion of triphalangeal thumb and triplication. *J Hand Surg Am.* 2008;33:373-377.
3. Oberg KC, Feenstra JM, Manske PR, Tonkin MA. Developmental biology and classification of congenital anomalies of the hand and upper extremity. *J Hand Surg Am.* 2010;35:2066-2076.
4. Baek GH, Gong HS, Chung MS, et al. Modified Bilhaut-Cloquet procedure for Wassel type-II and III polydactyly of the thumb. *J Bone Joint Surg Am.* 2007;89:534-541.
5. Dijkman RR, Selles RW, Hülsemann W, et al. A matched comparative study of the Bilhaut procedure versus resection and reconstruction for treatment of radial polydactyly types II and IV. *J Hand Surg Am.* 2016;41:e73-e83.
6. Stutz C, Mills J, Wheeler L, et al. Long-term outcomes following radial polydactyly reconstruction. *J Hand Surg Am.* 2014;39(8):1549-1552.
7. Dijkman RR, van Nieuwenhoven CA, Selles RW, Hovius SER. Comparison of functional outcome scores in radial polydactyly. *J Bone Joint Surg Am.* 2014;96:463-470.

Index Finger Pollicization for Hypoplastic Thumb

Amir H. Taghinia, Brian I. Labow, and Joseph Upton

DEFINITION

- The thumb is the functional keystone of the hand. The basic hand unit has three main elements: a thumb, a web space, and a prehensile post. Severe hypoplasia or aplasia of the thumb leads to significant functional impairment.
- Index finger pollicization is the procedure of transposing the index finger into the position of the thumb. It is the quintessential operation of hand surgery, incorporating key principles and requiring meticulous technique and execution.
  - The methods outlined herein include further refinements[1] to the techniques initially proposed, developed, and refined by D. Buck-Gramcko[2] and J. W. Littler.[3]

ANATOMY

- The normal thumb is perfectly adapted for pinch and grasp. It is broad with osseous and articular structures that move in multiple planes. Its intrinsic muscles provide a short moment arm, powering the movement enabled by the osseoarticular column.
- The normal first web space has a gentle curve spanning from the thumb metacarpophalangeal (MP) joint to the index finger MP joint.
- A thumb is considered hypoplastic if any of its osseous, musculotendinous, or articular components is deficient or if the web space that it forms with the index finger is shallow.
- The modified Blauth[4] classification system provides a surgically useful basis for categorizing thumb hypoplasia. Most surgeons agree that Blauth types I, II, and IIIA thumbs can be reconstructed, whereas Blauth types IIIB, IV (*pouce flottant*), and V (aplasia) hypoplastic thumbs require index finger pollicization.
- The differentiating factor between Blauth type IIIA and IIIB thumbs is the presence (IIIA) or absence (IIIB) of a functional carpometacarpal (CMC) joint.
- The preoperative state of the index finger is the greatest determinant of long-term postoperative function after pollicization.[1,5] Patients with normal index fingers will have the best function. Abnormal index fingers are typically seen in patients with radial longitudinal deficiency. Abnormalities include stiffness, joint hypoplasia, incomplete intrinsic muscles and/or extrinsic tendons, and hypoplastic or anomalous vessels and nerves.

PATHOGENESIS AND NATURAL HISTORY

- Thumb hypoplasia occurs as a result of multiple potential factors, including genetic (associated syndromes), environmental, teratogenic (thalidomide), and idiopathic causes.

- It is considered to be a malformation, based on the Oberg, Manske, and Tonkin classification of 2010.[6]
- Thumb hypoplasia occurs in 1 out of 100 000 live births.
- A large number of patients with thumb hypoplasia have associated conditions such as cardiac or hematologic anomalies.

PATIENT HISTORY AND PHYSICAL FINDINGS

- Patients are usually seen in infancy. In severe cases such as type IV or type V, the diagnosis is clear. Nevertheless, the difference between type IIIA and IIIB can be difficult to ascertain in a newborn. The integrity of the CMC joint is sometimes not obvious on plain film radiographs. Functional differentiation can be made by allowing the child to grow and watching the toddler at play—if the thumb is not used, the joint is likely nonfunctional.
- Indeed, most children with severe thumb hypoplasia will scissor pinch using the index and middle fingers in lieu of the nonfunctional thumb. With time, the web space between the index and middle fingers widens and the index finger starts to pronate. These patients are ideal candidates for pollicization.
- The hand surgeon should be aware of the conditions associated with thumb hypoplasia, and have a low threshold to refer if suspicions arise.
  - In particular, roughly 50% of patients with Fanconi anemia (an inherited defect in DNA repair leading to bone marrow failure and premature malignancy) manifest thumb hypoplasia, along with a variety of other anomalies. The diagnosis of Fanconi anemia can be made via a blood test early in life.
  - Other associated conditions include Holt-Oram syndrome, VACTERL association, radial longitudinal deficiency, and thrombocytopenia-absent radius (TAR).

IMAGING

- Plain radiographs help to determine the status of the CMC joint, any abnormalities of the index finger, and the status of the distal radius and ulna (presence of radial longitudinal deficiency).
- The authors do not routinely perform angiography.

DIFFERENTIAL DIAGNOSIS

- Differentiate type IIIA and IIIB thumbs by functional assessment of the child.

SURGICAL MANAGEMENT

- The authors perform index finger pollicization in toddlers around 2 years of age, but the timing is more dependent on size, weight, and other medical comorbidities that may delay intervention.
  - The procedure is technically easier if performed in a toddler, rather than an infant.
  - Manske[5] has shown that pollicization can be functional and effective even if performed later in childhood.
- The main objective of the operation is to shorten and reposition the index finger into a recessed, pronated, and palmarly abducted position, as well as to simultaneously create a well-contoured web space.
- The main steps of the procedure are as follows:
  - Make incisions in a modified Y to V fashion that will allow the index finger to be recessed and rotated.
  - Isolate the index finger as a neurovascular island.
  - Disinsert and isolate the intrinsic muscles of the index finger.
  - Excise the metacarpal, ablate the metacarpal growth plate, and secure the metacarpal head in a hyperextended position into the cut metacarpal base.
  - Rebalance the extensor tendons.
  - Rebalance the intrinsic muscles.
  - Adjust skin flaps to create an aesthetically pleasing outcome.

- Almost always, there is sufficient skin to transpose the index finger and close all the wounds without needing skin grafts.
  - Any open wounds or flaps under tension are the result of poor incision planning or execution.
- Simultaneous bilateral index finger pollicization is not performed.

Preoperative Planning

- Again discuss risks, benefits, and expectations with parents on the day of surgery.
  - Specifically outline the risks of flap loss (partial or complete), ischemia of the digit, poor positioning, and suboptimal function and the potential need for revisional or adjunct procedures later in childhood.
- The surgeon needs fine surgical instruments and vessel loops for tagging and dissection of important structures.

Positioning

- The patient is positioned supine with the arm out on a small hand table.

Approach

- Incisions are planned carefully prior to use of the tourniquet. Dorsal and palmar approaches are needed.

TECHNIQUES

■ Index Finger Pollicization

Markings and Dissection

- Place two small round marks, one at the base of the index finger and the other at the position where the new thumb base will be placed. Mark a racquet-shaped incision around the base of the index finger. Extend these markings onto the proposed new thenar flexion crease; this will be the recession incision.

- The markings for the incisions should be planned so they extend through the round marks (**TECH FIG 1A,B**).
- The back-cut incision is not made until the ray has been transposed.
- Exsanguinate the upper extremity and inflate a tourniquet in the upper arm.
- Incise transversely on the dorsum of the index finger (**TECH FIG 1C**). (Note that the patient shown in the clinical photographs has radial longitudinal deficiency and a stiff index finger.)

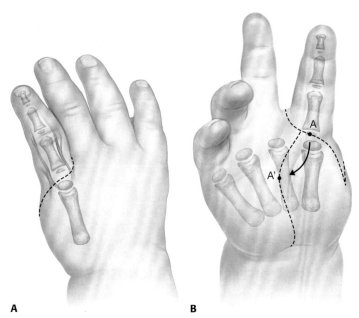
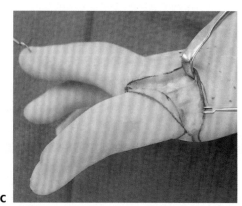

TECH FIG 1 • **A,B.** Dorsal and palmar markings. A racquet-shaped incision is planned around the index finger. The index finger will be recessed into the proposed thenar flexion crease incision. **C.** Dorsal incision is made, and veins are identified and dissected. One sizeable vein should be present on either side of the extensor tendon.

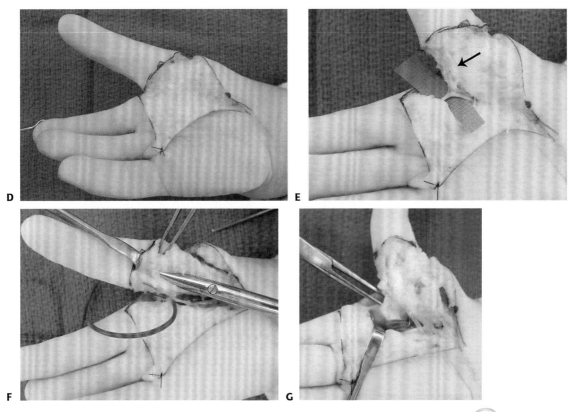

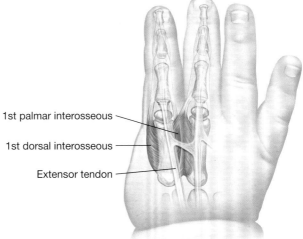

TECH FIG 1 (Continued) • **D.** The palmar incision is made and a flap raised on the palmar fascia. The flap is reflected and tacked back for the remainder of the case. **E.** The ulnar contribution of the common digital artery to the index-middle web is isolated (on the green background). The ulnar digital nerve of the index finger is visualized (*arrow*). **F.** The A1 pulley is exposed and ready to be divided. The scissor tip is underneath the pulley. **G.** The fine-tipped clamp is underneath the intermetacarpal ligament. The retractor is pulling the lumbrical muscle to the middle finger. The artery and nerve are free with the index finger. **H.** First dorsal and volar interosseous muscles. These muscles will be rebalanced to mimic the intrinsic muscles of the new thumb.

- Upward traction on the skin will reveal the longitudinally oriented veins on either side of the extensor tendon at the MP joint level. These veins run in the plane between the superficial (small globular) fat and the deep (large lobular) fat.
  - Dissect these veins proximally beyond the mid-dorsum of the hand.
  - Place blue vessel loops around these veins to help with dissection and subsequent identification.
- Incise the remaining volar markings and raise a volar skin flap just above the palmar fascia up to the middle finger (**TECH FIG 1D**).
- Identify and dissect the neurovascular bundle in the index-middle web, and isolate the middle finger

contribution of the common digital artery (**TECH FIG 1E**). Ligate this branch.
- Separate the nerves. Intraneural loops may be present and should be carefully dissected.
- Divide the A1 pulley (**TECH FIG 1F**).
- Isolate the intermetacarpal ligament and divide it sharply (**TECH FIG 1G**).
- Dissect and isolate the intrinsic muscles of the index finger—the first dorsal interosseous and the first volar interosseous (**TECH FIG 1H**).
  - The first dorsal interosseous may have two heads; each should be isolated. A small lumbrical may also be present.
- Dissect and isolate the extensor tendons.

Metacarpal Preparation and Osteosynthesis

- Incise and strip the periosteum off the diaphysis of the metacarpal.
- Cut the metacarpal head at the level of the growth plate (**TECH FIG 2A**). This can usually be done with a blade.
- Cut the metacarpal base in a volar oblique fashion using a saw. The angle of this cut determines the degree of palmar abduction of the neothumb. Ideal is about 60 degrees of palmar abduction.
- Measure the length of the removed metacarpal (**TECH FIG 2B**). This measurement approximates the length of extensor to shorten.
- Ablate the growth plate using a blade (**TECH FIG 2C**). Avoid injuring the collateral ligaments.
- Affix the metacarpal head to the metacarpal base (**TECH FIG 2D**).

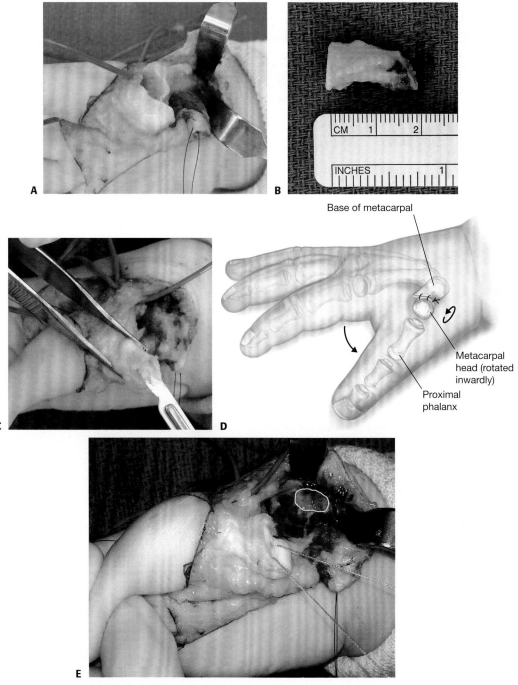

TECH FIG 2 • A. The metacarpal head is divided. The metacarpal has been stripped of its periosteum. The first dorsal interosseous muscle is seen retracted with a black suture at its insertion. A volar oblique osteotomy is planned at the base of the metacarpal (*purple* markings). **B.** The removed metacarpal. Figure left is distal; figure top is dorsal. The length of the excised bone approximates the shortening of the extensor tendons. **C.** Use a blade to ablate the metacarpal physis. **D.** The metacarpal head should be placed at its base with the joint in hyperextension. The angle of the base osteotomy determines the degree of palmar abduction. **E.** Suture osteosynthesis gives more control for accurate positioning of the metacarpal head. The base is outlined in white.

- The metacarpal head should be pronated and flexed so its cut surface aligns with the cut surface of the base. The MP joint should be hyperextended.
  - If placed in a neutral or flexed position, the MP joint will hyperextend naturally with time. Placing it initially in hyperextension prevents this problem.
- Place a braided nonabsorbable, double-armed suture (3-0 Ethibond) in a mattress fashion into the metacarpal head (**TECH FIG 2E**). Insert the needles from inside the cut surface of the metacarpal base dorsally and tie. Additional sutures to the nearby soft tissues help to secure the fixation. Wires are not needed.

Dorsal Flap Placement

- Make the back-cut incision. Advance the dorsal hand skin flap and assess a position on the digit where the dorsal flap will inset (**TECH FIG 3A**).

- Design a straight, longitudinal incision on the dorsum of the transposed digit. The incision typically stops just proximal to the PIP joint. Incise the skin and spread down to the extensor tendon to separate the veins and subcutaneous tissue (**TECH FIG 3B**).
- Dissect the lateral bands from the extensor mechanism for subsequent attachment to the intrinsic muscles on each side of the new thumb (**TECH FIG 3C**).
- Release the tourniquet and watch for vascularity of the fingertip (**TECH FIG 3D**).

Tendon Repair

- Rebalance the extensor tendons. Dissect and separate the extensor indicis proprius (EIP) from the extensor digitorum communis (EDC). On occasion, the interval between these two tendons can be difficult to ascertain.

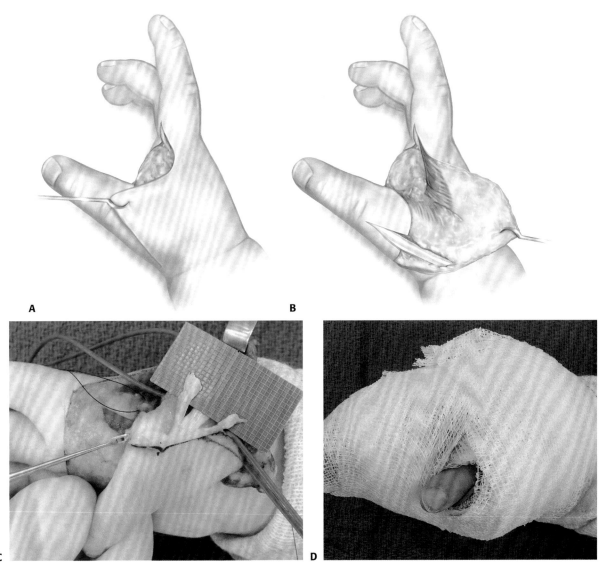

TECH FIG 3 • A. Once the osteosynthesis is complete, the dorsal flap is advanced and the location of the cut back incision on the index finger is determined. **B.** An incision is then made, and the veins and subcutaneous structures are separated. **C.** The lateral bands on either side of the extensor are delineated. **D.** Releasing the tourniquet allows one to assess vascularity of the digit. Furthermore, any bleeding sites can be addressed at this time.

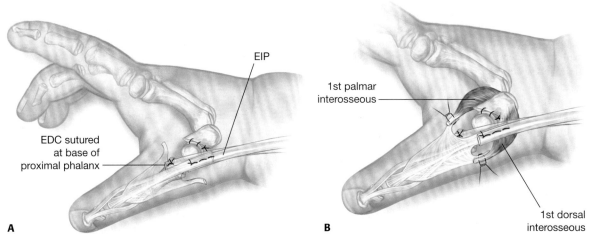

TECH FIG 4 • A. The EIP is shortened and secured with a side-to-side tenorrhaphy. The EDC is shortened and attached to the ulnar base of the proximal phalanx. **B.** The first dorsal interosseous and volar interosseous are sutured to the lateral bands. If the first dorsal interosseous has two heads, one head can be directly attached to the periosteum on the radial side of the middle phalanx.

- Shorten the EIP by approximately the length of bone removed. Side-to-side tenorrhaphy works well (**TECH FIG 4A**). The digit should hold an extended posture. The EIP becomes the new extensor pollicis longus.
- Disconnect the EDC, shorten it, and reattach it to the ulnar base of the index finger proximal phalanx (see **TECH FIG 4A**). Attaching it to the ulnar base of the proximal phalanx enhances pronation. The EDC becomes the new abductor pollicis longus.
- Reattach the first dorsal interosseous to the radial lateral band and the first volar interosseous to the ulnar lateral band (**TECH FIG 4B**). The first dorsal interosseous will mimic the abductor pollicis brevis, and the first volar interosseous will mimic the adductor pollicis muscle.

- If the first dorsal interosseous has two heads, one head can be attached to the periosteum of the radial middle phalanx. The digit should hold an extended posture but be easily flexed down with gentle finger pressure.

Completion

- Inset the proximal neothumb skin flap into the proximal corner of the thenar crease incision.
- Close the web space with 6-0 chromic sutures.
- Inset the remaining skin flaps and close (**TECH FIG 5**).
- Apply antibiotic-impregnated gauze to all incisions and cover with sterile gauze.
- Wrap loosely and apply a well-padded long-arm cast. Keep the tip of the neothumb exposed for vascular checks postoperatively.

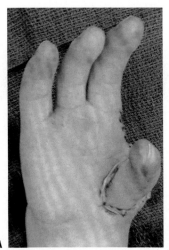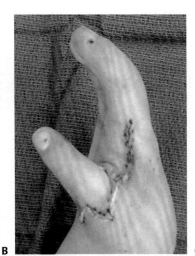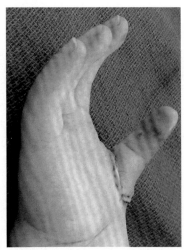

TECH FIG 5 • A–C. The final outcome after insetting of the skin and closure of the web space. (As mentioned previously, this patient had radial longitudinal deficiency.)

PEARLS AND PITFALLS

Physical findings	■ It may be difficult to differentiate between type IIIA and IIIB thumbs in an infant. Allow the child to grow. With time, the functional differentiation becomes more apparent.
Technique	■ The more common, and more difficult, vascular problem that occurs is venous insufficiency. Be most cautious with the veins during the initial dissection. Although it may oppose common practice, using a blade (instead of scissors) to sharply lift the dorsal skin flap off the veins works well at avoiding venous injury. ■ Neural loops around the arteries can be difficult to separate especially in smaller children. Do not hesitate to employ a microscope or microinstruments for this purpose. ■ Obtain careful hemostasis and close the skin while the tourniquet is down so hematoma is avoided.
Postoperative	■ Because the flexor tendon is not routinely shortened, it takes up to 6 months for digit to start actively flexing.
Therapy	■ Early on, a few children will avoid use of the new thumb and instead start pinching with the middle and ring fingers. To discourage this behavior, consider buddy taping the middle and ring fingers together.

POSTOPERATIVE CARE

- Remove the cast after 3 to 4 weeks of immobilization.
- Fashion a thumb spica thermoplast splint that can be worn for 2 to 3 weeks at night for protection.
- Start range-of-motion exercises with hand therapy.

OUTCOMES

- Functional outcomes of pollicization depend mostly on the preoperative status of the index finger. Those patients with normal index fingers will have the best results, whereas those with stiff or abnormal index finger (eg, radial longitudinal deficiency) will have suboptimal results.[1,5]
- The new thumb is a suboptimal replica of a normal thumb. It lacks the broadness, strength, and osteoarticular integrity of a normal thumb. Under the best of circumstances, one can expect about 50% pinch strength as compared to an unaffected contralateral side.

COMPLICATIONS

- Positional problems include the new thumb being too long or not adequately pronated and/or abducted. Both of these complications make the thumb appear like a shortened finger, the former because it is too long and the latter because it is in the same plane as the fingers.
- Inadequate web space is mainly a problem of poor incision planning or excessively thinned/ischemic flaps.
- Hematoma is most commonly seen on the dorsum where it can cause ischemia of the dorsal skin (via pressure and direct toxicity) or of the new thumb (via pressure on the draining veins).

- Vascular insufficiency is a dreaded complication and can be arterial or venous in origin. Fortunately, these complications are rare.
  - Arterial insufficiency is less commonly due to kinking and compression and more commonly due to direct injury. Once the injury is recognized, it should be promptly repaired using the operating microscope.
  - Venous insufficiency can be due to direct injury, kinking, or compression. Ensure that veins are adequately dissected proximally, that they lie tension-free without kinking, and that there is no hematoma or site of compression.
- Opposition weakness is commonly seen in the long term. Opponensplasty with abductor digiti minimi transfer (Huber) can provide additional power. If needed, this procedure is performed several years after the pollicization.

REFERENCES

1. Taghinia AH, Littler JW, Upton J. Refinements in pollicization: a 30-year experience. *Plast Reconstr Surg.* 2012;30:423e-433e.
2. Buck-Gramcko D. Pollicization of the index finger: method and results in aplasia and hypoplasia of the thumb. *J Bone Joint Surg Am.* 1971;53:1605-1617.
3. Littler J. The neurovascular pedicle method of digital transposition for reconstruction of the thumb. *Plast Reconstr Surg.* 1953;12:303-319.
4. Manske PR, McCarroll HR Jr, James M. Type III-A hypoplastic thumb. *J Hand Surg [Am].* 1995;20:246-253.
5. Manske PR, Rotman MB, Dailey LA. Long-term functional results after pollicization for the congenitally deficient thumb. *J Hand Surg [Am].* 1992;17:1064-1072.
6. Oberg KC, Feenstra JM, Manske PR, Tonkin MA. Developmental biology and classification of congenital anomalies of the hand and upper extremity. *J Hand Surg [Am].* 2010;35:2066-2076.

67 CHAPTER

Second Toe-to-Thumb Transfer for Hypoplastic Thumb

Amir H. Taghinia, Brian I. Labow, and Joseph Upton

DEFINITION

- Toe-to-thumb transfer for congenital conditions is usually indicated in cases in which the carpometacarpal joint and (at least) the proximal part of the metacarpal are intact and functional but the remainder of the thumb is absent or diseased.[1]
- Either the great toe or the second toe is typically used for thumb reconstruction. Although the modified great toe looks more like a thumb, the length of first metatarsal that can be harvested without functional loss in the foot is quite limited.
- In congenital patients,[2] toe-to-thumb transfer is most commonly performed for amniotic constriction bands, symbrachydactyly (atypical cleft hand), transverse failure of formation, (typical) cleft hand, and highly select cases of type IIIB thumb hypoplasia.
  - The congenital conditions in which the thumb is diseased include macrodactyly and vascular anomalies.

ANATOMY

- The second toe is smaller than the normal thumb. It has a lower width to pulp depth ratio, thus appearing more clubbed and bulbous. It has three phalanges and a metatarsophalangeal joint, which, in the foot, functions as a hyperextension joint rather than a flexion joint as in the thumb.
- The arterial anatomy of the second toe can be variable. The dorsalis pedis artery is the main proximal blood supply. It gives rise to the first dorsal metatarsal artery (FDMA) and the first plantar metatarsal artery (FPMA) via anastomosis with the medial plantar artery, a branch of the posterior tibial arterial system of the foot.
- There are three common branching patterns (**FIG 1**)[3]:
  - The FDMA lies superficial to the first dorsal interosseous muscle.

- The FDMA lies within or deep to the first dorsal interosseous muscle.
  - The FDMA is diminutive or absent.
- The more plantar the dominant system, the more difficult is the dissection.
- The venous anatomy provides abundant large veins. Venous branches of the second toe reside in the dorsal subcutaneous plane; a vein on either side of the toe drains to the lesser saphenous (lateral) or great saphenous (medial) veins.
- The second toe has two extensor tendons—extensor digitorum longus and brevis—and two flexor tendons—flexor digitorum longus and brevis. The extensors approach the second ray in an oblique fashion, from lateral to medial. Two plantar digital nerves travel below the transverse metatarsal ligament and arrive on either side of the toe to provide sensation to the pulp.
- Unlike the first ray of the foot where the metatarsal is crucial for gait, the second ray's metatarsal is expendable and its entire length may be harvested if needed. The goal should be to construct a new thumb of normal length. In full adduction, a normal thumb extends to the proximal interphalangeal (PIP) joint of the adjacent index finger.
- In congenital conditions where the foot is also affected, the surgeon may carefully consider harvesting an anatomically abnormal toe. Investigation of arterial anatomy under these special circumstances is, at a minimum, important to avoid vascular compromise of the toe transfer—or worse, the other toes.
- In cases of amniotic constriction bands, the proximal anatomy of the hand is usually normal. However, in other conditions such as symbrachydactyly or transverse failure, the anatomy of the hand may not be normal.

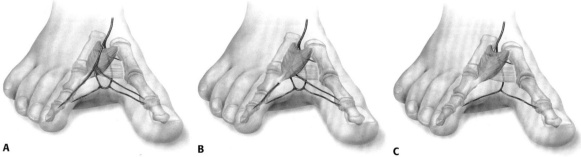

A   **B**   **C**

FIG 1 • Variations in arterial anatomy of the first web space of the foot. As it reaches the base of the first and second metatarsals, the dorsalis pedis artery can continue on dorsally as the first dorsal metatarsal artery (FDMA) and send a plantar branch, the first plantar metatarsal artery (FPMA). **A.** The FDMA may be the dominant blood supply to the second toe and may lie superficially to the first dorsal interosseous. **B.** Alternatively, the FDMA may lie within or deep to the first dorsal interosseous. **C.** Last, the FDMA may be diminutive or completely absent.

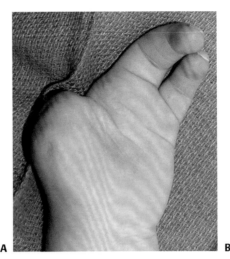
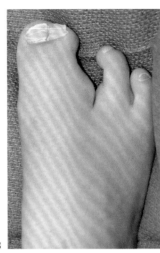

FIG 2 • This 3-year-old patient with typical cleft hand/cleft foot syndrome (the example case throughout) has two ulnar fingers but no thumb **(A)**, as well as webbed great and second toes **(B)**.

■ Variations in anatomy tend to be the rule and include deficient or missing tendons, nerves, muscles, and arteries. These variations may only become evident during the operation, and so the surgeon should be prepared with multiple contingency plans. Angiography is used more liberally in these patients.

PATIENT HISTORY AND PHYSICAL FINDINGS

■ A full history and physical examination should be obtained to define and document deficient anatomy, assess current functional use, ascertain associated conditions, and set goals for reconstruction.
■ Physical examination of the hand (**FIG 2A**)
  ▪ The skin is inspected for suppleness, turgor, and pliability.
  ▪ The soft tissue around the thumb is inspected for presence of intrinsic muscles.
  ▪ Dimples in the skin may indicate underlying tendons.
  ▪ Pulse examination and an Allen test are necessary to assess the blood supply to the hand and presence of palmar arch.
■ Physical examination of the foot (**FIG 2B**)
  ▪ General appearance of the foot and/or toe may indicate presence of any anatomic abnormalities. In amniotic constriction bands, the toes may also be affected.

▪ Pulses are examined. A pencil Doppler probe can be used to ascertain the presence of an FDMA by tracing its course on the dorsum of the foot.

IMAGING

■ Plain radiographs of the hand and foot are required (**FIG 3**).
■ Routine angiography is debatable; nevertheless, it is the authors' practice to obtain angiography of the hand and foot on most patients (**FIG 4**).
  ▪ Angiography helps to create a road map and a plan for the operation. Questions such as the need for vein grafting (foot), end-to-side vs end-to-end anastomoses (hand), and residual vascularity of the foot after flap harvest can be answered preoperatively. This planning is essential in cases where a team approach with multiple surgeons is undertaken. Certainly for patients with abnormal foot anatomy (**FIG 5**), angiography helps with preoperative planning to ensure a viable flap.

SURGICAL MANAGEMENT

■ The time to perform the toe transfer should not be an arbitrary age but rather tailored to the individual child.
  ▪ Although it is important to perform the transfer as early as possible to take advantage of brain plasticity and enhanced nerve regeneration, the child has to be of appropriate size to allow a technically feasible operation.

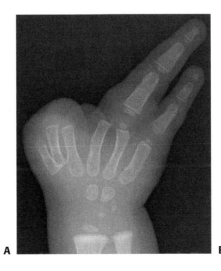
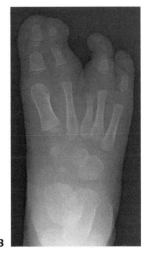

FIG 3 • Radiography of the example case shows three metacarpals on the radial side of the hand **(A)** and separate skeletal structures in the foot despite webbing of the great and second toes **(B)**. Note that there are only two phalanges in the second toe. The epiphysis of the second metatarsal is not present in this early radiograph, but it is distally located in subsequent films (see **TECH FIG 7A**), indicating that this is indeed a phylogenetic second toe rather than a preaxial synpolydactyly.

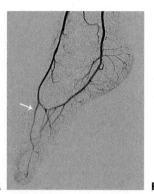 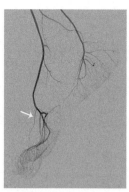 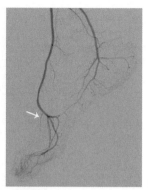 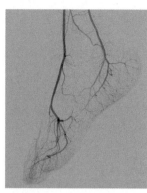

A   **B**   **C**   **D**

FIG 4 • Angiographic variation in arterial anatomy of the foot (FDMA indicated by *white arrow*). The variations outlined in **FIG 1** are seen in the angiograms, with a large, dominant FDMA **(A)**; a thinner, intramuscular FDMA **(B)**; a diminutive FDMA **(C)**; and no FDMA **(D)**. The plantar system is dominant in **B** to **D**.

- Specifically, the vessels tend to be too small for a predictable operation in most children under the age of 2.
- The decision-making process for the parents (and the child) often requires substantial discussion. The sacrifice of part of a foot for improved function of the hand can be a difficult decision, especially when there is a small risk that the toe may not survive or that the function may not be optimal.
    - Thorough preparation of the parents for this process, including an honest explanation of the risks and expected outcomes, is a crucial preoperative step.
- Radiographs, preoperative and postoperative photographs, molds, and movies of other patients can help with the decision-making.
- Jones advocates arranging for parents to meet the families of previous patients with toe transfers.[1]
- Multiple toe transfers are possible and can be performed reliably. Reconstruction of a thumb and finger(s) usually requires separate toes from both feet.
    - In contrast, multiple toes from the same foot can be used to reconstruct fingers.
- Preparation of the hand recipient site with the addition of skin and soft tissue as a first-stage procedure is rarely needed in congenital cases.
    - However, in cases in which there is a paucity of soft tissue and skin (eg, where the base of the thumb is very short), transfer of skin via pedicled (eg, groin or lower abdomen) or free (eg, anterolateral thigh) should be considered at least 6 to 9 months before definitive toe transfer.

- Skin grafting is often necessary and is much better tolerated on the hand than on the foot.

Preoperative Planning

- Simultaneous dissection of the donor toe and the recipient site requires two surgical teams. This approach minimizes time of surgery and anesthesia and ensures that the critical portions of the operation take place during times when operating room staffing is optimal.
- A careful analysis of deficient length is critical to ensure optimal function in the future. Plan the length of the thumb needed and the appropriate length of the second ray to harvest to achieve this length.
- The surgeon will need fine instruments for toe and hand dissections, loupe magnification, microsurgical instruments, a microscope, a handheld Doppler probe, and an adhesive-backed, disposable finger pulse oximetry monitor for postoperative monitoring of the toe transfer. In addition, automatic clip appliers and vascular loops greatly enhance the dissection.

Positioning

- The patient is positioned supine with the arm out on a small hand table. A small gel roll under the ipsilateral hip can help orient the foot into a more pronated position for dissecting the toe. The lower abdominal area for the skin graft is squared off with Steri-Drapes.
- Incisions are planned carefully prior to use of the tourniquet.

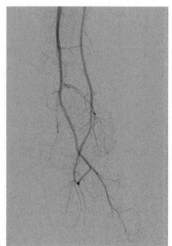 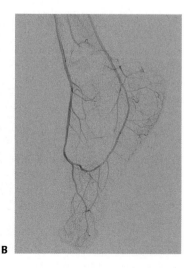

A   **B**

FIG 5 • Angiography of the foot of example case reveals an FDMA deep to the first dorsal interosseous supplying a single diminutive common dorsal and a single large common plantar artery. The dominant (plantar) vessel to the tibial, webbed toes lies in the web space and extends distally to the tips, sending branches along the way to both toes **(A)** anteroposterior view, **(B)** lateral view. The entire vessel was harvested with the second toe.

■ Second Toe Flap

Markings and Incision

- Identify and mark the path of the dorsalis pedis and FDMA, if present, using a handheld Doppler probe.
- Squeeze the ankle and milk the soft tissue distally to allow the dorsal foot veins to engorge. Mark these veins.
- Draw a wedge-shaped incision around the second toe (**TECH FIG 1A,B**).
  - In the case of abnormal foot anatomy, the incisions will need to be modified (**TECH FIG 1C,D**).
- Exsanguinate the extremity and inflate a mid-thigh tourniquet.
- Incise the dorsal markings and extend the incision along the path of the FDMA.

Soft Tissue Dissection

- Identify, dissect, and follow the superficial veins to the large dominant veins. Clip and divide all tributaries. Place blue vessel loops around the dominant veins and free them proximally.
- Identify and tag any dorsal sensory branches of the superficial peroneal nerve coursing to the second toe.

- Identify and dissect the extensor digitorum communis (EDC) tendon until enough length is achieved; transect it.
- Identify the short extensor tendon, which has a distal muscle belly and a thin tendon. Divide the tendon.
- Dissect proximal to the first and second metatarsal bases and identify the vascular pedicle. Place loops around the dorsalis pedis artery and its venae comitantes (**TECH FIG 2A**).
  - Usually, two comitant veins are present, but only one is suitable for microvascular anastomosis.
- Trace the pedicle distally to the FDMA, if present. The FDMA may lie dorsal to the first dorsal interosseous, may lie within or deep to the first dorsal interosseous, or may be absent (see **FIG 1**).
- Incise the first and second web space and plantar markings and dissect the soft tissues.
- Splay the great and third toes with a Gelpi retractor. This maneuver provides ample retraction and allows great visualization of the web space (**TECH FIG 2B**).
- Identify the neurovascular bundle on the fibular side of the great toe and the tibial side of the second toe in the first web space. Clip and divide the fibular digital artery to the great toe and sweep the vessels in the fibular direction (**TECH FIG 2C**). Similarly, clip and divide the tibial digital artery to the third toe, if present.

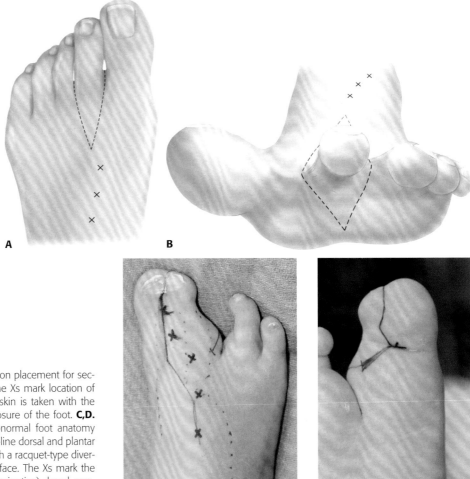

A B C D

TECH FIG 1 • A,B. Typical incision placement for second toe flap on a normal foot. The Xs mark location of audible Doppler pulses. Minimal skin is taken with the toe to allow tension-free linear closure of the foot. **C,D.** Modified incision planning for abnormal foot anatomy seen in the example case. Straight-line dorsal and plantar incisions were planned distally, with a racquet-type diversion proximally on the plantar surface. The Xs mark the path of the (deep) FDMA and (diminutive) dorsal common digital artery.

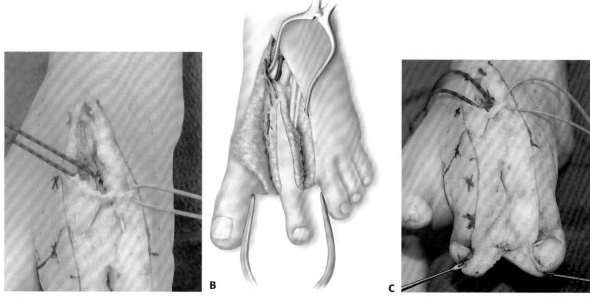

TECH FIG 2 • A. A dorsal superficial vein (*blue loop*) and the dorsalis pedis and its venae comitantes (*red loop*) have been identified and tagged. The muscle next to the artery, the extensor hallucis brevis, has been divided to expose the underlying vessels. **B.** Typical second toe dissection, dorsal view. Gelpi retractors help with exposure. A dorsal dominant arterial system is shown. The extensors to the second toe take an oblique course medially. The extensor hallucis brevis muscle (next to the artery) has been divided. **C.** The first web space has been exposed. The dominant, plantar common digital artery is shown with a clip on the great toe branch that has been divided. The entire common digital artery was kept with the second toe.

- Follow the artery proximal. The FDMA may have a communicating branch to the FPMA that passes anterior to the intermetatarsal ligament (see **FIG 1**).
- Isolate and divide the intermetatarsal ligament.

Artery and Nerve Dissection

- At this point, the plantar and dorsal systems are outlined and the dominance of the arterial system should be clear, even if an angiogram was not obtained.
- Select the dominant arterial system, and divide communicating branches as needed. The first dorsal interosseous may need to be divided; there are many small branches from the main pedicle to the bone and the muscle in this area.
- If the dominant system is plantar, the surgeon can avoid performing the tedious plantar dissection by using a vein graft to bridge the gap. The authors' practice, however, is to perform the full plantar dissection and avoid vein grafting.
  - Early osteotomy and elevation of the second metatarsal will help with exposure if the system is plantar dominant.
- Trace the artery all the way to the dorsalis pedis system. There is a hub of multiple arterial and venous branches at the base of the first and second metatarsals. Substantial additional length on the pedicle can be obtained if these branches are divided, and the dorsalis pedis system proper is used as the feeding vessel to the toe.
- Dissect the fibular and tibial digital nerves of the second toe to the common digital nerves in the respective proximal web spaces. These nerves are short and additional length is always necessary (**TECH FIG 3**).

- Use microinstruments to gently tease the nerves to the second toe from the common digital nerve on both sides. Perform the intraneural dissection as far proximal as needed.
- Transect the digital nerves and mark them with either small clips or sutures.
- Identify the flexor digitorum longus and brevis tendons (see **TECH FIG 3**); dissect and divide these as far proximally as possible.

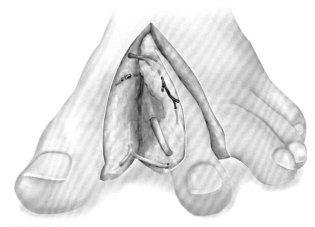

TECH FIG 3 • Typical second toe dissection, web space view. A dorsal dominant system is shown with the dorsal digital branch to the great toe clipped and divided. The proper digital nerves usually require intraneural dissection to obtain adequate length. The flexor system to the second toe should be divided as far proximal as possible.

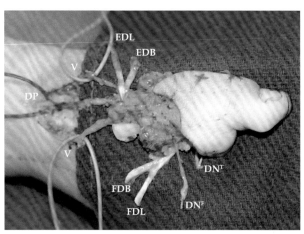

TECH FIG 4 • The second toe has been fully dissected and remains attached to the foot via its blood supply, the dorsalis pedis (*DP*) and two superficial veins (*V*). The extensor digitorum longus (*EDL*) and brevis (*EDB*), the flexor digitorum longus (*FDL*) and brevis (*FDB*), and the tibial (*DN^T^*) and fibular (*DN^F^*) are outlined. The FDMA was deep to the first DI in this case.

Metatarsal Osteotomy and Flap Placement

- Incise the periosteum over the second metatarsal, retract the vessels and tendons dorsally, and cut the metatarsal at the preplanned location.
  - Even though there is temptation to leave redundant bone length on the flap, trimming the bone when the flap is free and all the structures are loose is tedious and can be dangerous. It is best to get the ballpark length right the first time and make only small adjustments during the transfer.

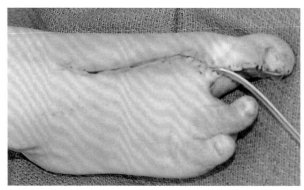

TECH FIG 5 • Foot closure is complete. The fibular side of the great toe has been covered with a full-thickness skin graft.

- Isolate the flap as a vascularized island (**TECH FIG 4**) and release the tourniquet.
  - Apply papaverine to the vessels and warm saline-soaked sponges to the wounds.
  - Assess the perfusion to the flap. If a difficult plantar system is encountered, the dissection may require a second, albeit shorter, tourniquet run.

Closure

- Close the foot wound by suturing the intermetacarpal ligaments attached to the first and third metatarsals, thus closing the gap in the first web space.
- Close the skin wound using absorbable sutures.
- A skin graft may be used if needed, but it is imperative to avoid skin grafts on the plantar surface. A thin drain may be used for a few days (**TECH FIG 5**).
- Apply a well-padded leg cast.

■ Preparation of the Hand for Toe Transfer

- The steps for the hand are dependent on the given anatomy.
- Placement of the incisions is likely to differ for each case (**TECH FIG 6A**).
  - If the incisions for inset are distant from appropriate vessels (most cases), a separate dorsal/radial transverse wrist incision provides ample access to large dorsal veins and the dorsal branch of the radial artery in the anatomic snuffbox.
- Exsanguinate the arm and inflate a tourniquet.

- Make the incisions and raise flaps.
- Identify and tag two large dorsal veins and the dorsal branch of the radial artery. The authors prefer to use at least two veins for microanastomosis.
- Dissect, isolate, and tag the intrinsic muscles of the proposed new thumb.
- Identify the extrinsic extensor and flexor tendons. Multiple tendons may be present, in which case the best flexor and extensor should be chosen (**TECH FIG 6B**).
- Dissect, isolate, and tag the digital nerves.
- Prepare the bone for osteosynthesis. Options include Kirschner wires, 90-90 interosseous wiring, or plate and screws for fixation.

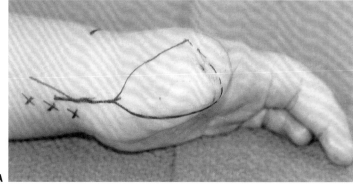

TECH FIG 6 • **A.** Markings for hand dissection. An ulnarly based skin flap is planned to partially cover the tibial portion of the second toe flap. A volar wrist incision exposes the radial artery. A dorsal transverse wrist incision exposes large dorsal veins.   **A**

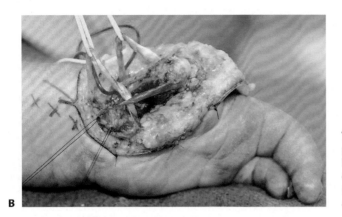

B

TECH FIG 6 (Continued) • **B.** Recipient hand has been prepared. Of the three radial metacarpals, the middle one has been preserved for osteosynthesis while the other two adjacent ones have been removed. Long extensor and flexor tendons are retracted (*yellow loops*). The intrinsic muscles of the thumb base are reflected (*black sutures*).

■ Transfer of Toe to Hand

- Assess the length of the toe on the new thumb, and adjust the size by cutting the bone with a saw.
    - The fully adducted, normal thumb tip extends to the level of the index finger PIP joint.
- Perform the osteosynthesis of choice (**TECH FIG 7A**).
- The positioning of the thumb is critical for function. The CMC joint and the proximal metacarpal are already set; however, the surgeon does have control over the degree of pronation and radial/ulnar angulation of the new thumb. Ensure that the new thumb rests in an appropriate position of function.
- Gauge the tension on the flexor and extensor tendons. Balance these so that the toe rests in near full MP joint extension and minimal flexion of the toe PIP and DIP joints. Repair the extensor tendon and then the flexor tendon using side-to-side tenorrhaphies.

- Perform the arterial and venous anastomoses using an operating microscope and microinstruments. Ideally, an end-to-side arterial anastomosis is performed to the radial artery to avoid compromise of the palmar arch (**TECH FIG 7B**).
- Perform the neurorrhaphies using the microscope; these repairs can be augmented by wrapping with neural conduit and/or topical tissue sealant.
- Close the skin. Avoid pressure on the vessels. Use full-thickness skin grafts from the lower abdomen to close any remaining open wounds (**TECH FIG 7C,D**).
- Apply a bulky protective dressing and a stable sugar-tong splint with the elbow at 90 degrees with just enough of the toe exposed for monitoring.
- Wrap a pulse oximeter–adhesive probe around the toe for continuous monitoring.

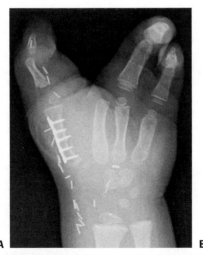

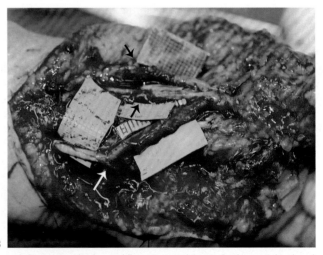

A   B

TECH FIG 7 • **A.** Osteosynthesis is complete. Of the three radial metacarpals, the middle metacarpal forms the base of the thumb; the other two adjacent metacarpals have been removed. Plate and screws provide rigid fixation. **B.** The vascular anastomoses in the example patient demonstrate an end-to-side arterial anastomosis to the radial artery (*white arrow*) and two separate end-to-end venous anastomoses (*black arrows*).

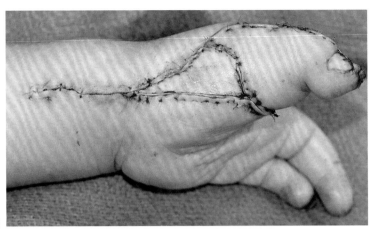 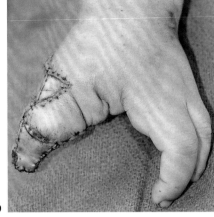

TECH FIG 7 (Continued) • **C,D.** Radial and ulnar views, respectively, of the example case after skin closure. The ulnar-based flap has been trimmed and inset. The open wounds have been covered with full-thickness skin grafts from the lower abdomen.

PEARLS AND PITFALLS

Surgical management	▪ Have low threshold to obtain angiogram in cases where the foot anatomy may not be normal, eg, congenital cleft.
Technique	▪ Exposure of a plantar-dominant system is made easier by performing the metatarsal osteotomy early on.
	▪ Meticulous closure and protection of the donor site helps to avoid wound-related problems that can take weeks to heal. Skin grafts are much better tolerated on the hand than the foot.
	▪ Once the toe is disconnected from the foot, a lot of preparation work is needed prior to performing the vascular anastomosis. Ensure that as much of this preparation as possible is performed prior to introducing ischemia. Do not rush through this part, as the osteosynthesis and balancing of tendons are critical for future function.
	▪ Although some surgeons prefer to avoid skin grafting directly over vessels, sometimes this practice is unavoidable after toe transfer. The authors have performed this practice many times without any untoward consequences.
Postoperative monitoring	▪ There are multiple options for postoperative monitoring: these include clinical assessment of capillary refill and warmth as well as handheld or implantable Doppler probe assessment of pulses. The authors prefer using a continuous pulse oximeter as a monitor as its use is simple and its monitoring of vascularity is reliable.

POSTOPERATIVE CARE

▪ Admit the patient to a high-level care unit and monitor the toe once per hour, assessing capillary refill, turgor, and warmth.
   ▫ A small opening can be left in the dressing where a site distal to the anastomosis can be monitored with a handheld Doppler.
   ▫ A continuous pulse oximeter is cheap, accurate, widely available, and highly reliable. Pulse wave changes are indicative of arterial compromise, whereas saturation changes may signal venous compromise.[4]
▪ Adequate pain control is important postoperatively. Regional anesthesia with indwelling catheters can provide both pain control and sympathetic block, which may help with perfusion.
▪ The authors use aspirin for 30 days routinely to avoid unwanted platelet aggregation.

▫ No other anticoagulants are used unless there are problems with the anastomosis or abnormal clotting early on.
▪ After several days, the dressings and splint are removed and a well-padded cast is applied. The patient can then be discharged.
▪ No weight bearing should be undertaken with the lower extremity for 3 weeks.
▪ The casts are removed after 3 to 4 weeks; weight bearing, hand therapy, and range-of-motion exercises commence at this time.

OUTCOMES

▪ Outcomes after toe transfer for congenital absence of the thumb are very good.
   ▫ Patients with amniotic constriction bands and a stable CMC joint with solid metacarpal base tend to have the best outcomes because the proximal structures are normal and present.

- Those with congenital absence do not have as good outcomes because structures may be abnormal or absent proximally.
- In large series of toe transfers,[1,5–8] most investigators have found that mobility and sensation are satisfactory and function and appearance show significant improvement.
  - The toe does grow, though not to the same extent as a normal thumb.
  - Most parents and patients are very satisfied with function and appearance.

COMPLICATIONS

- Vascular compromise can be due to arterial or venous problems. In most series, about 5% to 10% of patients require take-back for vascular compromise, but most of these toes are salvaged with prompt return to the operating room.
  - The main steps to minimize vascular compromise are in the setup prior to performing the anastomoses.
  - These include atraumatic dissection, appropriate pedicle length, avoiding vein grafts (if possible), and minimizing sharp turns, kinks, and external pressure from tightly closed wounds.
- Wound complications can occur, especially on the foot. Meticulous technique in harvesting, tension-free skin closure, and adequate postoperative immobilization can minimize these issues.

- Long-term functional problems can include poor growth, flexor/extensor imbalance, inappropriate length, problematic positioning, and poor sensory or motor return. Tendon transfers, osteotomies, and other operations can alleviate some of these problems, but they can be challenging to perform.

REFERENCES

1. Jones NF, Kaplan J. Indications for microsurgical reconstruction of congenital hand anomalies by toe-to-hand transfers. *Hand.* 2013;8:367-374.
2. Jones NF, Hansen SL, Bates SJ. Toe-to-hand transfers for congenital anomalies of the hand. *Hand Clin.* 2007;23:129-136.
3. Upton J. Direct visualization of arterial anatomy during toe harvest dissections: clinical and radiological correlations. *Plast Reconstr Surg.* 1998;102:1988-1992.
4. Jones NF, Gupta R. Postoperative monitoring of pediatric toe-to-hand transfers with differential pulse oximetry. *J Hand Surg [Am].* 2001;26:525-529.
5. Foucher G, Medina J, Navarro R, Nagel D. Toe transfer in congenital hand malformations. *J Reconstr Microsurg.* 2001;17:1-7.
6. Kay S, McGuiness C. Microsurgical reconstruction in abnormalities of children's hands. *Hand Clin.* 1999;15:563-583.
7. Kay SP, Wiberg M, Bellew M, Webb F. Toe to hand transfer in children. Part 2: functional and psychological aspects. *J Hand Surg Br.* 1996;21:735-745.
8. Upton J, Guo L. Pediatric free tissue transfer: a 29-year experience with 433 transfers. *Plast Reconstr Surg.* 2008;121:1725-1737.

Reconstruction of Amniotic Constriction Bands

Amir H. Taghinia

DEFINITION

- Amniotic constriction band (ACB) refers to the clinical manifestation of an unknown insult that results in predictable phenotypic patterns including bands around limbs and digits, oligodactyly, acrosyndactyly, lymphedema, and other conditions.
- The etiology, terminology, and nosology of this condition have been debated in the literature for years, resulting in no less than 34 different names for this condition.[1] As some others do,[1,2] the author prefers *amniotic constriction band*, as this terminology conveys the most accurate description and most widely accepted etiology.

ANATOMY

- Extremity anatomy can be quite variable, and in fact, no two cases are the same.
  - The bands may be circumferential (rings) or incomplete, and the anatomic presentation may include amputation, hypoplasia, nail deformities, joint deviations, stiffness, and coalescence of the digits termed *acrosyndactyly*.
  - Usually, the anatomy proximal to the constriction band is normal.
- Patterson[3] classified the extremity findings:
  - Type 1—mild digital groove with normal distal extremity
  - Type 2—deeper ring with distal deformity, including atrophy or lymphedema
  - Type 3—syndactyly with fusion of the distal parts, termed acrosyndactyly or fenestrated syndactyly
  - Type 4—amputation distal to the constriction band
- Syndactyly in this condition is different from developmental syndactyly, which is caused by failure of apoptosis and is always present proximally. In typical syndactyly, the involvement proceeds proximal to distal and the digits are normal length, whereas the opposite is true in ACB.
- Constriction bands can affect underlying muscles, tendons, nerves, and vessels.
  - Urgent release is indicated in cases of ischemia or severe (or worsening) lymphedema.

PATHOGENESIS

- The cause of this condition is unknown, and potential etiologies are still debated. Three main theories have been proposed[2]:
  - The intrinsic theory implicates a germline developmental abnormality. It helps to explain the craniofacial, body wall, and internal organ anomalies seen but fails to sufficiently explain the patterns of limb findings.
  - The vascular theory advocates that a traumatic insult may disrupt development by disrupting blood flow, with the timing during gestation determining the anomaly.
  - The extrinsic theory best explains the limb manifestations. It maintains that a rupture of the amniotic sac creates mesodermal bands of tissue that entangle limbs and cause the characteristic findings.

NATURAL HISTORY

- ACB occurs in 1200 to 15 000 live births.
- It is more common in females and is likely to occur more frequently in African Americans as compared to Caucasians.
- It is not considered a familial condition.

PATIENT HISTORY AND PHYSICAL FINDINGS

- Newborns who need relatively urgent care can present with either progressive limb ischemia or lymphedema due to a tight band. Ischemia is a surgical emergency, and the band should be treated quickly to avoid limb loss. Worsening lymphedema should also be treated quickly because it can go on to cause ischemia if treatment is delayed.
- Infants who present electively should be evaluated for limb involvement. Digits and limbs involved, depth, presence of syndactyly, stiffness, joint deviation, and distal manifestations should be documented (**FIG 1**).
- Other potentially associated conditions should also be noted, especially those that impact the general health of the child and may influence anesthetic safety.

IMAGING

- Plain radiographs are the study of choice, though they are not needed in mild cases where the distal limb is normal (**FIG 2**).
  - For complex syndactyly cases, plain radiographs with multiple views are critical for surgical planning of separation.
- Other imaging modalities may be needed if nerve, vessel, tendon, or muscle compression is suspected.

DIFFERENTIAL DIAGNOSIS

- Differential diagnosis includes symbrachydactyly, cleft hand, and transverse deficiency.
- Another condition that can mimic ACB is ectrodactyly, ectodermal dysplasia, and cleft lip and palate (ECC) syndrome.

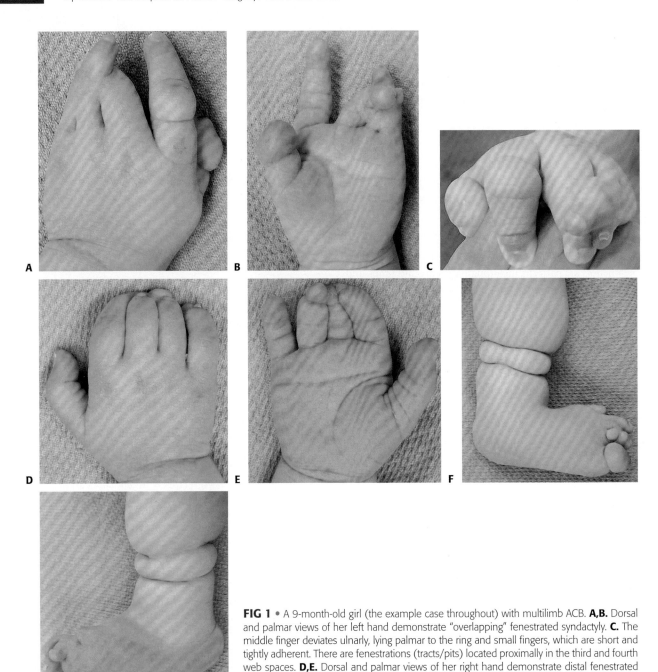

FIG 1 • A 9-month-old girl (the example case throughout) with multilimb ACB. **A,B.** Dorsal and palmar views of her left hand demonstrate "overlapping" fenestrated syndactyly. **C.** The middle finger deviates ulnarly, lying palmar to the ring and small fingers, which are short and tightly adherent. There are fenestrations (tracts/pits) located proximally in the third and fourth web spaces. **D,E.** Dorsal and palmar views of her right hand demonstrate distal fenestrated syndactyly. **F,G.** Medial and lateral views of her left lower extremity show significant involvement. The leg has two adjacent deep bands, and there are multiple bands around the toes.

NONOPERATIVE MANAGEMENT

- Minor bands may not need operative intervention. This determination is subjective and based on the experience of the surgeon.
  - As the infant grows and becomes more ambulatory, the subcutaneous fat that accentuates the band gets absorbed and most minor bands improve significantly in appearance.

SURGICAL MANAGEMENT

- Urgent intervention is needed in cases of vascular compromise or worsening lymphedema soon after birth. For other cases, usual time of surgery is around late infancy or early childhood. In treating bands, the surgeon should take advantage of extra subcutaneous tissue and elastic skin in the young child.
- The treatment of this condition includes repair of the band and the fenestrated syndactyly. The main goals of treatment are to improve appearance and function.
- Multiple approaches have been advocated for repair of the band. These include a variety of rearrangement schemes of skin and subcutaneous tissue. Many of these options are effective at releasing the band.
- The author advocates the adipofascial advancement technique first proposed by Upton.[4] The band is excised and skin flaps are elevated; extra fat is removed, and adipofascial flaps are elevated and closed as a separate, distinct layer underneath the skin.

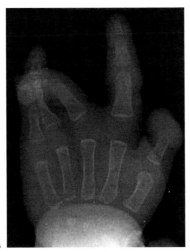 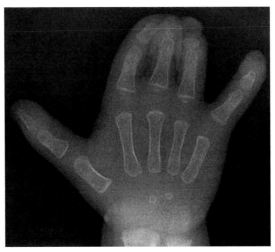

FIG 2 • Plain film radiographs of the example case demonstrate ulnar deviation of the middle finger of the left hand **(A)** and foreshortened digits on the right hand **(B)**.

■ Similar to others,[5] the author prefers to avoid Z-plasties, especially in narrow bands where excellent contour can be obtained with flap advancement and linear closure. In cases where the band is wide and adequate contour cannot be obtained (see Technique section), Z-plasties can be placed on the lateral and medial aspects of the limb/digit.[4]

■ In most cases, it is safe to repair circumferential bands in one stage, especially if the band is not too deep.

  ▪ In general, however, the deeper and more distal the band, the less safe it is to perform a circumferential repair. Circumferentially releasing deep bands in the digits may predispose to venous insufficiency as dermal drainage may become impaired.

  ▪ Another indication to perform staged repair is when two bands are in close proximity.

■ In most cases of fenestrated syndactyly, there are no flexion or extension creases in the area of the syndactyly. As such, there is little need to do zigzag incisions.

  ▪ The author releases most cases using straight-line incisions and covers the wounds with full-thickness skin grafts.

■ If bands are released at the same operation, one can consider using discarded skin from the bands for skin grafting. However, this skin tends to be somewhat thicker, and it does not take as well as thinner grafts from the lower abdomen.

Preoperative Planning

■ Review radiographs again.

■ In cases of deep bands that seem fixed to the underlying bone, one should consider assessing distal blood flow with a Doppler probe. An Allen test is important in cases of deep distal forearm bands.

Positioning

■ The patient is positioned supine with the arm out on a small hand table.

■ The lower abdominal area is squared-off with Steri-Drapes for skin grafts, if needed for treating fenestrated syndactyly.

■ Incisions are planned carefully before the tourniquet is applied.

■ Adipofascial Advancement

Markings and Flap Creation

■ The markings dictate where flaps will advance. Push the edges of the band together and mark the area of skin excision (**TECH FIG 1A**).

■ The operation is easier and results are better when there is ample subcutaneous tissue and when the band is narrow rather than wide (**TECH FIG 1B,C**).

■ Make the skin incisions and remove the intervening skin but leave all of the subcutaneous fat. Any tendon adhesions or nerve or vessel compression can be relieved at this point.

■ Elevate skin flaps proximally and distally.

■ Elevate adipofascial flaps in the areolar plane just above the extensor mechanism or fascial plane.

■ Excise and discard any excess fat.

Advancing Flaps and Creating Z-Plasties

■ Suture the adipofascial flaps together. Use a horizontal mattress technique so as to evert the edges and create additional tissue redundancy under the skin incision (**TECH FIG 2**).

■ Plan and create Z-plasties to gain additional circumference for the closure (**TECH FIG 3**).

  ▪ Plan these so the transverse limb falls in the midlateral aspect of the limb or digit.

Closure

■ Close the skin with everting horizontal mattress 6-0 chromic gut sutures for the digits (**TECH FIG 4A–D**).

■ More proximal limb bands are repaired using deep dermal and running intradermal absorbable sutures (4-0 and 5-0 Monocryl) (**TECH FIG 4E**).

■ Immobilize with a long extremity cast for 3 weeks.

T
E
C
H
N
I
Q
U
E
S

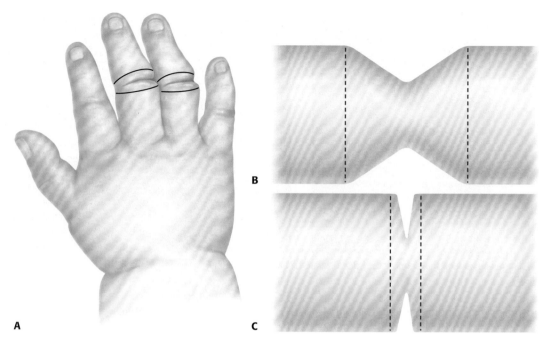

TECH FIG 1 • **A.** Incision planning for bands. The surgeon can push the edges together and draw one line where the edges meet. When the edges are allowed to retract, two lines result where the incisions should be made. **B,C.** Narrow vs wide bands. To achieve normal contour, wide bands **(B)** require a larger section of the band to be removed (*dashed lines*) as compared to narrow bands **(C)**.

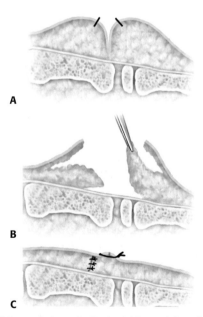

TECH FIG 2 • Technique of adipofascial flap and skin advancement for correction of bands. The band is excised **(A)** and separate skin and adipofascial flaps are raised **(B)**. Unnecessary fat is excised and the adipofascial flaps are advanced and closed. **C.** The skin is closed as a separate layer away from the adipofascial flap closure line.

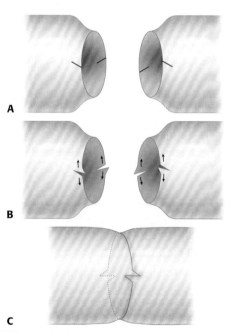

TECH FIG 3 • Theoretical basis of using Z-plasties for treatment of amniotic constriction bands. Z-plasties performed at the edge increase the circumference of the band. **A.** This is useful in wide bands where the entire band cannot be excised but unnecessary for narrow bands. Z-plasties are performed (only two are shown in **B**, but multiple can be performed), lengthening the circumference and allowing improved contour **(C)**.

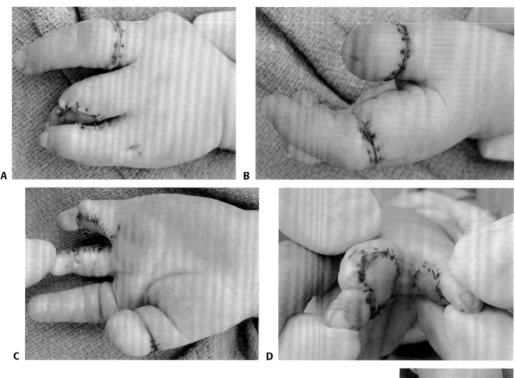

TECH FIG 4 • Immediate postoperative clinical images of the example case showing dorsal **(A)**, radial **(B)**, palmar **(C)**, and web space **(D)** views after correction of thumb and index finger constriction bands and release of third web space fenestrated syndactyly and coverage with full-thickness skin grafts. **E.** Anterior view after repair of medial leg band. These were two adjacent deep bands, and thus a staged approach was undertaken. The medial bands were treated in one stage by removing the intervening skin between the two bands. The lateral bands were treated in a second stage, preserving the intervening skin, because the band was wider on the lateral aspect.

■ Release of Fenestrated Syndactyly

- Release the fenestrated syndactyly using straight-line longitudinal incisions. In most cases, there are no functional joints in the area where the fingers are joined.
  - Accordingly, the surgeon should not worry about flexion contractures due to straight-line incisions.
- In cases where the syndactyly is distal, the resulting wounds can be closed or skin grafted (**TECH FIG 5**).
- In more proximal cases, the fenestration can be a narrow tract that communicates dorsal and palmar pits (see **FIG 1A,B**). Place a lacrimal probe into this tract.
- Release the syndactyly up to this tract. This degree of release is sufficient in most cases; however, if the tract is too distal, additional release can be performed with standard commissure flaps and full-thickness skin grafts.
- Apply skin grafts to the open wounds (see **TECH FIG 4C,D**).
- Apply a standard syndactyly release dressing with antibiotic-impregnated gauze, moist cotton, and gauze wrap.
- Immobilize with a well-padded long extremity cast.

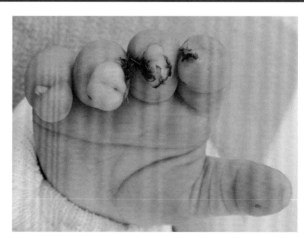

TECH FIG 5 • Postoperative image after release of fenestrated syndactyly of the right hand. The wounds were small and could be closed primarily.

PEARLS AND PITFALLS

Surgical management	■ The older infant or younger toddler is an ideal candidate for repair because there is ample subcutaneous fat and highly elastic skin. ■ Mild, shallow bands can be treated conservatively and usually improve with observation as the child grows. ■ If releasing the band is done to improve appearance (as in most cases), by performing the operation, the surgeon and patient are choosing to trade one appearance for a better one. This issue should be kept in mind, as sacrifices in technique and approach may be necessary to maximize overall appearance. For example, it may be worthwhile to accept a small bit of contour depression to avoid multiple zigzag incisions in a conspicuous area.
Technique	■ In treating bands, the primary focus should be to improve contour. Overall appearance is much more influenced by contour than by scar. ■ Be meticulous about hemostasis as hematoma under advanced skin flaps can cause ischemia and tissue loss. ■ The proximal tract in fenestrated syndactyly may be located too distally—in these cases, plan a standard syndactyly release using commissure flaps and skin grafts. Make sure to excise the epithelial tract.

POSTOPERATIVE CARE

■ Remove the cast in 3 weeks.
■ Start range of motion exercises
■ In cases of syndactyly release, refer the patient to hand therapy for fabrication of splint and web space pressure conformer to be used at night for about 1 month.

OUTCOMES

■ Functional outcomes after treatment of this condition are fully dependent on the preoperative degree of involvement. Function is much more likely to be determined by the presence of any congenital amputations as compared to minor bands or syndactyly.

■ Because each patient is different, comparative functional outcomes are difficult to standardize.
■ Aesthetic outcomes are dependent on the preoperative status of the bands and the technical execution of the repair (**FIG 3**).
■ Unfavorable outcomes include contour depression, significant scarring, and contractures.

COMPLICATIONS

■ In repair of bands, complications include flap ischemia or distal limb ischemia. Flap ischemia occurs as a result of overzealous undermining, too much tension, or hematoma. Venous insufficiency can occur when deep circumferential digital bands are treated in one stage.

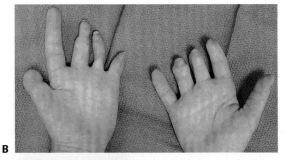
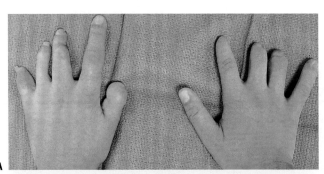
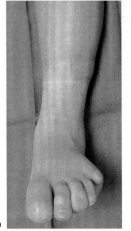
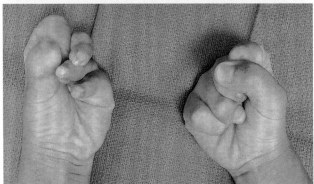

FIG 3 • Long-term postoperative photographs of the example case. **A,B.** Dorsal and palmar view of the hands. **C.** The digits of the left hand are short and stiff, as shown in the clenched fist view. **D.** The leg shows significant improvement in contour of the leg (note one medial scar and two lateral scar; see **TECH FIG 4E**) and toes after two-stage correction. The patient is fully ambulatory.

- Typical complications after syndactyly repair can be seen. These include flap ischemia, skin graft loss, and web creep. Careful planning and meticulous execution can avoid these complications.

REFERENCES

1. Rayan GM. Amniotic constriction band. *J Hand Surg [Am]*. 2002;27(6):1110-1111.

2. Goldfarb CA, Sathienkijkanchai A, Robin NH. Amniotic constriction band: a multidisciplinary assessment of etiology and clinical presentation. *J Bone Joint Surg Am*. 2009;91(suppl 4):68-75.

3. Patterson TJ. Congenital ring-constrictions. *Br J Plast Surg*. 1961;14:1-31.

4. Upton J, Tan C. Correction of constriction rings. *J Hand Surg [Am]*. 1991;16(5):947-953.

5. Habenicht R, Hülsemann W, Lohmeyer JA, Mann M. Ten-year experience with one-step correction of constriction rings by complete circular resection and linear circumferential skin closure. *J Plast Reconstr Aesthet Surg*. 2013;66(8):1117-1122.

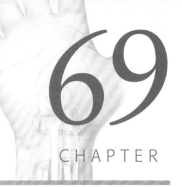

Centralization for Radial Longitudinal Deficiency

Amir H. Taghinia, Brian I. Labow, and Joseph Upton

DEFINITION

- Radial longitudinal deficiency (RLD) is a congenital condition characterized by hypoplasia of the radial side of the hand, wrist, and forearm. The bony, articular, and soft tissue structures can be affected in various degrees.
- RLD encompasses a spectrum of conditions ranging from minimally affected radius and normal hand to complete absence of radius and thumb. In some instances, other digits on the affected limb can also be involved—most significantly the index finger, which can be hypoplastic.
  - The degree of severity lessens with progression from the radial to ulnar side of the hand.

ANATOMY

- The radius can be mildly foreshortened, significantly hypoplastic, or completely absent. In the most severe cases, the radius, radial carpal bones (scaphoid and trapezium), and thumb are absent. Elbow and (to a lesser extent) shoulder abnormalities can also be present.
- The most common manifestation is an absent radius or a small proximal remnant. In these cases, a tough fibrous anlage is present that connects the proximal radius to the carpal region and distal ulna (**FIG 1**).
- The ulna may be bowed, and its distal end is widened.
- The absence or hypoplasia of the radial structures is accompanied by radial deviation and radial-palmar displacement of the wrist. This positioning weakens flexion power of digits and wrist.
- When the thumb is severely affected, the index finger is usually stiff and hypoplastic. This is clear on physical examination as the finger is usually thinner, slightly flexed with poorly developed flexion and extension creases.
- The ulnar digits and ulnar muscles tend to be normal, so children manipulate objects with their ulnar digits.
- The flexor carpi radialis and extensor carpi radialis brevis and longus may not be distinctly present. They are usually joined together to form a single set of muscles dubbed "dorsoradial muscle mass." These radial extensors of the wrist may be poorly developed or nonfunctional. In contrast, the ulnar-sided flexors and extensors are usually present and functional (see **FIG 1**).
- The radial nerve usually ends proximally around the elbow. The median nerve is radially and dorsally displaced, lying superficially on the radial aspect of the wrist.
  - During surgical exposure, the median nerve is superficial over the radial incision and is often mistaken for a tendon. One must recognize and protect this cordlike structure, the median nerve, during surgery. In addition to providing sensation to the radial palm, this nerve also supplies

sensation to the usual areas of radial nerve distribution. For this reason, it is often dubbed the "radian" nerve.
  - The radial artery is absent or hypoplastic, but a median artery is present instead.
- RLD is classified based on the degree of involvement. The original Bayne and Klug classification remains widely accepted (**FIG 2**), though a few modifications have been introduced. Types III and IV are the most common.
  - Type I—Minimal radial shortening of 2 mm as compared to ulna. The elbow is normal and the thumb is present, though possibly hypoplastic.
  - Type II—Radius is hypoplastic ("radius in miniature"), wrist is deviated, ulna is bowed, and thumb and radial carpal bones are absent.
  - Type III—The radius is partially absent, usually the distal two-thirds. The thumb and radial carpus are severely affected. A fibrous anlage is associated with flexion and pronation of the wrist.
  - Type IV—The radius is absent and the wrist is severely deviated—sometimes beyond 90 degrees. The thumb is usually absent. Often a small remnant of proximal radius will ossify during the adolescent growth spurt.

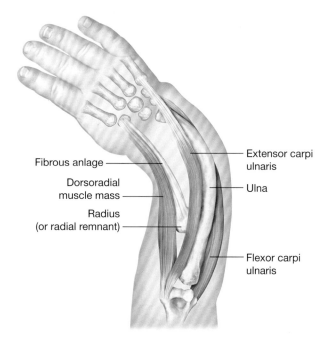

FIG 1 • Wrist and forearm anatomy in radial longitudinal deficiency (type III is shown). The fibrous anlage, a remnant of the radius, tethers the wrist radially. The radial wrist extensors and flexors fuse into a "dorsoradial muscle mass." The radial carpal bones are absent as is the thumb.

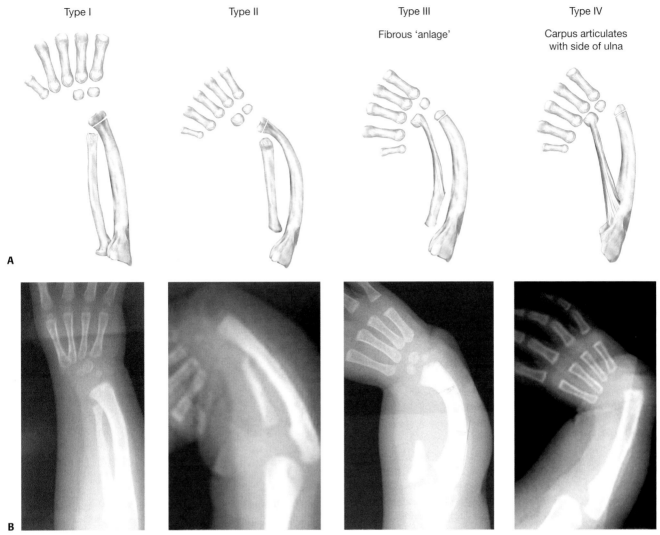

FIG 2 • Bayne and Klug classification of RLD. **A.** Radial deviation and palmar subluxation are worse with increasing hypoplasia of the radius. **B.** Representative radiographs of RLD types I to IV.

- Modifications to the original classification system includes introduction of three additional types:
  - Type N—Thumb hypoplasia with normal radius
  - Type 0—Absent or hypoplastic carpal bones with normal radius
  - Type V—Humeral abnormalities

PATHOGENESIS

- RLD occurs in 1 in 30 000 to 1 in 100 000 live births. Bilateral and unilateral cases occur in equal frequency.
- The cause of RLD is unknown. Environmental and genetic factors are likely responsible for developmental anomalies in the apical ectodermal ridge (AER) between the 4th and 7th weeks of gestation. Animal models with radial deficiencies can be created by ablation of the radial section of the AER.
- RLD is considered to be a malformation, based on the Oberg, Manske, and Tonkin classification of 2010.[1]

NATURAL HISTORY

- If untreated, radial deviation usually worsens and the wrist develops stiffness.

- Radial deviation usually recurs to some extent even after surgical correction unless the ulnocarpal joint has been fused.
- Although the forearm does grow, it usually grows slower than the normal forearm and ends up about 60% of normal length.

PATIENT HISTORY AND PHYSICAL FINDINGS

- The infant's shoulder, elbow, and wrist should be examined.
- The degree of wrist deviation and the capacity for passive correction should be noted and recorded.
- The status of the thumb and the radial fingers should be noted, especially in terms of intrinsic muscle development, passive motion of the joints, flexion and extension creases, and the presence of contractures.
- RLD is frequently associated with other conditions (70%–90%) and the likelihood increases with severity.[2] Bilateral involvement increases the likelihood of associated conditions by over 30%.
  - Although a long list of possible conditions can occur with RLD, the most common are the VACTERL association, Holt-Oram syndrome, craniofacial microsomia, and Fanconi anemia.

IMAGING

- Plain radiographs delineate the degree of involvement and help with classification.
- The hand-forearm angle (HFA) and the hand-forearm position (HFP) should be measured on the anterioposterior radiograph (**FIG 3**).
  - HFA is the angle between the longitudinal axes of the long finger and the distal ulna.
  - HFP is the shortest distance between a line drawn through the longitudinal axis of the distal ulna and the proximal pole of the fifth metacarpal.
- These measures can be followed over time and growth to assess long-term success of surgical correction vs nonoperative treatment.

DIFFERENTIAL DIAGNOSIS

- Thrombocytopenia-absent radius (TAR) syndrome is a genotypically distinct entity, although the treatment is similar.
- Patients have hypomegakaryocytic thrombopenia with a completely absent radius. In contrast to RLD with absent radius (type IV), patients with TAR have thumbs.
- TAR is an autosomal-recessive condition linked to a defect in chromosome 1q21.1.
- Clinical findings include bruising, hemorrhage, and cardiac and renal anomalies.
- The thumb is biphalangeal and contains varying degrees of skeletal and thenar muscle hypoplasia.

NONOPERATIVE MANAGEMENT

- For most patients, nonoperative management with splinting and stretching is instituted early in infancy.
  - This type of treatment maybe a long-term solution for those with mild RLD (types 0, I, and II) or a short-term "bridge" solution in preparation for subsequent surgery (types III and IV).
- The family performs stretching about 8 to 10 times per day by applying longitudinal traction and ulnar deviation.
  - A form-fitting radial gutter splint is then used to keep the wrist in the corrected position.

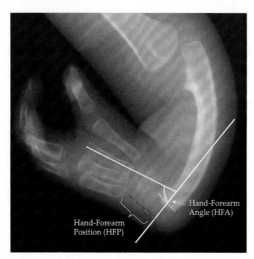

FIG 3 • Measuring hand-forearm angle (HFA) and hand-forearm position (HFP) on the plain radiograph.

- Early on, as the family strives for a neutral wrist, the splint will need to be worn at all times and will need frequent revisions. Once the wrist is passively correctable to neutral, the splint can be weaned to night use only.
- Splinting is also a critical postoperative adjunct to keep the wrist in neutral; as the natural history of this condition is progressive radial deviation of the wrist with growth.
- Treatment may not be indicated at all in the following:
  - Adults who have adapted well
  - Patients who cannot tolerate stretching and splinting (eg, develop hygiene problems such as rash)
  - Patients in whom operative treatment poses unnecessary medical risk
  - Patients whose function will worsen with a straight wrist (eg, patients with stiff elbows who may be unable to wipe or feed themselves with the hand).

SURGICAL MANAGEMENT

- Types 0, I, and II RLD are usually treated with stretching and splinting. In rare instances where these measures are ineffective, surgical management can include tendon transfers and/or distraction lengthening.
- Types III and IV RLD can be treated with stretching and splinting first, as a "bridge" intervention, to bring the wrist into neutral prior to formal repair. However, this intervention alone is usually not sufficient to allow the carpus to translate beyond the distal ulna.
- In most cases, preoperative soft tissue distraction is necessary to achieve satisfactory positioning.[2] This procedure involves application of a (usually) uniplanar distractor without an osteotomy. Once slow distraction (1 mm/d) moves the carpus beyond the distal ulna, formal centralization or radialization can be performed (**FIG 4**).
- In early reports, centralization involved resection of the distal ulna, but this led to early growth arrest. Thereafter, carpal resection was introduced (carving a notch in the carpus to accommodate the distal ulna), which helped with alignment and avoided growth arrest, but led to stiffness and recurrence.
- To remedy these issues, Buck-Gramcko introduced radialization, which involves:
  - Stabilization of the radial carpal column onto the distal ulna without carpal resection.
  - Transfer of the dorsoradial muscle mass ulnarly to counteract the deforming forces and provide long-lasting correction.
- There is debate about what constitutes centralization vs radialization.
  - Traditionally, centralization involves carving of a carpal notch for insertion of the ulnar head and alignment of the base of the third metacarpal with the central carpus and the distal ulna (**FIG 5A**).
  - In contrast, radialization involves alignment of the second metacarpal with the radial carpus without carpal resection (**FIG 5B**).
- There continues to be disagreement about which of these options is best. Some argue that stabilization of the wrist (radialization) without a carpal notch does not provide a stable equilibrium, whereas others prefer to preserve motion and avoid shortening.
- Nevertheless, most surgeons agree that for the operation to be effective:
  - The fibrous anlage and dense soft tissues should be released or excised.

Normal

Centralized or
Radialized

Stretched or
Distracted

Preoperative
Type IV

FIG 4 • The process of soft tissue distraction is demonstrated. The deficient forearm reaches about 60% of the length of a normal one.

- The dorsoradial muscle mass should be transferred to the ulnar wrist.
- Alignment should be maintained with a pin that is kept in for several months, if not longer.
- Microvascular free toe joint transfer involves transfer of vascularized osseous structural support to stabilize the radial column of the wrist. Soft tissue distraction is usually necessary to align the wrist and create a "space" into which the toe will be placed. The metatarsal and proximal phalanx of the second toe are transferred with their growth centers and attached to the distal ulna.
  - Although technically demanding, the operation provides the advantage of avoiding injury to the distal ulnar physis and preservation of wrist motion.
- The time to perform corrective surgery is about 1 year of age, barring small patient size and/or associated comorbidities.

Preoperative Planning

- Review risks, benefits, and expectations with parents on the day of surgery. Specifically outline the risks of possible wrist stiffness, poor growth, and persistent or recurrent deviation.
  - The long-term outcomes and natural history of this condition should be discussed well before the operative date.
- Fluoroscopy, drills, and pins will be required for the procedure.

Positioning and Approach

- The patient is positioned supine with the arm out on a small hand table.
- Incisions are planned carefully prior to use of the tourniquet.
- A transverse dorsoulnar approach is usually undertaken. There is usually no need to extend incisions along the entire dorsal forearm.

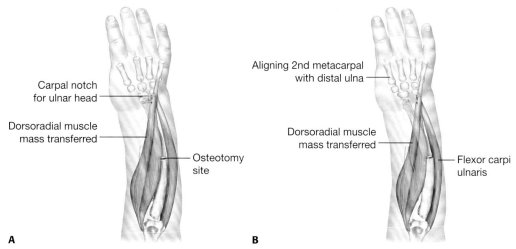

Carpal notch
for ulnar head

Dorsoradial muscle
mass transferred

Osteotomy
site

Aligning 2nd metacarpal
with distal ulna

Dorsoradial muscle
mass transferred

Flexor carpi
ulnaris

A   **B**

FIG 5 • Centralization vs radialization. **A.** For centralization, a transverse distal wrist incision is made, the "radian" nerve identified, and the tight radial fibrous anlage released. All tethering soft tissues must be release. A small notch is carved into the carpus to allow introduction of the ulnar head. The wrist is reduced and stabilized with a pin aligning the third metacarpal with the ulnar head. The ECU is advanced. The dorsoradial muscle mass is transferred to the ulnar wrist extensors. A corrective osteotomy of the ulna may be necessary if the bowing is significant. Excess skin on the ulnar side of the wrist is excised. **B.** In radialization, the maneuvers are similar to those for centralization except that the carpal bones are not excised. Instead, the carpus is stabilized over the distal ulna and held there with a pin. The hand is more ulnarly deviated to provide a better moment arm for the musculature to keep the wrist in the proper posture. The pin aligns the second metacarpal with the distal ulna.

■ Preoperative Soft Tissue Distraction

- Consult manufacturer instructions for application of distractor of choice.
  - The authors prefer a uniplanar distractor as it is easy to apply and manage and effective at achieving the desired result.
- If the wrist is not passively correctable to 50 to 60 degrees of radial deviation (**TECH FIG 1A,B**), a concomitant releasing procedure may be necessary to obtain adequate alignment for placement of the distractor.
  - In this case, plan a transverse incision dorsally on the ulnocarpal joint for exposure of the radial fibrous anlage and tethered soft tissues.
- Plan small longitudinal incisions over the third metacarpal and the proximal ulna. Plan the length of these incisions based on the length of the distractor clamp that will house the pins. Assemble the apparatus and obtain all needed parts before the tourniquet is inflated.
- Exsanguinate the upper extremity.

- If performing a release, make the dorsal wrist incision and expose the fibrous anlage from the dorsal approach (**TECH FIG 1C**).
  - Take care to avoid injury to the "radian" nerve and the extensor tendons.
  - Release the tough radial soft tissues (**TECH FIG 1D**).
- Incise over the third metacarpal and the proximal ulna. Spread the soft tissues; retract and protect any longitudinally running vital structures (tendon, muscle) until down to bone.
- Insert one pin into the metacarpal and another into the ulna.
- Arrange the distractor clamps onto the pins and tighten slightly. Apply the lengthening bar while manually distracting the wrist; secure the clamps onto the bar.
- Insert another pin into the metacarpal and one more into the ulna, each into the second seat of the respective distractor clamp.
- Loosen the clamps from the bar. Distract the soft tissues as much as possible and secure the clamps back onto the bar tightly.

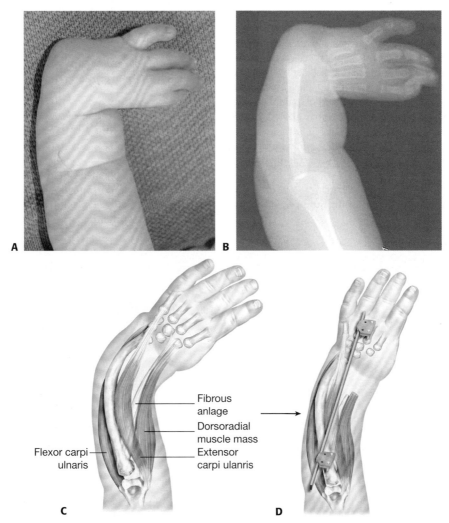

TECH FIG 1 • Preoperative clinical **(A)** and radiographic **(B)** images of 6-month-old girl with type IV RLD. **C.** If the wrist is tight and significantly radially deviated, the fibrous anlage and tough tethering tissues should be released prior to placing the distractor. **D.** Releasing these structures allows proper alignment of the distractor and makes the process of distraction smoother.

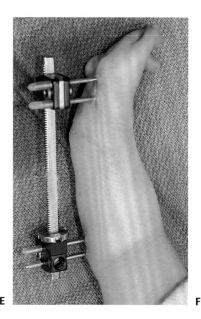
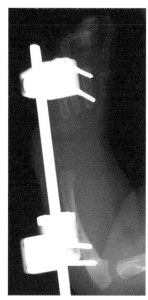

TECH FIG 1 (Continued) • **E,F.** After soft tissue distraction and immediately prior to centralization, the deviation and subluxation of the wrist has been corrected.

- Close all the wounds and apply a soft dressing.
- The family can start distraction at 1 mm/d in about 3 to 4 days.
  - Instruct the family on how to perform pin-site care to avoid infection. Provide written instructions and a timetable or turning the screw, and mark the distance between the pins so they can see the progress (and avoid turning the wrong way).

- It helps if they send weekly pictures via e-mail so the surgeon can monitor the progress.
- Once the carpus has translated beyond the distal ulna, leave the distractor on without distracting for another several weeks.
  - At that point, the patient will be ready for formal centralization or radialization (**TECH FIG 1E,F**).

■ Centralization or Radialization

- If preoperative distraction has been performed, the distractor can be removed at the time of the centralization or radialization procedure.
- A transverse dorsoulnar incision is planned over the ulnocarpal joint. Extra skin should be reserved until the end where the exact amount can be carefully assessed prior to removal.
- The authors do not routinely employ local Z-plasty or transposition flaps. The use of preoperative soft tissue distraction has virtually eliminated any problems with skin deficiency.
- Exsanguinate the extremity.
- Incise the skin; identify and protect any veins that can be saved. Identify the fibrous anlage, the radian nerve, the dorsoradial muscle mass, the extensor tendons to the digits, and the extensor carpi ulnaris tendon.
- The radian nerve is usually radiodorsally translated and located just under the skin on the radial aspect of the wrist (**TECH FIG 2A–C**).
- Release the fibrous anlage and the dorsoradial muscle mass. Release any other tight investing fascia.
- Release the extensor carpi ulnaris from its attachment on the fifth digit metacarpal. This tendon will be advanced to provide more ulnar pull.
- Incise the wrist capsule transversely.

- If performing traditional centralization, carve a small notch into the carpus to accommodate the distal ulna. Otherwise, no carpal resection is needed.
  - Align the third metacarpal (centralization; see **FIG 5A**) or second metacarpal (radialization; see **FIG 5B**) with the distal ulna.
  - A 0.062-in. Kirschner wire can now be passed anterograde through the wrist entering the base of the chosen metacarpal. The authors prefer to insert the pin obliquely to avoid the metacarpophalangeal joint. Thus, the pin would come out of either the first (if second metacarpal) or second (if third metacarpal) web space.
- Insert the distal ulna into the carpal slot (centralization) or stabilize the carpus over the distal ulna (radialization). Drive the K-wire down the ulna in retrograde fashion.
- If necessary, perform an opening wedge ulnar osteotomy to correct any bowing of the ulna and drive the pin further proximally to secure this osteotomy.
- Close the wrist capsule securely.
- Advance the extensor carpi ulnaris and reattach to the base of the fifth digit metacarpal. Transfer the dorsoradial muscle mass to the extensor carpi ulnaris tendon to provide additional ulnar moment arm to the wrist.
- Excise any redundant skin and close using absorbable sutures. Apply antibiotic-impregnated gauze to all incisions and cover with sterile gauze. Wrap loosely.
- Apply a long-arm cast.

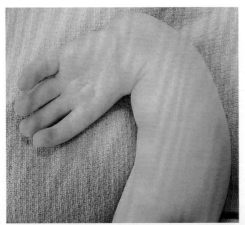

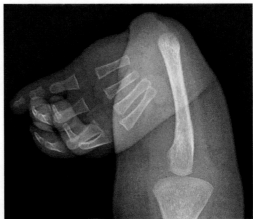

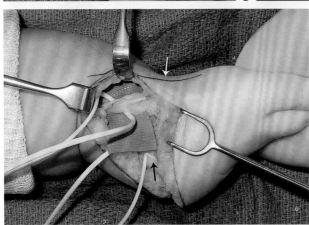

TECH FIG 2 • Preoperative clinical **(A)** and radiographic **(B)** images of an 8-month-old boy with type IV RLD showing significant deviation. His family declined preoperative soft tissue distraction but did perform stretching and splinting such that the wrist could be passively corrected to 20 degrees of radial deviation. The "radian" nerve is the most superficial structure on the radial side of the wrist. **C.** It is demonstrated here under the green background. A smaller dorsal sensory branch (sensory radial nerve equivalent) is looped and visible dorsally (*black arrow*). The expected path of the nerve was marked on the skin preoperatively (*white arrow*).

PEARLS AND PITFALLS

Technique	▪ The pins may be left in for a long time; in fact, some surgeons leave the pins in for a year or longer. Although this may increase stability, it decreases range of motion and can result in physeal injury and hardware failure. ▪ The "radian" nerve is the most superficial structure on the radial side of the wrist; the surgeon should be cautious to avoid injury while dissecting in this area.
Postoperative	▪ Cast immobilization time should be limited, only to allow the soft tissues to heal. These children have short forearms and can easily escape from their casts.
Therapy	▪ It is critical to instruct the parents to move the fingers passively during preoperative soft tissue distraction. This action prevents stiffness and contractures.

POSTOPERATIVE CARE

▪ Remove the cast after 2 or 3 weeks and apply a thermoplast splint. Range-of-motion exercises of the digits can be started at this time.
▪ Leave the pin in for 8 to 10 weeks.

OUTCOMES

▪ Long-term outcomes for the two cases depicted are shown in **FIG 6**.
▪ The main unfavorable outcome seen after centralization or radialization is recurrence of the deviation. The recurrence appears to be related to the preoperative degree of deviation and amount of correction achieved postoperatively.[2]

▪ Rigorous compliance with night splinting may decrease the risk of recurrence (**FIG 7**).
▪ Despite the leveling and realignment of skeletal support from the remaining carpus and hand, the muscular imbalance across the wrist remains the primary cause for recurrent deviation.
▪ Despite the risk of recurrence, Kotwal et al.[3] showed that surgical treatment of RLD is sensible. He compared patients who had undergone surgery to those who had not, showing that surgical treatment of RLD improves appearance and function, and leads to better performance in daily activities.
▪ Although the focal point of treatment is correction of the radial deviation, the importance of this concern has been

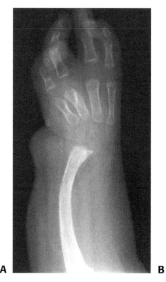 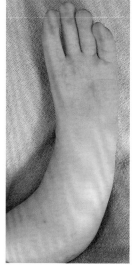 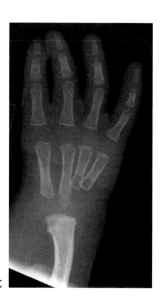

FIG 6 • A. The case in TECH FIG 1 year after radialization. **B,C.** Long-term post-operative images after centralization for the case in TECH FIG 2. A carpal notch was required to adequately reduce the wrist.

questioned. Recent studies have shown that wrist and digit range of motion as well as grip strength and forearm length may be better than wrist angulation in predicting functional outcomes in RLD.[4]

- Hence, it may be worthwhile to avoid carpal resection, thereby sacrificing some loss in position of the wrist in favor of better motion.

COMPLICATIONS

- Infections during soft tissue distraction are frequent and range from minor pin-tract infections to cellulitis and, rarely, deep bone infection. These problems are avoided with good pin-site care and close follow-up.
- Other complications with the distraction include inadequate distraction by the parents, device malfunction or

malalignment requiring repair, and stiffness and/or contracture of the digits. These problems can be avoided with good parent education and support as well as passive range-of-motion exercises.

- Complications of centralization or radialization include wound infections and hardware problems. Because the pin has to be in place for many weeks, it may migrate, dislodge, or break.
- One of the most concerning complications is early growth arrest of the distal ulna, since it will cause additional shortening of an already short forearm.
  - This issue can be avoided by earlier removal of the pin and minimal manipulation of the distal ulna during the corrective operation.
  - Physeal damage may also occur with rapid, aggressive distraction in young children.

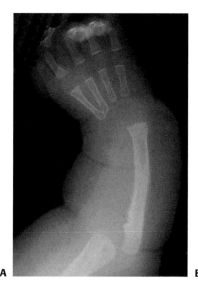 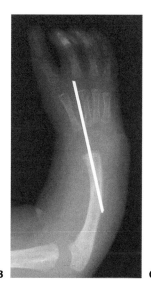 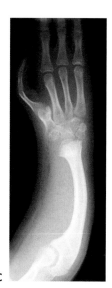

FIG 7 • Long-term result after centralization. **A.** Initial radiograph showing type IV RLD. After centralization and 12 weeks of pin fixation **(B)** and 14 years later **(C)**. At long-term follow-up, the wrist maintained adequate alignment. This child was compliant with nightly splint use. Note the index finger has been pollicized.

REFERENCES

1. Oberg KC, Feenstra JM, Manske PR, Tonkin MA. Developmental biology and classification of congenital anomalies of the hand and upper extremity. *J Hand Surg [Am]*. 2010;35(12):2066-2076.
2. Taghinia AH, Al-Sheikh AA, Upton J. Preoperative soft-tissue distraction for radial longitudinal deficiency: an analysis of indications and outcomes. *Plast Reconstr Surg*. 2007;120(5):1305-1312.
3. Kotwal PP, Varshney MK, Soral A. Comparison of surgical treatment and nonoperative management for radial longitudinal deficiency. *J Hand Surg Eur Vol*. 2012;37(2):161-169.
4. Ekblom AG, Dahlin LB, Rosberg H-E, et al. Hand function in adults with radial longitudinal deficiency. *J Bone Joint Surg Am*. 2014;96(14):1178-1184.

Excision of Vascular Malformation of the Hand

Amir H. Taghinia

70

CHAPTER

DEFINITION

- Vascular anomalies fall into two main categories: tumors and malformations. Tumors, such as hemangiomas, exhibit cellular hyperplasia. In contrast, malformations represent a localized defect in vascular morphogenesis.
- Vascular malformations can be broadly classified into slow-flow and fast-flow lesions.
  - Slow-flow lesions include capillary, lymphatic (LM), and venous (VM) malformations or mixed lesions.
  - Fast-flow lesions include arteriovenous malformations (AVM).

ANATOMY

- Vascular anomalies can occur anywhere in the hand and upper extremity, and can involve all components of soft tissue, bone, and joint. When present, they can alter or distort the normal anatomy.

PATHOGENESIS

- The exact etiology of vascular anomalies is the subject of intense scientific investigation.

- Somatic activating mutations in the phosphatidylinositol-3-kinase (PIK3CA)/mammalian target of rapamycin (mTOR) pathway appear to underlie a number of overgrowth phenotypes with vascular anomalies.[1]

NATURAL HISTORY

- Hemangiomas have a biphasic growth phase with proliferation early in life and subsequent involution.
- Malformations have a propensity to slowly expand throughout life.

PATIENT HISTORY AND PHYSICAL FINDINGS

- With a few exceptions, hemangiomas are usually absent at birth or present as a small stain.
  - Patients present with a growing, vascular, high-flow lesion in early infancy.
  - These lesions have a deep red appearance and strong Doppler signals throughout.
- Vascular malformations can present any time in life. Although they are likely present at birth, they may be clinically silent for years. They usually present with a combination of discoloration, disproportionate growth, swelling, and pain (**FIG 1**).

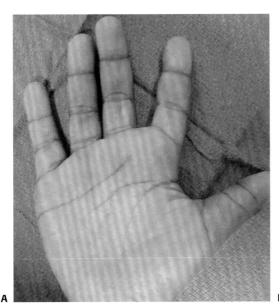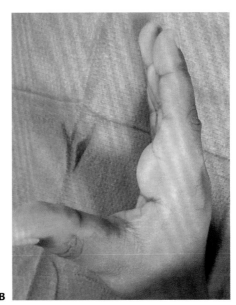

FIG 1 • A,B. AP and lateral views of a growing, painful mass on the palm of a 7-year-old boy (the example case throughout).

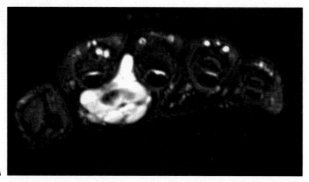
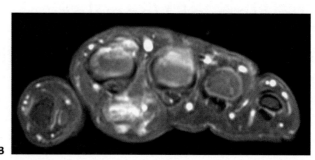

FIG 2 • T2-weighted **(A)** and T1-weighted postgadolinium **(B)** MRI images of the lesion.

- LMs may also develop drainage or infections, and AVMs can develop paradoxical ischemia and ulceration.
- Most vascular malformations can be correctly diagnosed by physical examination. A multidisciplinary approach to diagnosis and treatment gives the best outcomes.

IMAGING

- Ultrasonography is the best initial radiological examination for these lesions. It can be done in the clinic room during the first multidisciplinary visit. The type and extent of the lesion can be determined quickly and easily.
- For surgical planning purposes, however, more extensive imaging is usually required. An MRI is the best soft tissue imaging tool for these lesions (**FIG 2**). Angiography is helpful for high flow AVMs.

DIFFERENTIAL DIAGNOSIS

- The myriad of multiple overlapping conditions that include vascular malformations can be confusing. Although these lesions can be solitary, the presence of associated conditions is often the rule rather than the exception. For an extensive list of associated conditions, the reader is referred to other readings.[2]
- Differential diagnosis includes overgrowth conditions, malignancies, and a variety of other benign conditions. When in doubt, biopsy is recommended.

NONOPERATIVE MANAGEMENT

- Hemangiomas are often treated conservatively with no intervention or with medical therapy including steroids and beta-blockers. Surgery has a minimal role in the treatment of these lesions.
- Most malformations are amenable to interventional radiological treatments, which involve sclerotherapy and embolization. Certain lesions cannot be treated this way—notably, microcystic lymphatic malformations—and thus require surgery.
- In the hand and upper extremity, the authors advocate against sclerotherapy of lesions close to neurovascular structures unless surgical resection is deemed to be too morbid. Sclerotherapy around major upper extremity nerves can cause numbness, motor deficit, and chronic pain.

SURGICAL MANAGEMENT

- The indications for surgical intervention are pain, functional compromise (impending or extant), rapid or persistent growth, ischemia, and ulceration in lesions that are not suitable for treatment by interventional radiologists.
- A few key principles are outlined here[2]:
  - Plan extensively. Outline the extent of the resection and abide by it.
  - Place incisions thoughtfully. Often multiple debulking procedures may be necessary.
  - Use magnification.
  - Approach the lesion from known to unknown.
  - Avoid vascular compromise. When a critical arterial segment to an extremity is removed, it should be reconstructed.
  - Avoid intraneural dissection. Dissection within nerves often leaves neuromas-in-continuity with disruption of distal sensory or motor function.
  - Avoid partial dissections. Removal of an entire involved area is preferred as it avoids future challenging dissection in a scarred bed.
  - Replace abnormal or ischemic skin; use flaps or skin grafts.
  - Use drains liberally.
  - Amputate if needed. Ischemic, nonfunctional, painful, and parasitic digits or limbs should be removed.
  - Follow patients long term.
- The purpose of surgery should be clearly outlined. In large or complex cases, the goal of surgery is relief of pain and improvement of function. With the exception of small lesions, total eradication of most lesions is impossible. These lesions are not malignant, and so a wide excisional approach that sacrifices normal functioning structures is ill advised.

Preoperative Planning

- Again discuss risks, benefits, and expectations with parents and patient on the day of surgery.

Positioning and Approach

- The patient is positioned supine with the arm out on a hand table.
- Incisions are planned carefully prior to use of the tourniquet.
- In infants and toddlers, an Esmarch bandage is used as a tourniquet because it is more effective at providing a bloodless field in small arms. In older children, a standard pneumatic tourniquet is used.

Excision of Palmar Venous Malformation

- Mark a palmar incision that incorporates the thenar flexion crease (**TECH FIG 1A**).
  - Exposure will be needed beyond the area of malformation to fully expose all the vital neurovascular structures—away from the lesion.
  - Design the incision so that distal or proximal extension of the wounds will be possible.
- Raise skin flaps over the palmar fascia.
- Venous malformations tend to become much smaller when the limb is exsanguinated and the tourniquet is inflated.
- Incise the palmar fascia sharply and explore to find the nerves and vessels proximal to the lesion.
- Isolate the arteries and nerves with vessel loops (**TECH FIG 1B**). Dissect these structures off the venous malformation.
  - For lesions of the palm, it is easier to dissect the ulnar and radial aspects of the lesion first. This way, any vital longitudinal structures that traverse the lesion can be identified, protected, and dissected more easily.
- Use vessel loops not only for identification but also to place traction on vital structures so they can be dissected along their native paths.
- Venous malformations of the digits and distal palm will often arise from the venae comitantes of the digital arteries and thus run along the arteries. Isolate the venous malformation completely with the arteries that traverse it on either side (**TECH FIG 1C,D**).

- Avoid sacrificing arteries. Dissection of the venous malformation off the digital arteries is possible and should be attempted.
  - Perform the dissection with magnification using an operating microscope and micro instruments (**TECH FIG 1E**).
  - Use an ultrafine bipolar forceps (on a low setting) to cauterize all of the branches of the arteries that feed the venous malformation.
- Release the tourniquet and obtain hemostasis.
  - To avoid bleeding postoperatively, the best strategy is to remove all the venous malformation.
  - If subtotal excision is too difficult, the second best strategy is to prophylactically (ie, during the excision procedure) tie or clip the entire portion of the venous malformation that will be left behind.
  - The least favorable (though not always avoidable) strategy is to sharply remove some of the venous malformation and leave some behind with channels wide open. These will bleed a lot and are very hard to control with the tourniquet down. Bleeding should controlled with a combination of prolonged direct pressure, tissue sealants, and local clotting enhancers.
- Use drains liberally. The author prefers the TLS drain system for digital and palmar lesions. The suction tube can be changed once it is one-third full or every 4 hours.
- A soft gauze dressing is applied followed by a well-padded cast. The cast is bivalved if there is any concern about postoperative bleeding or swelling.

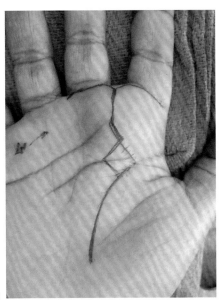 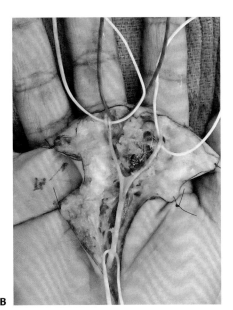

A   B

TECH FIG 1 • A. Incision markings. The proximal incision extends into the thenar flexion crease. This incision is made proximal to the lesion to identify the digital nerves and branches of the superficial palmar arch. A Y-type pattern at the distal extension in the web is versatile as this incision can be extended into the digits via midlateral or oblique incisions while keeping the flaps wide-based for optimal vascularity. **B.** The common digital nerve to the second web space and its branches have been mobilized (*yellow loops*). Proximal incision extension was made to find the superficial palmar arch, which was absent in this patient. The venous malformation is decompressed under tourniquet control.

TECHNIQUES

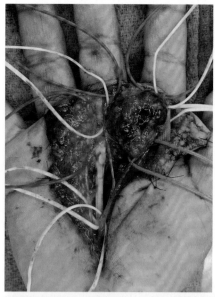

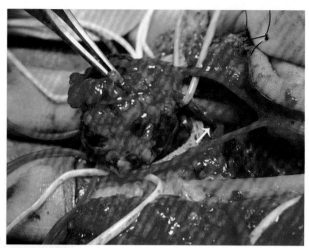

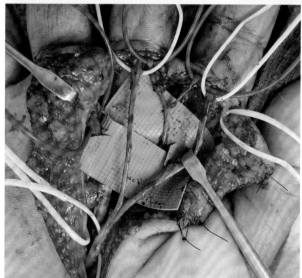

TECH FIG 1 (Continued) • **C.** The venous malformation has been completely mobilized—the green background sits underneath it. The ulnar digital artery to the index finger and the radial digital artery to the middle finger have been identified and looped. These vessels emerge from the malformation. The *blue loop* is around the common digital artery to the second web space. **D.** The common digital artery (*arrow*) can be seen emerging from (the deep arch) underneath the flexor tendon to the index finger and piercing the venous malformation. **E.** The venous malformation can be safely dissected away from the common and proper digital arteries using the operating microscope and microinstruments. The vessels are shown after the lesion has been removed.

PEARLS AND PITFALLS

Diagnosis	▪ A multidisciplinary approach is the best way to take care of these patients, especially in more complicated cases.
Nonoperative management	▪ Avoid sclerotherapy of palmar venous malformations.
Technique	▪ Keep meticulous hemostasis during the case. Once important structures become bloodstained, they can be much more difficult to identify and dissect.
Technique	▪ Use fine instruments, especially in children who have smaller vital structures in the hand than do adults.

POSTOPERATIVE CARE

- For VMs, the drain can be removed within 24 hours, once the threat of bleeding has faded. For LMs, the drain should be in until drainage has abated significantly. If the fluid collects in the wound, it can coalesce into firm scar and added bulk.
- Immobilize with a cast or a splint for 2 to 3 weeks.
- Discontinue immobilization and start hand therapy.

OUTCOMES

- Outcomes are variable and highly dependent on the initial degree of involvement. In patients with joint and or tendon/muscle contractures, surgery may result in limited improvement.
- For patients with painful VMs, removal usually results in significant improvement in symptoms.[3]

COMPLICATIONS

- The most common complications are bleeding and skin flap compromise.
  - Bleeding and hematoma can be avoided with meticulous hemostasis and liberal use of drains and hemostatic agents.

- Skin flap compromise may be caused by inherent disease (vascular steal) or attributed to poor planning and execution. Ischemic flaps should be debrided and replaced with healthy flaps or skin grafts.
- Recurrence and persistent growth are common problems, especially in extensive lesions.
- Distal ischemia is a dreaded complication, especially after treatment of AVMs when the arterial feeders have to be divided.
  - In these cases, it is wise to have a backup plan to bypass with vein grafts if needed.

REFERENCES

1. Kurek KC, Luks VL, Ayturk UM, et al. Somatic mosaic activating mutations in PIK3CA cause CLOVES syndrome. *Am J Hum Genet.* 2012;90(6):1108-1115.
2. Upton J, Taghinia A. Special considerations in vascular anomalies: operative management of upper extremity lesions. *Clin Plast Surg.* 2011;38(1):143-151.
3. Upton J, Coombs CJ, Mulliken JB, et al. Vascular malformations of the upper limb: a review of 270 patients. *J Hand Surg [Am].* 1999;24:1019-1035.

71

CHAPTER

Lumps and Bumps of the Hand and Wrist

Paymon Rahgozar and Kevin C. Chung

DEFINITION

- Ganglion cysts
  - Ganglion cysts are the most common soft tissue tumor of the hand.
  - Though not a true cyst because the lack of an epithelial lining, ganglion cysts are mucin-filled lesions with collagen-lined walls, usually attached to an underlying joint capsule, tendon, or tendon sheath.[1]
  - Ganglion cysts are a frequent cause of hand and wrist pain. Sixty to seventy percent of ganglion cysts appear in the dorsal wrist, whereas 18% to 20% of ganglions can be found in the volar wrist.[1]
- Mucous cysts
  - Mucous cysts are primarily found in the dorsal distal interphalangeal (DIP) joint and have been referred to as mucous cysts of the finger, mucoid cysts, mucinous pseudocyst, myxomatous cutaneous cyst, synovial cyst, periarticular fibroma, periungual ganglion, epidermal cyst, nail cyst, dorsal cyst, digital myxoid cyst, and cutaneous myxoid cyst.[2]
  - The lesions may be associated with osteoarthritis of the joint (degenerative mucous cyst).

- Giant cell tumors
  - Giant cell tumors are benign, slow-growing tumors of the tendon sheath, and have also been referred to as fibrous xanthoma, pigmented villonodular tenosynovitis, or localized nodular synovitis.
  - After ganglion cysts, giant cell tumors are the second most common tumor of the hand.

ANATOMY

- Ganglion cysts
  - Ganglion cysts consist of a solitary or multilobulated cyst sac filled with a clear jellylike mucinous fluid. They are composed of hyaluronic acid, glucosamine, albumin, and globulin.[1]
  - The lesion originates from an underlying joint or tendon sheath and maintains communication to the cyst sac via a tortuous stalk (**FIG 1**).
  - Dorsal ganglion cysts typically originate at the scapholunate ligament, whereas volar ganglion cysts often originate from the radiocarpal or scaphotrapeziotrapezoidal joint, flexor carpi radialis tendon, or A1 pulley.[3]
  - Volar wrist ganglions may be intertwined with branches of the radial artery, complicating surgical dissection.

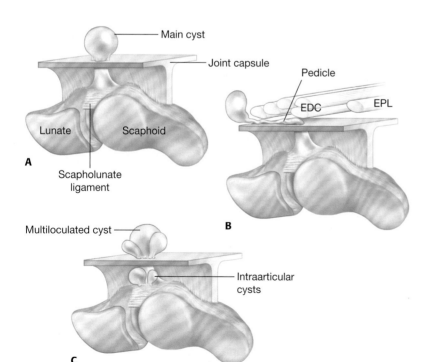

FIG 1 • A. Communication of a dorsal ganglion through the joint capsule to the underlying scapholunate ligament. **B.** In cases where the ganglion cyst is not directly overlying the scapholunate ligament, it is still connected via a long pedicle. **C.** A multicystic ganglion with intra-articular cysts.

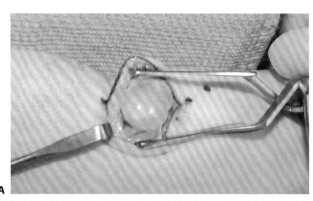 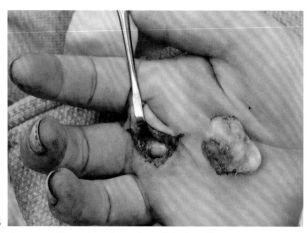

A **B**

FIG 2 • **A.** Volar ganglion cyst in situ. **B.** Giant cell tumor of the tendon sheath removed from the volar surface of the long finger.

- Grossly, the lesions are smooth, well circumscribed, white, and translucent (**FIG 2A**).
- Microscopically, the cysts have dense fibrous connective tissue without any true cellular lining. The outer surface is irregular and fibrillated, composed of disorganized collagen fibers.[4]
- Mucous cysts
  - Mucous cysts typically originate at the DIP joint with its stalk passing between the extensor insertion and the collateral ligament.
  - The microscopic appearance is similar to ganglion cysts.
- Giant cell tumors
  - Giant cell tumors are yellow- to brown-colored rubbery lesions that may present with joint involvement or bone erosion (**FIG 2B**).
  - The tumors are typically found on the volar surfaces of the radial three digits of the hand, though dorsal involvement is also common.[5]
  - A type I tumor is a single round or multilobulated tumor entirely surrounded by one pseudocapsule. Type II tumors consist of two or more distinct tumors not joined or surrounded by a pseudocapsule.[6]
  - Histologically, giant cell tumors contain multinucleated giant cells, histiocytes, and hemosiderin deposits.

PATHOGENESIS

- There are multiple theories for the cause of ganglions and mucous cysts. It had been thought that synovial herniation resulted in mucoid degeneration. However, the lack of a cellular lining argues against this theory.
- Another theory is that a stress-induced stretching of capsular and ligamentous joint structures stimulates increased mucin production. The mucin collects in the form of capsular ducts and lakes that eventually coalesce into a main cyst.[7]
- The pathogenesis of giant cell tumors is not completely understood. The most widely accepted hypothesis is that of an inflammatory process leading to a reactive or regenerative hyperplasia.[8]

NATURAL HISTORY

- Ganglion cysts
  - Ganglion cysts typically arise spontaneously and are most frequently found in women between the second and fourth decades of life.

- Though a history of trauma is rare, local injury may make the patient aware of the presence of the tumor.
- The size of ganglion cysts may fluctuate with use of the extremity, enlarging with increased activity and shrinking with rest.
- Ganglion cysts may rupture or disappear without treatment. However, there is no known marker to reliably predict which cysts will resolve spontaneously and which will persist.
- Spontaneous resolution is more commonly seen in the pediatric population.[9]
- Mucous cysts
  - Mucous cysts primarily occur between the fifth and seventh decades in the DIP joint of the index and long fingers.
  - The lesions are typically associated with osteoarthritis of the joint.
  - An open or draining cyst can become infected leading to septic arthritis of the underlying DIP joint.[1]
- Giant cell tumors
  - A giant cell tumor begins as a single nodule but may become multinodular as it enlarges over time.
  - Malignant transformation has not been reported.[10]

PATIENT HISTORY AND PHYSICAL FINDINGS

- Ganglion cysts
  - Patients often present with an asymptomatic 1- to 2-cm well-circumscribed, slightly mobile, fluid-filled mass.
  - Patients typically report that the mass has been present for months to years with fluctuations in size.
  - Dorsal wrist ganglions most often present with the mass overlying the dorsal scapholunate interval (**FIG 3A**).
  - Volar wrist ganglions commonly appear with a mass between the extensor tendons and the flexor carpi radialis (**FIG 3B**).
  - Volar retinacular cysts involve the tendon sheath overlying the A1 or A2 pulleys and may appear fluctuant or firm with palpation. Though typically asymptomatic, patients may complain of discomfort with forceful grip. Although on examination these lesions may be slightly mobile, they do not typically glide with tendon movement.
  - Patients often seek medical attention for ganglion cysts due to aesthetic concerns.
  - Pain or sensory symptoms secondary to ulnar or median nerve compression can occur. The pain is typically a dull ache and is most pronounced with active hand use.
  - Weakness of grip may be a complaint, particularly with dorsal wrist ganglions.

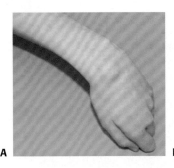
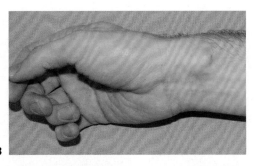

FIG 3 • A. Clinical appearance of dorsal ganglion cyst. **B.** Clinical appearance of volar ganglion cyst.

- The fluid within ganglion cysts will transilluminate light, whereas other solid lesions will not.
- Frequently, there is no history of antecedent trauma. However, if there is a dorsal ganglion in the presence of trauma, the exam should include a complete evaluation of carpal stability.
- Mucous cysts
  - Mucous cysts are commonly found over the DIP joint of the long or ring finger as a painless mass lateral to midline on either the dorsal radial or ulnar side of the joint with extension into the eponychial fold.
  - Mucous cysts may make the overlying dermis thin, causing rupture of the skin and drainage.
  - Longitudinal nail grooving or Heberden nodes with DIP joint osteoarthritis can be present in mucous cysts.
- Giant cell tumor
  - Giant cell tumors present as a painless, firm, nodular, nontender, slow-growing subcutaneous nodule.
  - Patients may present with sensory deficits secondary to nerve compression.
  - It typically presents in females in the fourth to sixth decade and is often found on the volar surfaces of the hand, though dorsal involvement is not infrequent. Most often, it is found in the radial three digits and the DIP joint.
  - The lesion is firmer than a ganglion cyst and will not transilluminate light.

IMAGING

- Radiographs are required if the patient complains of pain or there is a history of trauma.
- Plain films are useful in identifying intraosseous ganglion cysts.
- An arthrogram can demonstrate communication between the cyst and the joint space.
- MRI is used to identify an occult ganglion cyst or to localize the site of origin for preoperative planning.
- Mucous cysts often have radiographic osteoarthritic changes in the joint with Heberden nodes
- On plain radiographs, giant cell tumors may demonstrate erosion of bone secondary to mass effect. Although bony erosion may indicate a higher risk of recurrence, bony indentation does not.[6]
- Ultrasonography can aid in detecting giant cell tumor satellite lesions.[11]

DIFFERENTIAL DIAGNOSIS

- Ganglion and mucous cysts
  - Lipoma
  - Synovial cyst
  - Epidermal inclusion cyst or sebaceous cyst
  - Giant cell tumor of tendon sheath

- Giant cell tumor
  - Tendon sheath fibroma
  - Synovial hemangioma
  - Tophaceous gout
  - Periosteal chondroma

NONOPERATIVE MANAGEMENT

- Ganglion cysts can be treated nonsurgically with rest, splinting, oral analgesics, or aspiration. The injection of lidocaine, hyaluronidase, or steroids can also be employed during aspiration.
- Aspiration treatments yield recurrence rates as high as 59%.[12]
- Volar retinacular cysts that are not associated with a stenosing tenosynovitis have a better response to aspiration/injection, and surgical excision can often be avoided.
- Traumatic rupture with a book (ie, Bible) is only of historical significance.
- Aspiration of nondraining mucous cysts may be performed, but repeat aspiration is not advised to avoid joint infection.
- There is no role for nonoperative management for giant cell tumors.

SURGICAL MANAGEMENT

- For ganglion and mucous cysts, excision is indicated for symptomatic patients and for those who have failed conservative measures.
- Draining mucous cysts should be excised because of the risk of infection, which can ultimately lead to septic arthritis.
- Surgery is indicated for giant cell tumors for appearance, loss of function, or neuropathy.
  - A marginal excision with identification and excision of satellite lesions is necessary.

Preoperative Planning

- Appropriate preoperative imaging should be performed to identify the extent of the lesion, presence of any satellite lesions, or involvement of any vital structures.
- In cases of volar wrist ganglions, an intact palmar arch must be confirmed with a preoperative Allen test.
- Patients with giant cell tumors must be informed of the high recurrence rates.

Positioning

- The patient is positioned supine on the operating table, and the extremity is positioned on a hand table.
- The extremity is prepped and draped circumferentially.
- The appropriate anesthesia is administered (general, regional block, digital block) and an appropriate tourniquet is applied (upper arm or digit).
- The location of the lesion dictates the technique and the approach chosen.

■ Dorsal Wrist Ganglion

- Exsanguinate the extremity and apply an upper arm tourniquet.
- Make a 2-cm transverse incision centered over the dome of the ganglion (**TECH FIG 1A**).
- Dissect the subcutaneous tissues, taking care to identify and protect the dorsal radial and ulnar sensory nerve branches.
- Identify the extensor pollicis longus (EPL) and extensor digitorum communis (EDC) tendons and retract them. Use a self-retaining retractor for exposure. The ganglion is typically in the interval between the third and fourth extensor compartments (**TECH FIG 1B**).
- Free the cyst circumferentially using blunt dissection. If possible, avoid rupturing the capsule, so that it is easier to trace the ganglion to the stalk, which is attached to the dorsal retinaculum (**TECH FIG 1C,D**).
- Identify the stalk connecting the main cyst to the joint. It usually can be found on the dorsal aspect of the scapholunate interosseous membrane just proximal to the dorsal scapholunate ligament.

- Tangentially excise the ganglion with the capsular attachments, without disrupting the scapholunate ligament. A mucin-filled duct piercing the fibers of the scapholunate ligament connecting the joint with the cyst can be identified (**TECH FIG 1E**). One should not cut into the scapholunate ligament.
- If the ganglion is large, it should first be decompressed. With a no. 15 blade, excise the base of the stalk with a rim of the dorsal wrist capsule.
- To minimize recurrence, cauterize the site of origin of the cyst and the edge of the wrist capsule with bipolar cautery.
- Release the tourniquet, confirm hemostasis, and close the wound in multiple layers. The skin is closed with a nonabsorbable monofilament suture.
- Capsular closure should be avoided to prevent joint stiffness. Place the wrist in slight flexion postoperatively.
- Place the hand in a bulky dressing with a neutral palmar splint. Remove the dressing and sutures in 7 to 10 days.

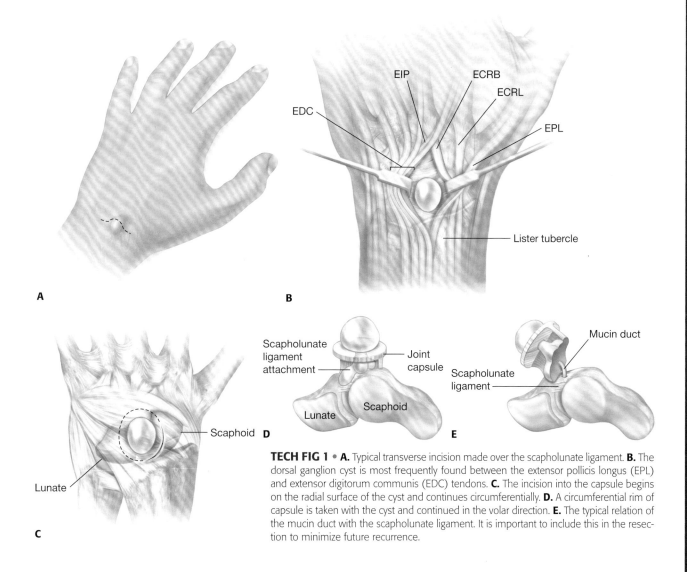

TECH FIG 1 • A. Typical transverse incision made over the scapholunate ligament. **B.** The dorsal ganglion cyst is most frequently found between the extensor pollicis longus (EPL) and extensor digitorum communis (EDC) tendons. **C.** The incision into the capsule begins on the radial surface of the cyst and continues circumferentially. **D.** A circumferential rim of capsule is taken with the cyst and continued in the volar direction. **E.** The typical relation of the mucin duct with the scapholunate ligament. It is important to include this in the resection to minimize future recurrence.

■ Volar Wrist Ganglion

- Perform a preoperative Allen test to evaluate for radial dominant circulation.
- Make an incision centered over the cyst. This incision is most commonly in the interval between the first extensor compartment and the flexor carpi radialis (FCR) tendon (**TECH FIG 2A**).
- Create skin flaps and place a self-retaining retractor for exposure. Incise the underlying forearm fascia longitudinally.
- While taking care to protect the branches of the lateral antebrachial cutaneous nerve and the radial artery, identify the capsule and trace the pedicle to the volar joint capsule (often the radiocarpal or the scaphotrapezial ligament) (**TECH FIG 2B**).
- If extension into the carpal canal is necessary, avoid injury to the palmar cutaneous branch of the median nerve by not straying ulnar to the FCR tendon.

- In a fashion similar to the dorsal wrist ganglion, open the joint and excise all the capsular attachments along with the cyst (**TECH FIG 2C**).
- If the cyst is adherent to the radial artery, a small cuff may be left behind to avoid arterial injury. It is particularly important to avoid dissecting the ganglion away from the radial artery because a shared wall may be indistinct and injuring the radial artery is likely. Therefore, one should decompress the ganglion and leave the cyst wall attached to the artery. Then trace the ganglion to the wrist joint for resection and cauterization of the stalk.
- After excision of the cyst, digitally compress the surrounding tissue to rule out additional mucin-filled pockets requiring excision.
- Release the tourniquet, obtain hemostasis, and close the wound with a nonabsorbable monofilament suture. Avoid capsular closure.
- Place a bulky dressing. Remove sutures approximately 7 to 10 days after surgery.

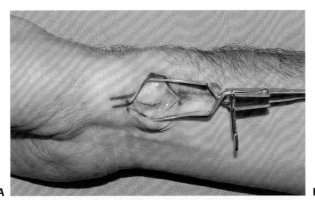

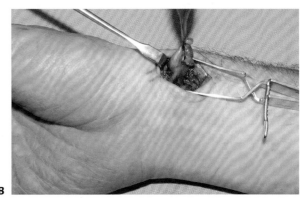

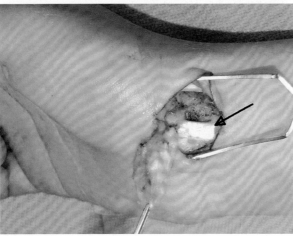

TECH FIG 2 • A. A longitudinal incision spanning from the proximal portion of the cyst to its distal extent. If additional distal exposure is necessary, the incision may be carried out into the carpal tunnel. **B.** Identification of the cyst pedicle toward the volar joint capsule. **C.** Excision of ganglion with all the capsular attachments. (*Arrow* indicates the FCR tendon.)

■ Mucous Cyst

- Apply a finger tourniquet after obtaining digital block anesthesia.
- If the overlying skin is of good quality, make a gentle curving transverse incision centered over the DIP joint.
- If there is involved overlying skin, make a longitudinal elliptical incision including the overlying skin to be excised (**TECH FIG 3A**).

- Mobilize the cyst and trace it to the joint capsule, excising it with the capsule and any involved skin (**TECH FIG 3B**).
- Often, it will be necessary to excise all the soft tissue between the collateral ligament and the extensor tendon, leaving the DIP joint exposed.
- It is imperative to avoid injury to the germinal nail matrix, the insertion of the extensor tendon, and the collateral ligament.

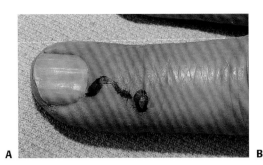

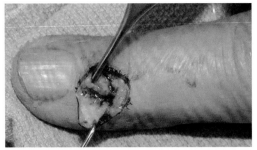

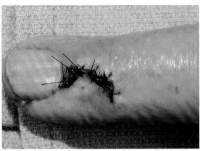

TECH FIG 3 • A. An elliptical incision is used to include the overlying skin when it is involved with the mucous cyst. **B.** The cyst is identified and traced down to the joint capsule. **C.** Closure of defect with nonabsorbable monofilament suture. Sutures are typically removed 7 to 10 days after surgery.

- With the extensor tendon retracted dorsally, explore the opposite side and excise any occult cysts or thickened synovial tissue.
- Excise osteophytes and hypertrophic synovial tissue with a rongeur to minimize recurrence.
- Release tourniquet and achieve hemostasis.

- Close the defect primarily with nonabsorbable monofilament suture (**TECH FIG 3C**).
- If the skin defect is excessive, a long rotational flap or full-thickness skin graft may be necessary. No excess tension should be placed on the closure.
- Place the distal joint in a splint, and remove sutures in 7 to 10 days.

■ Giant Cell Tumor

- Perform initial exposure using an appropriate incision based on the anatomic location of the mass, and isolate the neurovascular bundle proximal and distal to the mass.
- After identifying the pseudocapsule, use a Freer elevator to bluntly dissect the surrounding tissue from the lesion (**TECH FIG 4A**).
- Excise the tumor in total with a margin of normal tissue. If necessary, a portion of the tendon sheath may be excised and the area cauterized with bipolar electrocautery.[1]

- Meticulously examine the local area and excise any satellite lesions to minimize recurrence (**TECH FIG 4B**).
- If there is joint involvement, perform a capsulotomy and inspect the joint, debriding any pigmented soft tissue. If there is bony erosion, local curettage is necessary. If joint involvement is extensive, arthrodesis may be necessary to ensure complete excision.
- If the extensor tendon is involved, a portion may need to be excised. In rare cases, a tendon reconstruction can be performed if necessary.
- Close primarily and place hand in a bulky dressing.

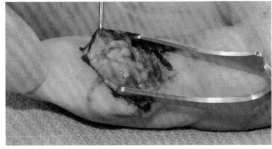

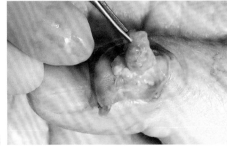

TECH FIG 4 • A. The giant cell tumor is dissected with a margin of normal tissue after identifying the neurovascular bundle proximal and distal to the mass. **B.** The local area must be closely inspected to identify and excise any satellite lesions. Failure to do so will inevitably lead to a high likelihood of recurrence.

PEARLS AND PITFALLS

Ganglion cyst	■ Adequate excision requires removal of a small cuff of the joint capsule. ■ Do not cut into the scapholunate ligament to avoid inadvertent injury. ■ Cauterize the edge of the capsule before releasing the tourniquet. It will be very difficult to adequately cauterize it subsequently. ■ Do not repair the capsule to avoid joint stiffness. ■ Always identify the deep and superficial branches of the radial artery when excising volar wrist ganglion cysts. It may be adherent to the artery.
Mucous cyst	■ Adequate excision requires debridement of joint osteophytes and any occult cysts. ■ Great care must be taken to avoid nail bed injury even if a small amount of cyst must be left behind. ■ Avoid injury to extensor tendon or collateral ligament to prevent postoperative extensor lag or DIP joint instability. ■ Evaluate both sides of the extensor tendon and the entire DIP joint to rule out occult cysts. ■ Do not close skin flaps under excess tension.
Giant cell tumors	■ Satellite lesions must be identified and excised to lower the likelihood of recurrence. ■ Perform capsulotomy if there is joint involvement to adequately resect all involved tissue. ■ Take care to identify and protect the neurovascular bundles because the lesion can displace or envelop the neurovascular structures

POSTOPERATIVE CARE

■ For ganglion and mucous cyst excisions, the hand is placed in a neutral wrist splint. Early hand elevation and early finger motion are encouraged. The splint and sutures are removed at 7 to 10 days postoperatively, and range-of-motion exercises begin at this time.

■ After excision of a giant cell tumor, range-of-motion exercises should be started immediately. Sutures can be removed after 7 to 10 days.

OUTCOMES

■ Ganglion cysts: The recurrence rates following open surgical excision is 21%.[12]

■ Mucous cysts: Recurrence rates are as low as 2% with complete osteophyte excision at the time of surgery.[2]

■ Giant cell tumors: Recurrence rates range from 5% to 50%.[1]
  ■ Factors predictive of high recurrence include incomplete excision, bony invasion, type II tumors, cellularity and mitotic activity on histology, and absence of nm23 gene expression on immunohistochemistry.[6,10]

COMPLICATIONS

■ Ganglion cysts: The most common complications include wound complications (painful or hypertrophic scar, infection, neurapraxia) or early recurrence.
  ■ Recurrence is secondary to incomplete excision or a missed occult cyst.
  ■ Pain may persist postoperatively despite complete resection.
  ■ Stiffness can occur as a result of capsular closure or delayed postoperative movement.

■ Mucous cysts: Excisions can result in extensor lag, joint stiffness, DIP joint deformity, nail plate deformity, pain, or infection.

■ Giant cell tumors: In addition to recurrence, postoperative complications may include transient numbness or infection.

REFERENCES

1. Nahra ME, Bucchieri JS. Ganglion cysts and other tumor related conditions of the hand and wrist. *Hand Clin.* 2004;20(3):249-260.
2. Kasdan ML, Stallings SP, Leis VM, Wolens D. Outcome of surgically treated mucous cysts of the hand. *J Hand Surg [Am].* 1994;19(3):504-507.
3. Henderson MM, Neumeister MW, Bueno R Jr. Hand tumors: I. Skin and soft-tissue tumors of the hand. *Plast Reconstr Surg.* 2014;133(2):154e-164e.
4. Loder RT, Robinson JH, Thomas Jackson W, Allen DJ. A surface ultrastructure study of ganglia and digital mucous cysts. *J Hand Surg [Am].* 1988;13(5):758-762.
5. Briet JP, Becker SJ, Oosterhoff TC, Ring D. Giant cell tumor of tendon sheath. *Arch Bone Jt Surg.* 2015;3(1):19-21.
6. Al-Qattan MM. Giant cell tumours of tendon sheath: classification and recurrence rate. *J Hand Surg Br.* 2001;26(1):72-75.
7. Angelides AC, Wallace PF. The dorsal ganglion of the wrist: its pathogenesis, gross and microscopic anatomy, and surgical treatment. *J Hand Surg [Am].* 1976;1(3):228-235.
8. Fotiadis E, Papadopoulos A, Svarnas T, et al. Giant cell tumour of tendon sheath of the digits: a systematic review. *Hand.* 2011;6(3):244-249.
9. Wang AA, Hutchinson DT. Longitudinal observation of pediatric hand and wrist ganglia. *J Hand Surg [Am].* 2001;26(4):599-602.
10. Grover R, Grobbelaar AO, Richman PI, Smith PJ. Measurement of invasive potential provides an accurate prognostic marker for giant cell tumour of tendon sheath. *J Hand Surg Br.* 1998;23(6):728-731.
11. Suresh SS, Zaki H. Giant cell tumor of tendon sheath: case series and review of literature. *J Hand Microsurg.* 2010;2:1-5.
12. Head L, Gencarelli JR, Allen M, Boyd KU. Wrist ganglion treatment: systematic review and meta-analysis. *J Hand Surg [Am].* 2015;40(3):546-553.e8.

Excision of Glomus Tumors

Paymon Rahgozar and Kevin C. Chung

DEFINITION

- Glomus tumors are benign hamartomas of the glomus body typically found in the reticular layer of the dermis in the distal phalanx or the subungual region.
- Glomus tumors account for 1% to 5% of all hand tumors.[1]

ANATOMY

- The glomus body normally regulates blood flow in the reticular dermis in response to local temperature changes, functioning as an arteriovenous shunt.
- Glomus bodies are found throughout the body but are most numerous in the fingertips and the nail bed.
- Subungual involvement is found in 25% to 65% of cases, typically seen as discoloration or deformation of the nail plate.[2]
- Histologically, glomus cells, smooth muscles, blood vessels, and nonmyelinated nerve fibers are found within the glomus tumor. There are three distinct histologic types that can occur with the possibility of having multiple histologic tumors simultaneously.[3]
  - Type I: mucoid hyaline type
  - Type II: solid type (classic glomus tumor)
  - Type III: angiomatous type
- The solitary glomus tumor is a well-encapsulated lesion with numerous small lumina, most commonly found in the subungual region.
  - Multiple tumors, on the other hand, are not encapsulated and rarely subungual.

PATHOGENESIS AND NATURAL HISTORY

- Glomus tumors occur as a result of hyperplasia of the neuromyoarterial glomus body.[3]
- They can be solitary or multiple. Solitary tumors often present with chronic extremity pain, frequently leading to initial misdiagnosis and inappropriate treatment.[1]

PATIENT HISTORY AND PHYSICAL FINDINGS

- Glomus tumors typically present in women 30 to 50 years old.
- Solitary glomus tumors have been associated with a classic triad of paroxysmal pain, pinpoint tenderness, and cold intolerance. The lesions can present with nail plate ridges, a pulp nodule, and/or bluish discoloration of the nail bed.[4]
- Often patients present with years of pain before definitive diagnosis. The tumor is often misdiagnosed because of its rarity, lack of the triad symptoms in the early course of the tumor, and several differential diagnoses.[1,5]
- Multiple glomus tumors tend to present earlier in life than solitary glomus tumors, and are usually asymptomatic.
- Diagnostic tests include the following:

- Love's pin test—severe pain reproduced with direct pressure
- Hildreth's test—relief of pain with tourniquet application followed by subsequent return of pain with tourniquet release
- Cold sensitivity test—immersion in an ice bath or application of a refrigerant spray elicits pain.

IMAGING

- If there is doubt about the diagnosis or the specific location of the tumor, MRI is helpful in identifying glomus tumors as small as 2 mm in the fingertip.
  - There will be high signal intensity on T2 images with strong enhancement following gadolinium infusion on T1 images.
  - The appearance of a high signal central dot surrounded by a zone of less signal intensity is characteristic[3,5,6] (**FIG 1**).
- In long-standing glomus tumors, a plain x-ray may show pressure atrophy of the distal phalanx.[1]
- Doppler ultrasonography can identify low signals within a hypoechogenic mass as small as 2 mm.[6]

DIFFERENTIAL DIAGNOSIS

- Leiomyoma
- Eccrine spiradenoma
- Cavernous hemangioma
- Sarcoma
- Neuroma
- Chronic paronychia
- Calcinosis
- Ganglion/mucous cyst
- Epithelial inclusion cyst

NONOPERATIVE MANAGEMENT

- Although excision is the only known cure for glomus tumors, nonsurgical treatment with prostaglandin inhibition, sclerotherapy, laser, or radiation have been described with mixed results.[5,6]

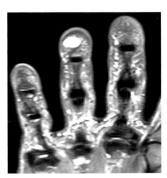

FIG 1 • MRI of glomus tumor of the ring finger. Note the high signal intensity of the tumor.

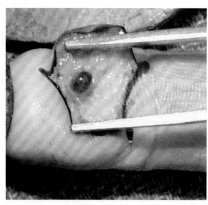

FIG 2 • A clean bloodless field permits easy visualization of the glomus tumor and the surrounding normal tissue.

SURGICAL MANAGEMENT

- A bloodless field is necessary during excision to delineate the tumor from surrounding tissues. Poor visualization increases the likelihood of inadequate resection and future recurrence (**FIG 2**).
- Subungual tumors require elevation of the nail plate and excision of the mass from the nail bed, followed by nail bed repair.
- If no gross tumor is found at exploration, remove a wedge of tissue from the area of maximum patient discomfort.[5]
- If the tumors have invaded the underlying bone, perform a partial bone excision or curettage.[1]

Preoperative Planning

- Preoperative imaging, if necessary, should be performed to identify the extent of the lesion and the involvement of any local vital structures.

Positioning

- The patient is positioned supine on the operating table, and the extremity is placed on a hand table.
- The extremity is prepped and draped circumferentially.
- The appropriate anesthesia is administered (general, regional block, digital block), and a tourniquet is applied (upper arm or digit). Typically, a digital nerve block is sufficient.

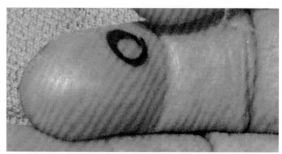

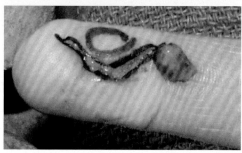

FIG 3 • **A.** The tumor is palpated and marked for excision. This corresponds to the area of most tenderness on examination. **B.** The volar digital glomus tumor was resected through a zigzag incision.

Approach

- The location of the lesion dictates the approach. Subungual tumors are excised through either a transungual or a midaxial incision.
  - Although the transungual approach provides the best visualization, it can lead to nail bed injury and postoperative nail deformity leading to an unsatisfactory cosmetic result. Careful excision and precise placement of sutures to repair the nail bed are essential.
  - The midaxial incision does not risk injury to the nail bed, but a flap needs to be developed under the periosteum, making the approach more challenging. Also, there is a risk of digital nerve injury.
- Mark the specific location of the tumor based on palpation or the area of most tenderness (**FIG 3A**).
- Volar digital tumors are resected with a zigzag incision (**FIG 3B**).

T E C H N I Q U E S

■ Transungual Approach

- Identify the area of most tenderness or discomfort. This is particularly important in lesions that are not grossly evident on examination (**TECH FIG 1A**).
- Inject digital anesthesia and apply a tourniquet. Limit exsanguination to elevation of the extremity because the tumors lose color in a bloodless field, making it more difficult to distinguish tumor from normal surrounding tissue.[5]
- Elevate the nail plate (**TECH FIG 1B**).
- Fold the nail over or remove it completely for adequate exposure if necessary (**TECH FIG 1C**).
- If additional exposure is necessary, make incisions over corners of the nail fold in an oblique angle to avoid contracture (**TECH FIG 1D**).

- With a no. 15 blade, make a longitudinal incision into the nail matrix directly over the tumor. Dissect the tumor from the surrounding nail matrix.[3]
- Free the lesion circumferentially to the level of the phalanx and excise it completely by leaving a defect in the nail bed (**TECH FIG 1E**).
- Curette the portion of the phalanx involved with the lesion.
- Close the nail bed defect with 6-0 plain gut suture meticulously by reapproximating the edges of the incision to minimize nail deformity (**TECH FIG 1F**).
- Replace the nail into the eponychial fold to act as a protective stent for the nail bed.
- Close the corner incisions primarily.
- Place a bulky dressing.

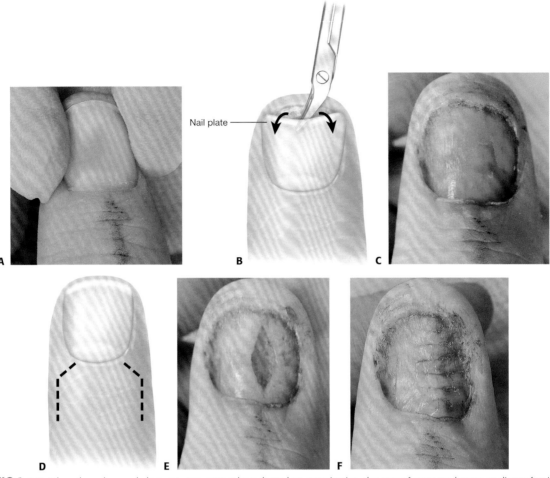

TECH FIG 1 • A. When the subungual glomus tumor cannot be palpated on examination, the area of most tenderness or discomfort is identified and marked. **B.** Elevation of the nail plate for exposure of a subungual glomus tumor. **C.** The nail is removed for exposure of the nail matrix. **D.** Incisions along the corners of the nail fold can provide additional proximal exposure if needed. **E.** The tumor is removed from a longitudinal incision in the nail matrix. **F.** Repair of the nail matrix is typically done with a 6-0 absorbable suture.

◾ Lateral Approach

- This approach is more suitable for more proximal subungual lesions to avoid violating the nail matrix.
- Make a longitudinal midaxial incision dorsal to the digital neurovascular bundle and volar to the lateral nail germinal matrix on the side of the digit closest to the lesion (**TECH FIG 2A**).
- Dissect sharply to the level of the distal phalanx.

- Create a composite dorsal subperiosteal flap with a sharp elevator. The flap consists of skin, nail, germinal tissue, and the nail plate as a unit[7] (**TECH FIG 2B**).
- Identify the lesion and excise it or remove it with a curette. Inspect for any additional lesions to excise.
- Replace the flap and close the incision primarily with an interrupted permanent suture.
- Place a bulky dressing.

TECHNIQUES

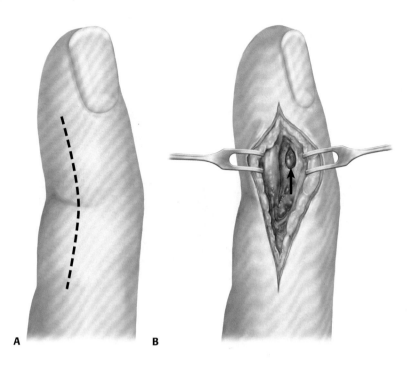

TECH FIG 2 • A. Incision for the lateral approach. **B.** Exposure is obtained by raising a dorsal subperiosteal flap exposing the glomus tumor (*arrow*).

PEARLS AND PITFALLS

Approach	▪ Transungual approach will give the widest view of the tumor.
	▪ The lateral approach has less incidence of nail deformity.
Outcomes	▪ Early postoperative recurrence of symptoms is typically from an incomplete resection.
	▪ A delayed recurrence is likely the development of a new tumor.

POSTOPERATIVE CARE

- The patient remains in the bulky dressing for 1 to 2 weeks.
- Sutures are removed at 10 to 14 postoperative days.
- Early range of motion and return to normal activity is encouraged.

OUTCOMES

- Recurrence rates range from 15% to 24%.[7]
- Early recurrence is typically from an incomplete excision, whereas late recurrence is likely from the formation of a new tumor.

COMPLICATIONS

- A nail bed deformity is described in 3.3% to 10% of cases with transungual excision.[7]
- There is always a risk of digital nerve injury with the lateral subperiosteal approach.

REFERENCES

1. Lee W, Kwon SB, Cho SH, et al. Glomus tumor of the hand. *Arch Plast Surg.* 2015;42(3):295-301.
2. Walsh JJ, Eady JL. Vascular tumors. *Hand Clin.* 2004;20(3): 261-268.
3. McDermott EM, Weiss APC. Glomus tumors. *J Hand Surg [Am].* 2006;31(8):1397-1400.
4. Van Geertruyden J, Lorea P, Goldschmidt D, et al. Glomus tumours of the hand: a retrospective study of 51 cases. *J Hand Surg Br.* 1996;2(21): 257-260.
5. Rohrich R, Hochstein L, Millwee R. Subungual glomus tumors: an algorithmic approach. *Ann Plast Surg.* 1994;33(3):300-304.
6. Netscher DT, Aburto J, Koepplinger M. Subungual glomus tumor. *J Hand Surg [Am].* 2012;37(4):821-823.
7. Vasisht B, Watson HK, Joseph E, Lionelli GT. Digital glomus tumors: a 29-year experience with a lateral subperiosteal approach. *Plast Reconstr Surg.* 2004;114(6):1486-1489.

Excision of Hemangioma of the Hand

Paymon Rahgozar and Kevin C. Chung

DEFINITION

- Hemangiomas are the most common benign tumor of infancy, with approximately 15% found on the upper extremities.[1,2]
- The lesion is a vascular tumor consisting of plump endothelial cells with a rapid turnover and a three-phase growth cycle[3]:
  - Rapid cell proliferation and growth
  - Slow growth and maturation
  - Involution

ANATOMY

- Histologically, there are two types of infantile hemangiomas.
  - The capillary type is nonvascular with a spongy appearance.
  - The cavernous type has plump endothelial cells and many mast cells lining large vessels with small lumina.[1,2]
- During the proliferative phase, the lumina widen and the endothelium flattens. As the hemangioma enters the involution phase, there is increased mast cell infiltration and progressive fibrosis of the mass.[1]
- Infantile hemangiomas will stain positive for GLUT-1 in all phases, differentiating them from other hemangiomas.[2]

PATHOGENESIS

- Hemangiomas occur as a result of endothelial cell proliferation.
- Congenital hemangiomas are caused by a failure of proper differentiation of vascular channels during embryonic development.
- Studies have shown that children with hemangiomas have increased estrogen levels that resolve after treatment. That, along with a female predominance, suggests a hormonal association.[1,3]

NATURAL HISTORY

- Although only 30% of hemangiomas are visible at birth, 70% to 90% are apparent by 4 weeks of age.
- The rapid cell proliferation phase outpaces the growth of the child, whereas the slow growth phase is more proportional to the child's growth.[1]
- About 50% will involute by age 5 and 90% involute by age 9 years.[2]
- Thirty percent of hemangiomas ulcerate with superficial bleeding.[3]

PATIENT HISTORY AND PHYSICAL FINDINGS

- Hemangiomas of the hand are found most commonly on the palm because it is the richest vascular area of the hand.[4]
- Superficial hemangiomas appear as a raised red papule, nodule, or plaque (**FIG 1A,B**). Deeper hemangiomas have a bluish hue (**FIG 1C**).
- An area of pallor with telangiectasias may be a precursor lesion identifiable at birth.[2]
- Children with a propensity to suck their fingers may present with ulcerations and paronychia.
- Other clinical findings may include pain, infection, bleeding, or congestive heart failure in very large lesions. Pain is most notable when the extremity is held in a dependent position secondary to venous engorgement.
- Platelet trapping within the hemangioma can lead to gross thrombocytopenia and consumptive coagulopathy, known as Kasabach-Merritt syndrome.
- Upper extremity growth and function is typically unaffected with hemangiomas.

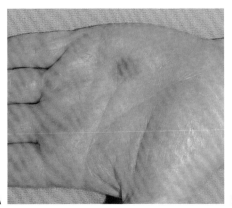 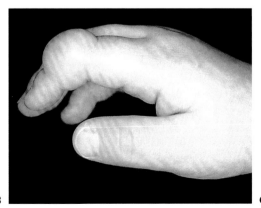 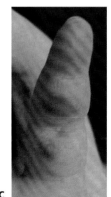

A　　　　　　　　　　**B**　　　　　　　　　　**C**

FIG 1 • **A,B.** Superficial hemangiomas typically appear as a raised red-colored papule. **C.** Deeper hemangiomas typically have a bluish hue.

IMAGING

- Plain radiographs rarely show small, smooth, round calcifications, termed phleboliths, but otherwise are of limited value.[4,5]
- Hemangiomas appear as a well-circumscribed mass on MRI with gadolinium enhancement.
  - The T1 signal is low and the T2 signal is high with an appearance of heterogeneity due to the variable feeding and draining vessels.[1]
- Ultrasound is also a valuable preoperative tool to determine the depth of the lesion.
- Angiograms will show a well-circumscribed lesion with a blush, as well as tributary feeding and draining vessels. It can be used for diagnosis and treatment if embolization is planned.

DIFFERENTIAL DIAGNOSIS

- Arteriovenous or lymphatic malformation
- Glomus tumor
- Angiosarcoma
- Hemangioendothelioma
- Pyogenic granuloma

NONOPERATIVE MANAGEMENT

- In the absence of systemic hematologic symptoms (thrombocytopenia), the initial treatment for hemangiomas is observation.
- Other modalities including steroids, propranolol, vincristine, laser ablation, and treatment with interferon alpha have been described.
- Propanolol is thought to increase apoptosis of endothelial cells and induce adipogenesis of hemangioma stem cells.[2]

SURGICAL MANAGEMENT

- Surgery is rarely indicated except for cases of mass effect, uncontrollable bleeding, or lesions refractory to conservative measures.
- Presence of a pseudocapsule during the proliferative phase simplifies excision as compared to surgery during the maturation or involution phases when the margins are more difficult to define.[3]

Preoperative Planning

- Appropriate radiographic studies should be performed to identify the extent of the lesion and involvement of any vital structures.
- Complete knowledge of the vascular anatomy is crucial, including assessment of the superficial palmar arch with an Allen test.

Positioning

- The patient is positioned supine on the operating table, and the extremity is positioned on a hand table.
- The extremity is prepped and draped circumferentially.
- Anesthesia is administered and a tourniquet is applied.

Approach

- The location of the lesion dictates the approach to provide adequate visualization for excision.
- Digital lesions are best approached with mid-axial or zigzag incisions, taking care to avoid crossing the flexion creases.
- Similarly, palmar lesions are best excised with zigzag incisions by avoiding placement of the incision at 90-degree angles to flexion creases.

TECHNIQUES

■ Incision and Dissection

- Apply a tourniquet without exsanguinating the extremity so that the entire tumor mass can be better identified for excision.[4]
- Make an incision to provide adequate access for excision of the hemangioma (**TECH FIG 1A,B**).
  - If ulceration is present, use an elliptical incision to excise the affected skin.
  - Take care to incise only to the depth of the dermis, avoiding the subdermal layer with any potential dilated plexuses.

- Identify the dilated subdermal vessels and ligate with suture or, if small enough, with electrocoagulation.
- Circumferentially dissect the tumor (**TECH FIG 1C,D**).
  - Between the surrounding fat will be septal structures with capillary networks that must be identified and coagulated with bipolar cautery.
  - Any reddish or purple fat particles within the tumor should not be disturbed to avoid significant bleeding.[6]
- Carefully dissect through the subcutaneous tissue to identify and ligate the proximal and distal tributary vessels (**TECH FIG 1E**).

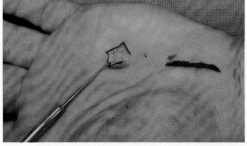
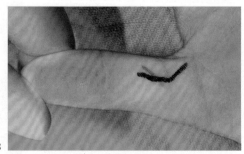

A **B**

TECH FIG 1 • A. Hemangioma of the palm of the hand. Note the zigzag incision for exposure. **B.** Hemangioma of the volar thumb. The incision provides adequate exposure and does not cross the flexion creases avoiding the risk of scar contracture.

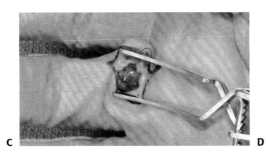

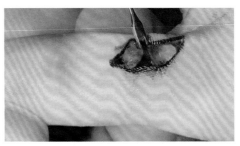

TECH FIG 1 (Continued) • **C,D.** Identification and circumferential dissection of the tumor. Take care to avoid injury to the tributary vessels prior to ligation. **E.** The tributary vessels feeding and draining the hemangioma should be ligated as far from the tumor as possible.

▇ Excision

- Identify all local neurovascular structures to confirm that the tumor is not wrapped around a nerve or vessel.
- Occasionally, the tumor may arise from vessels within striated muscle. Perform careful dissection and take a small cuff of muscle if necessary.[4]
- Excise the hemangioma and confirm that the resection is complete with margins (**TECH FIG 2A,B**).

- Inspect to confirm there is no injury to surrounding neurovascular structures (**TECH FIG 2C**).
- Release the tourniquet and obtain hemostasis.
- Perform primary closure if possible (**TECH FIG 2D**). If skin is excised due to dermal involvement and primary skin closure is not possible, the resultant defect may be closed with a skin graft or local flap.

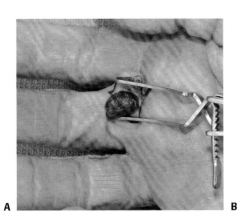

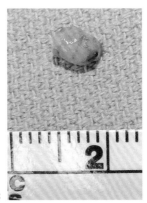

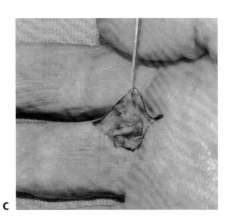

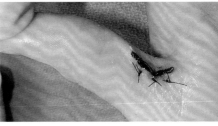

TECH FIG 2 • **A.** Excision of the specimen. **B.** Resected specimen. Hemangiomas can vary in size from millimeters to multiple centimeters in size. **C.** Inspection reveals that the digital neurovascular bundle remains intact. **D.** Primary closure following excision of a thumb hemangioma.

PEARLS AND PITFALLS

Management	■ Most lesions can be managed with observation.
Operative	■ Surgical excision is easiest in the proliferative phase because of the presence of a pseudocapsule making it easier to identify tumor margins.
	■ Apply the tourniquet without exsanguination.
	■ Ligate the tributary vessels as far as possible from the lesion.
	■ The lesion may be encasing a neurovascular structure. Meticulous dissection is crucial.

POSTOPERATIVE CARE

- A bulky dressing is applied for approximately 1 week and sutures are removed at 10 to 14 days after surgery.
- If a skin graft or flap is required, the appropriate dressing and wound care should be performed.

OUTCOMES

- Diffuse lesions have higher recurrence rates.
- Amputation may be necessary if there are multiple recurrences despite repeated excisions.
- Deep cavernous hemangiomas are the only type found to recur due to its intramuscular location, high vascularity, and proximity to neurovascular structures.[5]
- Most recurrences manifest by 2 years but can appear as long as 6 years after the primary excision.[7]

COMPLICATIONS

- Although rare, the most common complications are wound related (infection, dehiscence, contracture).

- Postoperative hematoma or bleed can best be avoided with meticulous hemostasis.

REFERENCES

1. Jacobs BJ, Anzarut A, Guerra S, et al. Vascular anomalies of the upper extremity. *J Hand Surg [Am]*. 2010;35(10):1703-1709; quiz 1709.
2. Willard KJ, Cappel MA, Kozin SH, Abzug JM. Congenital and infantile skin lesions affecting the hand and upper extremity, part 1: vascular neoplasms and malformations. *J Hand Surg [Am]*. 2013;38(11):2271-2283.
3. Walsh JJ, Eady JL. Vascular tumors. *Hand Clin*. 2004;20(3):261-268.
4. Palmieri TJ. Subcutaneous hemangiomas of the hand. *J Hand Surg [Am]*. 1983;8(2):201-204.
5. Canavese FS, Soo BC, Chia SK, Krajbich JI. Surgical outcome in patients treated for hemangioma during infancy, childhood, and adolescence: a retrospective review of 44 consecutive patients. *J Pediatr Orthop*. 2008;28(3):381-386.
6. Fujino T, Yamamoto K, Kuboto J, et al. Microsurgical technique in resection of hemangioma in infants. *Ann Plast Surg*. 1985;14(3):190-204.
7. Tang P, Hornicek FJ, Gebhardt MC, et al. Surgical treatment of hemangiomas of soft tissue. *Clin Orthop*. 2002;86(399):205-210.

Excision of Metacarpal Enchondroma

Paymon Rahgozar and Kevin C. Chung

DEFINITION

- Enchondromas are benign, intramedullary, cartilaginous lesions that are the most common primary bone tumors of the hand.

ANATOMY

- Enchondromas are typically white to blue-gray solitary lesions found in the diaphysis of tubular hand bones with varying degrees of calcification.
- The lesions are most often found in medullary cavities of the metacarpals and the phalanges.

PATHOGENESIS AND NATURAL HISTORY

- Enchondromas are thought to arise from displaced chondrocytes left behind in the metaphysis and diaphysis as the epiphysis moves through the process of enchondral growth.[1]
- Typically, they are found incidentally, but they can occasionally present with pathologic fractures.
- Although incidental enchondromas can be observed, those presenting with a fracture or radiographically at risk for a fracture can be treated surgically with a low likelihood for recurrence.[2]
- Rarely, an enchondroma may transform to chondrosarcoma.
- Malignant transformation is more likely in patients with enchondromatosis. However, malignancy occurs more often in the long bones rather than in the hand.[3]

PATIENT HISTORY AND PHYSICAL FINDINGS

- Enchondromas are typically asymptomatic and found incidentally.
- Bony deformities can be present with pathologic fractures.
- Patients may complain of painful swelling if bone distension is present.
- Multiple enchondromas are found in patients with Ollier disease (multiple enchondromatosis) and Maffuci syndrome (multiple enchondromatosis with multiple soft tissue hemangiomas).

IMAGING

- An appearance of a well-defined lobulated lytic lesion in the diaphysis or metadiaphysis on plains films is characteristic (**FIG 1**).

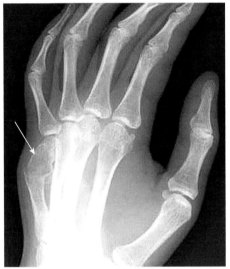

FIG 1 • Radiograph of fifth metacarpal enchondroma presenting with pathologic fracture (*arrow*).

- There may be calcifications or endosteal scalloping.[2]
- Findings concerning for malignant degeneration include progressive cortical bone destruction, replacement of the mineralized portion by a nonmineralized component, bone proliferation, or a soft tissue mass.[2]

DIFFERENTIAL DIAGNOSIS

- Chondrosarcoma
- Chondroblastoma
- Unicameral bone cyst
- Giant cell tumor of bone
- Chondromyxoid fibroma
- Fibrous dysplasia
- Bone infarct

NONOPERATIVE MANAGEMENT

- Incidental enchondromas can be observed if radiographic assessment suggests a benign, nonaggressive lesion.
- It is imperative to determine the risk of pathologic fracture, given the patient's activity level. Any concern for the possibility of pathologic fracture should prompt excision.

- The patient must be made aware of the rare but present risk of malignant degeneration with observation.
- Routine follow-up radiographs should be performed for at least a 2-year period to confirm stability of the lesion.[2]
- There should be a low threshold to re-evaluate a patient should symptoms develop.

SURGICAL MANAGEMENT

- Enchondromas that present with a pathologic fracture should be treated after a period of immobilization to allow fracture healing.
- If the fracture requires acute treatment with an open approach, immediate treatment of the enchondroma should be considered.[4]
- The first step in surgical management is an open biopsy with frozen section analysis to confirm the presence of cartilage tissue and rule out chondrosarcoma. If there is a concern for malignancy, the wound should be closed and further treatment deferred until permanent section analysis is performed.[2]

- The bony defect can be filled with bone autograft, bone allograft, a bone substitute such as calcium-based cement, or left unfilled with relatively comparable results.[4-7]

Preoperative Planning

- Radiographic imaging will reveal the location and extent of the lesion.

Positioning

- The patient is positioned supine on the operating table, and the extremity is positioned on a hand table.
- The extremity is prepped and draped circumferentially.
- The appropriate anesthesia is administered (general, regional block, digital block), and a tourniquet is applied.

Approach

- Metacarpal lesions are best approached through a dorsal incision.
- A longitudinal incision is preferable to facilitate future limb-sparing surgery if malignancy is identified on pathology.

TECHNIQUES

■ Enchondroma Excision and Bone Grafting

- Make a dorsal longitudinal incision overlying the involved metacarpal (**TECH FIG 1A**).
- Reflect the periosteum and identify the metacarpal bone (**TECH FIG 1B**).
- Create a cortical bone window with the use of a blade, rongeur, curette, or drill.
- Send a sample to pathology for frozen section to confirm the diagnosis of a benign enchondroma.
  - If there is any question of a malignancy, definitive treatment must be deferred until a final diagnosis is made on permanent pathologic analysis.

- Once diagnosis of enchondroma is confirmed, enlarge the bone window and curette the lesion (**TECH FIG 1C**).
  - It is imperative that there is adequate exposure to confirm complete excision.
- Pack the resultant cavity with preferred bone grafting material (autograft, allograft, or synthetic bone substitute; **TECH FIG 1D**).
- Confirm complete excision and adequate grafting with intraoperative radiographs.
- Close the incision primarily (**TECH FIG 1E**).
- Apply a bulky dressing and a protective splint.

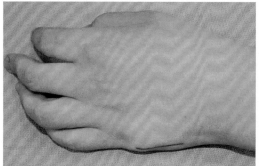
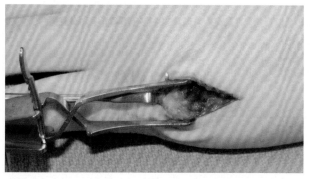

TECH FIG 1 • A. Dorsal longitudinal incision for a fifth metacarpal enchondroma. **B.** Soft tissue dissection reveals the periosteum of the metacarpal.

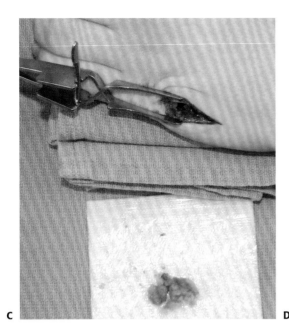

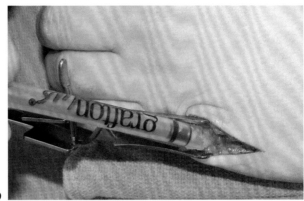

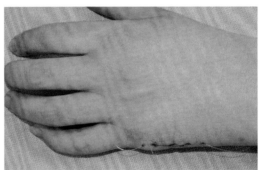

TECH FIG 1 (Continued) • **C.** An appropriately sized bone window will give access to curettage the enchondroma specimen, which has been removed in this photo. **D.** Placement of allograft in the bone defect. **E.** Primary closure of incision.

PEARLS AND PITFALLS

Presentation	■ In cases of pathologic fracture, allow healing of the fracture site before definitive treatment because fixation of the fracture can be difficult in the thin bone surrounding the tumor. ■ If found incidentally, the lesion can be observed if no malignant features are present.
Diagnosis	■ Plain films will show characteristic features. ■ Malignancy must be ruled out before proceeding with definitive excision. Consult a pathologist in advance.
Operative	■ Make the "bone window" approximately 2/3 the size of the lesion for adequate visualization of the lesion and the cavity. ■ Confirm complete excision with imaging before leaving the operating theater.

POSTOPERATIVE CARE

■ Continue protective splinting for 6 weeks after surgery but begin range-of-motion exercise at 7 to 10 days after surgery with supervised therapy.

■ Obtain surveillance radiographs at 6 months, 1 year, 2 year, and subsequently if symptoms develop.

OUTCOMES

■ Recurrence after curettage is between 2% and 15%.[2,7]

■ A malignant process must be considered and ruled out in all cases of recurrences, prompting a thorough review of the radiographs and histology.

COMPLICATIONS

■ Enchondromas may lead to extensor tendon adhesions, nonunions, metacarpal shortening, decreased range of motion, or postoperative fracture.

■ Complication rates are higher with excision of recurrent lesions.[7]

REFERENCES

1. Milgram JW. The origins of osteochondromas and enchondromas: a histopathologic study. *Clin Orthop Relat Res.* 1983;(174):264-284.
2. O'Connor MI, Bancroft LW. Benign and malignant cartilage tumors of the hand. *Hand Clin.* 2004;20(3):317-323.

3. Liu J, Hudkins PG, Swee RG, Unni KK. Bone sarcomas associated with Ollier's disease. *Cancer.* 1987;59(7):1376-1385.

4. Haase SC. Treatment of pathologic fractures. *Hand Clin.* 2013;29(4): 579-584.

5. Bachoura A, Rice IS, Lubahn AR, Lubahn JD. The surgical management of hand enchondroma without postcurettage void augmentation: authors' experience and a systematic review. *Hand.* 2015;10(3):461-471.

6. Lin SY, Huang PJ, Huang HT, et al. An alternative technique for the management of phalangeal enchondromas with pathologic fractures. *J Hand Surg [Am].* 2013;38(1):104-109.

7. Sassoon AA, Fitz-Gibbon PD, Harmsen WS, Moran SL. Enchondromas of the hand: factors affecting recurrence, healing, motion, and malignant transformation. *J Hand Surg [Am].* 2012;37(6): 1229-1234.

Excision of Peripheral Nerve Schwannoma

Paymon Rahgozar and Kevin C. Chung

DEFINITION

- Schwannomas, also termed neurilemmomas are the most common benign nerve tumors of the hand.
- The lesions are peripheral nerve sheath tumors arising from Schwann cells within the endoneurial layer.
- Schwannomas do not result in neural dysfunction. As a result, if it is not considered in the differential for an upper extremity mass, inadvertent nerve injury may result during excision.

ANATOMY

- Schwannomas grow eccentrically from the nerve sheath and are well encapsulated. As a result, nerve fasciculi cannot enter the lesions.
- The tumors are typically found on the volar surface of the forearm or the hand and are usually less than 2.5 cm in diameter.[1]
- On histology, there are interlacing fascicles of spindle cells with large oval nuclei in a palisade appearance, referred to as Antoni type A. Areas that are less well defined with fewer cells and less extracellular ground substance are termed Antoni type B.[1,2]

PATHOGENESIS

- Schwannomas are a result of a benign proliferation of differentiated Schwann cells of a single nerve funiculus that surround the nerve.[3]
- Malignant transformation is rare.[4]
- Neurofibromas also arise from Schwann cells but can easily be differentiated from schwannomas due to growth within the substance of the nerve, making enucleation impossible.

NATURAL HISTORY

- Schwannomas are quite rare and have a variable presentation, frequently leading to an incorrect clinical diagnosis.
- Multiple schwannomas of the large peripheral nerve trunks may be found in patients with neurofibromatosis type 1 (von Recklinghausen disease).
- Patients with neurofibromatosis type 2 develop bilateral acoustic schwannomas.

PATIENT HISTORY AND PHYSICAL FINDINGS

- Schwannoma typically presents in the middle decades of life as a well-circumscribed, firm, painless, slow growing tumor. It is rarely associated with a neurologic deficit.
- Typically, schwannoma is a mass that appears in line with the nerve trunk. Therefore, it is mobile in the transverse direction but not in the longitudinal plane.[2]
- Although schwannomas are usually solitary, they have been found to occur as multiple lesions. These tumors usually have no mass effect or ischemic effect of the involved nerve.[5]
- On exam, it can appear to have a cystic consistency often being misdiagnosed as a ganglion.[3,5]
- Intraoperatively, the tumor can easily be shelled out, distinguishing it from other nerve tumors (**FIG 1A**).
- Schwannomas appear within the digital nerve approximately half the time. However, it is uncommon to find one distal to the proximal interphalangeal joint of the fingers or distal to the interphalangeal joint of the thumb (**FIG 1B**).[3]

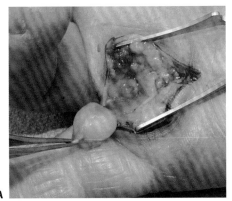 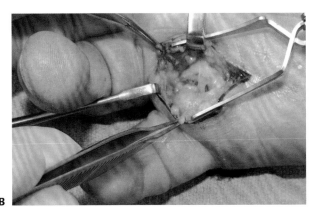

FIG 1 • A. Schwannomas are well-circumscribed tumors that can easily be enucleated from the involved nerve. **B.** Approximately half of schwannomas are found within digital nerves.

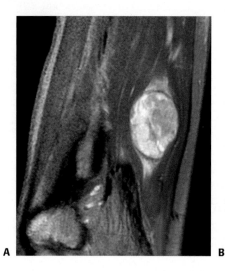
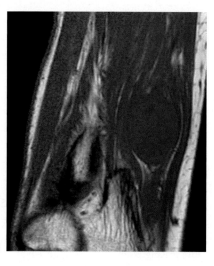

FIG 2 • MR images of an ulnar nerve schwannoma. **A.** T2-weighted image with bright appearance of the schwannoma. **B.** T1-weighted image has an intermediate signal intensity due to the presence of fat within the tumor.

IMAGING

- MRI is the standard to localize the tumor and delineate the surrounding anatomy for surgical planning.
- The lesion appears bright on T2-weighted images though the presence of adipose tissue within the lesion will give an intermediate signal intensity on T1-weighted images (**FIG 2**).
- The similar appearance on MRI makes it difficult to distinguish between a schwannoma, neurofibroma, and a malignant nerve sheath tumor.
- High-frequency ultrasound will show schwannomas as masses of low echogenicity with distal enhancement.[2]

DIFFERENTIAL DIAGNOSIS

- Ganglion cyst
- Neurofibroma
- Giant cell tumor
- Lipoma
- Epidermal inclusion cyst

NONOPERATIVE MANAGEMENT

- For asymptomatic schwannomas, observation is acceptable.
- Any malignant features on MRI imaging should prompt a discussion with the patient for surgical excision.

SURGICAL MANAGEMENT

- Surgery is indicated for definitive diagnosis, for symptom control, or to exclude malignancy.
- An excisional biopsy is performed by enucleation of the tumor following an intraneural dissection.

- Schwannomas are noninfiltrative and can be freed from adjacent fascicles without injury.[3]
- If the tumor is adherent to the surrounding tissue or is not well encapsulated, the diagnosis should be questioned.
  - An incisional biopsy should be performed with definitive treatment delayed until after a permanent pathologic examination.[1]

Preoperative Planning

- Preoperative imaging, typically MRI, can be used to identify the extent of the lesion and its proximity to other vital structures.
- The possibility of postoperative neurologic deficit, though uncommon, must be discussed with the patient.

Positioning

- The patient is positioned supine on the operating table, and the extremity is positioned on a hand table.
- The extremity is prepped and draped circumferentially.
- The appropriate anesthesia is administered (general, regional block, digital block) and a tourniquet is applied.

Approach

- The location of the lesion dictates the technique and the approach chosen.
  - Palmar lesions are best approached with a zigzag incision.
  - A midaxial approach is most effective for digital nerve lesions for best visualization and protection of the adjacent digital vessel.
  - Median nerve lesions should be excised with an open carpal tunnel incision.

■ Schwannoma Enucleation

- Expose the involved nerve and its nerve fascicles proximal and distal to the tumor. Fascicles will be seen draping over the mass and may have a multilobulated or pedicled appearance.
- Completely inspect the nerve to determine the location where there is a splaying of fascicles that would be the best resection plane (**TECH FIG 1A**).
- Incise the nerve sheath longitudinally, taking care to avoid injury to the fascicles and vessels running within the epineurium.
- Carefully peel away the fascicles from the tumor circumferentially until the tumor can be shelled out from the nerve (**TECH FIG 1B**).

- Following resection, inspect the nerve to confirm fascicular continuity (**TECH FIG 1C**).
- In cases of digital nerve, an operating microscope is needed to preserve axons.
  - Identify normal nerve fibers proximally.
  - Trace axon bundles distally and carefully dissect them free from the mass.
- The specimen should have no nerve fascicles within it (**TECH FIG 1D**).
- Close the incision with interrupted 4-0 nylon sutures and place a bulky dressing.

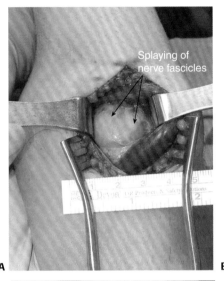
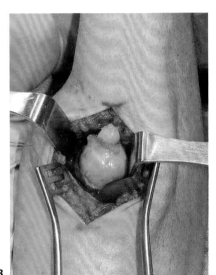
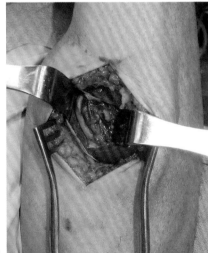
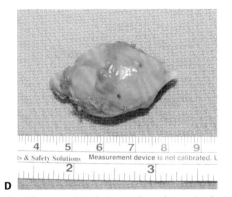

TECH FIG 1 • Schwannoma of the ulnar nerve. **A.** Splaying of the nerve fascicles around the lesion. A clean plane exists between the mass and the fascicles. **B.** The mass is shelled out carefully between the splayed fascicles. **C.** Following resection of the schwannoma, all nerve fascicles remain intact. **D.** Schwannoma specimen.

PEARLS AND PITFALLS

Indications	▪ Diagnosis—exclude malignancy
	▪ Symptom control
Diagnosis	▪ Misdiagnosis is common—often confused with a ganglion.
	▪ MRI is the best imaging modality.
Surgical approach	▪ Loupe magnification or an operative microscope will facilitate microdissection to minimize axonal injury.
	▪ If the mass is adherent to the nerve, question the preoperative diagnosis and consider malignancy.

POSTOPERATIVE CARE

▪ A bulky dressing is typically adequate. Early hand elevation and early finger motion are encouraged.
▪ The sutures are removed at approximately 10 days and range-of-motion exercises begin at this time.

OUTCOMES

▪ Recurrence is very rare.
▪ Transient paresthesias are common, but long-term nerve dysfunction is very uncommon.

COMPLICATIONS

▪ Incidence of postoperative neurologic deficit is 4%.[4]
▪ Inadvertent nerve resection can occur if the diagnosis is not considered preoperatively.

REFERENCES

1. Forthman CL, Blazar PE. Nerve tumors of the hand and upper extremity. *Hand Clin.* 2004;20(3):233-242.
2. Kehoe N, Reid R, Semple J. Solitary benign peripheral-nerve tumours: review of 32 years' experience. *J Bone Joint Surg Br.* 1995;77(3):497-500.
3. Rockwell GM, Thoma A, Salama S. Schwannoma of the hand and wrist. *Plast Reconstr Surg.* 2003;111(3):1227-1232.
4. Donner TR, Voorhies RM, Kline DG. Neural sheath tumors of major nerves. *J Neurosurg.* 1994;81(3):362-373.
5. Phalen GS. Neurilemmomas of the forearm and hand. *Clin Orthop Relat Res.* 1976;(114):219-222.

Excision of Malignant Skin Tumors

Paymon Rahgozar and Kevin C. Chung

CHAPTER 76

DEFINITION

- Basal cell carcinoma (BCC), the second most common cutaneous malignancy of the hand, arises from the basal layer of the epithelium or from the external root sheath of the hair follicle.
- Squamous cell carcinoma (SCC) is the most common malignant cutaneous tumor of the hand.
- Melanomas are aggressive tumors of the epidermis that account for 3% of all hand tumors.
- Both SCC and melanoma can invade locally, involve regional lymph nodes, or metastasize to distant sites.

ANATOMY

- BCCs most often occur in sites with higher concentrations of pilosebaceous follicles.
  - Up to 87% of the tumors appear on the dorsum of the hand between the wrist crease and the metacarpal heads.[1]
- SCC derives from the epidermal keratinocyte cell layer but can also develop in the nail matrix.
  - Although dorsal hand involvement is common for SCC, the tumors can also be found on the nails, fingers, interdigital skin, or dorsal wrist with relative frequency.[1,2]
- Melanoma is from a neural crest origin developing from the dendritic cell within the epidermis. The melanocytes can migrate to both cutaneous and noncutaneous locations, such as the nail matrix.
  - Subtypes include superficial spreading (most common), nodular (most aggressive), lentigo maligna, acral lentiginous, and amelanotic melanoma.
  - Skin tumors found in the palm are most commonly the acral lentiginous subtype.[1,3]

PATHOGENESIS

- Malignant tumors of the hand are rare, often leading to a delay in diagnosis and treatment.
- Risk factors for malignant skin tumors are similar and include sun/ultraviolet exposure, fair skin, male gender, or advancing age.
- Although basal cell cancer is the most common cutaneous malignancy, only 2% to 3% of all BCC appear in the upper extremities.[2] Therefore, in the hand, squamous cell cancer is the most common cutaneous malignancy.
- A history of severe burns, chronic ulcers, or immune compromise can lead to SCC.
- Those with a personal history of skin cancer, family history of melanoma, history of a changing mole, or exposure to coal tar, arsenic compounds, or radiation have an increased risk of melanoma.

NATURAL HISTORY

- Basal cell carcinoma
  - In comparison to SCC or melanoma, BCC does not arise from malignant changes of pre-existing structures. It originates from the basal layer of the epithelium or the root sheath of a hair follicle.[2]
  - High-risk lesions include the superficial, micronodular, morpheaform, and infiltrative subtypes.[3] Nodular BCC is the most common low-risk subtype.
  - The metastatic rates in BCC are as low as 0.1%, presumably because the reticular dermis functions as a relative barrier to its spread.[2,4]
- Squamous cell carcinoma
  - Seventy-five percent of skin cancers that appear in the hand are SCC with a male-to-female ratio of 4:1.[5]
  - SCCs originate from the spindle cell layer of the epithelium.[2] The tumor will typically begin as a nodule and will progress to develop areas of necrosis.
  - High-risk lesions are those with a diameter greater than 2 cm, vertical depth greater than 4 mm, rapid growth, perineural invasion, or presence of poorly differentiated cells.[4,5]
  - The risk of metastases involving the extremities is 2% to 5%.[6]
- Melanoma
  - The incidence of melanoma is increasing at a rapid rate, nearly doubling every 8 to 10 years.[3,6]
  - The lifetime probability of developing melanoma is 1 in 49 for males and 1 in 73 for females.
  - Prognosis is dependent on the vertical thickness (Breslow classification) or the anatomic level of invasion (Clark classification).

PATIENT HISTORY AND PHYSICAL FINDINGS

- Basal cell carcinoma
  - BCCs are characteristically found in middle-aged and elderly light-skinned individuals who report a history of multiple skin malignancies.
  - The typical appearance is that of a raised maculopapular lesion in the setting of skin atrophy, skin discoloration, and telangiectasias, with raised pearly borders and eventual ulceration (**FIG 1A**).
- Squamous cell carcinoma
  - SCC may appear as a slow-growing, verrucous, exophytic lesion or as a rapid-growing, nodular, indurated lesion with raised borders and early ulceration (**FIG 1B**).
  - The slow-growing variety has a higher propensity to metastasize.

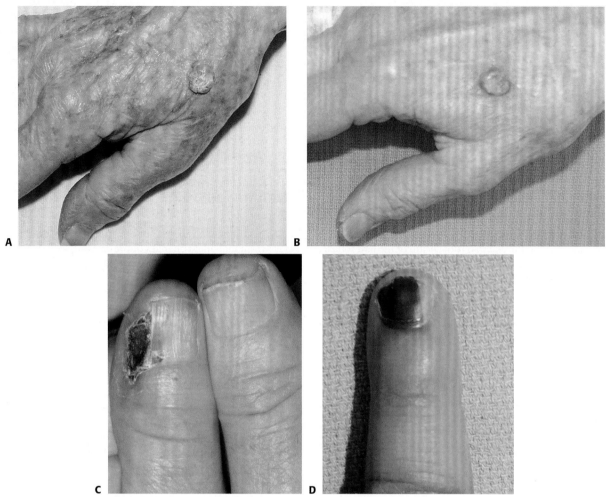

FIG 1 • A. Basal cell carcinoma on the dorsum of the hand. Note the raised pearly borders. **B.** Squamous cell carcinoma of the dorsum of the hand with ulceration. **C.** Squamous cell carcinoma with nail involvement. Often, this is misdiagnosed as a chronic paronychia or other benign pathology. **D.** Subungual melanoma with a Hutchinson sign, extension of pigment from the nail bed to the proximal nail fold.

- With time, most untreated SCCs will eventually become an inflamed, indurated lesion with central ulceration.
- The frequency of lesions on the dorsum of the hand is consistent with its association with sun exposure.
- It can be distinguished from basal cell cancer by the lack of a well-defined edge when placing stretch on the tumor with two hands.[5]
- Involvement of the nail unit presents as a chronic ulcer and is often misdiagnosed as a chronic paronychia, pyogenic granuloma, or verruca vulgaris[5] (**FIG 1C**).
- Similar to melanoma, regional lymph nodes should be evaluated to evaluate for lymphadenopathy.
- Melanoma
  - Evaluation involves the ABCs (asymmetry, borders, color) with regard to a changing mole.
  - Critical findings include asymmetry, irregularity, diameter greater than 6 mm, or presence of satellite lesions.
  - Regional lymph nodes must be examined to evaluate for metastasis.
  - Subungual melanoma may present with a Hutchinson sign (extension of brown/black pigment from the nail bed onto the cuticle or nail fold) (**FIG 1D**). It can also appear as a pigmented streak of the nail bed that is wider than 3 mm.

IMAGING

- Plain films can reveal bony involvement, particularly with nail bed involvement.
- Other imaging studies are typically performed to rule out distant disease (CT, PET, MRI).

DIFFERENTIAL DIAGNOSIS

- Hemangioma
- Dermatofibroma
- Blue nevus
- Seborrheic keratosis
- Kaposi sarcoma
- Metastasis
- Subungual lesions: chronic paronychia, pyogenic granuloma, onychomycosis, glomus tumor, hematoma

NONOPERATIVE MANAGEMENT

- Basal cell carcinoma
  - Small or superficial lesions can be considered for treatment with electrodessication and curettage, cryotherapy, radiotherapy, or CO_2 laser.

- Nonoperative management is contraindicated in morpheaform or sclerosing subtypes.
- Squamous cell carcinoma
  - Small, low-risk, or in situ squamous cell lesions can be managed conservatively in patients who are high-risk operative candidates with electrodessication and curettage, cryosurgery, or 5-FU.
  - Radiation therapy may also be used to treat inoperable lesions or recurrences.
- Melanoma
  - There is no role for nonoperative management in melanoma.

SURGICAL MANAGEMENT

- Basal cell carcinoma
  - Small (no more than 2 cm) BCCs should be resected with at least 4-mm margins.
  - Large (over 2 cm) BCCs or those with high-grade features require a 6-mm margin or the use of Mohs micrographic surgery to maximize preservation of uninvolved tissue.
  - Mohs micrographic surgery should be applied in the setting of tumors with aggressive malignant features and for morpheaform or sclerosing subtypes.[2]
- Squamous cell carcinoma
  - Because of the more aggressive nature of SCC, a wider margin of resection is typically necessary as compared to BCC.
  - A 3- to 10-mm margin of disease-free tissue should be maintained.
  - Mohs micrographic excision results in the highest cure rate and the best preservation of uninvolved tissue. It should be performed for high-risk lesions.
  - If the nail matrix is involved, amputation at the DIP joint is necessary.
- Melanoma
  - The depth of the lesion (Breslow thickness) dictates margin of resection:
    - In situ tumors: 0.5-cm margin
    - Less than 1 mm deep: 1-cm margin
    - 1 to 4 mm deep: 2-cm margin
    - More than 4 mm deep: 2- to 3-cm margin
    - For melanomas deeper than 0.76 mm, treatment includes intraoperative lymph node mapping with sentinel lymph node biopsy, followed by completion of lymphadenectomy if positive.

- For nail matrix melanomas, the digit should be amputated proximal to the DIP joint.
- In proximal digital melanomas with perineural invasion or bone involvement, a complete digital amputation or ray amputation is typically necessary.
- Large excision reconstruction can involve primary closure, skin graft, locoregional flap, or free flap (**FIGS 2** and **3C**).

Preoperative Planning

- Preoperative imaging, if necessary, should be performed to identify the extent of the lesion and the involvement of any vital structures.
- In cases of malignancy, the extremity should not be exsanguinated with the use of an Esmarch bandage to avoid a theoretical risk of seeding malignant cells.

Positioning

- The patient is positioned supine on the operating table, and the extremity is positioned on a hand table.
- The extremity is prepped and draped circumferentially, including the axilla if sentinel lymph node biopsy is planned.
- The appropriate anesthesia is administered (general, regional block, digital block), and an appropriate tourniquet is applied (upper arm or digit).

Approach

- The location of the lesion dictates the technique and the approach chosen.
- Wide local excision involves excision of the lesion with a predetermined perimeter of normal tissue (**FIG 3A**).
  - It is important to mark the specimen to orient the pathologist (**FIG 3B**).
  - If any margins are positive, the pathology will dictate the location for repeat excision.
- To facilitate primary closure, if the anatomy and the size of the lesion permit, the excision should be an ellipse.
- The incision for a biopsy should be designed longitudinally so that the biopsy site can be resected at the time of definitive treatment.
- Mohs micrographic surgery has good results for BCC and SCC. A Mohs-trained surgeon can excise the lesion and perform immediate pathologic analysis for critical areas where tissue preservation is important.

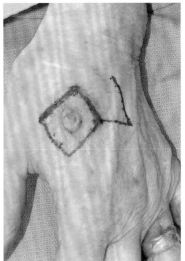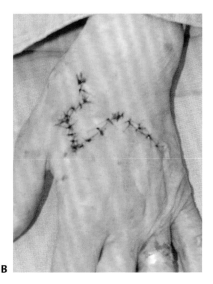

FIG 2 • SCC excision requiring a local flap for closure. **A.** Preoperative markings for a rhomboid flap for reconstruction. **B.** Closure after advancement of the flap.

A   B

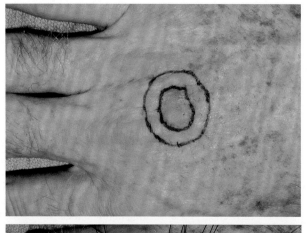

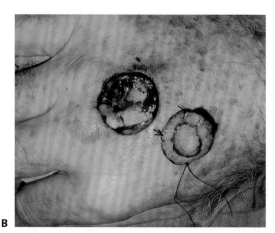

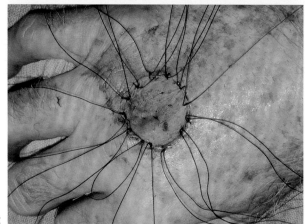

FIG 3 • Wide local excision of a SCC. **A.** The inner circle represents the boundaries of the lesion and the outer circle is the excision of a margin of normal tissue. **B.** The specimen is marked with sutures for pathologic orientation. **C.** Closure of dorsal hand defect with a split-thickness skin graft.

Mohs Micrographic Surgery

- Remove all evidence of gross tumor.
- Excise a thin 2- to 3-mm margin with the tissue (**TECH FIG 1A**). Bevel the peripheral skin edge such that it is in the same horizontal plane as the deep margin.
- Using a color-coded three-dimensional orientation, map the tissue for reference (**TECH FIG 1B**).

- Examine the deep and peripheral margin by frozen section analysis to determine the precise anatomic location of any residual tumor (**TECH FIG 1C**).
- Re-excise any residual tumor and repeat pathologic evaluation until margins are negative (**TECH FIG 1D–F**).

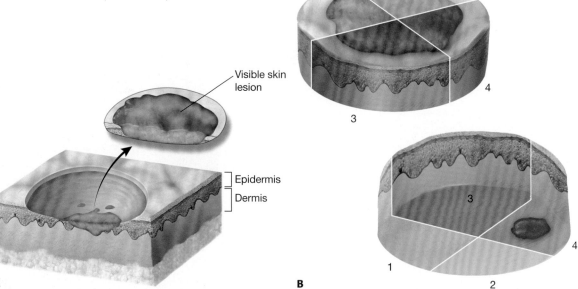

TECH FIG 1 • Mohs micrographic surgery. **A.** Gross tumor with a thin margin is excised. **B.** The sample is divided and mapped with color to help pinpoint any areas of residual tumor with frozen section analysis.

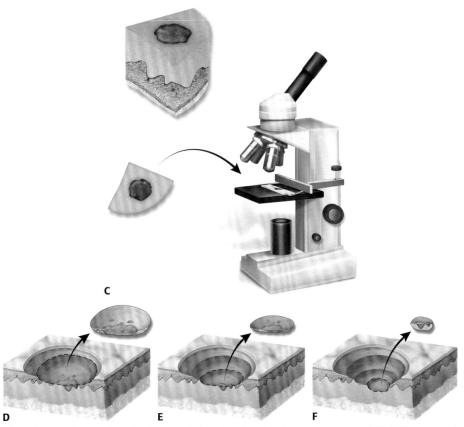

TECH FIG 1 (Continued) • **C.** Microscopic evaluation reveals that there is residual tumor in segment 4. **D–F.** The process is repeated, focusing on re-excision of the involved quadrant until all clear margins are obtained.

PEARLS AND PITFALLS

Incision	▪ Be certain of diagnosis before committing to a transverse incision for resection. This will make a limb-sparing incision more challenging for definitive resection if the lesion is malignant.
Basal cell carcinoma	▪ Telangiectasias with raised pearly borders are characteristic.
Melanoma	▪ Always consider amelanotic melanoma as part of the differential of a nonpigmented skin lesion. ▪ Before committing to a definitive reconstruction, perform temporary coverage until the final pathology confirms negative margins. ▪ Sentinel lymph node biopsy is often part of the management algorithm.
Squamous cell carcinoma	▪ Biopsy tissue in a chronic or nonhealing skin or nail matrix lesion
Mohs micrographic surgery	▪ Very low recurrence rates for BCC and SCC

POSTOPERATIVE CARE

- The hand is placed in a bulky dressing from the proximal forearm to the MP joints. Early hand elevation and early finger motion are encouraged.
- The splint and sutures are removed at 1 week, and range-of-motion exercises begin at this time.
- In cases of melanoma, the patient should follow up at regular 3-month intervals for 2 years, 6-month intervals for the following 2 years, and annually thereafter.

OUTCOMES

- Basal cell carcinoma
  - Cure rates for primary BCC treated with Mohs surgery have been reported as high as 99%.[2]
  - Recurrence rates are higher for lesions with increasing size or for those with more aggressive clinical subtypes.
- Squamous cell carcinoma
  - The risk of metastasis and recurrence is higher on the upper extremity than SCC at other locations on the body.
  - Excision with Mohs micrographic surgery has recurrence rates as low as 2.4%. However, periungual lesions have comparatively higher recurrence rates.[4]
  - The histologic risk factors associated with recurrence include degree of cellular differentiation, depth of tumor invasion, and presence of perineural invasion.[2]
- Melanoma
  - Prognosis is dependent on depth of tumor invasion, presence of nodal disease, and presence of metastatic disease.
  - The approximate 5-year survival rate for a melanoma less than 0.76 mm thick is 98%. Survival drops to 30% with nodal involvement and less than 10% if there are metastases.[6]

COMPLICATIONS

- Incomplete resection on final pathology warrants re-excision.
- With lymphadenectomy, there is a risk of hematoma, seroma, lymphocele, or lymphedema. Although the risk is also present with sentinel lymph node biopsies, it is much less commonly encountered.

REFERENCES

1. Maciburko SJ, Townley WA, Hollowood K, Giele HP. Skin cancers of the hand. *Plast Reconstr Surg.* 2012;129(6):1329-1336.
2. TerKonda SP, Perdikis G. Non-melanotic skin tumors of the upper extremity. *Hand Clin.* 2004;20(3):293-301.
3. Kakar S, Endress R. Skin cancer of the hand. *J Am Acad Orthop Surg.* 2015;23(5):307-316.
4. Henderson MM, Neumeister MW, Bueno R Jr. Hand tumors: I. Skin and soft-tissue tumors of the hand. *Plast Reconstr Surg.* 2014;133(2):154e-164e.
5. Sobanko JF, Dagum AB, Davis IC, Kriegel DA. Soft tissue tumors of the hand. 2. Malignant. *Dermatol Surg.* 2007;33(7):771-785.
6. Perdikis G, TerKonda SP. Pigmented skin lesions of the upper extremity. *Hand Clin.* 2004;20(3):283-291.

Index